BSAVA Manual of Canine and Feline Oncology

Third edition

Editors:

Jane M. Dobson
MA BVetMed DVetMed Diplomate ECVIM-CA(Onc) MRCVS

European and RCVS Specialist in Veterinary Oncology
Department of Veterinary Medicine, University of Cambridge
Madingley Road, Cambridge, CB3 0ES

and

B. Duncan X. Lascelles
**BSc BVSc PhD CertVA DSAS(ST) Diplomate ECVS
Diplomate ACVS MRCVS**

Comparative Pain Research Laboratory and Surgery Section
Department of Clinical Sciences, College of Veterinary Medicine
North Carolina State University, 4700 Hillsborough Street
Raleigh, NC 27606, USA

Published by:

British Small Animal Veterinary Association
Woodrow House, 1 Telford Way, Waterwells
Business Park, Quedgeley, Gloucester GL2 2AB

A Company Limited by Guarantee in England.
Registered Company No. 2837793.
Registered as a Charity.

First published 1991
Second edition 2003
Third edition 2011
Copyright © 2011 BSAVA

GW00537676

Illustrations in Figures 2.16, 6.7, 11.2, 13.6 and 15.27 were drawn by S.J. Elmhurst BA Hons (www.livingart.org.uk) and are printed with her permission.

A catalogue record for this book is available from the British Library.

ISBN 978 1 905319 21 3

The publishers, editors and contributors cannot take responsibility for information provided on dosages and methods of application of drugs mentioned or referred to in this publication. Details of this kind must be verified in each case by individual users from up to date literature published by the manufacturers or suppliers of those drugs. Veterinary surgeons are reminded that in each case they must follow all appropriate national legislation and regulations (for example, in the United Kingdom, the prescribing cascade) from time to time in force.

Printed by: Replika Press Pvt. Ltd, India
Printed on ECF paper made from sustainable forests

Other titles in the BSAVA Manuals series:

Manual of Canine & Feline Abdominal Imaging
Manual of Canine & Feline Abdominal Surgery
Manual of Canine & Feline Advanced Veterinary Nursing
Manual of Canine & Feline Anaesthesia and Analgesia
Manual of Canine & Feline Behavioural Medicine
Manual of Canine & Feline Cardiorespiratory Medicine and Surgery
Manual of Canine & Feline Clinical Pathology
Manual of Canine & Feline Dentistry
Manual of Canine & Feline Dermatology
Manual of Canine & Feline Emergency and Critical Care
Manual of Canine & Feline Endocrinology
Manual of Canine & Feline Endoscopy and Endosurgery
Manual of Canine & Feline Gastroenterology
Manual of Canine & Feline Haematology and Transfusion Medicine
Manual of Canine & Feline Head, Neck and Thoracic Surgery
Manual of Canine & Feline Infectious Diseases
Manual of Canine & Feline Musculoskeletal Disorders
Manual of Canine & Feline Musculoskeletal Imaging
Manual of Canine & Feline Nephrology and Urology
Manual of Canine & Feline Neurology
Manual of Canine & Feline Rehabilitation, Supportive and Palliative Care: Case Studies in Patient Management
Manual of Canine & Feline Reproduction and Neonatology
Manual of Canine & Feline Thoracic Imaging
Manual of Canine & Feline Ultrasonography
Manual of Canine & Feline Wound Management and Reconstruction
Manual of Exotic Pets
Manual of Farm Pets
Manual of Ornamental Fish
Manual of Practical Animal Care
Manual of Practical Veterinary Nursing
Manual of Psittacine Birds
Manual of Rabbit Medicine and Surgery
Manual of Raptors, Pigeons and Passerine Birds
Manual of Reptiles
Manual of Rodents and Ferrets
Manual of Small Animal Fracture Repair and Management
Manual of Small Animal Ophthalmology
Manual of Wildlife Casualties

For information on these and all BSAVA publications please visit our website: www.bsava.com

Contents

Contributors

Nicholas J. Bacon MA VetMB CertVR CertSAS Diplomate ECVS Diplomate ACVS MRCVS
Clinical Assistant Professor in Surgical Oncology, Department of Small Animal Clinical Sciences,
College of Veterinary Medicine, University of Florida, Gainesville, FL 32610-0126, USA

Laura Blackwood BVMS PhD MVM CertVR Diplomate ECVIM-CA (Oncology) MRCVS
European and RCVS Specialist in Veterinary Oncology
Senior Lecturer in Oncology, Small Animal Teaching Hospital, University of Liverpool,
Leahurst Campus, Chester High Road, Neston, Wirral CH64 7TE

Jonathan Bray MVSc MACVSc CertSAS Diplomate ECVS MRCVS
European and RCVS Specialist in Small Animal Surgery
Centre for Companion Animal Health, Institute of Veterinary, Animal and Biomedical Sciences,
Massey University, Palmerston North 4471, New Zealand

Malcolm J. Brearley MA VetMB MSc(Clin Onc) Diplomate ECVIM-CA(Oncology) FRCVS
European and RCVS Specialist in Veterinary Oncology
Principal Clinical Oncologist, Department of Veterinary Medicine, University of Cambridge,
Madingley Road, Cambridge CB3 0ES

William S. Dernell DVM MS Diplomate ACVS
Professor and Chair, Department of Veterinary Clinical Sciences, College of Veterinary Medicine,
Washington State University, PO Box 646610, Pullman, WA 99164-6610, USA

Jane M. Dobson MA BVetMed DVetMed Diplomate ECVIM-CA (Oncology) MRCVS
European and RCVS Specialist in Veterinary Oncology
Department of Veterinary Medicine, University of Cambridge, Madingley Road, Cambridge CB3 0ES

David Gould BSc(Hons) BVM&S PhD DVOphthal Diplomate ECVO MRCVS
RCVS and European Veterinary Specialist in Ophthalmology
Director, Davies Veterinary Specialists, Manor Farm Business Park, Higham Gobion,
Hitchin, Herts SG5 3HR

Stuart C. Helfand DVM Diplomate ACVIM (Oncology and Small Animal Internal Medicine)
Professor of Oncology, College of Veterinary Medicine, Oregon State University, Magruder Hall,
Corvallis, OR 97331, USA

Kieri Jermyn BVSc CertSAS MRCVS
Assistant Professor of Small Animal Surgery, College of Veterinary Medicine, Department of Clinical
Sciences, North Caroline State University, 4700 Hillsborough Street, Raleigh, NC 27606, USA

Susan E. Lana DVM MS Diplomate ACVIM
Associate Professor, Animal Cancer Center, Department of Clinical Sciences,
Colorado State University, Fort Collins, CO 80523, USA

B. Duncan X. Lascelles BSc BVSc PhD CertVA DSAS(ST) Diplomate ECVS Diplomate ACVS MRCVS
Comparative Pain Research Laboratory and Surgery Section, Department of Clinical Sciences,
College of Veterinary Medicine, North Carolina State University, 4700 Hillsborough Street,
Raleigh, NC 27606, USA

Christopher L. Mariani DVM PhD Diplomate ACVIM(Neurology)
Assistant Professor of Neurology, Department of Clinical Sciences, College of Veterinary Medicine,
4700 Hillsborough Street, North Carolina State University, Raleigh, NC 27606, USA

Richard Mellanby BSc(Hons) BVMS PhD DSAM Diplomate ECVIM-CA MRCVS
The Royal (Dick) School of Veterinary Studies, The University of Edinburgh, Easter Bush, Midlothian EH25 9RG

Reto Neiger DrMedVet PhD Diplomate ACVIM Diplomate ECVIM-CA
Klinik für Kleintiere, Justus-Liebig Universität Giessen, Frankfurter Strasse 126, 35392 Giessen, Germany

Amy F. Pruitt DVM PhD Diplomate ACVR(Radiation Oncology)
College of Veterinary Medicine, North Carolina State University, 4700 Hillsborough Street, Raleigh, NC 27606, USA

Bernard E. Rollin
University Distinguished Professor, Professor of Philosophy, Professor of Animal Sciences, Professor of Biomedical Sciences, University Bioethicist, Department of Philosophy, Colorado State University, Fort Collins, CO 80523-1781, USA

Korinn Saker DVM Diplomate ACVN
Associate Professor, Nutrition, Department of Molecular Biosciences, College of Veterinary Medicine, North Carolina State University, 4700 Hillsborough Street, Raleigh, NC 27606, USA

Timothy J. Scase BSc BVM&S PhD DipACVP MRCVS
Director, Bridge Pathology Ltd, Courtyard House, 26 Oakfield Road, Bristol BS8 2AT

J. Catharine R. Scott-Moncrieff MA Vet MB MS Diplomate ACVIM (SA Internal Medicine) Diplomate ECVIM-CA
Professor, Small Animal Internal Medicine, School of Veterinary Medicine, Purdue University, Lynn Hall, 625 Harrison Street, West Lafayette, IN 47907-2026, USA

Donald E. Thrall DVM PhD Diplomate ACVR (Radiology, Radiation Oncology)
Professor, Department of Molecular Biomedical Sciences, College of Veterinary Medicine, North Carolina State University, 4700 Hillsborough Street, Raleigh, NC 27606, USA

Brian J. Trumpatori DVM Diplomate ACVS
Veterinary Specialty Hospital of the Carolinas, 6405 Tryon Road #100, Cary, NC 27518, USA

David M. Vail DVM Diplomate ACVIM (Oncology)
Professor of Oncology, Director, Center for Clinical Trials and Research, School of Veterinary Medicine, University of Wisconsin–Madison, 2015 Linden Drive, Madison, WI 53706, USA

Henrik von Euler DVM MSc PhD Diplomate ECVIM-CA(Oncology)
Associate Professor, Small Animal Internal Medicine, Head of Center of Clinical Comparative Oncology (C3O), Department of Clinical Sciences, Swedish University of Agricultural Sciences (SLU), PO Box 7054, 750 07 Uppsala, Sweden

Richard A.S. White BVetMed PhD DSAS DVR Diplomate ACVS Diplomate ECVS FRCVS
ACVS, RCVS and European Recognised Specialist in Small Animal Surgery; RCVS Specialist in Veterinary Oncology
Dick White Referrals, Station Farm, Six Mile Bottom, Newmarket CB8 0UH

Robert N. White BSc(Hons) BVetMed CertVA DSAS(Soft Tissue) Diplomate ECVS MRCVS
RCVS Specialist in Small Animal Soft Tissue Surgery; European Specialist in Small Animal Surgery
Willows Veterinary Centre and Referral Service, Highlands Road, Shirley, Solihull B90 4NH

Foreword

Cancer is the leading cause of death in dogs (and likely cats) in most countries. As many as two out of three Golden Retrievers and former racing Greyhounds in the US die of cancer. However, cancer, unlike chronic kidney or heart diseases, is the only common chronic disease in small animals where a relatively early diagnosis frequently leads to either a cure or a prolonged period of remission, with very good to excellent quality of life.

This new edition of the very well known and widely used *BSAVA Manual of Canine and Feline Oncology* is a great contribution to the literature, providing easy-to-understand, practitioner-oriented information in a clear and concise matter. An all-star cast of seasoned clinicians and investigators, lead by Drs Dobson and Lascelles, both excellent clinicians, provides the latest on cancer diagnosis and treatment, in an appealing format. The chapters are well laid out and illustrated, and the information is easy to find.

Chapters are succinct, yet they provide valuable right-to-the-point information, easily applied to the clinical case the practitioner is reading about.

The inclusion of chapters such as Bernie Rollin's 'When to treat animals with cancer' provides an extra dimension rarely found in clinically oriented books. The chapter on pain management, by two of the main authorities in the field, should be of tremendous value to the practicing veterinarian.

In brief, a 'must-have' for any veterinary student or practitioner interested in small animal oncology. Practitioners frequently inquire as to what oncology book they should purchase for their clinic library; this Manual is at the top of my list!

C. Guillermo Couto DVM Diplomate ACVIM
The Ohio State University Veterinary Medical Center

Preface

In this, the third edition of the well established *BSAVA Manual of Canine and Feline Oncology*, we have sought to marry the best of the old with the new. A selection of new international authorities in fields of oncology have updated or rewritten the majority of chapters, with a view to making this new edition even more practical and user-friendly whilst keeping the content at the forefront of veterinary oncology – reflecting some of the significant advances in this field over the past 8 years.

The overall layout of the Manual remains the same, and will be familiar to those who have been using the second edition in their practice. However, the rapidly changing field of veterinary oncology demands that this Manual reflect the dynamism of the subject and the increasing interest in the subject in practice.

The first few chapters (on making a diagnosis) have been rearranged to be more easily applicable to practising veterinarians. Additionally, new to this edition, we have included the very important discussion of 'When to treat', including discussion of the interplay between therapy, quality of life and euthanasia decisions. Vital to the success of cancer therapy are the principles of surgery, chemotherapy, radiation therapy, and areas of nutrition and pain management. These chapters remain and have been thoroughly updated and expanded.

There has been a significant amount of new information produced since the last edition regarding treatment modalities for various tumours. Accordingly, the chapters dealing with oncology of various body systems have been carefully updated, with new information highlighted, again guiding the clinician to the most effective therapies. Throughout the Manual, we have tried to illustrate the chapters carefully, with appropriate and clinically useful tables, flow diagrams, drawings and images.

We hope you find this new edition useful to you in your work in diagnosing, treating and supporting the veterinary cancer patient – the most rewarding of disciplines.

Jane Dobson
Duncan Lascelles
October 2010

Introduction: cancer in cats and dogs

Jane M. Dobson

Introduction

Cancer is a major health concern in cats and dogs. It is estimated that one in four cats and dogs will die from cancer or cancer-related disease.

What is cancer?

'Cancer' is an umbrella term that describes a seemingly diverse range of conditions (Figure 1.1).

Term	Definition
Tumour	Literally 'swelling'. Tends to be used generically to describe any mass and can be qualified as benign or malignant
Neoplasia	Literally 'new growth'. Correct scientific term for the pathological process of abnormal cell growth
Cancer	Refers to malignant tumours or neoplasms
Oncology	The study of all of the above

1.1 Terms and definitions.

Features that these conditions have in common are the uncontrolled growth and proliferation of host cells, often to the detriment of the host itself. It is generally accepted that the majority of naturally occurring cancers arise from the transformation of a single precursor or stem cell (Figure 1.2). Although the events that lead to this neoplastic transformation are not fully understood, it is known that the basic change is related to disruption of the normal genetic mechanisms that control cell growth/division and cellular differentiation. Cancer is thus a genetic disease of somatic cells.

The key features of cancer are as follows.

- Cancer cell proliferation is uncontrolled and occurs independently of the requirement for new cells.
- The process of cellular differentiation is impaired in cancer cells: they are often 'immature'.

Two classes of genes, whose normal function is to control the intricate sequence of events by which a cell grows and divides, play major roles in triggering cancer:

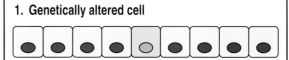

1. Genetically altered cell

A cell within a normal population sustains a genetic mutation that increases its tendency to proliferate when it would normally rest.

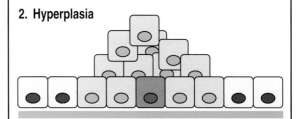

2. Hyperplasia

The altered cell proliferates; its progeny continue to look normal but also proliferate. Over time one of these cells suffers another mutation which drives further uncontrolled cell growth.

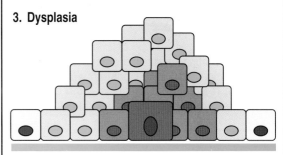

3. Dysplasia

The progeny of this cell start to appear abnormal in shape and in orientation. Over time another mutation occurs that alters cell behaviour.

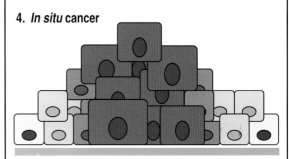

4. *In situ* cancer

The progeny of the mutated cell become still more abnormal in growth and in appearance and display features of malignancy. At this point the tumour has not become invasive and is still contained by the basement membrane.

1.2 Tumour development. (continues) ▶

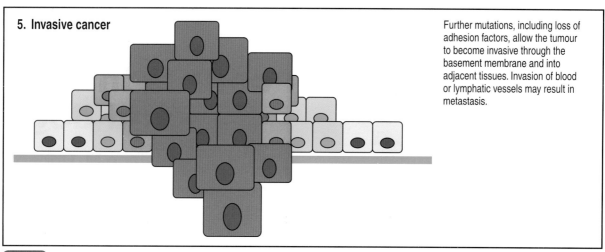

5. Invasive cancer

Further mutations, including loss of adhesion factors, allow the tumour to become invasive through the basement membrane and into adjacent tissues. Invasion of blood or lymphatic vessels may result in metastasis.

1.2   (continued) Tumour development.

- **Proto-oncogenes**, whose aberrant or excessive action promotes neoplastic growth, often by driving over-production of growth factors or causing over-stimulation of cellular growth stimulatory pathways
- **Tumour suppressor genes**, whose normal action prevents proliferation of genetically damaged cells. When inactivated by mutations there is a resulting loss of suppressor proteins and a failure to stop inappropriate growth; and genetically damaged cells are allowed to multiply.

Altered forms of other classes of genes may participate in carcinogenesis, for example by enabling the cell to become invasive or capable of metastasis. Thus, the development of cancer depends not on a single genetic mutation but on a series of mutations that accumulate over a period of time. It is thought that at least six genetic alterations are necessary for development of most cancers (Hanahan and Weinberg, 2000). As a result of these mutations the cancer cell acquires the capabilities outlined in Figure 1.3.

Acquired capability	Example of mechanism
Self-sufficiency in growth signals	*Ras* genes transmit stimulatory signals from growth factor receptors; hyperactive, mutant ras proteins are found in about 25% of all human cancers
Insensitivity to anti-growth signals	Evasion of actions of transforming growth factor beta (TGF-β), a substance that can stop growth of normal cells through inactivation of cell surface receptors or loss of *p15* gene
Limitless potential to replicate	Activation of the enzyme telomerase confers an immortal phenotype on cancer cells
Evasion of apoptosis	Inactivating mutations in tumour suppressor genes, e.g. *p53*
Sustained angiogenesis	Production or induction of vascular endothelial growth factor (VEGF)
Tissue invasion and metastasis	Altered binding specificities of cadherins, cellular adhesion molecules and integrins

1.3   Acquired capabilities of cancer cells.

What causes these genetic changes?

Although there are some germ line genetic abnormalities that confer an increased risk of cancer (see below), the aetiology of most cancers is probably multifactorial. Spontaneous genetic abnormalities occur in cells throughout life; in addition there are some external agents that may damage DNA and lead to genetic mutations:

- Viruses (e.g. retroviruses)
- Radiation (e.g. therapeutic, diagnostic or background environmental)
- Ultraviolet light (e.g. skin cancer related to sunburn)
- Chemical carcinogens (e.g. aromatic amines, azo dyes, alkylating agents).

Heritable cancer

In some cases there may also be an inherited, genetic predisposition to some cancers, where an abnormal gene is present in the germ line. For example:

- Familial breast cancer in women has been associated with mutations of the genes *BRCA1* (chromosome 17) and *BRCA2* (chromosome 13).
- The Li-Fraumeni families with *p53* (a tumour suppressor gene) mutations are associated with breast cancer, leukaemia, gliomas, adrenocortical carcinomas and soft tissue sarcomas.

Whilst breed predispositions for cancer in dogs are well documented (see below), the genetic basis for these has yet to be elucidated.

In the majority of cancers a sequence of several such genetic events or interactions, often occurring over a number of years, may be necessary before neoplastic transformation occurs and a 'cancer' develops.

Prevalence of cancer

The human population of the UK is estimated to be around 60 million, in which there are around 289,000 new cases of cancer diagnosed each year (one new

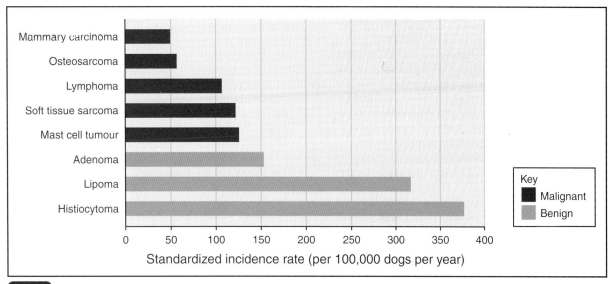

1.4 Incidence of specific types of canine neoplasia.

case every 2 minutes). According to Cancer Research UK, in 2006 in the UK there were 154,162 cancer deaths, representing roughly one in four (27%) of all human deaths. Such is the importance and impact of cancer in the human population.

Cancer is also an important disease in companion animals: it is one of the major causes of death reported in insured dogs (Bonnett *et al.*, 1997; Michell, 1999) and in geriatric cats. Accurate figures for the incidence of tumours in cats and dogs are hard to come by but a study of insured dogs in the UK showed that skin and soft tissues were the most common sites for tumour development, with a standardized annual incidence rate of 1437 per 100,000 dogs, followed by mammary, urogenital, lymphoid, endocrine, alimentary and oropharyngeal sites. Canine cutaneous histiocytoma was the most common single tumour type, followed by lipoma, adenoma, mast cell tumour, soft tissue sarcoma and lymphoma (Figure 1.4) (Dobson *et al.*, 2002).

Very few epidemiological studies of the incidence of cancer in cats have been published, but clinical observation suggests that the frequency of benign skin and soft tissue tumours is much lower than in dogs. Lymphoid tumours appear to be by far the most common malignancy in cats, accounting for nearly 30% of all tumours in one study, followed by tumours of the skin (22%), mammary gland (16%), connective tissue and alimentary system (Dorn *et al.*, 1968).

In the absence of reliable tumour registries, it is difficult to know whether the prevalence of cancer in dogs and cats is actually increasing, but a number of factors may contribute to an increase in the diagnosis of cancer in cats and dogs. As a result of improvements in health and welfare, animals are living longer and cancer is generally a disease of older age. Advances in veterinary medicine, particularly diagnostics and higher expectations of the pet-owning public, are likely to result in an increased rate of diagnosis.

Comparative aspects

Many spontaneously occurring cancers in cats and dogs share similar characteristics and behaviour to their human counterparts but their natural history is shorter, due to animals' shorter lifespans. Companion animals may be considered as sentinel species, sharing their environment and lifestyle with their owners. It is interesting to compare the incidence of human cancer with that seen in companion animals, as there are both some striking similarities and differences.

Breast cancer is the most common malignancy in women and the mammary gland is a common site for tumour development in bitches, though the risk is reduced in bitches spayed at a young age, demonstrating the importance of endogenous hormones in the development of this disease. However, carcinomas of the prostate, a very common condition in men and also associated with hormonal stimulation, are relatively rare in dogs and occur with equal frequency in entire and neutered animals. Carcinomas of the lung and large bowel, the most common human tumours excluding breast and prostate, do not feature highly in the canine or feline population, whereas soft tissue sarcomas, rare in humans, are relatively common in both species.

Spontaneous cancers are also good models for human disease in terms of therapy. With cats and dogs, their body size is more akin to that of humans than that of mice or rats, and their shorter lifespan means that therapeutic trials may be conducted and completed in a much shorter time frame than is possible in human patients. Animals bearing spontaneously occurring neoplasms are thus a potential resource for research into cancer aetiology, epidemiology, pathogenesis and genetics, and also represent potential models for therapeutic trails.

In dogs there are several good models of predictable metastatic disease:

- Osteosarcoma in large-breed dogs: with amputation alone, average survival time is 3–6 months; 'failure' is due to development of pulmonary metastatic disease in 90% of patients
- Oral malignant melanoma, an aggressive and highly metastatic disease: the primary tumour may be controlled by surgery/radiotherapy, giving average survival times in the order of 6 months, with failure due to metastasis
- Splenic haemangiosarcoma: following splenectomy, average survival times are less than 6 months, due to development of metastases.

In cats the majority of oral and pharyngeal tumours are squamous cell carcinoma and similar to human head-and-neck cancers. These tumours respond poorly to conventional therapy (especially when lingual) and in the absence of an effective means of therapy these feline patients would be ideal candidates for new approaches.

Breed predilections

In dogs it is well recognized that differences exist between different breeds regarding their risk of developing certain types of cancer, but there are few large-scale epidemiological studies on the incidence of different types of cancer in the canine population and its variation between breeds. In a study of rates and causes of death in insured dogs in Sweden, Bonnett *et al.* (1997) found that the Bernese Mountain Dog, Irish Wolfhound, Flat-coated Retriever, Boxer and St Bernard were the five breeds with the highest mortality from tumour-related death. In Denmark, Bernese Mountain Dog, Flat-coated Retriever, Golden Retriever and Rottweiler were the top four breeds, with over 20% of deaths due to cancer (Proschowsky *et al.*, 2003).

These population-based studies provide useful indicators to breeds at risk of cancer, but should not be regarded as completely definitive. The outcome often depends on the structure of the population at risk with respect to breed, which explains the differences found in studies from different countries. However, the fact that there are undoubtedly breed-related predispositions to development of cancer has important implications in understanding the aetiology of cancer, as it suggests a possible genetic, heritable component.

Some breeds of dog have been associated with specific types of tumour, such as Bernese Mountain Dog (systemic and malignant histiocytosis) and Irish Wolfhound (osteosarcoma); others, such as Boxer, Golden Retriever and Rottweiler, are associated with a higher risk of tumours in general. This observation also has important genetic implications, suggesting that the situation in some breeds may be like the rare human Li-Fraumeni syndrome where a germ line mutation in a tumour suppressor gene (*p53*) results in a hereditary predisposition to certain forms of cancer (Tabori and Malkin, 2008); whereas other breeds may have a more specific genetic abnormality leading to a particular type of tumour.

Far less is published about breed predilections in cats. Siamese cats appear to have a predilection for lymphoma. Early-onset mediastinal lymphoma has been reported in FeLV-negative Siamese-type breeds, suggesting a possible genetic predisposition to this condition. Siamese cats have been reported to respond more favourably than other breeds to chemotherapeutic treatment of lymphoma (Teske *et al.*, 2002).

Treatment of cancer

The last 20 years have seen many changes in the attitude and approach of the pet-owning public and of the veterinary profession to the diagnosis and treatment of cancer in cats and dogs, with the result that the demand for both basic and specialist treatment of animals with cancer has continually increased. However, while knowledge of the basic disease process has advanced hugely in the past two decades, this has yet to make a major impact on the clinical management of cancer in pet animals. Thus surgery, radiotherapy and chemotherapy remain for the time being the main weapons in the fight against cancer.

Surgery is and remains the most effective method of treatment for many 'solid' tumours such as mast cell tumours, low-grade sarcomas and low-grade carcinomas. The development of surgical techniques to allow adequate margins of excision for such tumours can frequently result in surgical cure.

The increasing availability of radiotherapy facilities, firstly in North America and then in the UK and Europe, has led to an increasing application of radiation, either as a primary treatment for brain and nasal tumours, for example, or in conjunction with surgery for the more invasive mast cell tumours and sarcomas.

Chemotherapy remains the treatment of choice for systemic diseases, particularly lymphoma, and is increasingly used as an adjunct to surgery for those tumours with a high risk of metastasis. With the exception of osteosarcoma, however, the latter indication has yet to be validated by clear demonstration of efficacy in controlled clinical trials.

Future directions

New technology is having an impact on the veterinary approach to the cancer patient. In terms of diagnostics, the use of monoclonal antibodies to immunophenotype tumours such as lymphoma and leukaemia has been shown to be of prognostic value, and immunocytochemistry has become more widely used in the diagnosis and classification of this and other forms of cancer. Increased availability of advanced imaging techniques such as advanced ultrasonography, computed tomography and magnetic resonance imaging is starting to revolutionize the ability to detect and determine the true extent of some tumours, allowing better planning for surgical approaches and radiotherapy.

Some novel methods of treatment have become available. For example, photodynamic therapy is being used for the treatment of superficial squamous cell carcinomas and other head and neck tumours. A novel immune system modulator, imiquimod, which possesses both antiviral and anti-tumour activity, has been used with variable degrees of success in human patients with cutaneous tumours, including basal and squamous cell carcinoma and epitheliotrophic lymphoma, and has also been used in veterinary practice.

In recent years much more targeted methods of cancer therapy have met with success in human medicine, such as the small molecule tyrosine kinase inhibitor imatinib (Gleevec, Novartis), which targets cells with activating mutations in KIT for treatment of chronic myeloid leukaemia and gastrointestinal stromal tumours (GISTs). It has been shown that 20–30% of canine mast cell tumours have mutations in the juxtamembrane region of c-kit, implicating KIT tyrosine kinase in the pathogenesis of these tumours. Tyrosine kinase inhibitors have been shown to have some efficacy in the treatment of non-resectable mast cell tumours in dogs (London *et al.*, 2003; Hahn *et al.*, 2008) and two such agents – masitinib (Masivet, AB Science) and toceranib phosphate (Palladia, Pfizer) – have recently been authorized for treatment of canine mast cell tumours.

Specific growth factor receptors are another potential target for newer therapeutic approaches. The antibody targeting the human epidermal growth factor receptor (HER-2), 'Herceptin', has proven to be effective in the treatment of HER-2-positive breast cancer. Antibodies have also been developed to target other receptors involved with cell signalling: CD20 is a transmembrane protein that regulates early steps in the activation of cell cycle initiation and differentiation. The antigen is expressed on most B-cell non-Hodgkin's lymphomas but is not found on stem cells, pro-B cells, normal plasma cells or other normal tissues. Rituximab, an anti-human CD20 antibody, is approved for treatment of B-cell lymphoma in adults. Further humanized anti-CD20 antibodies, some carrying radiopharmaceuticals, are in development for treatment of B-cell lymphoma.

Whilst there is much to be learnt from comparative oncology, these advances cannot be directly translated into veterinary medicine. For rational application of such targeted cytostatic treatments in veterinary cancer medicine the targets need to be defined, and so research is required to determine which cell surface receptors are expressed in different tumours and what signalling pathways are functional or dysfunctional in the neoplastic cells. Work already in progress in these areas offers a promising start to an exciting future.

References and further reading

Bonnett BN, Egenvall A, Olson P and Hedhammar A (1997) Mortality in insured Swedish dogs: rates and causes of death in various breeds. *Veterinary Record* **141**, 40–44

Dobson JM, Samuel S, Milstein H, Rogers K and Wood JLN (2002) Canine neoplasia in the UK: estimates of incidence rates from a population of insured dogs. *Journal of Small Animal Practice* **43**, 240–246

Dorn CR, Taylor DO, Schneider R, Hibbard HH and Klauber MR (1968) Survey of animal neoplasms in Alameda and Contra Costa counties, California. II. Cancer morbidity in dogs and cats from Alameda County. *Journal of the National Cancer Institute* **40**, 307–318

Hanahan D and Weinberg RA (2000) The hallmarks of cancer. *Cell* **100**, 57–70

Hahn KA, Oglivie G, Devauchelle P *et al.* (2008) Masitinib is safe and effective for the treatment of canine mast cell tumours. *Journal of Veterinary Internal Medicine* **22**, 1301–1309

London C, Hannah AL, Zadovoskaya R *et al.* (2003) Phase I dose escalating study of SU11654, a small molecule receptor tyrosine kinase inhibitor, in dogs with spontaneous malignancies. *Clinical Cancer Research* **9**, 2755–2768

Michell AR (1999) Longevity of British breeds of dog and its relationships with sex, size, cardiovascular variables and disease. *Veterinary Record* **145**, 625–629

Proschowsky HF, Rugbjerg H and Ersboll AK (2003) Morbidity of purebred dogs in Denmark. *Preventive Veterinary Medicine* **58**, 53–62

Tabori U and Malkin D (2008) Risk stratification in cancer predisposition syndromes: lessons learned from novel molecular developments in Li-Fraumeni syndrome. *Cancer Research* **68**, 2053–2057

Teske E, van Straten G, van Noort R and Rutteman GR (2002) Chemotherapy with cyclophosphamide, vincristine and prednisolone (COP) in cats with malignant lymphoma: new results with an old protocol. *Journal of Veterinary Internal Medicine* **16**, 179–186

2

How to make a diagnosis

Timothy J. Scase and Jane M. Dobson

Introduction

Obtaining an accurate pathological diagnosis is an essential requirement for optimizing the treatment of the individual cancer patient and for providing the client with an assessment of likely cancer behaviour and likely prognosis. An accurate diagnosis provides a rational starting point for selecting the best treatment for the cancer patient. Without an accurate pathological diagnosis, the clinician can only rely on empirical evidence to decide how best to treat the patient. At the most basic level, differentiation of neoplasia from non-neoplastic disease is likely to greatly increase the chance of therapy success.

With the increasing sophistication of techniques available to the diagnostic pathologist, there is much greater potential for obtaining an accurate diagnosis from submitted tissue samples. It is also expected that, with the refinement of diagnostic techniques, methodologies and classification schemes, the requirement to obtain an accurate and highly specific diagnosis for treatment and prognosis will increase in the future.

This chapter discusses the optimum strategies for achieving a pathological diagnosis, how to interpret a pathology report and what to expect from the pathologist in terms of diagnostic quality, margin examination and special stains. All of these factors can increase or decrease the likelihood of achieving the true pathological diagnosis, and from there the more likely it is that rational therapies can be chosen.

Choosing the correct biopsy modality for any particular tumour type can present a challenge to the clinician when trying to optimize the cost/benefit ratio of the extent of any investigations into the tumour prior to treatment. In some cases, if an excisional biopsy is chosen as the primary diagnostic modality and if a benign tumour has been excised with complete tumour-free surgical margins, the diagnostic and treatment modality have been the same and no money will have been used in the diagnostic work-up of the case. However, if histopathology shows a mast cell tumour (MCT) or soft tissue sarcoma that has been incompletely removed, the best chance of surgical cure has been lost. Thus in many cases the clinician will wish to have some idea as to what tumour type they are dealing with prior to further biopsy or treatment. In many cases, choosing an aspirate or smear as the first diagnostic procedure will enable rational decision making for choosing the subsequent diagnostic modality.

Cytology

Cytological examination of tissue samples is a quick and simple technique, requiring a minimum of equipment, that can easily be performed in the general practice setting. Many commercial clinical pathology laboratories will report on cytological samples and, with practice, most veterinary surgeons should be able to use cytology to discriminate between reactive and neoplastic lesions and even to diagnose some particularly characteristic tumours, such as MCTs.

Fine-needle aspirates or impression smears from solid tumours and the cytological examination of the cellular content of fluids collected from organs or body cavities can provide a great deal of information about the lesion and in most cases will enable differentiation between inflammatory and neoplastic processes. In the hands of an experienced clinical pathologist, it can be a highly rewarding diagnostic technique that can greatly assist in choosing the most appropriate subsequent diagnostic or therapeutic decision (Figure 2.1). In inexperienced hands, however, or if the samples are taken using poor technique or handled inappropriately, cytology can be either unrewarding or, at worst, misleading and result in the wrong diagnostic or therapeutic choices being made.

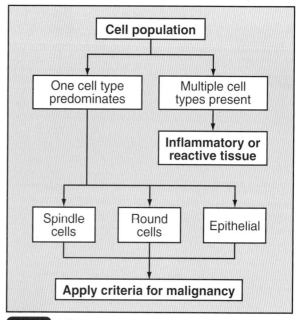

2.1 Decision tree for cytological diagnosis.

The morphology of neoplastic cells will also often provide an indication of the likely nature of a tumour and its degree of malignancy (Figures 2.2 and 2.3).

Cytological features	
Cell population	Pleomorphism Presence of mitoses, especially abnormal or bizarre forms
Cellular features	Large cell size/giant cells (anisocytosis) Poorly differentiated, anaplastic cells High nuclear to cytoplasmic ratio
Nuclear features	Large nuclear size, nuclear pleomorphism (anisokaryosis) Multiple nuclei (often of variable size) Hyperchromatic nuclei with clumping or stippling of chromatin Prominent and often multiple nucleoli of variable size and shape
Histological features	
Cellular features	As above
Tumour architecture	Lack of structural organization of cells into recognizable form
Relationship with adjacent tissues	Invasion of cells into adjacent normal tissues
Evidence of metastatic behaviour	Tumour cells invading or present within lymphatics or venules

2.2 Cytological and histological features of malignancy. (Adapted from Morris and Dobson, 2001, with permission of the publisher)

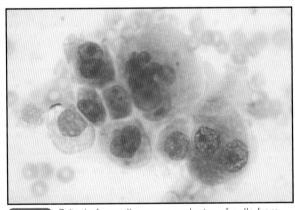

2.3 Criteria for malignancy: a cluster of cells from an aspirate of a prostatic carcinoma. The cells are displaying marked anisocytosis and anisokaryosis. In some cells the nuclear to cytoplasmic ratio is increased. There are bi- and even multinucleated cells. The nuclei contain prominent, often multiple, nucleoli. (Modified Wright's stain, original magnification X1000)

Cytology is undoubtedly a useful diagnostic technique in the investigation of neoplasia, but it is important to be aware of its limitations:

- Cytology often will not provide a definitive tumour diagnosis. For instance, in some solid tumours, neoplastic cells may not exfoliate sufficiently to provide enough cells for diagnosis. This may occur with any tumours that produce considerable stromal components, such as a fibroma or osteoma

- Cytology cannot be used to 'grade' most tumours, as grading is largely dependent on consideration of the relationship of the neoplastic cells with the surrounding normal tissues, and other factors such as the mitotic rate, the degree of inflammation and necrosis, all of which can be difficult or impossible to assess on cytological examination alone

- Some tumours, such as mammary tumours, have a very complex architecture and examination of histological tissue sections is required to make a diagnosis. In these cases, cytology is much less useful, as it may not be able to distinguish between different mammary tumour types (Figures 2.4 and 2.5).

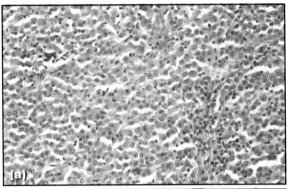

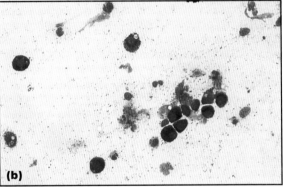

2.4 Mast cell tumour. **(a)** Histological section from a well differentiated MCT, showing homogenous sheets of mast cells; tumour architecture is not important in diagnosis. (H&E, X20 objective) **(b)** A fine-needle aspirate from such a tumour is likely to yield a similar population of tumour cells. (Giemsa, X40 objective)

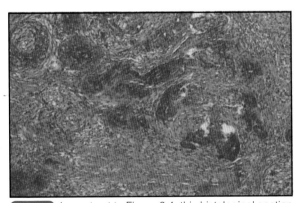

2.5 In contrast to Figure 2.4, this histological section from a mixed mammary tumour shows the architectural arrangement of the cells, forming lobules and ducts. This is an important aspect of diagnosis and cannot be represented cytologically. (Giemsa, X20 objective)

Cytology techniques

Impression smears

Impression smears can be performed with the mass *in situ*, or using biopsy specimens from the mass.

1. Pat the cleanly incised surface dry with gauze (sterility dependent on whether the impression smear is taken *in situ* or not) to remove excess blood that would otherwise swamp the cytology preparation.
2. Dab a clean glass slide on to the cut surface if the mass is *in situ,* or dab the cut face of a sample on to a slide (Figure 2.6), and allow to air dry.

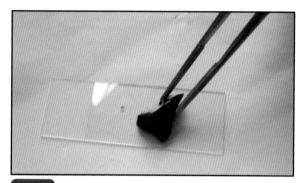

2.6 Making an impression smear.

To increase the likelihood of a diagnostic preparation being achieved, multiple slides should be prepared. Multiple impressions can be placed on a single slide if the surface area of the tissue is small.

Performing impression smears from the tissue in-house prior to submission of a biopsy for histological examination can be rewarding for the practitioner, as it enables direct correlation of the in-house cytological diagnosis with the final histological diagnosis and allows the practitioner to pit themselves against the pathologist.

Fine-needle aspiration

Fine-needle aspiration (FNA; Figure 2.7) is the cytological technique of choice for those situations where a provisional diagnosis is required prior to incisional/excisional biopsy or where an aspirate can be obtained via imaging-guided techniques rather than requiring surgical intervention, such as when sampling an intra-abdominal mass using ultrasound guidance. FNA is frequently used for diagnosis and staging of lymphoma, as the neoplastic cells exfoliate well and it is usually diagnostic without resorting to more invasive surgical biopsy techniques.

1. Prepare the skin. In most cases, the skin does not need clipping or preparing other than wetting the fur with alcohol. In those cases where the FNA sample might be cultured, it is good practice to clip and prepare the skin as for a surgical biopsy, in order to reduce the possibility of contaminating the sample with cutaneous microorganisms. In some cases, where a fluctuant mass is being aspirated, it is similarly prudent to prepare the skin further in order to reduce the chance of contamination of the fluid within the mass/cavity.

This might be particularly important where the fluid-filled structure is close to a joint or body cavity (for instance, aspiration of a perineal mass that could represent a perineal hernia), where there is a possibility of communication between the mass and a body cavity.

2. Prepare a needle (20–25 G, starting with 1-inch 23 G) and syringe (5–10 ml). Insert the needle into the mass and reposition using a stabbing action three to five times. This can be done either with negative pressure generated by pulling back on the syringe plunger, or with no negative pressure. In some cases, excessive negative pressure on the aspirated cells can result in cell damage and thereby reduce the diagnostic utility of the sample.

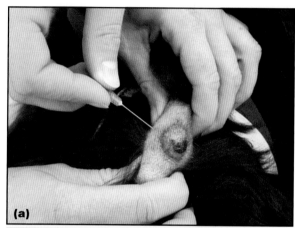

(a)

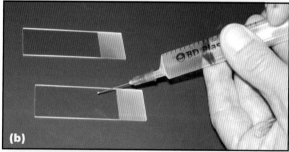

(b)

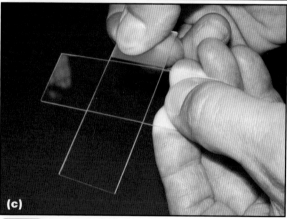

(c)

2.7 FNA technique for a subcutaneous nodule. **(a)** The lesion is located and held firmly while the needle is inserted. **(b)** An air-filled syringe is connected to the hub of the needle and the contents blown on to a clean glass slide. **(c)** A second clean glass slide is placed gently on top of the sample, allowing the film to spread between the slides, which are then gently drawn apart. See text for full details.

3. Release any pressure on the syringe plunger and withdraw the needle and attached syringe from the patient. Detach the syringe from the needle hub (any aspirated cells will be in the hub/needle). Air is drawn into the syringe. Reattach the syringe to the needle hub.
4. Place a clean slide on a horizontal surface, and press the plunger down firmly to expel the needle/needle-hub contents on to the slide. A single FNA may be enough to make two or three slide preparations.
5. To make the smears, and to prevent the preparation being too thick to examine microscopically, place a second clean slide at right angles on top of the first and smoothly and gently smear out to the edge. No extra pressure should be exerted on the slide beyond that required to move it over the slide beneath. Excessive pressure will result in extensive rupture of the aspirated cells and render the preparation impossible to interpret (Figure 2.8).
6. The smears are then air dried prior to submission or in-house staining.

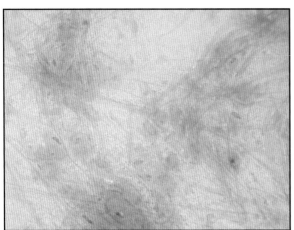

2.8 Poor smearing technique: the stringy blue streaks reflect DNA material from ruptured cells. (Modified Wright's stain, original magnification X400) (Courtesy of Clinical Pathology Laboratory, Department of Veterinary Medicine, University of Cambridge)

Cytospins of body fluids/effusions

For any body cavity, or indeed any fluid-filled mass, cytological examination of cells exfoliating into the fluid may enable a diagnosis to be made and in particular may provide evidence for the presence or absence of a neoplastic process. As the cells are often present at low density within the fluid, a concentrating technique is usually required in order to provide enough cells on a slide to make a confident diagnosis. This is most easily achieved by using a cytospin machine – a specialized centrifuge where one or more drops of the fluid are placed in a holder attached to a glass slide, and the cells are precipitated on to the slide by the spinning of the centrifuge arm. Once the arm has stopped spinning, the slide is detached and left to air dry and the cytospin preparation is stained routinely (Figure 2.9). In most cases cytospin preparations will be performed at a diagnostic laboratory rather than in a practice laboratory.

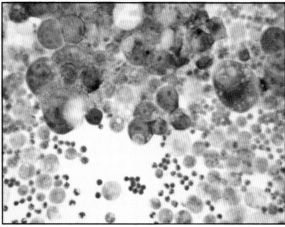

2.9 Cytospin preparation of pleural fluid from a cat with a mediastinal mass. (Giemsa, X100 objective)

Bone marrow sampling

Aspiration: Specialized needles with stylets to prevent cortical bone blocking the end of the needle are required for bone marrow aspiration. The 'Klima' needle (Figure 2.10) is one example but other types (e.g. Jamshidi; see Figure 2.13) and disposable versions are available.

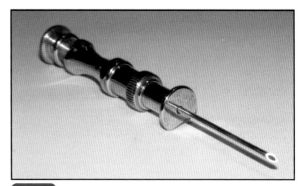

2.10 Klima needle for bone marrow aspiration.

In the dog, bone marrow can be collected from any of the larger long bones, the pelvis or the ribs. Different clinicians have their preferred approaches: the dorsal wing of the ileum is an easy site to sample provided the patient is not overweight (Figure 2.11); other people prefer the cranial aspect of the proximal humerus. In the cat the femur is usually the preferred site and the procedure is often performed under general anaesthetic.

1. In the dog: with the patient sedated and local anaesthetic infiltrated into the surrounding skin, muscle and periosteum, insert the Klima needle (with stylet in place) into the dorsal wing of the iliac crest using a twisting action (Figure 2.12.a).
2. Once the needle is deeply seated within the bone, remove the stylet, connect a 10 ml syringe and apply suction, resulting in a sample of bone marrow bubbling into the syringe (Figure 2.12b).
3. Withdraw the syringe and needle from the bone as one unit and apply drops of bone marrow to 5–10 clean glass slides positioned at about 45 degrees

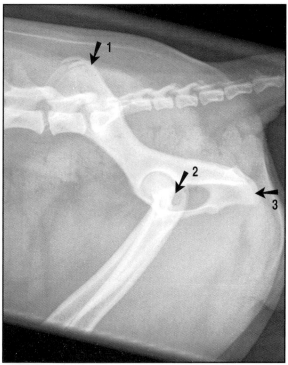

2.11 Bone marrow sampling sites. (1) The dorsal wing of the iliac crest is one of the most common sites used in medium to large dogs. (2) The femur may be sampled via the trochanteric fossa (dog and cat, anaesthesia required). (3) The caudal ischium may be more easily located in overweight dogs.

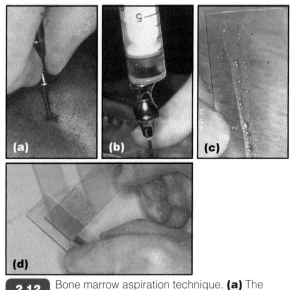

2.12 Bone marrow aspiration technique. **(a)** The needle is inserted, using a twisting action.
(b) Bone marrow bubbles into the syringe. **(c)** Globules of fat and flecks of marrow are visible in the sample.
(d) Making the smear. See text for full details.

to vertical. This allows the excess blood to run down the slide, thus reducing the haemodilution of the sample. In a good sample of bone marrow, it should be possible to see globules of fat and flecks of marrow (Figure 2.12c).
4. Use a second clean glass slide, drawn perpendicularly across the first, to make the smear (Figure 2.12 d). Speed is important here to prevent the marrow from clotting before the

smear is made (some people advocate use of anticoagulants, e.g. ACD, in the syringe prior to suction, but in the authors' experience tilting the slides allows excess blood to run off, thus preventing haemodilution of the sample, and prompt and adept smearing gives good results). The sample is then air dried and sent to the laboratory for fixation and staining.

Biopsy: The same approach and positioning may be used with a Jamshidi needle (Figure 2.13) to collect a core of bone marrow. This will require fixation in formalin and processing by standard histological methods.

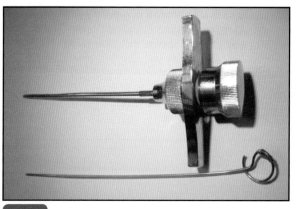

2.13 Jamshidi biopsy needle.

Submission of cytological specimens

It is imperative that cytological specimens, in particular smears, do not come into contact with formalin fumes. Exposure to formalin markedly decreases the intensity and microscopic appearance of standard cytological stains, rendering examination of the smears almost impossible. This is mostly a problem when cytological preparations and histological specimens are submitted in the same packaging to a diagnostic pathology laboratory. If at all possible, the cytological preparations should be sent to the laboratory in separate packaging to prevent formalin exposure, as even tightly closed specimen containers containing formalin can emit small amounts of formalin fumes, sufficient to destroy the cytological detail on the smears.

Surgical biopsy techniques

Histological examination of a biopsy sample is the most accurate method of cancer diagnosis and is likely to lead to a more definitive diagnosis than sampling for cytological diagnosis alone. In general, larger tissue specimens will be obtained, enabling the neoplastic cells to be observed with the surrounding tissue architecture. This also has the advantage that histological examination of the tumour may allow identification of invasive features, such as invasion of blood vessels or lymphatics, and may allow grading of the tumour. In many cases, the smaller the sample of tissue submitted for examination, the greater the chance of the tissue sections being non-representative, or of the pathologist being unable to make an accurate diagnosis. This is one reason why post-mortem examination is the ultimate diagnostic modality.

Excisional *versus* incisional biopsy

In the majority of cases it is useful to determine the likely type and grade of tumour prior to definitive surgery, so that the definitive surgical approach can be optimized. An incisional biopsy is therefore most appropriate in many cases, such as when approaching a large cutaneous or subcutaneous mass, or a mass in a surgically challenging location. However, biopsy prior to surgery is not necessary if prior knowledge of tumour type and grade will not affect the surgical approach, e.g. with splenic, renal or canine mammary tumours.

The variety of biopsy techniques that may be used to collect tumour samples includes:

- Punch
- Needle core
  o Tru-cut (soft tissue)
  o Jamshidi (bone)
- Grab
- Incisional
- Excisional.

Selection of technique will depend upon the size, site and nature of the suspected tumour. Careful thought should be given to the biopsy procedure in order to ensure that a representative sample of tissue is collected, without predisposing to local tumour dissemination or compromising future therapy (Figure 2.14).

Objective	Considerations
Procure a representative sample of the tumour	Avoid superficial ulceration, areas of inflammation or necrosis Ensure adequate depth of biopsy, particularly for oral tumours Try to include tumour/normal tissue boundary in the biopsy sample
Procedure should not predispose to local tumour recurrence or local dissemination	Minimize handling of tumour by adequate surgical exposure Ensure adequate haemostasis Minimize trauma to tumour and normal tissues Avoid contamination of normal tissue by surgical instruments
Do not compromise subsequent therapy	Any biopsy procedure should be sited well within the margins of future excision, as the biopsy tract will potentially be contaminated with tumour cells

2.14 Biopsy considerations. (Adapted from Morris and Dobson, 2001, with permission of the publisher)

Punch biopsy

Punch biopsy is suitable for collecting samples from superficial lesions (e.g. skin or any external relatively superficial tumour). It can also be used at laparotomy for organs such as liver or spleen.

1. Clip and surgically prepare the site and infiltrate local anaesthetic into the area to be sampled.

2. Press the circular blade of the punch (Figure 2.15) on to the surface of the lesion and rotate under gentle pressure to the required depth to collect a cylindrical specimen within the punch. One or more sutures may be required to close the wound.

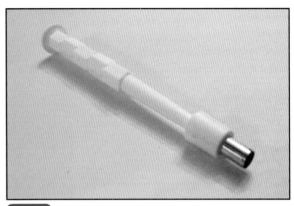

2.15 Skin biopsy punch.

The punch does not penetrate deeply into the lesion and so care should be taken to collect representative tissue in cases where there is necrosis or inflammatory tissue (e.g. oral tumours). Additionally, if going through the skin to retrieve a sample from a subcutaneous mass, care must be taken to ensure that the punch biopsy instrument does not just fill with skin. In this scenario, it is best to make a small incision to allow the instrument to reach the mass.

Needle core biopsy

Needle core biopsy is suitable for collecting small cores of tissue from solid soft tissue lesions that can be located and fixed for sampling. This technique can be used with ultrasound guidance for sampling intra-abdominal (and certain intrathoracic) lesions.

1. Clip and surgically prepare the skin over the lesion. The patient should be sedated and local anaesthetic infiltrated into the skin and soft tissue in the region of the lesion.
2. The 'Tru-cut' biopsy needle (Figure 2.16) is most commonly used. Some types are manually operated: following introduction of the needle into the lesion, the central core is advanced further into the lesion and rotated to collect tissue in the specimen notch. The outer sleeve is then advanced, trapping the tissue in the notch. The needle is withdrawn and opened for collection of the biopsy sample. Spring-loaded versions of the 'Tru-cut' needle perform this procedure automatically and are particularly useful, as they allow the operator to have one hand free to stabilize the lesion.

The Tru-cut needle is not usually sufficiently robust to sample bony lesions. Specialized needles (e.g. Jamshidi, see Figure 2.13) are available for this purpose, as described in Chapter 13.

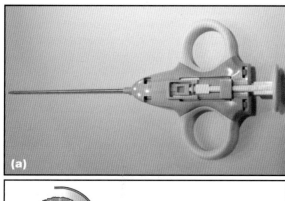

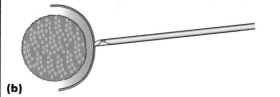

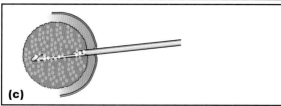

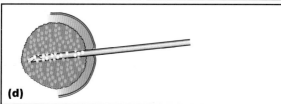

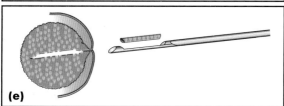

2.16 Needle core biopsy. **(a)** Tru-cut needle. **(b)** With the stylet retracted, the needle is advanced into the lesion. **(c)** The stylet is advanced to expose the specimen notch, which is then rotated to collect tissue. **(d)** The outer sleeve is advanced to cover the sample. **(e)** The sample is removed from the notch. (b–d reproduced from the *BSAVA Guide to Procedures in Small Animal Practice*).

Grab or pinch biopsy

Grab or pinch biopsy is suitable for collecting samples from mucosal surfaces (e.g. respiratory, alimentary and urogenital systems). This technique is often used in conjunction with endoscopy, allowing visualization of the surface to be sampled. Most endoscopes are equipped with biopsy cups (Figure 2.17), which collect mucosal samples through a biting action. General anaesthesia is usually required.

Whilst allowing access to hollow organ systems in a relatively non-invasive manner, the disadvantage of the grab or pinch biopsy technique lies in the superficial nature of the samples collected, which may not be truly representative of the pathology

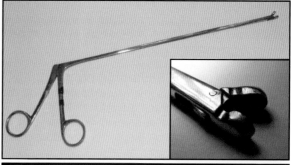

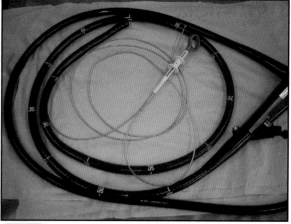

2.17 Grab biopsy equipment.

affecting the organ. Indeed, due to the nature of the biopsy technique and the size of the biopsy cup that may need to be used in a restricted space (for instance, when biopsying the urethra), the samples obtained may be extremely small. This may make a meaningful histopathological diagnosis very difficult to achieve.

Submission of histological samples

The whole sample should be sent in formalin wherever possible, as this allows the assessment of the entire tumour specimen, including surgical margins. For complex specimens, the tissue orientation should be marked if important. If it is necessary to send part of a large tissue mass (e.g. spleen), a number of representative portions from the periphery of the mass should be sent, avoiding areas of haemorrhage or necrosis. It is important to ensure a high ratio of formalin volume to tissue volume (e.g. 10:1) and not to force big samples into small containers.

If only part of the tumour is being submitted, necrotic or haemorrhagic areas (e.g. the centre of an ulcerated mammary gland mass or the centre of a suspected splenic haemangiosarcoma) should be avoided, as these areas often lack sufficient cellular detail for a diagnosis to be made.

If very small samples are to be submitted (e.g. endoscopic biopsies), it is imperative to avoid artefacts that are introduced during collection of the specimens. For instance, crush artefacts obscure cellular detail within the sections, as all the nuclei and cytoplasm are squeezed out of the damaged cells. Other artefacts to be avoided are those caused by cautery, especially at important tumour margins.

The accuracy of the diagnosis will be much greater where the clinician provides further information about the case, including signalment, lesion location and orientation (where appropriate) and any important clinical details such as evidence of metastasis, presence of invasion based on imaging studies, etc. The pathologist should then be able to provide an accurate diagnosis and prognostically useful information such as tumour grade, presence of vascular/lymphatic invasion, and extent of surgical excision. Where there is uncertainty in the diagnosis, it is useful for the pathologist to provide details of the degree of uncertainty and the likely differential diagnosis. The pathologist may recommend further diagnostic or prognostic assays, such as undertaking different histochemical stains or through the use of immunohistochemical staining.

Surgical margins

The evaluation of surgical margins as an indicator of the effectiveness of surgical excision can often present a challenge to clinicians, pathologists and histology technicians. Because the entire tissue cannot be easily examined, the evaluation represents a trade-off between what is most practical and what is most cost-effective for an individual case. For instance, if the entire specimen of an elliptical piece of skin measuring 3 × 2 × 1 cm was cut into 5 micrometre sections, it would take approximately 4000 histological sections to examine the entire tissue (Figure 2.18). Consequently any practical evaluation of surgical margins involves some pragmatism and degree of judgement as to which of the many orientations or planes of sections are the most likely to provide the information.

In human medicine, it has been recognized that it is very important to have a pathologist involved in the evaluation and dissection of a gross specimen right from its initial receipt into the laboratory. This should enable the most appropriate sections to be taken for subsequent microscopic evaluation.

There are set guidelines for how tissue specimens should be examined and processed in human medicine, provided by, for instance, the Royal College of Pathologists in the UK and the College of American Pathologists in the US. Yet even in human medicine there is a degree of controversy about how best to take the margins from any given tissue or tumour type, and indeed for some tissues the guidelines are much less stringent than for others.

The meaningful interpretation of the surgical margins of a tumour mass by the histopathologist is unfortunately not quite as straightforward as might be imagined. The most reliable way for the submitting clinician to be assured that the pathologist is examining the 'true' surgical margins of a specimen is for those margins to be marked. There are a number of different ways that this can be done.

Ink

The cut surgical margins of the unfixed specimen can be painted using one or more different inks. Drawing a diagram on the submission form with the

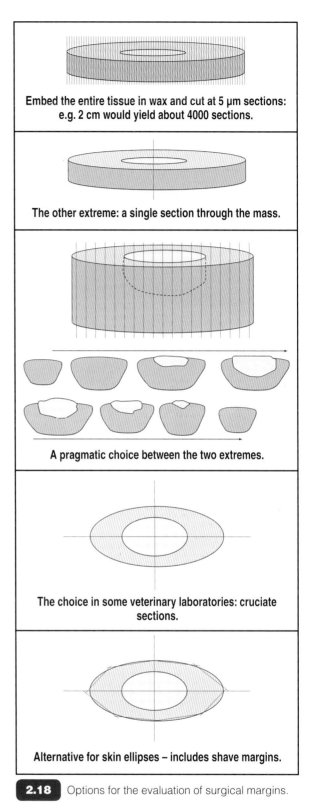

Embed the entire tissue in wax and cut at 5 μm sections: e.g. 2 cm would yield about 4000 sections.

The other extreme: a single section through the mass.

A pragmatic choice between the two extremes.

The choice in some veterinary laboratories: cruciate sections.

Alternative for skin ellipses – includes shave margins.

2.18 Options for the evaluation of surgical margins.

coloured margins indicated will also help the laboratory technician trimming the specimen. Painting the specimen is the most reliable method of margin identification and the use of different colours to paint different surgical margins can enable specific margins to be identified and individually assessed.

There are many different types and colours of commercially available surgical inks, but the cheapest and easiest method is to use one or more different colours of Indian ink. In order to ink the margins (Figure 2.19):

1. Pat the tissue dry with paper towels to remove the surface blood.
2. Paint the tissue with undiluted Indian ink over the margin surfaces as appropriate (for instance, over the subcutaneous fat over the deep border of a skin tumour). The tissue should be painted

with a soft brush or cotton-buds, rather than being immersed in the ink, as otherwise ink can percolate through small fissures in the tissue and result in ink accumulating on the tissue that is not actually the margin.
3. Immerse the painted tissue in 10% acetic acid (e.g. white vinegar) to stop it being washed away in the formalin.
4. Pat the tissue with a paper towel to remove the excess ink/acetic acid and then place it into formalin for submission to the laboratory.

For the pathologists at the microscope, prior inking of the tissues can make a huge difference to how easy it is identify the 'real' surgical margins from false margins.

Suture-tagging

Sutures can be placed at the appropriate margins that are of particular importance (e.g. a margin that grossly is close to normal tissue, or at an anatomically important site). This method works less well for broad tumour fronts or very large specimens, or where multiple surgical margins are being assessed. Because the sutures have to be removed prior to processing, it is often impossible to identify the specific margins again on the wet tissue should further sections be requested.

Separate surgical margins

Marginal tissue is taken from the tissue bed that is left behind in the animal and this tissue is submitted separately as representing the tissue margins. Particularly for large samples, this is a very good way of submitting margins. It reduces the chances of processing/trimming errors, allows the surgeon to submit the most anatomically relevant margins and may also be cheaper, as fewer blocks may need to be processed. In addition, when done in combination with the standard 'cruciate' sections through the main tumour mass, useful measurements can still be obtained for the tissue margin/tumour margin distance.

At the diagnostic laboratory, the tissue will be removed from the fixative and appropriate samples taken for processing and subsequent histological examination. In most veterinary diagnostic laboratories examination of margins may not be as thorough as it is in human medicine. Indeed, in the majority of commercial diagnostic practices, trimming of gross tissues will be performed by a technician rather than a pathologist. The 'standard' method for tissues, where it can be done, is to take 'cruciate' sections (north, east, south, west) (Figure 2.20) such that margins can be assessed around the tissue. However, this process does not work particularly well in all cases. Therefore, peripheral or tangential 'shave' sections may be more representative of the tissue margins in these cases, aided by pre-fixation inking. This is particularly appropriate where there are large specimens, specimens from anatomically complex sites (head/neck), tissues from an extremity (for instance, the ear pinna or tail) or tissue from a tubular organ (for instance the intestine).

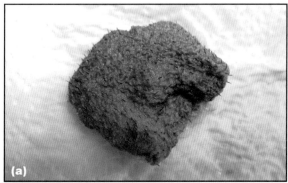
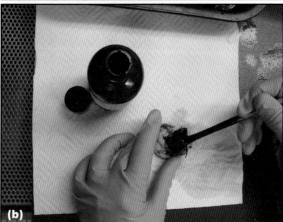
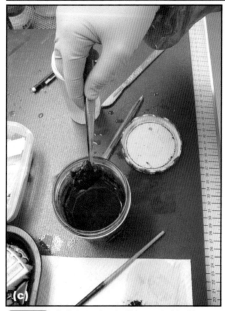

2.19 **(a)** A typical ellipse of skin from an excisional biopsy of a subcutaneous mass. **(b)** The subcutaneous tissues are dried with paper towels and painted with indian ink. **(c)** The tissues are then dipped in acetic acid (white vinegar) to precipitate the ink on to the tissue surface.

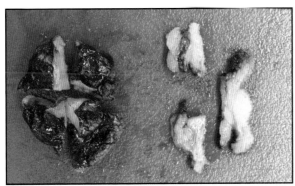

2.20 Gross tumour specimen showing cruciate sections for margins. Typical full-thickness cruciate sections are taken, and the tissue samples are placed into cassettes prior to processing into paraffin blocks.

Interpretation of tumour descriptions

As with any other diagnostic modality, the clinician should read the pathology report critically, i.e. does the histological diagnosis fit the clinical picture?

There are two main types of technique that pathologists use to describe tumours. The first, which is most widely used in the UK, is a free-form description. This method, although often more flowing, does not always provide sufficient information for a clinician to be able to assess the degree of differentiation, adequacy of margins, etc. It is one of the main reasons that oncologists might request a second opinion.

Many pathologists are now using a more standardized format that has been promoted by the Armed Forces Institute of Pathologists and the American and European Colleges of Veterinary Pathology. This descriptive technique mirrors the diagnostic process that a pathologist will go through. More importantly, it provides large amounts of information on the tumour specimen in a relatively concise form, with the majority of the most clinically relevant information being presented at the beginning (Figure 2.21). The aim of the approach is both to convey the descriptive information that enables a definitive histological diagnosis to be made (e.g. peripheral nerve sheath tumour) and to convey clinically important information (e.g. degree of differentiation).

By reading the histological description, the clinician can form a mental picture of the lesion. In particular, a good description should include both qualitative and quantitative detail that should enable diagnostically and prognostically useful information to be gleaned from it. For instance, enumeration of the mitotic index is prognostically relevant in canine cutaneous MCTs; where terms such as 'brisk mitotic activity' or 'small numbers of mitoses' are used, it can be impossible to obtain this information.

In some cases, if there is insufficient tissue available for examination it can be very difficult for a pathologist to reach a definitive diagnosis about the tissue. Other problems facing the pathologist include orientation of the tissue sample, artefacts introduced by crushing of small samples, and thermocautery of the tissue edges.

Line	Description	Significance
Line 1: Subgross description	Includes: subgross tissue location; size; shape; cell density; expansile or infiltrative; encapsulated or non-encapsulated; well demarcated or poorly demarcated; fully excised or not fully excised	The most important line of the description, giving some of the most clinically relevant information. For instance, is it infiltrating (carcinoma) *versus* expanding (adenoma); are the surgical margins tumour-free?
Line 2: Patterns of cells and types of stroma	The patterns in which the tumour cells are arranged, e.g. nests, packets, lobules, cords (carcinoma); acini, tubules (adenocarcinoma); streams, bundles, fascicles, storiform patterns (sarcoma); sheets, cords (round cell tumour). The amount and type of stroma are also assessed	Describes whether the tumour is of epithelial, mesenchymal or round cell origin. Provides a large amount of potentially useful prognostic and therapeutic information
Line 3: Cytological features	Individual cellular features, including cell size, shape, cytoplasm features	This line and the following lines give some indication as to the degree of differentiation of the neoplastic cells. In many cases, the less well the tumour is differentiated, the worse the prognosis
Line 4: Nuclear features	Details of nuclear shape, size, chromatin patterns, nucleoli features	Large, irregular nuclei with very prominent nucleoli are often a feature of aggressive tumours
Line 5: Unique features	Examples: presence of multinucleated cells; degree of anisokaryosis (variation in nuclear size) or anisocytosis (variation in cell size)	In general, the higher the degree of cellular and nuclear pleomorphism, the less well differentiated the tumour
Line 6: Mitotic activity	Usually expressed as numbers of mitotic figures per high power field (HPF) or per 3, 5 or 10 HPFs	The higher the mitotic rate, the more quickly the neoplastic cells are proliferating. A high mitotic rate is often associated with more aggressive tumour behaviour
Line 7: Evidence of malignancy	Evidence of capsular invasion, vascular invasion, lymphatic invasion, necrosis, haemorrhage	In general, the more invasive and infiltrative the tumour, the more likely it is that the tumour has already metastasized or will recur locally
Line 8: Anything else	Any other pathological feature related to, or unrelated to, the neoplastic process, e.g. ulceration or peritumoral inflammation	Many tumours will result in pathological changes within the adjacent tissues, e.g. inflammation in adjacent tissue, atrophy of adjacent skeletal muscle

2.21 Standardized pathology report format.

Immunohistochemistry

Immunohistochemistry (IHC) can enable the pathologist to confirm a histological diagnosis made from a standard stained section and to determine the cell of origin of poorly differentiated tumours. In addition, it can be used to aid in tumour prognostication. This can provide the clinician with useful information for deciding on the best treatment for the tumour and for helping to predict how the tumour is likely to behave. As the number of antibodies that can be successfully employed in veterinary diagnostic pathology is growing, IHC is increasingly being seen as an essential part of the pathologist's and clinician's armoury.

The technique involves the detection of antigen-specific antibodies binding to their antigen targets in a tissue section. An insoluble coloured precipitate forms at the antigen–antibody binding site and is visualized using a microscope. Positive and negative controls are used to aid interpretation and for quality control purposes. The extremely selective nature of antibody binding to its ligand is utilized to identify the extent and cellular localization of expression of the antibody, and its target antigen within a tissue (Figure 2.22).

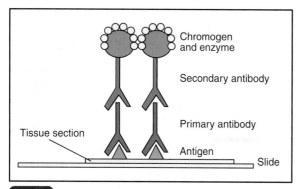

2.22 The basic principle of immunohistochemistry.

The main steps in performing IHC are as follows:

1. A tissue section is incubated with a specific dilution of a primary antibody that has been developed to bind to a single tissue antigen (such as a particular protein, or part thereof).
2. A secondary antibody that is linked to a marker enzyme (usually horseradish peroxidase) is incubated with the tissue and the primary antibody. This secondary antibody will bind to the non-antigen-binding end of the primary antibody molecule (for example, it might be a rabbit antibody that will bind specifically to all mouse antibodies).
3. A substrate is added to the final mixture, which undergoes a colour change and precipitates on to the tissue section when it is activated by the enzyme bound to the secondary antibody.
4. The sections are then counterstained with haematoxylin, coverslipped and examined under a microscope. Specific positive staining is identified where there is staining of the cells by the coloured enzyme substrate.

In practice there are many factors that can affect the quality and quantity of IHC staining. For instance, tissues that are inadequately fixed in formalin will often show very high levels of background staining, which can make it very difficult to assess the true staining characteristics and raises the possibility of false positive results. Conversely, tissues that have been exposed to formalin for extended periods of time may lose their ability to bind some antibodies, thereby creating false negative results. Fixation artefacts are some of the reasons that controls are so essential for the interpretation of IHC staining results.

Figure 2.23 lists some of the tumour markers that are commonly identified using IHC. In cancer diagnostics, the main use of IHC has been to aid the pathologist in determining the cell or tissue of origin of the neoplastic cell population. This has significant practical application: it can be very difficult to determine the exact cell of origin for some poorly

Marker (antigen)	Significance and usage
Vimentin	Identifies all mesenchymal cells. Often used to help confirm diagnosis of a tumour of mesenchymal origin, e.g. all sarcomas are positive for vimentin whereas most carcinomas are negative
Cytokeratin	Identifies most epithelial cells. Often used to help confirm diagnosis of a tumour of epithelial origin, e.g. most carcinomas are positive for cytokeratin whereas sarcomas are almost always negative
CD3	A marker of T-cell origin. Together with CD79a, used to help distinguish between T- and B-cell lymphomas, and essential in helping to apply the WHO–REAL lymphoma classification system
CD79a	A marker of B-cell origin. Used in a similar manner to CD3. Most plasma cells do not express CD79a, making it of less use in diagnosing plasmacytomas
CD18	A marker of leucocytes. Very useful in helping to diagnose tumours of monocyte/macrophage origin, such as histiocytic sarcomas
Desmin	A marker of muscle origin. Is expressed in most tumours of smooth muscle or striated muscle origin
S100	A marker of neuroectoderm origin. Is expressed in a number of different tumours, including peripheral nerve sheath tumours, melanomas, chondrosarcomas
Glial fibrillary acid protein (GFAP)	A marker of glial origin. Used for confirming the diagnosis of gliomas
CD117 (KIT)	A marker of mast cell origin or interstitial cells of Cajal
Mac387	A marker of macrophages. Can be used to help distinguish histiocytic tumours from granulomatous inflammation
Synaptophysin	A marker of neuroendocrine cells
Melan A	A specific marker of melanocyte differentiation. Can be used to help confirm a diagnosis of amelanotic melanoma

2.23 Tumour markers commonly identified using immunohistochemistry.

differentiated tumours based on routine light microscopy alone, and without IHC the amount of information that can be gleaned from examination of the specimens may be greatly limited.

Using a panel of antibodies against a range of intermediate filament proteins, the general tissue of origin can usually be identified and the tumour classified into the broad categories of epithelial/glandular *versus* mesenchymal. In general, the former tumour types often metastasize via lymphatics and frequently early in the course of disease, whilst the latter type often metastasizes haematogenously and later on in the disease course. Antibody panels can also help to distinguish mesenchymal tumours from the general category of 'round cell tumours', which are likely to have a different biological behaviour and to be sensitive to different treatment protocols. Intermediate filaments of a variety of different specific tissue types are found in all cells and range from 8 to 10 nm in diameter. For instance, cytokeratins are expressed by cells of epithelial origin and vimentin is expressed by mesenchymal cells, with only some cell types (e.g. mesothelium) expressing both. Vimentin is particularly useful because, as all mesenchymal cells express it, all tissues would be expected to contain some vimentin-positive cells within them. It therefore acts as a useful control to assess fixation artefacts: if no vimentin staining is identified, it is likely that the tissue is over-fixed, and

that the absence of positive staining using other IHC markers cannot be interpreted.

In order to classify tumours further, a range of tissue-specific proteins can be targeted using specific antisera raised against them. For instance, the intermediate filament protein desmin can be used to confirm a muscle origin of the tumour tissue. Then, using antibodies against a range of different actins and myoglobin, it is possible to characterize the cell of origin as smooth muscle, skeletal muscle or cardiac muscle.

In general, the most useful information for the clinician treating a cancer patient is likely to be provided by panels of antibodies that enable distinction between two tumours that, although they appear grossly and microscopically similar, are likely to have very different biological behaviours or responses to therapies.

However, it should be noted that in general when a tumour appears very poorly differentiated microscopically, it is likely that, whatever the cell of origin, the response to therapy and prognosis will be poor. Indeed, when neoplastic cells are very poorly differentiated, they can often exhibit aberrant expression of cellular proteins, such that it becomes very difficult to identify the cell of origin with certainty.

Some examples where IHC would be very useful to help to distinguish tumours of different prognosis/treatment options are given in Figures 2.24 and 2.25.

Histological differential diagnosis	Response to antibodies	
Amelanotic melanoma *versus* fibrosarcoma in oral cavity	*Amelanotic melanoma:* S100 +, Melan A +	*Fibrosarcoma:* S100 −, Melan A −
Osteosarcoma *versus* fibrosarcoma	*Osteosarcoma:* osteocalcin +	*Fibrosarcoma:* osteocalcin −
Synovial sarcoma *versus* histiocytic sarcoma	*Synovial sarcoma:* vimentin +, cytokeratin +, CD18 −	*Histiocytic sarcoma:* vimentin +, cytokeratin −, CD18 +
Nasal carcinoma *versus* lymphoma	*Carcinoma:* cytokeratin +, CD18 −, CD79a −, CD3 −	*Lymphoma:* cytokeratin −, CD18 +, CD79a/CD3 ±

2.24 Examples of use of immunohistochemistry in distinguishing certain tumours.

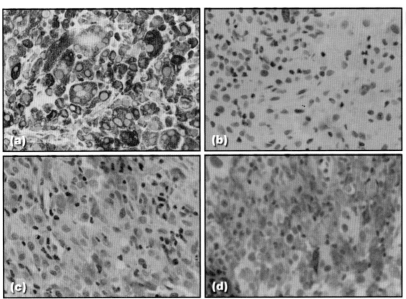

2.25 Histological sections showing IHC staining of a histiocytic sarcoma for: **(a)** vimentin; **(b)** cytokeratin; **(c)** lysosyme; **(d)** CD18. Note that the tumour is negative for cytokeratin.

Tumour markers and targeted treatment

The Holy Grail of cancer therapy is to identify tumour-specific targets that will allow tumour cells to be targeted and killed, leaving normal, non-neoplastic cells unharmed. IHC plays a vital role in a research setting to aid identification of novel targets; and in a diagnostic setting it is often the tool of choice to determine whether the individual case is likely to benefit from such targeted therapy. It is routinely used in human surgical pathology to determine the extent of HER-2/Neu expression in breast cancer to identify those women who would benefit from anti-HER-2/Neu antibody therapy (i.e. Herceptin). This protein is similarly expressed in some canine and feline mammary tumours and it is possible that, should the drug ever become affordable, it might be of potential use in a veterinary setting. Similarly, detection of oestrogen receptor expression in mammary tumours can be used to predict whether the patient will benefit from anti-oestrogen therapy.

In canine MCTs, the expression of the receptor tyrosine kinase KIT (CD117) may help to predict response to a new class of small-molecule tyrosine kinase inhibitors. KIT is expressed by normal mast cells, but is variably expressed in neoplastic mast cells. Those individual MCTs that express minimal or undetectable levels of KIT and other similar receptor tyrosine kinases would be predicted to respond less favourably to this class of drugs, compared with those that express high levels of the drug target. Although relative KIT expression levels can be determined by IHC, IHC cannot be used to identify whether KIT mutations are present. Rather, molecular methods such as PCR and nucleotide sequencing are required to identify the presence or absence of mutations.

Tumour grading

The specific histological/immunohistochemical diagnosis itself is likely to give the most important prognostic information for the clinician. For instance, a diagnosis of lymphoma *versus* soft tissue sarcoma is likely to result in very different treatments and a different prognosis. However, identifying various features of different subtypes of the same tumour (e.g. low-grade *versus* high-grade soft tissue sarcomas; grade I *versus* grade III MCTs) can also be used to direct therapy and to predict prognosis. Tumour grading can be further augmented by assessment of a variety of other markers of potential prognostic benefit, such as by measurement of proliferation markers.

Proliferation markers

One of the hallmarks of a neoplastic mass is uncontrolled growth. Several different techniques of measuring cell proliferation have been developed, the most robust and reliable of which are based on histochemical stains (AgNORs) and immunohistochemical stains (PCNA, Ki67).

AgNORs

Argyrophilic nucleolar organizing regions (AgNORs) are loops of DNA that contain ribosomal genes, and it is the NOR-associated proteins that bind the silver molecules of the stain. An increase in the number of AgNOR proteins indicates an increased demand for ribosomal biogenesis and therefore a higher metabolic activity. High AgNOR counts are associated with a shorter cell cycle and therefore a higher rate of cell proliferation. AgNOR counts are independent prognostic factors in many human tumours. In companion animal species, they are predictive of survival times in canine lymphoma and canine MCTs. However, only recently have the techniques for AgNOR staining and quantification been standardized, making comparisons between different studies difficult.

Ki67

This is an unidentified antigen to which the monoclonal antibody MIB-1 binds. Ki67 is a very large nuclear protein that is expressed exclusively by cells during the cell cycle; therefore, if a cell is expressing Ki67, it is actively replicating. Ki67 provides a measure of the growth fraction of a cell population. It is an independent prognostic factor in many human tumours and it has been shown to be an independent prognostic factor in canine MCTs. In general, the greater the proliferation index of a mast cell tumour, the more likely it is to recur locally and to metastasize, and hence the worse the prognosis.

PCNA

Proliferating cell nuclear antigen (PCNA) is the delta subunit of DNA polymerase I. PCNA expression is determined by immunohistochemistry. PCNA counts are expressed as the number of positively staining nuclei as a percentage of all neoplastic nuclei counted. It is an independent prognostic factor in a number of human tumours, but the role for it as a prognostic marker in canine and feline tumours is still unclear.

Summary

With the increased sophistication of clinical oncology in cats and dogs, obtaining an accurate diagnosis prior to embarking on therapy is becoming of ever greater importance. In most cases this will entail obtaining a tissue biopsy or cytology sample and submitting it to a qualified veterinary pathologist. The manner in which these samples are taken, and the associated information that the clinician provides to the pathologist, can greatly enhance or potentially detract from the diagnosis that can be made based on those samples. Therefore it is of utmost importance (if valuable resources, time and expense are not to be wasted) that thought is put into deciding what sampling modality will provide the best cost/benefit balance for the patient and the client.

It is incumbent on the pathologist to examine the samples in such a way as to provide the clinician with the most accurate and prognostically relevant information. In this way, a highly fruitful relationship can be developed between clinician and pathologist, such that patient care is optimized and the tissue samples obtained can be utilized and analysed to their full potential.

There are an increasing range of immunohisto-chemical staining techniques that can be used with canine and feline tissue and much research is being undertaken to use these techniques to distinguish previously indistinguishable tumours. By using these techniques, it is becoming increasingly possible to provide more accurate prognostic information to clinicians, enabling them to make the best treatment decisions for their patients. In addition, it is likely that application of these techniques will help to identify new therapeutic targets, which will further increase the arsenal of drugs that might be rationally applied to veterinary cancer patients.

References and further reading

McGavin MD and Zachary JF (2007) *Pathological Basis of Veterinary Disease, 4th edn.* Mosby Elsevier, St. Louis

Meuten DJ (2002) *Tumors in Domestic Animals, 4th edn.* Iowa State Press, Ames, Iowa

Morris J and Dobson JM (2001) *Small Animal Oncology.* Blackwell, Oxford

3

Clinical staging and the TNM classification

Jane M. Dobson

Introduction

The diagnostic evaluation of the patient is of paramount importance in the management of cancer. The initial approach to any patient with suspected cancer must be designed to achieve the following objectives to the extent that is appropriate for the individual owner:

- To make a histological/cytological diagnosis
- To grade the disease
- To determine the extent of the disease in terms of both local and distant spread
- To investigate and treat any tumour-related or concurrent complications that might affect the overall prognosis or the patient's ability to tolerate therapy.

Chapter 2 discusses methods for tumour diagnosis and histological grading, but the stage or extent of the tumour is equally important in determining treatment and prognosis. The stage of cancer at diagnosis is a powerful predictor of survival and often dictates treatment selection. This chapter covers techniques to evaluate the cancer patient as a whole and discusses what may be gained from such comprehensive approaches. Paraneoplastic syndromes are addressed in Chapter 4.

Appropriate clinical staging is largely informed by a knowledge of the biological behaviour of malignant tumours, their patterns of local growth and mechanisms of metastasis. Although it is not the remit of this chapter to delve into the fine detail of tumour biology, an understanding of the basic pathological behaviour of tumours is a prerequisite to the process of clinical staging.

Tumour biology

The processes that lead to tumour development are described briefly in Chapter 1. Two important facts must be borne in mind:

- A tumour does most of its growing before it can be detected
- The cells that make up a tumour mass are not identical.

A tumour cannot be detected by palpation, radiography or other imaging techniques until it reaches approximately 0.5–1 cm in diameter or 0.5–1 g in weight, by which time it contains approximately 10^8–10^9 cells (Figure 3.1).

Cancer cells continually modify their properties during the process of growth, largely through small mutations occurring during cell division. Hence, although the cells in the tumour mass may share some features of the original precursor cell, they may be different in other properties, such as the ability to

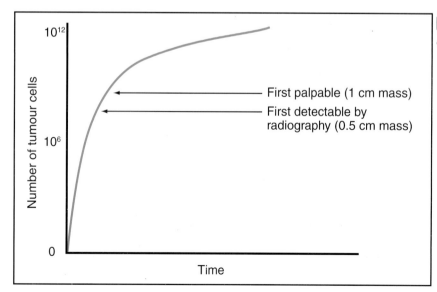

3.1 Tumour growth and clinical detection.

metastasize or to metabolize a cytotoxic drug. This variation is important in therapy because different cells within the tumour mass may be inherently more or less sensitive to cytotoxic drugs or to radiation.

Tumour behaviour

Tumours are traditionally classified as being benign or malignant, according to their growth and behavioural characteristics (Figure 3.2).

Although this division is useful for descriptive purposes, in reality tumours display a spectrum of behaviour, ranging from truly benign to highly malignant. Some (e.g. low-grade spindle cell tumours) have local characteristics of malignancy but rarely metastasize. Others (e.g. mast cell tumours (MCTs)) can display a wide spectrum of behaviour ranging from benign to malignant.

Histologically, a number of morphological features of a tumour can be used to predict its likely behaviour. The histological appearance or **grade** of

the tumour, in terms of relationship to adjacent normal tissues, mitotic rate, cellular and nuclear characteristics, is therefore important in prognosis (see Chapter 2).

Features of malignancy

Clinically, the most important features of malignancy are invasion and metastasis (Figure 3.3). These are closely allied processes, as in many cases invasion is the first step on the road to metastasis. Invasion and metastasis are very complex processes, the genetic and biochemical basis of which are still not fully understood. It is known that cell–cell adhesion molecules (notably members of the cadherin family) and integrins (which link cells to extracellular matrix substances) are involved in the process, as is proteolytic remodelling of the extracellular matrix, which allows tumour cells to move through connective tissue barriers.

Characteristic	Benign	Malignant
Rate of growth	Relatively slow. Growth may cease in some cases	Often rapid. Rarely ceases growing
Manner of growth	Expansive. Usually well defined boundary between neoplastic and normal tissues. May become encapsulated	Invasive. Poorly defined borders; tumour cells extend into, and may be scattered throughout, adjacent normal tissues
Effects on adjacent tissues	Often minimal. May cause pressure necrosis and anatomical deformity	Often serious. Tumour growth and invasion result in destruction of adjacent normal tissues, manifest as ulceration of superficial tissues, lysis of bone
Metastasis	Does not occur	Metastasize by lymphatic and haematogenous routes and transcoelomic spread
Effect on host	Often minimal but can be life-threatening if tumour develops in a vital organ (e.g. brain)	Often life-threatening by virtue of destructive nature of growth and metastatic dissemination to other (vital) organs

3.2   Characteristics of benign *versus* malignant tumours.

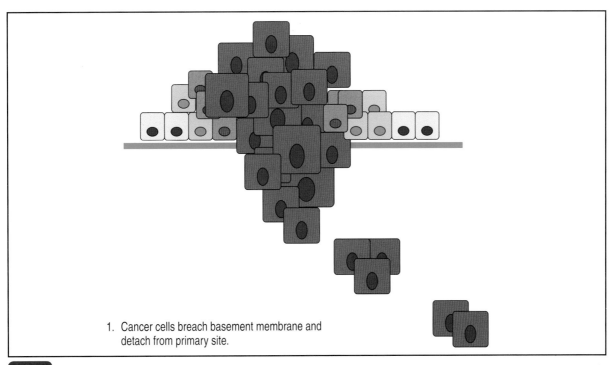

1. Cancer cells breach basement membrane and detach from primary site.

3.3   Invasion and metastasis. (continues)   ▶

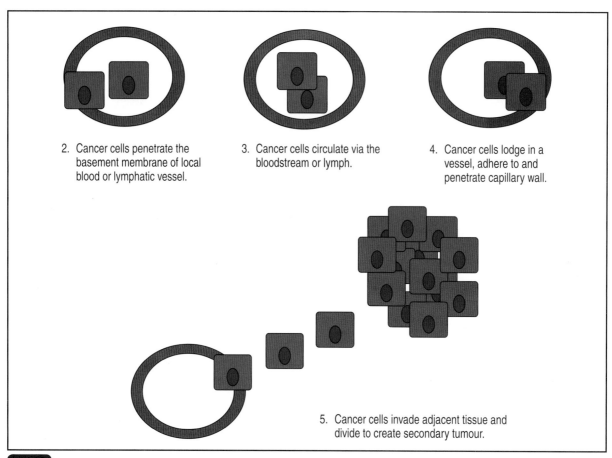

2. Cancer cells penetrate the basement membrane of local blood or lymphatic vessel.

3. Cancer cells circulate via the bloodstream or lymph.

4. Cancer cells lodge in a vessel, adhere to and penetrate capillary wall.

5. Cancer cells invade adjacent tissue and divide to create secondary tumour.

3.3   (continued) Invasion and metastasis.

Invasion

From the clinical perspective, tumour invasion into the wall of a hollow organ or into adjacent tissue compartments dictates the extent of surgical margin required to effect complete removal and thus the feasibility of a surgical cure (Figure 3.4).

Unfortunately, in the clinical setting it is very difficult to assess the pathological invasiveness of a particular tumour prior to surgical resection; thus, in clinical practice it is usual to rely on data generated from previous pathological studies of tumour invasion. For example, the requirement for wide margins of resection for grade II MCTs is well documented. A recent study of 23 cutaneous MCTs showed that 75% of 20 grade II tumours were completely excised at 1 cm and all were completely excised at 2 cm (Simpson *et al.*, 2004). The authors concluded that a 2 cm lateral margin and a deep margin of one fascial plane appear to be adequate for complete excision of grade I and grade II tumours and subsequently

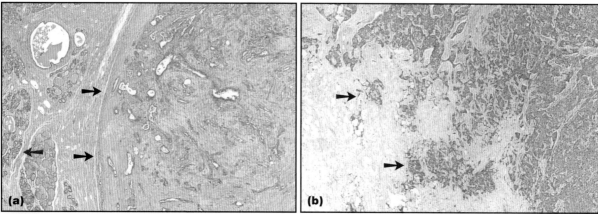

3.4   Microscopic comparison of well defined *versus* invasive tumours. **(a)** Well defined complex mammary adenoma from an 8-year-old female Staffordshire Bull Terrier. The black arrows show the clear demarcation between tumour and surrounding normal tissue. The red arrow shows normal mammary gland. **(b)** An invasive anal sac gland carcinoma from a 6-year-old Cocker Spaniel. In contrast to (a), there is no clear boundary between tumour and normal tissue, and lobules of tumour cells are seen invading the adjacent connective tissue (black arrows). (H&E, original magnification X40) (Images courtesy of Dr Fernando Constantino-Casas, Department of Veterinary Medicine, University of Cambridge)

confirmed this in a separate prospective study in 16 dogs (Fulcher *et al.*, 2006). Veterinary-specific data on other tumour types is relatively sparse.

Metastasis

The ability of malignant tumours to spread to and grow in distant organs is their most serious and life-threatening characteristic. Cancer metastases are the cause of 90% of human cancer deaths. The mechanisms involved in the process of metastasis are not fully understood. In order to form a meta-static growth, a cancer cell must detach from the pri-mary tumour, invade and move into the vasculature to travel to a new location, aggregate with platelets and fibrin to arrest at the new site, extravasate into surrounding parenchyma and establish growth (see Figure 3.3). During this process the cell must evade host defence mechanisms and survive in the circula-tion. Current theories suggest that only certain clones of cells within a tumour develop all the abili-ties required for metastasis but that these clones probably arise and disseminate in the early stages of that tumour's growth, often prior to the detection of the primary tumour.

Tumours may metastasize via the lymphatic route to local and regional lymph nodes, or via the haem-atogenous route, allowing secondary tumours to develop in any body organ. These two systems are widely interconnected and many tumours use these connections to spread through the body. Tumours may also disseminate through body cavities via haemor-rhage or effusions and may be spread on instruments.

In humans, different types of cancer show different target organ specificity for metastasis. For example:

- Prostatic carcinoma: bone
- Breast carcinoma: bone, brain, adrenal, lung, liver
- Cutaneous melanoma: liver, brain, bowel.

In small animals, the lungs are the most common site for the development of haematogenous second-ary tumours but other sites, including liver, spleen, kidneys, skin and bone, should not be overlooked.

- Carcinomas and MCTs usually metastasize first by the lymphatic route, before disseminating more widely.
- Sarcomas (soft tissue and bone) and melanomas metastasize by the haematogenous route.

However, tumours do not always follow expected patterns of behaviour and some may spread by both lymphatic and haematogenous routes.

Clinical staging of cancer

The clinical stage describes the anatomical extent of a tumour at a set point in time, i.e. it defines how much the cancer has spread. The clinical stage often takes account of the size of a tumour, how deeply it has penetrated the wall of an organ or other adjacent tissues, whether it has metastasized to local or regional lymph nodes and how many are affected, and whether it has spread to more distant organs.

Staging has several purposes:

- To define the local, regional and distant extent of disease
- To help to determine the optimum treatment
- To provide a baseline against which response to treatment can be assessed
- To provide prognostic information.

Cancer staging can be divided into a clinical stage and a pathological stage:

- **Clinical stage** is based on all of the information obtained by physical examination, imaging, endoscopy, biopsy, etc., prior to surgery
- **Pathological stage** adds additional information gained by microscopic examination of the tumour by a pathologist; this is a postoperative staging.

Clinical stage and pathological stage should be regarded as complementary. It is not unusual for there to be a difference between the clinical stage of a disease and the pathological stage, because it is not possible to detect microscopic tumour exten-sions or deposits by gross examination or with the imaging tools available to the clinician. The patho-logical stage is usually considered the 'truer' stage as it is informed by direct (microscopic) visualization of the tumour, whereas clinical staging is limited by the fact that the information is gained by indirect observation of a tumour that is still *in situ*. However, pathological staging can also be problematic, as it relies on the presence of malignant cells in the sec-tions of tissues examined and on the visual skills of the pathologist to identify maybe one or two cancer cells mixed with healthy cells on a slide. New, more sensitive, methods using molecular screening (reverse transcription polymerase chain reaction, RT-PCR) for cancer-specific proteins are being developed for use in human patients.

Many clinical staging systems have been described for use in human and veterinary patients with cancers at various sites in the body. The ideal staging system should be: easy to use and remem-ber; reproducible; not subject to inter- or intra-observer variation; and based on prognostically important factors. The World Health Organization's *TNM Classification of Tumours in Domestic Animals* (Owen, 1980) is one of the most widely used and adapted in veterinary medicine. Although it may not be appropriate or necessary for the practitioner to use the TNM or other staging nomenclature, the basic principle of determining the extent of a tumour in terms of local invasion and nodal and distant metastasis is vital to the work-up of any cancer case.

TNM classification

The TNM system is based on the anatomical extent of spread (Figure 3.5):

- **T** refers to the extent of the primary tumour
- **N** refers to the extent of nodal metastasis
- **M** refers to the presence or absence of distant metastasis.

T – primary tumour	
Tx	Primary tumour cannot be assessed
T0	No evidence of primary tumour
Tis	Carcinoma *in situ*
T 1–4	Increasing size and local extent of primary tumour
N – regional lymph nodes	
Nx	Regional nodes cannot be assessed
N0	No regional node metastasis
N 1–3	Increasing involvement of regional nodes
M – distant metastasis	
Mx	Distant metastasis cannot be assessed
M0	No distant metastasis
M1	Distant metastasis present

3.5 The TNM system. Two classifications can be described for each site: clinical (TNM) and pathological (pTNM).

Clinical assessment of the primary tumour (T)

Certain physical features of the primary mass may give important clues as to its degree of malignancy, feasibility of treatment and prognosis. A thorough assessment of the primary mass is obviously of paramount importance in planning surgery.

Physical examination

The size of the primary mass is important. For example, in mammary tumours, those < 3 cm in diameter generally carry a more favourable prognosis than larger ones (see Chapter 16).

The degree of infiltration or invasion of adjacent normal tissues by the primary tumour reflects its malignancy and affects both treatment and prognosis for local recurrence. This may be assessed by features such as how well circumscribed the mass appears, the degree of mobility, fixation of the lesion in one or more planes, adhesion to adjacent structures, or ulceration of overlying skin or epithelium.

These features should be assessed and recorded as part of the initial examination of the cancer patient. For superficial soft tissue tumours, physical examination may be all that is required for assessment of the primary tumour. For tumours at certain sites, (e.g. head and neck), close to or involving bone, or involving hollow organs, further investigations may be indicated. Endoscopy enables visual assessment of the extent of tumours of the upper and lower alimentary system, upper respiratory system (intranasal) and bladder. A biopsy sample may be taken at the same time.

Diagnostic imaging

Radiography: Radiography of, for example, intra-oral tumours, intranasal tumours or tumours affecting digits allows assessment of the degree of bony destruction and thus the invasiveness of the tumour. Whilst radiography is relatively low cost and readily available, its use for staging primary tumours of the head and neck and soft tissue sarcomas has largely been superseded by magnetic resonance imaging (see below).

Ultrasonography: Ultrasound examination has an important role in evaluation of the site, size and extent of any tumour mass in either body cavity. It is superior to radiography for assessment of abdominal organs and lesions and in cases with pleural or peritoneal effusions. It can also be used to assess soft tissue masses on limbs and in the neck. In all these situations ultrasound is very sensitive at locating lesions and in assessing their extent and relationship with adjacent structures; however, it is not specific for the aetiology of the lesion and cannot differentiate neoplastic from non-neoplastic lesions, nor benign from malignant. Cytology or histology are still required to make the diagnosis; and fine-needle aspiration or needle biopsy samples can be collected from lesions under ultrasound guidance.

High-quality ultrasonography can be very useful in assessment of tumours affecting organs such as the alimentary system and urogenital system as it allows visualization of the layers of muscle forming the walls of these organs and thus can give information on the depth of penetration of the tumour (Figure 3.6).

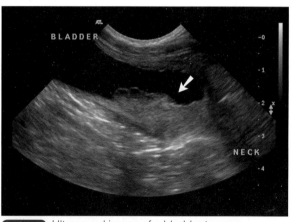

3.6 Ultrasound image of a bladder tumour (arrowed) showing layers of the bladder wall.

Computed tomography: CT uses ionizing radiation but images are acquired perpendicular to the body or body part. Spiral CT scanners allow these images to be reformatted in high detail with greatly increased tissue definition in comparison with radiography. CT is highly sensitive for fine bone detail, but soft tissue definition is not as good as with magnetic resonance imaging (MRI) and for this reason, in general, CT is used more for detection of metastatic disease than the staging of primary tumours. However, this also depends upon availability, cost and time. CT is considerably quicker than MRI and patients do not always need to be anaesthetized. CT-guided biopsy can be performed on, for example, lung masses, which cannot be imaged using ultrasound. In some centres CT is preferred for radiation planning, as the physical tissue density figures can be used by treatment planning computer programs.

Magnetic resonance imaging: MRI produces images in transverse, sagittal and dorsal planes. It provides excellent soft tissue detail and anatomical definition, but does not provide any detail of cortical bone. It is particularly sensitive for imaging the brain (Figure 3.7) and spinal cord (and has largely replaced myelography in human medicine) but is also very useful for pre-treatment assessment of soft tissue sarcomas and intranasal tumours (Figure 3.8) (see also relevant chapters). MRI can be used for imaging primary tumours of the head and neck, spine, dorsum and pelvis but, because of the need for the area of interest to remain still during acquisition of images, it is used less frequently for imaging lesions of the chest and abdomen in small animals. Gating systems can be applied to negate movement artefact, but CT is preferable for imaging tumours of these regions.

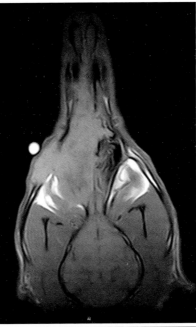
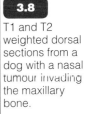

3.8 T1 and T2 weighted dorsal sections from a dog with a nasal tumour invading the maxillary bone.

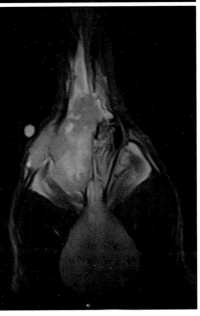

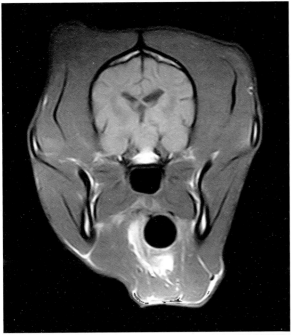

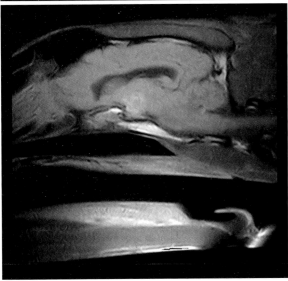

3.7 MRI transverse and sagittal sections of the brain in a dog with pituitary macroadenoma.

Clinical assessment of local and regional lymph nodes (N)

Lymph node metastasis is most common in carcinomas, melanomas and mast cell tumours; soft tissue sarcomas may occasionally metastasize by this route. The clinician should be familiar with the principal lymph nodes and patterns of lymphatic drainage (Figure 3.9).

Physical examination

The size, shape, texture and mobility of local and regional lymph nodes should be assessed as part of the initial patient appraisal. Gross enlargement, irregularity, firmness and fixation are all features indicative of neoplastic involvement. A more subtle lymphadenopathy may indicate a small metastatic deposit or may arise as a result of reactive hyperplasia.

Any degree of lymphadenopathy should be investigated further by collection of fine-needle

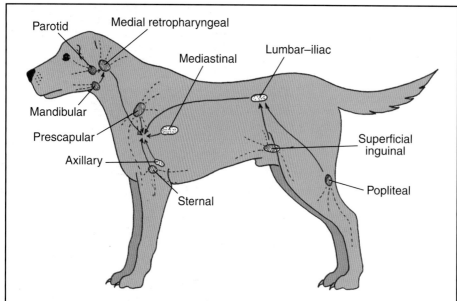

3.9

Principal lymph nodes and lymphatic drainage in the dog.

aspirates and cytology. Arguably, aspirates should be collected from even apparently normal lymph nodes from regions draining highly malignant tumours such as malignant melanoma.

Interpretation of lymph node cytology can be challenging in some cases, particularly in MCTs because mast cells can be found in lymph node aspirates from normal animals. Current recommendations are that metastasis of an MCT to a lymph node may be diagnosed on cytology if mast cells represent >3% of the cell population (Duncan, 1999). However, using this criterion, up to 25% of normal dogs would then be diagnosed with a metastatic MCT (Bookbinder *et al.*, 1992); therefore, results from lymph nodes draining a mast cell tumour must be treated with caution. Conversely, a fine-needle-aspirate 'negative' for mast cells does not completely exclude the possibility of metastasis. Excision and histopathology is the most secure method for evaluation of lymph nodes draining MCTs (see Chapter 12).

Imaging

Radiography: Whilst radiography is useful for screening for enlargement of intrathoracic or intra-abdominal lymph nodes, it can only detect gross changes in lymph node size, and other imaging methods are superior for staging lymph nodes.

Ultrasonography: Ultrasonography is a very sensitive method for detecting abdominal lymphadenopathy. It allows guided fine-needle aspirates to be collected for cytology, and measurement of lymph nodes for initial staging and treatment monitoring. It is less useful for assessment of thoracic lymphadenopathy because of the limitations of air-filled lung.

Computed tomography: CT is more sensitive than radiography for detection of mediastinal lymphadenopathy and would be the method of choice for assessment of an animal with a lung mass, as it is also more sensitive for detection of pulmonary

metastases. It can also provide good soft tissue definition of abdominal lymph nodes and can be used to guide fine-needle aspiration or needle biopsy, or surgical investigation at exploratory laparotomy.

Magnetic resonance imaging: Because of cost, the length of time required to acquire images, the need for anaesthesia and gating, MRI is not the method of choice for evaluation of thoracic or abdominal lymph nodes.

Clinical assessment of distant metastasis (M)

Malignant tumours may spread via the haematogenous route, giving rise to metastases in distant organs. Soft tissue sarcomas, osteosarcomas (OSAs) and malignant melanoma characteristically metastasize in this way but some carcinomas and MCTs also spread via the blood to distant sites.

Although the lungs are the most common site for the development of metastases in small animals, other potential sites for metastatic spread should not be overlooked. These include:

- Skin
- Bones
- Brain and spinal cord
- Internal organs, spleen, liver, kidneys, heart.

The detection of metastases is problematic: tumours only become large enough to detect at a relatively late stage in their development and micrometastases that are below the threshold of detection of imaging techniques may be present.

Physical examination

A thorough history may reveal signs indicative of a wider problem; for example, weight loss, anorexia, lethargy or pyrexia may raise the suspicion of metastatic disease. Clinical findings such as skin nodules, hepatosplenomegaly or bone pain would warrant further investigations.

To some degree the search for metastatic disease should be informed by the histology, type of tumour and its known metastatic behaviour. An all-encompassing 'met. check' is probably not appropriate for every cancer patient.

Imaging

Radiography: Routine thoracic radiography is a standard screening process for tumours that metastasize via the haematogenous route (e.g. OSA, haemangiosarcoma, malignant melanoma, mammary carcinoma and other carcinomas – thyroid, bladder) as the lungs are one of the first sites for development of metastases. Radiography is not a very sensitive means of detecting pulmonary masses. Sensitivity can be optimized by:

- Reducing movement blur
- Making the exposure on maximum inflation
- Taking appropriate views.

Right and left lateral thoracic radiographs are the minimum requirement for screening for pulmonary metastases, as contrast is optimized in the upper, air-filled lung, whilst the partial compression of the lower lung may obscure a soft tissue nodule. Whether a third dorsoventral or ventrodorsal view adds to sensitivity is debatable, though one study of canine haemangiosarcoma suggested that obtaining three views significantly reduced the false negative rate (Holt *et al.*, 1992). Even then an apparently clear thoracic radiograph does not rule out the presence of metastases.

Whilst survey abdominal radiographs are often not very helpful in assessing metastatic disease in organs such as the liver and spleen, survey skeletal films may be useful for those tumours that metastasize to or involve bone (e.g. multiple myeloma).

Ultrasonography: Ultrasound is very sensitive at detecting lesions in the liver, spleen and kidneys but, as above, is not specific for the nature of the lesion and often cannot distinguish benign nodular hyperplasia from more aggressive disease. Ultrasonography may be used to guide fine-needle aspiration from suspicious lesions, but the diagnostic yield is often low.

Contrast-enhanced ultrasonography using micro-bubble contrast media has been used to improve characterization between benign and malignant focal or multifocal lesions in the spleen (Rossi *et al.*, 2008).

Computed tomography: CT is more sensitive than radiography for detecting pulmonary nodules and may be indicated when the thoracic radiograph appearance is equivocal or in the case of tumours with a high risk of pulmonary metastases (e.g. OSA), as it has been shown to be superior to radiography for detection of pulmonary metastatic neoplasia (Nemanic *et al.*, 2006) (Figure 3.10)

CT may also be used for assessment of abdominal organs. Contrast-enhanced CT has been shown to provide significant differences in imaging characteristics between benign and malignant splenic

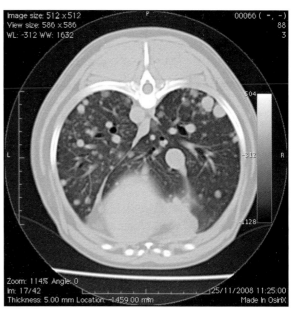

3.10 CT transverse section of canine thorax, showing multiple pulmonary metastases. (Image courtesy of Paddy Mannion, Cambridge Radiology Referrals)

lesions but, as with other imaging techniques, it does not provide a histological or cytological diagnosis (Fife *et al.*, 2004).

Magnetic resonance imaging: Although whole-body MRI is used in staging human cancer patients, its role in veterinary medicine is more directed at staging the primary tumour than assessing the patient for metastases.

Nuclear medicine (scintigraphy): The use of radioactive pharmaceuticals that localize to the area of interest to assess organ function and extent of disease is well established in human medicine but little used in veterinary small animal medicine. The most commonly used radioisotope is [99m]technetium, because it has a short half-life and is easily bound to localizing pharmaceuticals such as the bone-seeking methylene diphosphonate (MDP). This combination ([99m]TcMDP) is a sensitive and non-invasive method of evaluating the skeleton in animals suspected of having or being at risk from bone metastases, such as dogs with OSA (see Chapter 13).

Other investigations

Routine blood sampling

Assessment of haematological and biochemical parameters may be performed for many reasons in the animal cancer patient and can form part of the staging process. For example, in haematological malignancies it is important to know the degree of involvement in the peripheral blood and the presence of any cytopenias (see Chapter 19). Some tumours are associated with paraneoplastic syndromes such as hypercalcaemia and hypoglycaemia (see Chapter 4).

Bone marrow aspiration

Bone marrow aspiration is particularly useful in the diagnosis and staging of haematological malignancies (lymphoma, myeloma and leukaemia).

Some authorities also recommend that bone marrow evaluation is necessary for clinical staging of MCTs. Although systemic mastocytosis has been reported in dogs (O'Keefe *et al.*, 1987) this is a rare condition and the vast majority of dogs with cutaneous MCTs do not have circulating mast cells or evidence of bone marrow infiltration. Consequently, in the author's opinion such investigations are not warranted in the evaluation of dogs with solitary cutaneous MCTs.

Example of a clinical staging system

An example of the clinical staging system for tumours of the skin, applied to squamous cell carcinoma (SCC) of the nasal planum in the cat, is shown in Figures 3.11 and 3.12.

Tis, T1 and T2 tumours may be treated successfully by surgery, cryosurgery or radiotherapy, whereas T4 tumours are difficult to treat by any means other than radical surgery and even then carry a poor prognosis (see Chapter 18).

Clinical stage is particularly important in clinical studies, especially trials of a new drug or therapy where it is essential that like is compared with like. For example, a new treatment for SCC of the nasal planum in cats would not be given fair assessment if all cats receiving the new therapy bore T4 tumours and outcome was compared with cats with Tis and T1 tumours who received standard therapy.

Summary

Figure 3.13 summarizes clinical staging procedures and indications.

The principles of clinical staging are of paramount importance in general clinical practice, where knowledge of the likely behaviour of different tumour types forms the basis for selection of clinical investigations. Clinical staging and stage grouping are included where relevant in the following chapters for specific tumours and body systems.

T group	Description
Tis	Pre-invasive carcinoma (carcinoma *in situ*) (Figure 3.12a)
T1	Tumour, 2 cm maximal diameter, superficial or exophytic (Figure 3.12b)
T2	Tumour 2–5 cm maximal diameter, or with minimal invasion irrespective of size
T3	Tumour > 5 cm, or with invasion of the subcutis irrespective of size (Figure 3.12c)
T4	Invasion of other structures, e.g. fascia, muscle, cartilage or bone (Figure 3.12d)

3.11   Clinical staging system for tumours of epidermal origin (Owen, 1980).

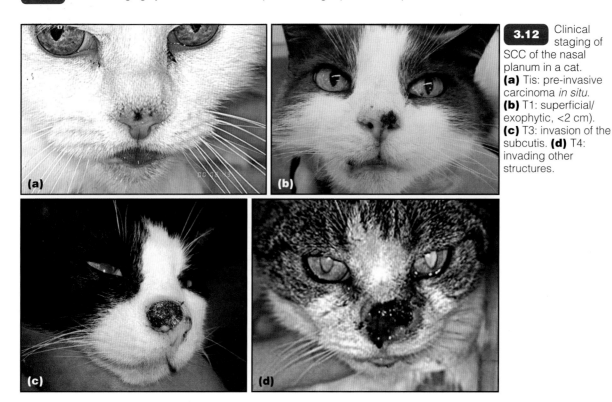

3.12   Clinical staging of SCC of the nasal planum in a cat. **(a)** Tis: pre-invasive carcinoma *in situ*. **(b)** T1: superficial/exophytic, <2 cm). **(c)** T3: invasion of the subcutis. **(d)** T4: invading other structures.

Technique	Indication
Physical examination	A detailed and thorough physical examination is mandatory for all cancer patients for staging of primary tumour and assessment of nodal and distant metastasis
Radiography	**T** – Primary site where tumours are adjacent to or involving bone **N** – Screening for thoracic and abdominal lymphadenopathy **M** – Right and left lateral thoracic radiographs for all malignant tumours likely to metastasize to the lungs
Ultrasonography	**T** – Primary tumours of soft tissues, abdominal organs **N** – Abdominal lymph nodes **M** – Assessment of abdominal organs in tumours likely to metastasize to liver/spleen, especially malignant mast cell tumours and gastrointestinal tumours
CT	**T** – Primary lung masses (also N and M) **N** – Thoracic and abdominal lymphadenopathy **M** – Most sensitive method for detection of pulmonary metastases. Animals with highly malignant tumours
MRI	**T** – Good for extent of head and neck tumours (including brain), presurgical assessment of soft tissue sarcomas
Scintigraphy	**M** – Assessment of bone metastasis. Evaluation of ectopic or metastatic thyroid tumours
Haematology / biochemistry	May help in staging haemopoietic malignancies
Bone marrow aspiration / biopsy	Important in staging haemopoietic malignancies

3.13 Summary of clinical staging procedures and indications.

References and further reading

Bookbinder PF, Butt MT and Harvey HJ (1992) Determination of the number of mast cells in lymph node, bone marrow and buffy coat cytological specimens in dogs. *Journal of the American Veterinary Medical Association* **200**, 1648–1650

Duncan J (1999) The lymph nodes. In: *Diagnostic Cytology and Haematology of the Dog and Cat, 2nd edn*, ed. RL Cowell *et al.*, pp. 9–103, Mosby, St. Louis

Fife WD, Samil VF, Drost WT, Matton JS and Hoshaw-Woodard S (2004) Comparison between malignant and non-malignant splenic masses in dogs using contrast-enhanced computed tomography. *Veterinary Radiology and Ultrasound* **45**, 289–297

Fulcher RP, Ludwog LL, Bergman PJ *et al.* (2006) Evaluation of a two-centimetre lateral surgical margin for excision of grade I and grade II cutaneous mast cell tumours in dogs. *Journal of the American Veterinary Medical Association* **228**, 210–215

Holt D, Van Winkle T, Schelling C *et al.* (1992) Correlation between thoracic radiographs and post mortem findings in dogs with hemangiosarcoma: 77 cases (1984–1989). *Journal of the American Veterinary Medical Association* **200**, 1535–1539

Nemanic S, London CA and Wisner ER (2006) Comparison of thoracic radiographs and single breath-hold helical CT for detection of pulmonary nodules in dogs with metastatic neoplasia. *Journal of Veterinary Internal Medicine* **20**, 508–515

O'Keefe DA, Couto GC, Burke-Schwartz C and Jacobs RM (1987) Systemic mastocytosis in 16 dogs. *Journal of Veterinary Internal Medicine* **1**, 75–80

Owen LN (1980) *TNM Classification of Tumours in Domestic Animals*. World Health Organization, Geneva

Rossi F, Leone VF, Vignoli M, Laddaga E and Terragni R (2008) Use of contrast-enhanced ultrasound for characterization of focal splenic lesions. *Veterinary Radiology and Ultrasound* **49**, 154–164

Simpson AM, Ludwig LL, Newman SJ *et al.* (2004) Evaluation of surgical margins required for complete excision of cutaneous mast cell tumors in dogs. *Journal of the American Veterinary Medical Association* **224**, 236–240

4

Paraneoplastic syndromes

Richard Mellanby

Introduction

Paraneoplastic syndromes result from indirect effects of tumours due to the production and release of biologically active substances such as hormones, growth factors and cytokines. Paraneoplastic syndromes are an extremely important consideration in the management of malignancies in small animal patients for a variety of reasons; the presence of clinical signs related to the paraneoplastic syndrome may be the first indication that an animal has an underlying neoplasia, and recurrence of the paraneoplastic syndrome may be the earliest indication that the tumour has recurred following treatment. In addition, paraneoplastic syndromes may be associated with a higher degree of morbidity and even mortality than the primary tumour itself and consequently may have important prognostic implications and/or may alter the therapeutic approach to the underlying malignancy.

Paraneoplastic syndromes tend to be classified according to the body system which is most affected. This chapter will review paraneoplastic syndromes involving the endocrine, haematological/ haemostatic, gastrointestinal, renal, cutaneous and neuromuscular body systems and will briefly discuss other less commonly observed paraneoplastic syndromes.

Endocrine system

Hypercalcaemia

Hypercalcaemia is one of the most common paraneoplastic syndromes diagnosed in small animal patients. Although parathyroid adenomas are well recognized in both dogs and cats as a cause of hypercalcaemia due to excessive production of parathyroid hormone, non-parathyroid tumours more commonly cause malignancy-associated hypercalcaemia in companion animals. The tumours that are associated with hypercalcaemia differ slightly between dogs and cats.

Dogs

The two most common tumours associated with hypercalcaemia in the dog are lymphoma and adenocarcinoma of the apocrine gland of the anal sac, but hypercalcaemia has been associated with a wide range of other canine tumours, including:

- Carcinomas such as nasal, mammary, bronchial and squamous cell neoplasms

- Multiple myeloma
- Leukaemia
- Thymoma
- Malignant melanoma.

Cats

In cats, lymphoma and squamous cell carcinoma are the most common tumour types associated with hypercalcaemia. Other feline tumour types reported to be associated with hypercalcaemia include:

- Leukaemia
- Osteosarcoma
- Bronchiogenic carcinoma
- Fibrosarcoma
- Undifferentiated sarcoma.

In contrast to dogs, adenocarcinoma of the apocrine gland has rarely been diagnosed in cats (Mellanby et al., 2002).

Clinical signs

Although the raised plasma calcium concentration in many dogs and cats with malignancy-related hypercalcaemia can cause significant clinical signs, in other cases the clinical signs may be related predominantly to the underlying neoplasia. For example, tenesmus in dogs with adenocarcinoma of the apocrine gland of the anal sac is a common presenting complaint. Hypercalcaemia in dogs tends to cause inappetence, polydipsia, polyuria and vomiting in the majority of cases, with muscle weakness or twitching occurring in a minority.

One of the most important effects of hypercalcaemia is the inhibition of antidiuretic hormone, which leads to an inability to concentrate urine and causes polyuria and polydipsia. Urine specific gravity may be isosthenuric or hyposthenuric. If the animal fails to drink enough water to compensate for the increased urinary water loss, dehydration will develop, with resultant prerenal azotaemia. Longstanding hypercalcaemia, especially if accompanied by hyperphosphataemia, may result in renal tubular damage and so an intrinsic renal azotaemia. Consequently, it is difficult to distinguish prerenal from renal azotaemia in animals with hypercalcaemia, since in both situations the urine specific gravity will be lowered.

In cats with hypercalcaemia the signs are more non-specific. Inappetence is recorded in most cases, with polydipsia and vomiting occurring less commonly than in dogs.

Parathyroid hormone-related protein

The main hormones involved in the regulation of calcium metabolism in healthy animals are:

- Parathyroid hormone
- 1,25-dihydroxyvitamin D (1,25(OH)$_2$D)
- Calcitonin.

However, a fourth hormone, namely parathyroid hormone-related protein (PTHrp), has been demonstrated to play an important role in calcium metabolism, particularly in malignant conditions in humans and companion animals (Rosol *et al.*, 1992; Mellanby *et al.*, 2006). PTHrp has a similar structure and function to parathyroid hormone and causes hypercalcaemia by increasing bone resorption and renal tubular resorption of calcium. In contrast to hypercalcaemia associated with primary hyperparathyroidism, which is typically due to the excessive production of parathyroid hormone by a parathyroid adenoma (Feldman *et al.*, 2005), the pathogenesis of hypercalcaemia associated with malignancies is usually due to ectopic production of PTHrp. Dogs with hypercalcaemia associated with chronic renal failure or primary hyperparathyroidism due to a parathyroid adenoma do not have a raised PTHrp concentration (Mellanby *et al.*, 2006).

PTHrp causes an increase in both total and ionized calcium concentrations. There is no correlation between PTHrp concentration and the degree of hypercalcaemia (either ionized or total calcium). However, it is important to acknowledge that hypercalcaemia associated with malignancy is not invariably caused by ectopic production of PTHrp by the tumour, since a minority of cases have a plasma PTHrp concentration within the reference range (Mellanby *et al.*, 2006).

A range of other cytokines and hormones have been implicated in causing hypercalcaemia-associated malignancy, such as ectopic production of 1,25(OH)$_2$D and interleukin-1, but little objective work has been done in this area in dogs and cats with spontaneous tumours. Parathyroid hormone tends to be within or below the reference range in animals with malignancy-related hypercalcaemia and raised plasma PTHrp concentrations.

PTHrp assay: A two-site immunoradiometric PTHrp assay has been clinically validated for both dogs and cats (Figure 4.1) (Bolliger *et al.*, 2002; Mellanby *et al.*, 2006). The assay uses two different antibodies to human PTHrp that are specific for different well defined regions of the PTHrp molecule. The two-site assays are generally considered to be superior to assays that detect only one region of the PTHrp molecule, since the two-site assays are more likely to measure intact PTHrp rather than PTHrp fragments. A radioimmunoassay has also been validated in the dog, but this assay is not currently commercially available (Rosol *et al.*, 1992).

PTHrp is a labile protein and care has to be taken in the transportation of the sample to the laboratory; it is advisable to discuss specific requirements with the laboratory. The usual requirement is to collect the sample into EDTA, separate the plasma immediately and store frozen (–20°C is adequate for short-term shortage). The frozen plasma should be delivered to the laboratory in special freezer packs, which are usually supplied by the laboratory.

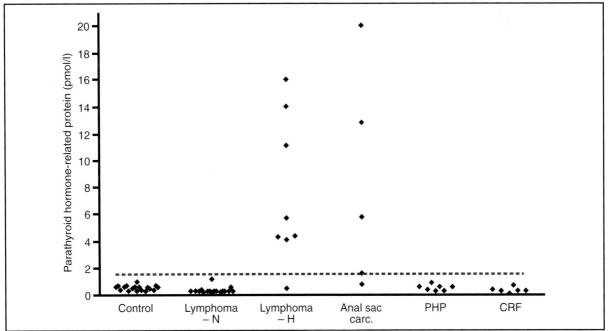

4.1 PTHrp concentrations in: healthy dogs (Control); dogs with lymphoma that were normocalcaemic (Lymphoma – N) and hypercalcaemic (Lymphoma – H); dogs with hypercalcaemia associated with an adenocarcinoma of the apocrine gland (Anal sac carc.); hypercalcaemic dogs with primary hyperparathyroidism caused by a parathyroid adenoma (PHP); and dogs with hypercalcaemia and chronic renal failure (CRF). The dotted line represents the upper limit of the reference range. Normal dogs and hypercalcaemic dogs with a non-malignant disease rarely have elevated PTHrp concentrations. In contrast, dogs with hypercalcaemia caused by neoplasia often (but not invariably) have elevated plasma PTHrp concentrations. (Data from Mellanby *et al.*, 2006).

Diagnosis

The diagnosis of hypercalcaemia-associated malignancy is usually straightforward, based on the clinical presentation and haematology, biochemistry, urinalysis and diagnostic imaging results. An approach to the evaluation of the hypercalcaemic patient (Figure 4.2) is detailed in the *BSAVA Manual of Canine and Feline Clinical Pathology*; differential diagnoses for hypercalcaemia in the dog and the cat are listed in Figure 4.3.

All hypercalcaemic animals should have their peripheral lymph nodes carefully palpated and dogs should have a rectal examination to assess for the presence of anal sac masses and sublumbar lymphadenopathy. In addition, in animals with hypercalcaemia where the underlying cause is not immediately apparent based on clinical examination, haematology, biochemistry, urinalysis and fine-needle aspiration/biopsy of lymph nodes or masses, further diagnostic imaging such as thoracic radiographs

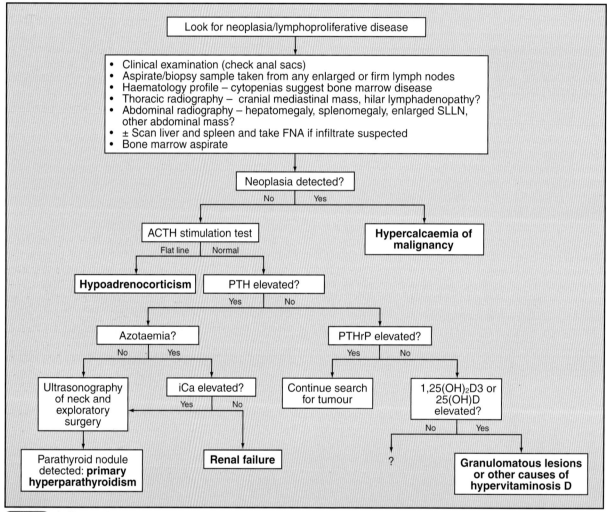

4.2   A diagnostic approach to hypercalcaemia. (Reproduced from *BSAVA Manual of Canine and Feline Clinical Pathology, 2nd edn*)

Dogs	Cats
Malignancy: • Lymphoma • Adenocarcinoma of the apocrine gland • Miscellaneous tumours (e.g. various carcinomas, multiple myeloma, leukaemia) Hypoadrenocorticism Chronic renal failure Primary hyperparathyroidism *Less common causes:* Granulomatous disease Hypervitaminosis D Juvenile dog	Malignancy: • Lymphoma • Squamous cell carcinoma • Miscellaneous tumours (e.g. various carcinomas, leukaemia, various sarcomas) Chronic renal failure Primary hyperparathyroidism

4.3   Differential diagnoses for hypercalcaemia in dogs and cats.

and abdominal radiographs/ultrasonography is advisable. An ACTH stimulation test should be undertaken if hypoadrenocorticism is suspected. Plasma electrophoresis should be considered if multiple myeloma is suspected. Measurement of PTH, PTHrp and vitamin D metabolites can also be helpful in the diagnostic evaluation of hypercalcaemic patients.

Treatment
The management of hypercalcaemia associated with malignancy is invariably based on treatment of the underlying neoplasia. However, supportive measures are important during the diagnostic evaluation process, particularly in dogs with elevated calcium and phosphate concentrations who are at risk of metastatic mineralization of soft tissues and irreversible renal damage.

Correction of fluid deficits and saline diuresis are the mainstay of therapy. Rehydration with intravenous fluids at two or three times maintenance (0.9% sodium chloride) and then continuing the aggressive fluid therapy once rehydrated is advisable in an effort to reduce the calcium concentration and to preserve renal function. Furosemide is also used to promote diuresis once the fluid deficits have been corrected. Glucocorticoids may increase the urinary excretion of calcium but make the diagnosis of some diseases, especially lymphoproliferative disorders, more difficult and so should not be used before a final definitive diagnosis has been made.

Salmon calcitonin has been used to treat hypercalcaemia in dogs, but its short half-life, high incidence of side effects and high cost have limited its clinical use (Dougherty *et al.*, 1990). Bisphosphonates decrease osteoclast activity and function and can be used to treat hypercalcaemia, particularly in cases of malignancy-related hypercalcaemia where the tumour is not amenable to treatment (Milner *et al.*, 2004). The bisphosphonate pamidronate has been used successfully to treat malignancy-related hypercalcaemia in dogs (Hostutler *et al.*, 2005). The oral bisphosphonate clodronate has also been used to treat hypercalcaemic dogs with unresectable tumours (Gould, 2001).

Hypoglycaemia
Hypoglycaemia is a well recognized paraneoplastic syndrome in dogs and cats. Insulinoma, which is an insulin-secreting islet cell neoplasm of the pancreas, is the most common cause of malignancy-associated hypoglycaemia. A range of non-islet cell tumours have also been associated with hypoglycaemia, including:

- Hepatocellular carcinoma
- Leiomyoma
- Leiomyosarcoma
- Haemangiosarcoma
- Multiple myeloma
- Renal adenocarcinoma
- Hepatoma.

The aetiology of the hypoglycaemia in insulinoma is excessive secretion of insulin, whereas in non-islet cell tumours associated with hypoglycaemia the pathogenesis of the low plasma glucose concentration is often unclear. Several theories have been proposed, such as hypersecretion of insulin or insulin-like substances, glucose utilization by a large tumour mass and failure of compensatory mechanisms. Hypersecretion of insulin by non-islet cell tumours is an unlikely explanation, since the majority of dogs with hypoglycaemia associated with non-islet cell tumours typically have low or normal insulin concentrations. Ectopic production of insulin-like factors is a more plausible explanation, which is supported by the case report of a dog with hypoglycaemia associated with a leiomyoma of the gastric wall that had elevated serum and intra-tumour concentrations of insulin-like growth factor II-like peptide (Boari *et al.*, 1995).

Clinical signs
Hypoglycaemia causes a range of clinical signs that include:

- Weakness
- Lethargy
- Inappetence
- Ataxia
- Blindness and seizures.

Treatment
Initial treatment is based on correction of the hypoglycaemic state by feeding complex carbohydrates or oral administration of syrups containing glucose/dextrose. Intravenous administration of glucose-containing fluids may be advisable if feeding is not practical or is ineffective. Glucagon and glucose infusions could also be considered for refractory cases.

Definitive treatment of non-islet cell tumour normally requires surgical excision of the tumour. Low-dose glucocorticoids can be valuable in the palliative management of hypoglycaemia where surgical excision is not possible.

Although not widely used, streptozocin has been administered to manage canine insulinomas medically (Moore *et al.*, 2002).

Miscellaneous endocrine paraneoplastic syndromes

Hyperadrenocorticism
Hyperadrenocorticism secondary to ectopic production of ACTH is a well described paraneoplastic syndrome in humans. This syndrome is associated with increased ACTH concentrations resulting in persistently raised plasma cortisol concentrations, which produces clinical signs such as polydipsia, polyuria and polyphagia. The diagnosis is based on the identification of a consistently increased plasma ACTH concentration in the absence of hypothalamic, pituitary and adrenal neoplasia and the identification of a primary neuroendocrine tumour. This condition has been infrequently recognized in companion animals (Galac *et al.*, 2005).

SIADH
The syndrome of inappropriate secretion of antidiuretic hormone (SIADH) is also a well recognized paraneoplastic syndrome in humans, leading to

hyponatraemia, serum hyposmolality and urine hyperosmolality in the absence of abnormalities in renal, adrenal and thyroid function. This paraneoplastic syndrome is extremely uncommon in companion animals but should be considered in patients with appropriate laboratory abnormalities.

Haematological/ haemostatic complications

Anaemia
Anaemia is one of the most common paraneoplastic syndromes diagnosed in companion animals. The clinical significance of malignancy-associated anaemia can be highly variable but in many cases it can have a marked negative impact on quality of life, response to treatment and survival. For example, dogs with lymphoma and anaemia at the time of diagnosis were found to have a shorter survival time than dogs that were not anaemic (Miller *et al.*, 2009). Anaemia may develop in companion animals with a malignancy through various mechanisms, including the following.

Anaemia of chronic disease
Anaemia of chronic disease is commonly observed in dogs and cats with neoplastic diseases. It is characterized by reduced erythrocyte lifespan, leading to a mild to moderate normocytic, normochromic, non-regenerative anaemia. It can occur secondary to a wide range of tumours and the aetiology is poorly understood; disordered iron metabolism is widely considered to be an important factor in the development of anaemia of chronic disease.

Immune-mediated haemolytic anaemia
Immune-mediated haemolytic anaemia is also a well recognized paraneoplastic syndrome (Figure 4.4). It is most commonly associated with lymphoid malignancies and less frequently with solid tumours.

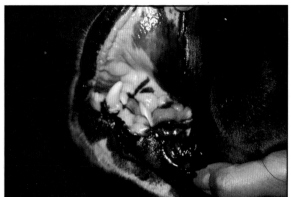

4.4 Pallor (shown here by the mucous membranes) is a common clinical finding in dogs with malignancy-associated immune-mediated haemolytic anaemia.

Chronic blood loss
Anaemia may result from blood loss due to a primary gastrointestinal tumour. It may also occur secondarily due to gastrointestinal ulceration in animals with mast cell tumours or gastrinomas.

Myelophthisis
In animals with myelophthisis, bone marrow invasion by tumour cells can directly reduce the production of red blood cells. This is most commonly seen in myelo- and lymphoproliferative disorders.

Microangiopathic haemolytic anaemia
Microangiopathic haemolysis occurs when red blood cells are fragmented within blood vessels by intravascular fibrin strands, for example in animals with splenic haemangiosarcoma (see Chapter 19).

Erythrocytosis (polycythaemia)
Paraneoplastic erythrocytosis is rarely diagnosed in companion animals. In contrast to primary erythrocytosis, which is a primary disorder of the erythroid cell lines, paraneoplastic erythrocytosis occurs due to inappropriately elevated erythropoietin concentrations. This may be due to ectopic production of erythropoietin by the tumour or due to induced excessive renal production of erythropoietin in response to hypoxia. Polycythaemia leads to an increase in blood viscosity and may induce clinical signs such as neurological signs, polydipsia, polyuria and retinopathies. Paraneoplastic erythrocytosis is treated by surgical excision of the tumour. Phlebotomy can be a useful temporary adjunctive therapy.

Leucocytosis
Increased peripheral granulocytosis without evidence of infection or leukaemia occurs infrequently in cats and dogs with a malignancy. The excessive leucocytes are normally mature neutrophils and clinical signs are rarely observed. Paraneoplastic neutrophilic leucocytosis has been reported in dogs with renal carcinoma, lymphoma, fibrosarcoma and pulmonary carcinoma. The diagnosis is made by exclusion of other causes of neutrophilia and resolution of the leucocytosis following successful treatment of the tumour.

Paraneoplastic eosinophilia has been rarely reported in companion animals. It may be difficult to distinguish paraneoplastic eosinophilia from eosinophilic leukaemia and hypereosinophilic syndrome.

Thrombocytopenia
Thrombocytopenia is commonly observed in companion animals with neoplasia and can develop through various mechanisms, including:

* Decreased platelet consumption
* Increased sequestration
* Increased consumption
* Immune-mediated platelet destruction.

The clinical significance of the thrombocytopenia varies widely, depending on the severity of the thrombocytopenia, the underlying tumour and concurrent illnesses. Severe thrombocytopenia can result in clinical signs such as petechiae and ecchymoses (Figure 4.5). The therapy of choice for paraneoplastic thrombocytopenia is definitive treatment of the underlying tumour.

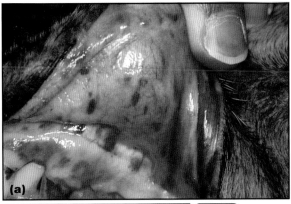

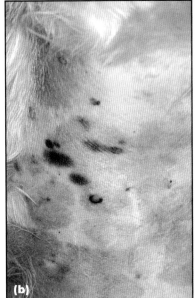

4.5

Severe thrombocytopenia can result in clinical signs such as **(a)** petechiae and/or **(b)** ecchymoses.

Pancytopenia

Pancytopenia is a well recognized complication of chemotherapy but can also occur as a paraneoplastic syndrome. The best described syndrome is in oestrogen-producing Sertoli cell tumours, which can result in anaemia, thrombocytopenia and leucopenia. The mechanism of oestrogen-related myelotoxicosis is incompletely understood and may be due to the oestrogen-induced production of a myelopoiesis inhibitory factor. The prognosis for dogs with myelotoxocity secondary to an oestrogen-producing Sertoli cell tumour tends to be poor; pancytopenia can persist even with successful removal of the primary tumour and supportive care.

Thrombocytosis

Thrombocytosis is an unusual paraneoplastic syndrome and has been described in animals with a range of tumours, including osteosarcoma, leukaemia and squamous cell carcinoma. It can be associated with thrombotic or haemorrhagic tendencies but in most cases is not associated with any clinical signs.

Coagulation disorders

Disseminated intravascular coagulation (DIC) is the most common malignancy-related coagulation disorder in dogs and cats. The diagnosis of DIC is made on the basis of clinical signs of a coagulopathy with laboratory findings of thrombocytopenia, hypofibrinogenaemia, increased fibrin degradation products and prolonged activated partial thromboplastin time (Figures 4.6 and 4.7). A wide variety of tumours has been associated with DIC, most notably haemangiosarcomas in dogs. Treatment of DIC is frequently challenging and prognosis is poor.

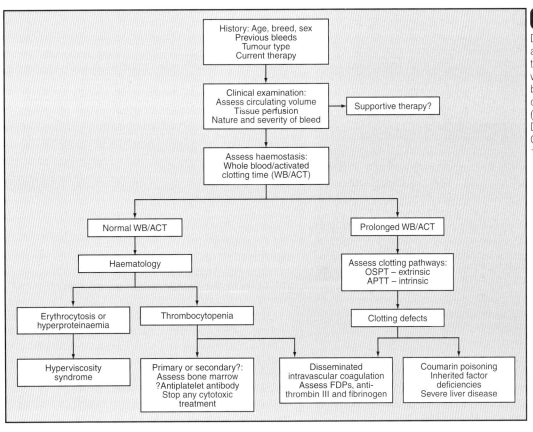

4.6

Diagnostic approach to the patient with a bleeding disorder. (Redrawn after Dobson and Gorman, 1993)

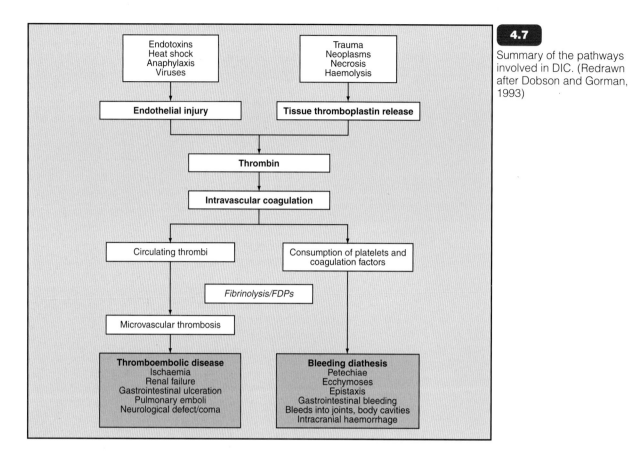

4.7

Summary of the pathways involved in DIC. (Redrawn after Dobson and Gorman, 1993)

Hyperproteinaemia

Paraneoplastic hyperproteinaemia can occur in cats or dogs diagnosed with multiple myeloma, leukaemia and lymphoma, resulting from excessive production of immunoglobulin (see Chapter 19). Increased concentrations of immunoglobulins can lead to clinical signs associated with serum hyperviscosity, such as retinopathies, ataxia, altered demeanour and seizures. Abnormalities in coagulation may also occur due to poor platelet aggregation or altered function of coagulation factors.

Gastrointestinal system

Gastrointestinal ulceration is a well recognized complication of primary gastrointestinal tumours in dogs and cats. It can also occur as a paraneoplastic syndrome secondary to mast cell neoplasia. Malignant mast cell tumours may secrete histamine, heparin and proteolytic enzymes, with hyperhistaminaemia regarded as the main factor contributing to gastrointestinal ulceration. Histamine is a potent secretagogue and acts on H-2 receptors in the parietal cells, leading to increased gastric acid secretion and potentially gastrointestinal ulceration. Histamine may also stimulate intestinal motility and blood flow. Consequently, gastroprotectant treatment should be considered in dogs with mast cell tumours, particularly in patients with clinical signs suggestive of gastrointestinal ulceration (see Chapter 12). Gastrinomas are rare pancreatic islet tumours that secrete excessive amounts of gastrin, which can lead to vomiting, lethargy and abdominal pain.

Renal system

Companion animals with a protein-losing nephropathy confirmed by concurrent evaluation of urine sediment and urinary protein:creatinine ratio should be thoroughly evaluated for an underlying disease, since tumour-related immune complexes may be deposited in the glomeruli resulting in excessive urinary protein loss. As highlighted in the section on malignancy-related hypercalcaemia (above), paraneoplastic hypercalcaemia can be damaging to renal function particularly if the hypercalcaemic state is associated with concurrent hyperphosphataemia.

Cutaneous system

A small number of cutaneous paraneoplastic syndromes have been reported in companion animals (Turek, 2003).

Nodular dermatofibrosis

Nodular dermatofibrosis is characterized by the development of multiple firm and well circumscribed cutaneous nodules in association with renal cystadenocarcinoma or cystadenoma. It is most commonly diagnosed in middle-aged German Shepherd Dogs where the disease is inherited in an autosomal dominant pattern. The cutaneous nodules are often non-pruritic, located in the dermis or subcutis, and are freely moveable. They tend to be located primarily on the extremities but the cutaneous lesions can be diffuse. Histologically, the nodules consist of irregular bundles of dense, well differentiated collagen fibres in the dermis or subcutis.

Most affected dogs present with the primary complaint of non-painful cutaneous nodules, but signs of renal pathology such as haematuria may also be present. There is no effective therapy for the underlying tumour. Palliative treatment by surgical excision of cutaneous nodules that are ulcerated or interfering with locomotion may be warranted in some cases.

Superficial necrolytic dermatitis (SND)

SND, also termed necrolytic migratory erythema or hepatocutaneous syndrome, is a well described cutaneous paraneoplastic syndrome in companion animals. The skin lesions associated with SND include erythema, crusting, exudation, ulceration and alopecia on the feet, pressure points such as the elbow and hocks, flank, perineal area, muzzle (Figure 4.8), facial mucocutaneous junction and/or oral cavity. Hyperkeratosis and fissuring of foodpads occur in many animals. Histopathological examination reveals epidermal parakeratosis, oedema and necrosis of keratinocytes in the stratum spinosum and hyperplastic basal cells.

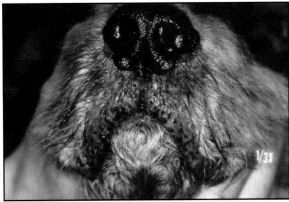

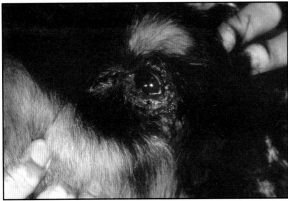

4.8 Superficial necrolytic dermatitis: skin lesions of crusting and exudation affecting the muzzle and the mucocutaneous junctions of the eyelid.

Underlying conditions in dogs with SND include glucagon-secreting pancreatic tumours, hepatic disease and diabetes mellitus. The pathogenesis of SND is unclear, though it has been postulated that hypoaminoacidaemia is important.

Feline paraneoplastic alopecia

Feline paraneoplastic alopecia presents as non-pruritic progressive symmetrical alopecia, which has been reported to occur mainly with pancreatic carcinoma and less commonly with biliary carcinoma. In the majority of cases, the disease has already metastasized at the time of diagnosis; however, successful resolution of paraneoplastic alopecia has been reported in a cat following surgical resection of a pancreatic mass (Tasker *et al.*, 1999).

Paraneoplastic exfoliative dermatitis

Paraneoplastic exfoliative dermatitis has been reported in cats in association with thymoma. Feline thymoma-associated exfoliative dermatitis begins as non-pruritic scaling and mild erythema on the head and pinnae, which may progress to a general distribution. Crusts and ulcers may develop in some cases.

Successful treatment of paraneoplastic exfoliative dermatitis has been reported following surgical excision of thymoma (Forster-Van Hijfte *et al.*, 1997).

Canine paraneoplastic alopecia

Bilateral symmetrical flank alopecia may occur as a paraneoplastic syndrome in dogs with testicular tumours. These are often Sertoli cell tumours and the alopecia is widely considered to be secondary to hyperoestrogenism.

Canine paraneoplastic pemphigus

Paraneoplastic pemphigus has been reported in a 7-year-old Bouvier des Flandres with mediastinal lymphoma which presented with erosive and ulcerative oral lesions (Lemmens *et al.*, 1998).

Neuromuscular system

Myasthenia gravis

Myasthenia gravis is a well recognized neuromuscular paraneoplastic syndrome in companion animals. Antibodies to acetylcholine receptors are commonly detected in dogs with myasthenia gravis, which result in a failure of transmission across the neuromuscular junction. Myasthenia gravis often occurs as a paraneoplastic syndrome in dogs with thymoma, but has also been reported to occur in association with osteosarcoma and bile duct carcinoma.

Typical clinical signs include intermittent mild to severe muscular weakness, exercise intolerance, dysphagia, megaoesophagus and aspiration pneumonia. Detection of circulating autoantibodies against the acetylcholine receptor and improvement of exercise tolerance following administration of edrophonium is supportive of a diagnosis of myasthenia gravis. Surgical removal of the underlying tumour is the treatment of choice, but myasthenia gravis does not invariably resolve even with successful excision of the thymoma.

Peripheral neuropathy

Peripheral neuropathy has been reported in association with a range of tumours, including multiple myeloma, lymphoma and various carcinomas and sarcomas. Clinical signs are weakness and progressive paraparesis to tetraparesis, characterized by lower motor neuron dysfunction.

Miscellaneous conditions

Hypertrophic osteopathy

Hypertrophic osteopathy in dogs is a well described condition that has been associated with a wide variety of malignant diseases, including primary and metastatic lung tumours, oesophageal tumours, rhabdomyosarcoma of the bladder, nephroblastomas and liver carcinoma. It can also occasionally be associated with non-malignant conditions.

It is characterized by progressive periosteal hyperostosis that occurs on the bones of distal extremities and occasionally on other long bones of the appendicular skeleton (Figure 4.9)

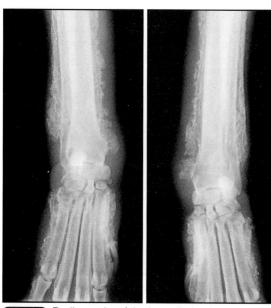

4.9 Radiographs of the lower limbs demonstrating periosteal new bone characteristic of hypertrophic osteopathy.

The causes of this condition remain ill-defined, though increased peripheral blood flow to the distal extremities stimulating connective tissue and periosteal proliferation have long been considered to be important. This may be due to increased vagal tone, since hypertrophic osteopathy can resolve following vagotomy.

The clinical signs of hypertrophic osteopathy are typically lameness and reluctance to move together with swollen and painful distal extremities, but clinical signs may also be related to the primary neoplastic disease. Diagnosis is based on identification of typical periosteal reaction on radiographs of the appendicular skeleton; the patient should then be followed up by additional diagnostic tests to identify the primary lesion. Therapy is based on treatment of the primary lesion in conjunction with analgesia and supportive care for the pain associated with the skeletal changes.

Hypertrophic osteopathy has only been rarely reported in cats.

Pyrexia

Fever can occur in companion animals with a variety of tumours. Typically, the pyrexia occurs due to the presence of a concurrent disorder such as an infection or adverse drug reaction, but it may also occur as a genuine paraneoplastic syndrome. The prevalence of fever as a genuine paraneoplastic disorder is unknown in dogs and cats. Animals with a neoplastic process and a fever should be carefully assessed for the presence of an inflammatory or infectious process and then treated appropriately.

Cancer cachexia

Cancer cachexia, defined as loss of both lean muscle mass and adipose tissue despite adequate nutritional intake, is an important and arguably the most common paraneoplastic syndrome diagnosed in dogs and cats. Cancer anorexia refers to weight loss due to poor nutritional intake.

Recent studies have found that, at the time of diagnosis, over 20% of dogs with neoplasia had lost more than 10% of their bodyweight. In addition, 15% had evidence of clinically relevant muscle wasting (Michel *et al.*, 2004). In a study of cats with neoplasms, 93% had evidence of muscle wastage and 44% had a body condition score of less than 5/9 (Baez *et al.*, 2007). Importantly, this study also demonstrated that cats with a body condition score of less than 5 had a shorter median survival period compared with cats with a body condition score of 5 or more.

References and further reading

Anderson GM, Lane I, Fischer J. and Lopez A (1999) Hypercalcemia and parathyroid hormone-related protein in a dog with undifferentiated nasal carcinoma. *Canadian Veterinary Journal* **40**, 341–342

Baez JL, Michel KE, Sorenmo K and Shofer FS (2007) A prospective investigation of the prevalence and prognostic significance of weight loss and changes in body condition in feline cancer patients. *Journal of Feline Medicine and Surgery* **9**, 411–417

Battaglia L, Petterino C, Zappulli V and Castagnaro M (2005) Hypoglycaemia as a paraneoplastic syndrome associated with renal adenocarcinoma in a dog. *Veterinary Research Communications* **29**, 671–675

Battersby IA, Murphy KF, Tasker S and Papasouliotis K (2006) Retrospective study of fever in dogs: laboratory testing, diagnoses and influence of prior treatment. *Journal of Small Animal Practice* **47**, 370–376

Beaudry D, Knapp DW, Montgomery T *et al.* (1995) Hypoglycemia in four dogs with smooth muscle tumors. *Journal of Veterinary Internal Medicine* **9**, 415–418

Bennett PF, DeNicola DB, Bonney P, Glickman NW and Knapp DW (2002) Canine anal sac adenocarcinomas: clinical presentation and response to therapy. *Journal of Veterinary Internal Medicine* **16**, 100–104

Boari A, Barreca A, Bestetti GE, Minuto F and Venturoli M (1995) Hypoglycaemia in a dog with a leiomyoma of the gastric wall producing an insulin-like growth factor II-like peptide. *European Journal of Endocrinology* **132**, 744–750

Bolliger AP, Graham PA, Richard V *et al.* (2002) Detection of parathyroid hormone-related protein in cats with humoral hypercalcemia of malignancy. *Veterinary Clinical Pathology* **31**, 3–8

Caywood DD, Klausner JS, O'Leary TP *et al.* (1988) Pancreatic insulin-secreting neoplasms: clinical, diagnostic, and prognostic features in 73 dogs. *Journal of the American Animal Hospital Association* **24**, 577–584

De Schepper J, van der Stock J and de Rick A (1974) Hypercalcaemia and hypoglycaemia in a case of lymphatic leukaemia in the dog. *Veterinary Record* **94**, 602–603

DiBartola SP and Reynolds HA (1982) Hypoglycemia and polyclonal gammopathy in a dog with plasma cell dyscrasia. *Journal of the American Veterinary Medical Association* **180**, 1345–1348

Dobson JM and Gorman NT (1993) *Cancer Chemotherapy in Small Animal Practice*. Blackwell Scientific Publications, Oxford

Dougherty SA, Center SA and Dzanis DA (1990) Salmon calcitonin as adjunct treatment for vitamin D toxicosis in a dog. *Journal of the*

American Veterinary Medical Association **196**, 1269–1272

Dunn KJ and Dunn JK (1998) Diagnostic investigations of 101 dogs with pyrexia of unknown origin. *Journal of Small Animal Practice* **39**, 574–580

Elliott J, Dobson JM, Dunn JK, Herrtage ME and Jackson KF (1991) Hypercalcaemia in the dog: a study of 40 cases. *Journal of Small Animal Practice* **32**, 564–571

Feldman EC, Hoar B, Pollard R and Nelson RW (2005) Pretreatment clinical and laboratory findings in dogs with primary hyperparathyroidism: 210 cases (1987–2004). *Journal of the American Veterinary Medical Association* **227**, 756–761

Foley P, Shaw D, Runyon C, McConkey S and Ikede B (2000) Serum parathyroid hormone-related protein concentration in a dog with a thymoma and persistent hypercalcemia. *Canadian Veterinary Journal* **41**, 867–870

Forster-Van Hijfte MA, Curtis CF and White RN (1997) Resolution of exfoliative dermatitis and *Malassezia pachydermatis* overgrowth in a cat after surgical thymoma resection. *Journal of Small Animal Practice* **38**, 451–454

Galac S, Kooistra HS, Voorhout G *et al.* (2005) Hyperadrenocorticism in a dog due to ectopic secretion of adrenocorticotropic hormone. *Domestic Animal Endocrinology* **28**, 338–348

Gaschen FP and Teske E (2005) Paraneoplastic syndromes. In: *Textbook of Small Animal Medicine*, ed. SJ Ettinger and EC Feldman, pp. 789–795. Elsevier Saunders, St Louis, Missouri

Gould SM (2001) The long term use of clodronate to control humoral hypercalcaemia of malignancy (HHM) in two dogs. *11th ESVIM Congress Proceedings*, p. 73

Hostutler RA, Chew DJ, Jaeger JQ *et al.* (2005) Uses and effectiveness of pamidronate disodium for treatment of dogs and cats with hypercalcaemia. *Journal of Veterinary Internal Medicine* **19**, 29–33

Kleiter M, Hirt R, Kirtz G and Day MJ (2001) Hypercalcaemia associated with chronic lymphocytic leukaemia in a Giant Schnauzer. *Australian Veterinary Journal* **79**, 335–338

Leifer CE, Peterson ME, Matus RE and Patnaik AK (1985) Hypoglycemia associated with nonislet cell tumor in 13 dogs. *Journal of the American Veterinary Medical Association* **186**, 53–55

Lemmens P, de Bruin A and de Meulemeester J (1998) Paraneoplastic pemphigus in a dog. *Veterinary Dermatology* **9**, 127–134

Matus RE, Leifer CE, MacEwen EG and Hurvitz AI (1986) Prognostic factors for multiple myeloma in the dog. *Journal of the American Veterinary Medical Association* **188**, 1288–1292

Mellanby RJ, Foale R, Friend E *et al.* (2002) Anal sac adenocarcinoma in a cat. *Journal of Feline Medicine and Surgery* **4**, 205–207

Mellanby RJ, Craig R, Evans H and Herrtage ME (2006) Plasma parathyroid hormone related protein concentrations in dogs with calcium metabolism disorders. *Veterinary Record* **159**, 833–838

Michel KE, Sorenmo K and Shofer FS (2004) Evaluation of body condition and weight loss in dogs presented to a veterinary oncology service. *Journal of Veterinary Internal Medicine* **18**, 692–695

Miller AG, Morely PS, Rao S *et al.* (2009) Anemia is associated with decreased survival time in dogs with lymphoma. *Journal of Veterinary Internal Medicine* **23**, 116–122

Milner RJ. Farese J, Henry CJ *et al.* (2004) Bisphosphonates and cancer. *Journal of Veterinary Internal Medicine* **18**, 597–604

Moore AS, Nelson RW, Henry CJ *et al.* (2002) Streptozocin for treatment of pancreatic islet cell tumors in dogs: 17 cases (1989–1999). *Journal of the American Veterinary Medical Association* **221**, 811–818

Pressler BM, Rotstein DS, Law JM *et al.* (2002) Hypercalcemia and high parathyroid hormone related protein concentration associated with malignant melanoma in a dog. *Journal of the American Veterinary Medical Association* **221**, 263–240

Rosol TJ, Nagode LA, Couto CG *et al.* (1992) Parathyroid hormone (PTH)-related protein, PTH, and 1,25-dihydroxyvitamin D in dogs with cancer-associated hypercalcemia. *Endocrinology* **131**, 1157–1164

Savary KC, Price GS and Vaden SL (2000) Hypercalcemia in cats: a retrospective study of 71 cases (1991–1997). *Journal of Veterinary Internal Medicine* **14**, 184–189

Sherding RG, Wilson GP and Kociba GJ (1981) Bone marrow hypoplasia in eight dogs with Sertoli cells tumors. *Journal of the American Veterinary Medical Association* **178**, 497–501

Skelly BJ and Mellanby RJ (2005) Electrolyte disorders. In: *BSAVA Manual of Clinical Pathology, 2nd edn*, ed. E Villiers and L Blackwood, pp. 113–134. BSAVA Publications, Gloucester

Strombeck DR, Krum S, Meyers D and Kappesser RM (1976) Hypoglycemia and hypoinsulinemia associated with hepatoma in a dog. *Journal of the American Veterinary Medical Association* **169**, 811–812

Tasker S, Griffon DJ, Nuttal TJ and Hill PB (1999) Resolution of paraneoplastic alopecia following surgical removal of a pancreatic carcinoma in a cat. *Journal of Small Animal Practice* **40**, 16–19

Turek MM (2003) Cutaneous paraneoplastic syndromes in dogs and cats: a review of the literature. *Veterinary Dermatology* **14**, 279–296

Weiss DJ, Evanson OA and Sykes J (1999) A retrospective study of canine pancytopenia. *Veterinary Clinical Pathology* **28**, 83–88

5

When to treat animals with cancer

Bernard E. Rollin

Trends in human medicine

The 20th century marked the transmutation of human medicine from a field perceiving itself as constituting a balance between art and science to one far more firmly ensconced in the sciences. Much of this was to the good, as the Flexner Report produced in the US noted (Flexner, 1910). Thus, for example, medicine moved from a situation of 'medical anarchism' with a bewildering array of therapeutic modalities competing for patient allegiance – homeopathy, hydrotherapy, naturopathy and the like – to a more uniform body of diagnostic and treatment modalities rooted (at least theoretically) in science and empirical verification.

Prolongation of life

The transition of medicine from art into science was not without costs. As medicine became 'applied biology' or 'biomedical science', certain key aspects of traditional medicine were suppressed. For example, as rational treatments for diseases such as cancer emerged, physicians marked their success by empirical parameters. Notable among these measures was additional life garnered by way of the treatments. Such a scoring system, however, entailed a neglect of quality of life considerations. While chemotherapy or radiation did indeed prolong life in many instances, medicine failed to ask at what cost. Qualitative considerations, such as the patient's subjective experience, became invisible to scientific medicine in the face of the assumption that more life was always better – a victory against the disease.

Social, cultural, idiosyncratic and moral dimensions of a person – features essential to being a person – came to be seen as irrelevant to the task of medicine, or as mystical or metaphysical and therefore outside the physician's purview. Thus physicians too often treated illnesses as bodily malfunctions and saw no need to be more than polite and competent applied scientists. A great deal has, of course, been written about the tendency of physicians to forget that patients are persons and to designate patients by such locutions as 'the kidney in room 422' or 'the osteosarcoma'. What is interesting to medicine as a science are the repeatable, universal features of bodies, not the individuality of people (Rollin, 1987).

Palliative care and euthanasia

'Palliative care' was forgotten in the zeal to preserve life. As recently as 1991, it was reported that although 90% of cancer pain was manageable with available modalities, 80% was not controlled (Ferrell and Rhiner, 1991). In the same vein, hospice was a concept developed almost wholly by nurses, not scientific physicians, to help to preserve patient quality of life. As one nursing dean stated, 'Physicians worry about cure; nurses worry about care.' If pain was ignored as scientifically unreal, what hope was there for other negative sequelae to treatment, such as loss of dignity? As the vast and international movement in favour of assisted suicide attests (laws in Belgium, the Netherlands and Oregon, the work of Dr Kevorkian, pleas for death with dignity) it became clear that many if not most patients fear pain, and the suffering and degradation that extreme pain inflicts on patients and families, more than they fear death.

It was the recognition of this point that led to the organization of a unique conference on euthanasia in 1980 in New York, sponsored jointly by the Columbus University College of Physicians and Surgeons and the Animal Medical Center, a major veterinary hospital. The idea of the planners was that the power of euthanasia as an ultimate modality for alleviation of suffering was well recognized in veterinary medicine, but insufficiently so in human medicine. This was well illustrated by the conundrum that a person who fails to euthanize a suffering animal is perceived societally as morally blameworthy, while a person who helps a suffering grandmother, begging to die, to end her life is also seen as blameworthy. The organizers felt that as companion animals become increasingly perceived as 'members of the family' and less like livestock, the moral imperative to end suffering might transfer to human medicine.

Trends in veterinary medicine

As the ensuing three decades evidenced, what subsequently took place societally was ironically the opposite: veterinary medicine became more like human medicine in the face of animals assuming greater familial significance as objects of love, and thus moved away from euthanasia as a powerful tool for alleviating suffering. This occurred by virtue of a number of synergistic and mutually reinforcing factors.

- In the first place, in the US more than half of marriages end in divorce. The UK has the highest divorce rate in Europe. Many divorced professionals with children live in urban environments, where the best jobs are to be found, where they are separated from extended family and making friends is notoriously difficult. Thus the animal assumes greater prominence in people's emotional lives, with upwards of 85% of the US public affirming that their animals are 'members of the family' (Harris Interactive, 2007). This strong emotional bond was well illustrated during Hurricane Katrina, where people refused rescue when told they could not bring their pets.
- There has been an explosion in veterinary specialty practices offering high-level complicated and aggressive treatment.
- At the same time, many companion animal owners will fight their animal's cancer as aggressively as they would fight their own. For such people, euthanasia is a last-resort option.

In some senses, these factors are salubrious. For example, the cost of treatment is far less of a deterrent to treating animal disease than it once was; therefore many animals who would historically have been euthanized now regain extended and good quality lives. It is in the field of oncology that this is most apparent.

But there is an offsetting negative side, again produced by converging factors. First of all, many academic oncologists are also researchers, who admirably utilize sick companion animals in their research, rather than creating disease in healthy animals. While this approach is inherently laudable, it also engenders some untoward effects, mainly the tendency to prolong treatment for reasons serving the science, not the individual animal. This obviously plays into natural owner reluctance to euthanize, sometimes resulting in extended unnecessary suffering.

Secondly, some clients simply cannot accept the need to euthanize their 'best friend' or 'family member'. The result is a willingness to 'try anything' to save the animal, however far gone or suffering it may be. A particularly pernicious consequence of this is the proliferation of evidentially baseless, unproven 'complementary' and 'alternative' therapies. Such modalities range from 'Bach flower essences' to homeopathy which, if true, invalidates basic principles of modern chemistry. Whether practitioners of alternative medicine are true believers or are simply bilking the gullible, access to the Internet assures that desperate clients can find an inexhaustible number of allegedly therapeutic modalities that they wish to pursue.

A particularly dangerous corollary to such an attitude can be represented by hospices for dying animals. In some cases, where an owner wishes to pursue palliative care and legitimate treatment for the cancer animal and has money but no time to provide care, the pet hospice can fulfil a valuable function. But just as often, the hospice can allow the owner to dodge the issue of euthanasia for untreated or untreatable suffering while endless new unproven and likely ineffective treatments are pursued. Of course, the same catering to an owner's unwillingness to let go can occur in general veterinary practice.

Thus, paradoxically, the rise of love for companion animals can result in new sources of uncontrolled suffering, buttressing the dictum that loving something is not sufficient in its own right to assure that one provides the beloved with good care.

Role of the veterinary surgeon

In the author's experience, the vast majority of veterinary surgeons, particularly companion animal practitioners, embrace the view of the veterinary surgeon as ideally analogous to a paediatrician rather than a garage mechanic. That is, in the case of competing obligations such as the owner electing to prolong suffering by pursuing useless therapies, the veterinary surgeon's primary obligation is to the animal and its wellbeing, not to the owner.

Plato sagely made this point with regard to the shepherd: in one's capacity as shepherd, one's primary role is to care for the sheep. What one earns doing this occurs in one's capacity as *wage-earner*, which is connected but subordinate to the shepherd role.

Obviously, given that animals are the property of owners, veterinary surgeons are not in a position to dictate treatments or, more relevant to this discussion, euthanasia to end suffering. Furthermore, we live in a society in which medical paternalism is a dirty word, and patient or client autonomy is a trendy slogan. Nonetheless, a powerful element of paternalism is alive and thriving, and can be deployed to good effect by veterinary surgeons.

That element is a practitioner's Aesculapian authority, the singular authority possessed by physicians and veterinary surgeons by virtue of being medical professionals (Rollin, 2002). To deploy such authority on behalf of the animal to end suffering is, in the author's view, not only permissible but obligatory under certain circumstances. When clients ask, 'What would you do if it were your dog, Doctor?', they are appealing to the practitioner's Aesculapian authority. Thus the dictum (sometimes pronounced in veterinary circles) that a practitioner should never suggest or advocate euthanasia, lest the client later blame the veterinary surgeon for 'killing' their beloved animal, should categorically be rejected.

Mental life of the animal

Inextricably bound up with successful deployment of such authority regarding the need for euthanasia to alleviate untreated or untreatable suffering is the issue of explaining to clients some fundamental differences between human and animal mental life that have major and radically distinct implications for quality of life in people versus companion animals. Human thought is irreducibly tied to language, which allows ingression into modes of thought closed to animals. Humans can think in very abstract terms (e.g. mathematics and logic); in negative terms ('there are no dragons in the library'); in conditional terms ('if it does rain, we will hold graduation indoors'); in future terms ('I wish to retire in Iceland someday'); in universal terms ('all triangles have three sides'); in fictional terms (writing novels); in counter-factual terms ('if Darwin had not discovered natural selection, someone else would have'). These are all made possible by being able to structure thought linguistically, which in turn allows linguistic syntax to transcend thought rooted in immediate experience.

The richness and moral relevance of animal mental life should not be denied. There is, however, a striking dissimilarity between humans and animals facing life-threatening illnesses, even as the tools of medicine dealing with such crises converge in the two areas. Human cognition is such that it can value long-term future goals and endure short-run negative experiences for the sake of achieving them. Examples are plentiful. Many people undergo voluntary food restriction, and the unpleasant experience attendant in its wake, for the sake of lowering blood pressure, or looking good in a bikini as summer approaches. They memorize volumes of boring material for the sake of gaining admission to veterinary or medical school. They endure the excruciating pain of cosmetic surgery in order to look better. And they similarly endure chemotherapy, radiation, dialysis, physical therapy and transplants to achieve longer life and a better quality of life than they would have without it, or, in some cases, merely to prolong the length of life to see their children graduate, or to complete an opus, or fulfil some other goal.

However, there is no evidence, either empirical or conceptual, that animals have the capability to weigh future benefits or possibilities against current misery.

To treat companion animals morally and with respect, their mentational limits need to be kept in mind. Paramount in importance is the extreme unlikelihood that they can understand the concepts of 'life' and 'death' in themselves, rather than the pains and pleasure associated with life or death. To the animal mind, in a real sense there is only quality of life, i.e. whether its experiential content is pleasant or unpleasant in all of the modes it is capable of – bored or occupied, fearful or not fearful, lonely or enjoying companionship, painful or not, hungry or not, thirsty or not, etc. There is no reason to believe that an animal can grasp the notion of extended life, let alone choose to trade current suffering for it.

This in turn demands a realistic assessment, as far as possible, of what animals are experiencing. An animal cannot weigh being treated for cancer against the suffering that this entails. An animal cannot affirm or even conceive of a desire to endure current suffering for the sake of future life; cannot choose to lose a leg to preclude metastasis. It must be remembered that an animal *is* its pain, for it is incapable of anticipating or even *hoping* for cessation of that pain. Thus when life-threatening illnesses afflict companion animals, it is not axiomatic that they be treated at whatever qualitative, experiential cost that may involve. The owner may consider the suffering that a treatment modality entails to be a small price for extra life, but the animal neither values nor comprehends 'extra life', let alone the trade-off this requires. The owner, in turn, may ignore the difference

between the human and animal mind and choose the possibility of life prolongation at any qualitative cost. It is at this point that the morally responsible veterinary surgeon is thrust into their role as animal advocate, speaking for what matters to the animal.

Quality of life

The best way to accomplish this sort of advocacy is to set up the type of relationship with a client from the outset that has both parties agreeing to keep the best interests of the animal in view as the paramount goal of treatment. In this way, the clinician can educate the client on the nature of animal mentation, suffering, and what matters to the animal. Such education should begin along with treatment, as should the veterinary surgeon's claim for advocacy for the animal's quality of life. Quality of life considerations should be introduced at the beginning of a relationship with the client, not suddenly sprung on them when treatment is over. The client (who, after all, knows the animal better than the veterinary surgeon) should be encouraged from the beginning to help to define quality of life for that animal.

Beginning with the onset of treatment for cancer, the veterinary surgeon should obtain from the client a list, as long as possible, of what makes the animal happy or unhappy, and how they know. This list, written down as part of the medical record, can serve to remind owners of their own criteria for quality of life at the point where treatment is failing, when wishful thinking and essentially selfish desires may replace objectivity. I used this method with a friend who asked me how to judge when it was time for euthanasia and how to avoid compromising his animal's quality of life by overly prolonging treatment. He later thanked me and told me that, was it not for his own encoded notes defining the animal's quality of life while the animal was still well, he would have rationalized trying a variety of modalities that would have greatly impaired the animal's quality of life. Unquestionably, he said, denial would have distorted his perception but for his own reflective, codified deliberations on that animal's quality of life which, even in extremis, was impossible to ignore.

The British Veterinary Association, in conjunction with the Universities Federation for Animal Welfare, held a groundbreaking seminar in 2006 on quality of life in animals. In the end, it is essential that veterinary medicine should learn from the mistakes of human medicine and not sacrifice quality of life for quantity.

This chapter is designed to assist veterinary surgeons in optimizing quality of life for cancer patients, through treatment and support. In treating and supporting their cancer patients, veterinary surgeons have a duty to be an advocate for the animal, and to assess the current situation from the perspective of the animal.

References and further reading

Ferrell BR and Rhiner M (1991) High-tech comfort: ethereal issues in cancer pain management for the 1990s. *Journal of Clinical Ethics* **2**, 108–115

Flexner A (1910) *Medical Education in the United States and Canada.* Carnegie Foundation for Higher Education, Princeton, New Jersey

Harris Interactive Inc. (2007) *Pets are 'Members of the Family' and Two-Thirds of Pet Owners Buy Their Pets Holiday Presents.* Harris Poll #120, December 4, 2007, www.harrisinteractive.com/harris-_poll/index.asp?PID=840

Marks RM and Sacher EJ (1973) Undertreatment of medical patients with narcotic analgesia. *Annals of Internal Medicine* **78**, 173–181

Polton G (2010) Patients with neoplastic disease. In: *BSAVA Manual of Canine and Feline Rehabilitation, Supportive and Palliative Care:* *Case Studies in Patient Management,* ed. S Lindley and P Watson, pp. 232–267. BSAVA Publications, Gloucester

Ramey DW and Rollin BE (2004) *Complementary and Alternative Medicine Considered.* Blackwell, Ames, Iowa

Rollin BE (1987) The rights of the dying person. In: *Principles of Thanatology*, ed. AH Kutscher, AG Carr and LG Kutscher, pp. 109–133. Columbia University Press, New York

Rollin BE (2002) The use and abuse of Aesculapian authority in veterinary medicine. *Journal of the American Veterinary Medical Association* **220**, 1144–1149

6

Principles of oncological surgery

Kieri Jermyn and B. Duncan X. Lascelles

Introduction

Oncological surgery is probably the most interesting and multifaceted surgery a veterinary surgeon can carry out. It encompasses aspects of soft tissue, orthopaedic and neurological surgery, and demands a comprehensive knowledge of anatomy and reconstructive procedures for resultant deficits. Boundaries are continually being pushed forward on the surgical procedures that can be employed to treat localized cancer in small animals. However, if oncological surgery is to be effective and successful, there are certain principles that must be adhered to, and these are outlined in this chapter.

Compared with other treatment modalities, surgery of localized tumours provides the possibility for an immediate cure, is not carcinogenic, is not immunosuppressive and does not have local toxic effects. With sensible and appropriate anaesthetic and analgesic protocols and adherence to the principles of oncological surgery, any morbidity associated with anaesthesia and surgery can be minimized and a successful outcome realized.

In order to carry out successful oncological surgery, surgeons require more than a comprehensive knowledge of anatomy, physiology and resection and reconstruction techniques for the specific area or organ involved. A thorough understanding of general tumour biology, the specific characteristics of the neoplasm involved, the stage of disease, and thus prognosis and the adjunctive therapies that may be appropriate, is essential in each case.

The decision to use surgery

Surgery in oncology is mainly used to facilitate diagnosis and for treatment of localized neoplasia. Prior to contemplating surgical management of a cancer, the patient and treatment options must be fully appraised to determine the most effective approach.

- The cancer must be characterized (type and grade). A surgical procedure (biopsy) may be involved in this process (see Chapters 2 and 3).
- The locoregional and systemic extent of the disease (stage) must be assessed using appropriate investigations, such as physical examination, blood evaluations, radiography, ultrasonography, or advanced imaging modalities (see Chapter 3).

- Complete patient evaluation is necessary to determine the options for surgical intervention. When indicated, the aim of surgery must be clearly recognized, i.e. curative intent, cytoreductive or palliative.
- Alternative treatment options, or a decision not to treat (see Chapter 5), must be fully assessed from a practical and prognostic standpoint, both individually and in combination with surgery.
- The owner must be fully informed of the intent of surgery, the adjunctive therapies available and the likely prognosis.

Primary surgery

The opportunity for the most favourable outcome exists when employing surgery for the first time; revision surgeries are less successful. The greatest chance of a cure lies with the primary surgery for a number of reasons:

- Untreated tumours tend to have more normal surrounding anatomy, which facilitates surgical removal
- Recurrent tumours may have seeded to previously non-involved tissue planes, hence increasing the required resection
- The most active and invasive parts of the tumour are at the periphery, where the blood supply is greatest, and subtotal resection may thus leave behind the most aggressive components of the tumour
- Patients with recurrence often have significant anatomical disruption and less normal tissue available for closure.

Preoperative planning

To optimize the likelihood of successful surgery, it is necessary to define precisely the role of the procedure whilst giving due consideration to the reconstructive aspects. Many tumour resections result in substantial tissue deficits. Apprehension about not being able to close the subsequent defect is a potent deterrent to following excision guidelines rigorously (Figure 6.1). Ideally, one individual should remove the tumour, adhering to the oncological principles on the margins required, and a second individual should then perform the reconstruction. This is rarely feasible and hence the surgeon must give full consideration to the reconstruction prior to embarking on the excision.

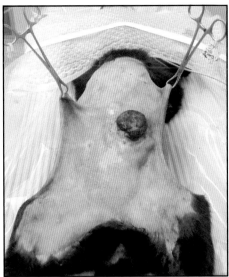
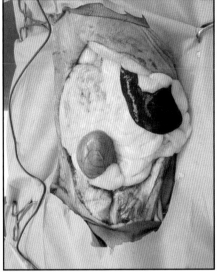

6.1 The sarcoma in this cat required wide resection margins, including full-thickness resection of the body wall. Apprehension about closing the resulting defect (almost complete resection of the ventral body wall) could result in the surgeon's compromising the resection margins in favour of being able to close the defect more easily.

Preoperative planning of the anaesthetic and analgesic regimen and the postoperative care will minimize perioperative morbidity.

Revision surgery

As previously stated, the first surgery has the best chance of a successful outcome. Excised tissue margins are examined histologically and further surgery may be indicated if the margins are positive for tumour cells or narrow (presence of tumour cells very close to the margin). Management of incompletely or closely excised tumours requires that the entire existing surgical scar and any drainage sites are considered 'contaminated'. The surgical margins indicated are then the same as for the initial surgery. Usually this results in a much wider resection than the original surgery (Figure 6.2).

The role of oncological surgery

Oncological surgery may have the following purposes:

- Prophylactic surgery
- Diagnosis and staging of neoplastic disease
- Definitive excision
- Cytoreduction of the tumour mass
- Palliative surgery
- Dealing with emergencies
- Support surgery
- Surgical treatment of metastatic disease.

Prophylactic surgery

Prophylactic oncological surgery can be defined as surgery that results in a reduction of either the anticipated incidence rate of a particular tumour type, or the rate of recurrence of a neoplastic disease after therapy. There are several common examples of prophylactic surgery in small animal surgery.

Mammary tumours in the bitch

Ovariohysterectomy performed prior to the first season is known to reduce the incidence of malignant mammary tumours to 0.05% of that which might be

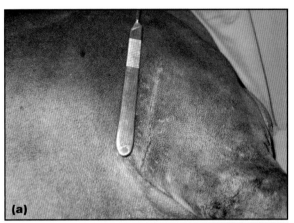
(a)

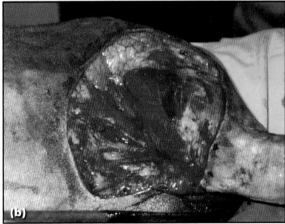
(b)

6.2 Management of an incompletely excised grade II mast cell tumour. **(a)** The entire surgical scar and any adherent tissue must be considered contaminated. **(b)** The surgical margins indicated for revision surgery on this tumour resulted in a much wider resection and subsequent tissue deficit than the original surgery.

expected in entire bitches (Schneider *et al.*, 1969). This relative risk rises quickly beyond the first oestrus. The incidence is 25% of that which might be expected in intact bitches for bitches spayed after the second season. The relative risk for queens is 9% and 14%, respectively. By the age of 2 years, little or no cancer-sparing effect can be expected in bitches.

Oestrogen receptor and/or progesterone receptor expression has been demonstrated in both benign (70%) and malignant (50%) mammary tumours. Expression of progesterone receptors appears to occur more frequently in benign tumours and may be of positive prognostic significance. Even late-stage ovariectomy can reduce the risk for benign tumours. There also appears to be a histological continuum in the progression of canine mammary tumours from benign to malignant, which would argue for prophylactic removal of benign neoplasms (see Chapter 16 for more information).

Benign vaginal tumours in the bitch

Ovariectomy is an effective means of preventing both the development and the recurrence of benign and possibly malignant vaginal tumours in the bitch, and this procedure should be considered an integral part of the surgical management of this disease along with local excision (Figure 6.3). Malignant vaginal tumours are not as hormonally influenced as benign tumours (see also Chapter 17).

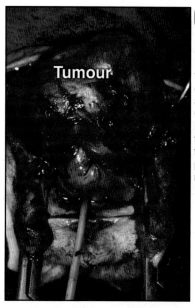

6.3

Local resection of a vaginal leiomyoma following an episiotomy approach. Ovariectomy is an important part of the approach to these tumours to prevent recurrence.

Testicular tumours in the dog

The incidence of testicular neoplasia is significantly greater (by about 14 times) in an undescended testicle over the incidence in a normal dog. This means that about 50% of cryptorchid testicles will develop neoplastic lesions. Neoplasia is also more common than expected in the descended testicle of cryptorchid dogs, probably due to genetic factors that predispose to the development of neoplasia. Sertoli cell tumours (60% of cryptorchid tumours) and seminomas are the most frequent tumour types associated with cryptorchidism. Bilateral elective orchidectomy prevents the development of such tumours in at-risk patients.

Castration of the non-cryptorchid male dog will also help to prevent perianal adenomas and testicular cancer. Although castration does not appear to precipitate development of prostatic neoplasia in dogs, it may favour tumour progression.

Dermal squamous cell carcinoma in the cat

Exposure of unpigmented skin to ultraviolet radiation can result in the development of squamous cell carcinoma (SCC). Often this is preceded by the development of a crusting erythematous pigmented premalignant lesion. The removal of this, together with any susceptible unpigmented area (e.g. resection of the complete pinna and vertical aural canal; nasal planum amputation) is highly successful in preventing the development of SCC (see also Chapters 12 and 18).

Colorectal tumours in the dog

Up to 18% of benign polypoid lesions and carcinoma *in situ* of the colon and rectum have demonstrated potential to undergo malignant transformation into carcinoma. Early wide local resection of these lesions is able to prevent some forms of rectal cancer.

Trauma/chronic inflammation

Chronic inflammation can lead to mutations that result in tissues undergoing neoplastic transformation. This process may play a role in development of digital SCC following chronic subungual infection/inflammation, aural sebaceous cell adenocarcinoma and feline injection site sarcomas, to name a few. The current recommendation from the Vaccine-Associated Feline Sarcoma Task Force is that masses that occur at sites following vaccination should be treated by surgical excision if the lesion is still evident more than 3 months after vaccination, if it is >2 cm or if it is increasing in size more than 4 weeks following vaccine administration.

Diagnosis and staging

Obtaining a diagnosis and clinical staging of suspected neoplasia are of paramount importance before determining treatment options. The histopathological diagnosis will influence prognosis and help to establish the most appropriate recommendations for surgical and adjunctive therapy (Figure 6.4). This will assist the veterinary surgeon and owner in making decisions about how to progress. With the exception of truly emergent cases, treatment without diagnosis will at best be speculative and can rarely be justified, even in the hands of an experienced oncologist.

Biopsy technique

There is a variety of biopsy techniques (see also Chapter 2):

- Cytology (fluid and exfoliative cell recovery, fine needle aspiration (FNA), impression smears)
- Needle core biopsy (Tru-cut, Menghini or Jamshidi type needles)
- Incisional biopsy (surgically removed pinch, punch or wedge samples)
- Excisional biopsy ('complete' postsurgical specimen).

The type of biopsy procedure chosen will depend on the information that the clinician requires. If the detection of individual neoplastic cells is sufficient, cytological techniques will suffice (e.g. for mast cell

Tumour presentation	Reason for performing biopsy prior to surgery
Subcutaneous mass on the lateral thorax/abdomen of a dog	Two possible diagnoses are a lipoma and a peripheral nerve sheath tumour (spindle cell sarcoma). The surgeries required to gain a cure are vastly different. The prognosis for the two tumours is very different, and the prognosis for differing grades of nerve sheath tumours is also very different. Grade I tumours can be cured by wide surgical resection. About 40% of grade III tumours will metastasize. This knowledge may well affect the owner's decision on treatment strategy. Removal of the whole mass to obtain a diagnosis may well result in a more difficult surgery being required later, with less chance of complete resection
A large cranial mediastinal mass	The distinction between lymphoma and thymoma is important. Lymphoma is best treated by chemotherapy, and thymoma best treated by surgery
A 2 cm diameter mass on the rostral mandible of a dog	The distinction between peripheral odontogenic fibroma (an epulis) and osteosarcoma is important. The epulis requires only narrow margins of resection; the osteosarcoma requires wide resection and carries a significantly worse prognosis. However, the prognosis for a mandibular osteosarcoma is much better than for an amelanotic melanoma

6.4 Some examples of when biopsy should be performed prior to surgery.

tumours (MCTs)). However, if a stromal tumour is suspected (e.g. a sarcoma), the tissue architecture will need to be examined and needle core or incisional biopsy techniques will be the minimum requirement. Also, if tumours are to be graded, needle core or incisional techniques are generally indicated. *Tumour type and grade are usually required to help to direct the surgeon towards the requisite or recommended resection margins.* Often a relatively non-invasive or simple procedure is used initially (e.g. FNA) followed by sequential employment of other techniques until sufficient is known about the neoplasm to allow formulation of the most effective surgical and adjunctive therapy protocol.

To avoid compromising future treatment, a few general principles of biopsy should be observed.

- The biopsy site should be positioned within the probable surgical or radiation field.
- The biopsy incision should be as small as is required, and oriented so as not to increase the size of the subsequent treatment area unnecessarily (usually along skin tension lines). For example, biopsy incisions on limbs should be oriented parallel to the long axis of the limb.
- Specimens should be handled carefully. Use of electrocautery to obtain the sample will distort tissue architecture and make it unreadable by the pathologist. Electrocautery may be used afterwards for haemostasis.
- Multiple samples should be obtained if possible and from different areas of the lesion. The tumour should be carefully examined prior to biopsy, and areas of inflammation and necrosis avoided, as the underlying neoplastic process may be masked by secondary tissue changes. Often the best area for biopsy is the junction of normal and abnormal tissue. Important exceptions to this are primary bone tumours; as they often have an extensive reactive process surrounding the primary lesion, samples should be obtained from the centre.
- The biopsy should result in minimal risk of local dissemination of the neoplastic disease. Uninvolved anatomical planes and compartments should not be breached and fresh instrumentation should be used for each site sampled.

- Adequate exposure is necessary for both incisional and excision biopsies to ensure minimal disruption of the tumour and adjacent tissues.

Use of biopsy
In the majority of instances, preoperative biopsy is indicated because the kind or extent of treatment will be altered by knowledge of the tumour type (Figure 6.4). The biopsy report will provide information on diagnosis and, where appropriate, grades that are major prognostic determinants and this provides the cornerstone for subsequent surgical planning. For example, soft tissue sarcomas, oral fibrosarcomas and MCTs (intermediate to high grade) have a high rate of local recurrence after conservative resection and thus require removal with much wider margins than benign or other low-grade tumours. Permanent local tumour control and survival are positively correlated, and preoperative knowledge of the tumour type will help in planning the correct definitive surgery and thus achieving a local cure.

In some instances, however, prior knowledge of the tumour type will not alter the surgical treatment plan. Examples of this include lobectomy for a solitary lung mass and splenectomy for localized splenic neoplasia. In many instances of aggressively destructive bony lesions the treatment plan will include amputation, regardless of the diagnosis. Conversely, the ability to obtain a diagnostic cytology with the assistance of imaging (such as ultrasonography and computed tomography) in a minimally invasive fashion is improving. For example, imaging-guided FNA can make a positive diagnosis in 89% of osteosarcomas (Britt *et al.*, 2007) and 65% of intrathoracic lesions (Zekas *et al.*, 2005). If the biopsy is as difficult as the postulated curative surgery, such as is true for the removal of brain tumours, information about the tumour type should be obtained after surgical removal.

In some instances, usually driven by owners and often on financial grounds, masses are removed without any preoperative knowledge of what the mass is. Examples include old dogs bothered by ulcerated cutaneous masses. *Communication is of paramount importance in these cases:* the owner must understand that the surgery being carried out may not be appropriate for this mass, could impact future treatment options and may not effect a local cure.

It is important to remember that tumour tissue itself often has a poor or absent nerve supply and so biopsy samples representative of the neoplastic process can be obtained using only the minimum of sedation and local analgesia; general anaesthesia is not necessarily required. The argument that 'it is just as much hassle to get the biopsy as to chop it off' is sometimes used against procuring a biopsy. This is not true.

Definitive excision

This refers to the use of surgery as the sole treatment, without adjunctive radiotherapy or chemotherapy, to achieve an outright cure – 'curative intent'. Surgical excision remains the dominant modality of curative therapy. This is possible with localized and occasionally with regionally confined neoplastic disease. The goal is complete removal of all neoplastic tissue, with clear negative margins and maximum preservation of function, in *one* surgery. Realistically, the definitive surgery probably does not remove every last tumour cell; instead, the animal's own local immune defence mechanism may well 'mop up' the remaining neoplastic cells. However, this process should not be relied on to correct compromised surgical technique. The incision, the surgical exposure and the surgical margin are the most important aspects of a definitive surgery.

The incision and surgical exposure

The placing of the incision should take into account the need to resect any scars that are a result of previous surgery or sites of biopsy. Such scars should be afforded the same margins as the bulk of the tumour due to contamination from the primary mass. These margins will have been decided on prior to surgery on the basis of the biopsy information. The incision should also allow adequate access to the tumour to avoid rough handling and fragmentation of the neoplastic tissue.

The surgical margin

The choice of the margin at surgery will profoundly affect the success of the surgery as a curative procedure. The apparently normal tissue surrounding malignant tumours is frequently infiltrated by neoplastic cells. Generally, the greater the likelihood of local infiltration, the wider the surgical margin must be because of the propensity for local, unappreciated spread (Figure 6.5). The magnitude of grossly normal tissue taken with the obvious 'primary' mass will depend on the histological type and grade of tumour, again emphasizing the need for establishing this information by biopsy preoperatively. The tumour and adjacent tissues need to be considered three-dimensionally with respect to margin determination, peripheral/circumferential and deep, all of which are equally important.

Although margins are usually described in terms of a specified measurable distance, consideration should also be given to the biological behaviour of the tumour in question. The most effective natural barriers to the spread of cancer are collagen-rich relatively avascular tissues, including fascia, tendons, ligaments and cartilage. Fat, subcutaneous tissue, muscle and other parenchymatous organs offer relatively little resistance to invading neoplastic cells. Peripheral margins are frequently referred to in terms of metric measurements and deep margins in terms of metric measurements or fascial planes. Fixation of the tumour to adjacent structures or fascial planes mandates removal of the adherent area in continuity with the tumour.

Tumour type and grade	Required margins to give 'good' chance of clean resection	Depth of resection needed
Peripheral odontogenic fibroma (POF) and ameloblastoma (epulides)	0.5 cm	Through tissue in all directions. Some surgeons will 'scrape' the POF from bone (they do not invade bone), but this can be associated with recurrence
Oral basal cell carcinoma (epulis)	1 cm	Through tissue in all directions
Grade I (low grade) MCT	1 cm	Down to and including the muscle or fascial plane below the tumour
Grade I soft tissue sarcomas (spindle cell sarcomas)		
Osteosarcomas that have not invaded soft tissues		
Well differentiated dermal SCC		
Grade II (intermediate grade) MCTs	2 cm	Down to and including the muscle or fascial plane below the tumour; or tissue in all directions (for oral tumours)
Most malignant oral tumours (fibrosarcoma, osteosarcoma, squamous cell sarcoma)		
Intermediate or poorly differentiated dermal SCC		

6.5 Guideline resection margins required for a range of tumours. These are guidelines only and do not guarantee complete resection.

Figure 6.6 outlines some natural barriers to tumour spread at different locations in the body. These are taken into consideration when deciding on the appropriate extent of resection.

There is substantial evidence to support the theory that a 'positive surgical margin' (presence of tumour cells at the edge of the excised tissue) has a negative impact on local recurrence rates, risk of metastatic disease, length of disease-free interval and disease-related death. Equally, margins excessively wide or too narrow may adversely affect quality of life. Significant debate remains as to the optimal excision margins. Excessively wide margins contribute to increased duration of hospitalization, cost, increased cosmetic disfigurement and wound complications. If margins are too narrow there will be increased incidence of recurrence, metastasis and mortality. Surgeons aim for a margin that is wide enough to remove the tumour completely for an acceptable percentage of time and narrow enough to minimize removal of excessive normal tissue.

One study in MCTs evaluated the presence of tumour cells in excised tissue at locations of 1, 2 and 3 cm from the primary mass (Simpson et al., 2004). For low-grade lesions, all were completely excised at a distance of 1 cm; intermediate grades achieved 75% complete excision at 1 cm and 100% at 2 cm. Another study demonstrated 91% complete excision of low- and intermediate-grade MCTs at a distance of 2 cm with no local recurrence during the follow-up period (Fulcher et al., 2006). Even with histologically complete excision, local recurrence is still possible (Weisse et al., 2002). The likelihood of recurrence following marginal excision varies with tumour type and histological grade.

It is also well recognized that the prognosis for certain tumours is impacted by tumour size and anatomical location, for example with MCTs and SCCs.

Intuitively this could be expected to influence the size of appropriate margins and, indeed, has been demonstrated to be correct for melanoma in human patients, where anatomical site and thickness are independent predictors of outcome. Current margin recommendations for melanoma are site- and size-dependent and vary from 1 to 2 cm to reflect this (Zitelli et al., 1997).

The ability to appreciate accurately the extent of the gross disease (particularly where it is not possible to palpate the entire tumour externally) and hence obtain adequate surgical margins is substantially improved by use of advanced imaging modalities (Wallack et al., 2002). Attempting to achieve a negative surgical margin in the case of metastatectomy still appears to be important, as some studies have demonstrated an impact on risk of disease recurrence and survival times.

The extent of the surgical margin can be categorized anatomically as:

- Local excision
- Wide local excision
- Radical local excision.

Local excision: This is the removal of the gross tumour with the minimal amount of surrounding normal tissue. This often means removal of the tumour through its natural capsule or immediate boundaries, usually leaving residual microscopic disease. Although an additional margin of normal tissue is usually removed, there are some instances when it is desirable not to exceed the boundary of the tumour, so as to preserve vital surrounding tissue (e.g. removal of feline thyroid tumours with preservation of the parathyroid tissue, or removal of central nervous system tumours with preservation of surrounding neuronal tissue).

Area of the body	Fascial or muscle structure that can be removed and may act as a ventral barrier to tumour spread [a]
Antebrachium	Antebrachial fascia covering the antebrachial muscles
Head	Fascia covering the temporalis muscles
Lateral thorax	Latissimus dorsi muscle. Although the muscle does not need to be sutured back together, dead space should be carefully closed to prevent seroma formation
Lateral abdomen	Abdominal muscles (e.g. external abdominal oblique). Once two of the three main abdominal muscles have been resected, the deficit should be closed or reinforced
Ventral abdomen	Rectus sheath. Deficits in the rectus sheath should be closed; if they cannot be closed, further deep muscle should be resected to allow apposition of the edges of the rectus sheath
Dorsum	Fascia over the dorsal spinal and paralumbar muscles. If tumours are attached to fascia that is in turn attached to spinous processes of vertebrae, these spinous processes should be removed
Crural region	There is no fascial sheath comparable to that in the forelimb. Although locally the fascia over muscles such as the cranial tibial muscle can be resected, and periosteum used as a deep margin, tumours in this area often can only be cytoreduced without amputation
Lateral thigh	Fascia over the biceps femoris. This is intimately associated with the biceps femoris muscle, and usually margins are gained by partial resection of the biceps femoris muscle

6.6 Examples of natural barriers to tumour spread. [a] If the tumour has infiltrated through this layer, it no longer acts as a barrier and the resection must go to *below the next uninvolved* fascial/muscle layer.

Tumour types suitable for local excision are:

- Lipoma
- Histiocytoma
- Sebaceous adenoma
- Thyroid adenoma.

Wide local excision: When a significant predetermined margin of surrounding tissue is removed together with the primary mass, the excision is termed 'wide local excision'. Again, preoperative knowledge of the tumour type and grade is essential for deciding on that appropriate margin. Figure 6.5 gives some guidelines as to the resection margins required, and how they differ for various tumour types and grades.

Anatomical considerations may dictate whether it is possible to resect the mass with the appropriate margin; if not possible, consideration should be given to the use of suitable adjunctive therapy. Very often, especially on the limbs, the appropriate depth of surgical margin cannot be obtained without significant functional consequence. In these circumstances use is made of the known biology of tumours. A collagen-rich fascial plane (e.g. a muscle sheath or aponeurosis) may act as a natural boundary to tumour spread. Figure 6.7 shows how grade and fascial plane involvement alter the resection required. This form of surgery (wide local resection) is probably the most difficult because it is so tempting to take less tissue than may be required in order to preserve tissue for closure. The required margins, when measured out in the patient, can often appear very large (Figure 6.8). Preoperative planning is essential in these cases.

For example, for a grade II MCT, the suggested margin of excision is 2 cm. On the antebrachium of a dog, 2 cm deep would take the surgeon down to bone, or even into bone. However, the thick antebrachial fascial sheath acts as a barrier to the ventral

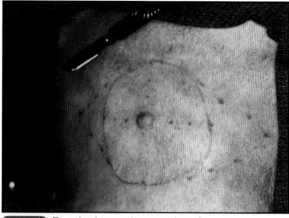

6.8 Required resection margins often seem very large. This skin tumour has 3 cm margins marked out.

spread of tumour cells; this is removed with the tumour and acts as the 'deep margin'. The fascia is removed over the same area as the skin resection. If there is any adhesion of the fascia to the underlying muscle or tissue, the next layer down should be removed also. Preoperative evaluation is therefore essential to plan for such findings. Other examples of natural barriers to spread of tumours are indicated in Figure 6.6; removal of indicated structures does not compromise function.

Radical local excision, supraradical excision, compartmental excision and amputation: Removal of the tumour with anatomically extensive margins of tissue, including fascial planes that are undisturbed by the primary growth of the tumour, is termed radical local, supraradical or compartmental excision. Sarcomas, in particular, extend along fascial planes rather than through them and this pattern of growth dictates removal of the entire anatomical

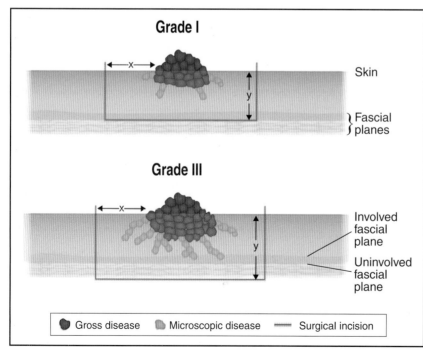

6.7 The degree of local tissue infiltration varies with the tumour grade. The central tumour mass is the grossly visible and palpable part. Invisible to the naked eye are strands, or tentacles, of neoplastic tissue penetrating out into normal tissue. It is this infiltration that determines the required margins of resection, and the degree of infiltration varies with tumour type and grade. Tumour grade is generally designated as I,II or III, with III usually being the most aggressive. Other terms used are low, intermediate and high grade and well differentiated through to poorly differentiated. *x* indicates the necessary peripheral or circumferential margin (usually a metric measurement) and *y* the deep margin (usually measured in terms of fascial planes, also can be measured metrically).

compartment rather than simply wide margins of tissue. One example of this is the resection of a single muscle group for small tumours involving muscle bellies where the outer fascial planes have not been breached. Resection to clean fascial planes on all sides necessitates removal of all blood vessels, nerves and lymphatics that lie within the affected compartment. In the limbs, muscles with their associated fascial capsules comprise individual compartments. Other examples of compartmental or supraradical resections include:

- Removal of the whole pinna and vertical ear canal for resection of SCC of the pinna
- Resection of the complete mandible and its muscle attachments for treatment of mandibular chondro- or osteosarcomas (OSAs)
- Amputation of a limb for appendicular OSA
- Hemipelvectomy for high hindlimb tumours
- Removal of the scapula and associated muscles for scapular tumours.

Examples of radical resections include:

- Excision of the eyelids and orbital contents for removal of invasive SCCs of the eyelid
- Total or partial orbitectomy for the treatment of periorbital tumours
- Radical chest wall resection or abdominal wall resection for the removal of sarcomas
- Radical resections of the nasal planum and rostral maxilla.

For margins equalling or exceeding 3 cm, surgery often involves resection of large compartments of tissue such as amputation, hemipelvectomy, extensive maxillofacial surgery, or abdominal and chest wall resections. Higher-grade tumours often travel extensively along fascial planes; hence surgeries such as amputation are indicated rather than local resection.

Examples of tumours that require radical excision (3 cm, down to and including an uninvolved muscle or fascial plane below the tumour) include the following, but these are only guidelines and unfortunately do not guarantee complete resection of the tumour:

- Grade III (high grade) MCTs
- Grade II and III soft tissue sarcomas (spindle cell sarcomas)
- OSAs that have invaded soft tissues
- Feline vaccine-associated sarcomas.

In summary, in order to formulate a surgical plan the surgeon must establish:

1. The local, regional and systemic extent of the tumour in the patient
2. The margins required for attempted definitive excision
3. How those margins will translate anatomically on to the patient in the area of the tumour
4. The impact on the patient and the anticipated postoperative care
5. Whether the surgeon has the requisite skill, facilities and comfort level to perform the procedure or will offer referral
6. What the owners' expectations are and whether they can be met or modified.

Dissection technique

A scalpel offers or provides the least traumatic form of tissue separation and is recommended for the skin incision and incisions into hollow viscera. Scissors and swabs should be used for the separation of fascial planes, the separation of adhesions and in body cavities where use of a scalpel may be dangerous. Blood vessels should be identified and ligated or cauterized prior to transection, and tissues should be placed under moderate tension as the dissection is carried out to facilitate the identification of fascial planes and tumour margins.

Reduction of tumour cell contamination within surgical field

There are many reports of tumour seeding after biopsy or surgical procedures in human patients, and veterinary cases of surgically induced tumour seeding have also been identified. The pseudocapsule around many tumours, especially sarcomas, has viable tumour cells on its surface. Manipulation and surgical exposure of the pseudocapsule promote tumour spread via exfoliated cells.

Although it is tempting to grasp a tumour using traumatic tissue forceps, this may lead to tissue fragmentation and dissemination of neoplastic cells; stay sutures, placed in normal surrounding tissue being resected, are the best way to manipulate a tumour. In body cavities, neoplasms should be isolated from surrounding viscera by large laparotomy pads to minimize contamination of normal tissue by exfoliated tumour cells.

It is often helpful to approach tumours as if they were abscesses or infected tissue, and the techniques and precautions used to prevent spread of bacteria will also help to minimize the spread of neoplastic cells through inadvertent tumour violation. However, there are some differences. With respect to adhesions between neoplastic tissue and adjacent structures, these adhesions represent direct tumour invasion in up to 57% of cases, and the tumour and the adhesions should be removed *en bloc* whenever possible. Seeded tumour cells appear to adhere to normal tissue via specific cell surface receptors, and routine wound or cavity lavage following removal is of little benefit in terms of 'washing out' remaining tumour cells. However, remaining tumour cells are not likely to be spread by lavage; thus, lavage is recommended to effect removal of blood clots, foreign material, necrotic tissue fragments and any unattached tumour cells. In human patients with inadvertent contamination of the surgical site following soft tissue sarcoma resection, it is possible to achieve similar outcomes when compared with those without contamination, but re-excision and wound irrigation is necessary (Virkus *et al.*, 2002). Gloves, instruments and drapes should be changed after tumour excision and lavage, as tumour cells will adhere to these inanimate objects and potentially be seeded to tissues as closure is carried out. Gloves and equipment should also be changed when performing multiple procedures in the same patient, to avoid mechanical contamination.

Avoidance of wound complications

Local cellular defence mechanisms and immuno-modulation may well be very important in the removal of residual tumour cells. The development of haematomas, seromas or sepsis will interfere with this function and these should be avoided by meticulous haemostasis, effective closure of dead space and appropriate use of drains and perioperative antibiotics. The use of drains is somewhat controversial amongst veterinary oncological surgeons, especially if the resection has been incomplete. There is potential for seeding of tumour cells along the tissues where the drain is placed (this may be decreased with the use of active *versus* passive drains), making further surgery or adjunctive therapy very much more difficult if there is recurrence. The author [KJ] does use drains, but positions their exits close to the incision so as not to compromise further adjunctive therapy that may be needed.

Vascular occlusion techniques

Vascular supply to the tumour, and venous and lymphatic drainage from it, should be ligated as early as possible during surgery. The predominant reason for vascular occlusion is improved intraoperative haemostasis and visualization but it is of notable importance where the probability of cell exfoliation is high, such as for tumours of ectodermal origin (e.g. SCCs, MCTs).

Management of local lymph nodes

The flow of lymph is directional; lymph nodes that are the first to receive drainage from any given location are called 'sentinel' lymph nodes. Sentinel lymph nodes have been mapped in humans using contrast, dyes and radioactive tracers; in human patients it is the 'sentinel' lymph nodes that are targeted for biopsy to stage disease, or for removal in the treatment of disease (Krag, 2000). Once the marker is injected, the first sentinel lymph node is identified and biopsy is performed. If that node is negative for the cancer, further dissection is avoided; if the sentinel node is positive, further dissection is performed.

In veterinary medicine such studies are limited and oncologists usually refer to the 'regional' lymph nodes. These nodes should be sampled (usually via FNA) as a component of routine oncological staging, as it is not possible to determine the presence, or absence, of micrometastasis through mere palpation. This is especially important if the decision regarding the use of adjunctive therapy is dependent on whether or not there is disease in the lymph nodes. Tumour grade and survival have been linked with the presence of micrometastasis in the lymph nodes, as detected by cytological assessment (Withrow and Vail, 2007; Krick *et al.*, 2009). Further studies, using contrast-enhanced imaging modalities, are starting to chart these lymph nodes and this

practice is likely to become more commonplace (Pereira *et al.*, 2008; Tang *et al.*, 2009).

Lymph nodes are only minimally effective barriers to the passage of tumour cells and their function is probably one of immunological surveillance and immune editing, rather than filtration of tumour cells. The immunological response of regional lymph nodes appears to be more effective early on in the course of disease. Local lymph node metastasis is common for malignant melanomas and most carcinomas, of intermediate frequency for sarcomas, respiratory tumours, cutaneous carcinomas and MCTs, and rare for nervous system tumours, skeletal tumours, nasal tumours and most endocrine tumours (e.g. thyroid carcinoma). Removing lymph nodes may interfere with local immune defence mechanisms in the postoperative period. There is also a potential increase in surgical morbidity related to the more extensive surgical procedure.

The practice of routinely removing the 'sentinel' or regional lymph nodes in both humans and animals prophylactically is a matter of continued controversy but is generally no longer recommended (Krag, 2000).

In general, although decisions must be made on a case-by-case basis, current recommendations are the non-destructive biopsy (FNA) of grossly normal local nodes, and removal of the node in the following situations:

- The node is histologically proven to contain tumour cells
- The node appears grossly abnormal at surgery
- The node is intimately associated with the tissue being removed and surgical margins dictate its removal (e.g. as part of a compartmental resection such as the inguinal lymph node during mastectomy)
- The node is sufficiently large and/or located in such an area as to cause some degree of functional impairment associated with space occupation.

One case where local lymph node removal is probably beneficial is the removal of the medial iliac lymph nodes (often erroneously referred to as the sublumbar lymph nodes) in patients with metastatic apocrine or anal sac gland adenocarcinomas of the perineum. Removal of these positive lymph nodes does not result in a cure, but can help to alleviate the paraneoplastic syndrome of hypercalcaemia and may help to prevent large bowel obstruction. It is recommended that, in critical areas (retropharyngeal, hilar, mesenteric), lymph nodes that have eroded through the capsule and become adherent to surrounding tissues are not removed, because attempting to do this would cause significant harm to the patient.

Reconstruction of the resulting deficit

There is often a great temptation to compromise excision margins through a lack of confidence in one's ability to reconstruct the resulting deficit. This compromise may result in failure of a single surgical procedure that could have produced a cure. It may also result in death of an animal that should have been cured. It is the resection of tumours involving the skin and associated structures that often results in substantial deficits, and a variety of techniques are available to deal with these deficits (see *BSAVA Manual of Canine and Feline Wound Management and Reconstruction*).

Primary skin closure: This is the coaptation of the wound edges at the time of the initial surgery without the need for extensive skin-releasing techniques. It is used mainly in the closure of smaller deficits or where there is a lot of loose skin. Towel clamps may be used temporarily to help to align skin edges and stretch skin, and 'walking' sutures should be used to bring skin edges together gradually. There are many other tension-releasing techniques that can be used to facilitate primary skin closure and in oncological surgery full consideration should be given to these prior to planning extensive flap techniques.

Secondary skin healing: This is the closure of the wound by the natural processes of wound contracture and epithelialization. It is particularly suited to contaminated wounds or where the reconstruction of the wound is prohibited by the lack of surrounding skin.

Pedicle flap closure of the skin: This is closure of wounds using sliding flaps of skin, e.g. local plasty techniques, skin meshing, advancement flaps, rotation flaps and transposition flaps. It also includes the use of axial (Figure 6.9) or island flaps. Such techniques can be used immediately after the excisional surgery.

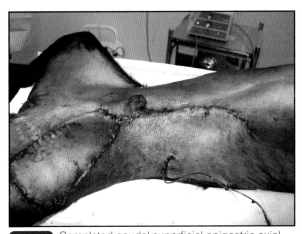

6.9 Completed caudal superficial epigastric axial pattern flap being used in a dog to close a skin deficit resulting from tumour resection.

Free skin grafts: This is particularly suited to the closure of skin deficits over the distal limbs where there is a lack of adjacent skin and axial or island flaps are not possible. These techniques will be delayed until after the excisional surgery to allow for the establishment of a good recipient granulation bed.

Local tissue augmentation: Omentum can be tunnelled, after appropriate extension, to most areas of the body to provide extra tissue to allow closure of dead space. Gastro-omental pedicle flaps can also be used to provide a source of extra tissue in the reconstruction of hollow viscera such as the bladder. Skin expanders can potentially be used to augment skin in the area of a tumour prior to resection.

Myocutaneous flaps: These may be harvested as muscle flaps or combined muscle and skin flaps for closure and support of larger structural defects such as those involving thoracic wall (Halfacree *et al.*, 2007).

Mesh implants: These can be used on their own, or combined with omental transfer techniques, to provide a scaffold for reconstruction of the thoracic and abdominal wall (Matthiesen *et al.*, 1992; Liptak *et al.*, 2008) (Figure 6.10). Cutaneous reconstruction techniques are then used to close the skin. As an alternative to the use of mesh to reconstruct the thoracic wall after resections, diaphragmatic advancement with or without caudal lung lobectomy can be used to obviate the necessity to reconstruct a thoracic wall (Matthiesen *et al.*, 1992).

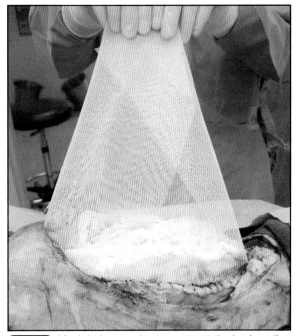

6.10 Mesh being used to reconstruct the body wall defect created in Figure 6.2.

Closure considerations

The oncological surgeon should be familiar with all of the above techniques. A suitable closure technique should be planned prior to resection of the tumour. Appropriate alternatives for closure must also be considered in the event the resection has to be more radical than originally planned. Most often primary closure techniques are used in veterinary oncology due to the fact that if elaborate cutaneous reconstructive techniques are used, there is potential for very wide tumour recurrence with incomplete resection. To minimize this potential for seeding, separate instruments should be used for the reconstructive part of the procedure.

Cytoreduction of the tumour mass

In some circumstances, definitive excisional curative surgery for solid tumours is not possible. The need to preserve vital structures (central nervous system, bladder, nasal sinuses) can often preclude complete excision. Also, second attempts at complete surgical excision of a tumour may be difficult due to distorted anatomy or lack of resectable tissue. Certain tumour types or grades are associated with significant rates of local recurrence even after radical surgery, and resection of such tumours should always be regarded as incomplete.

Such 'cytoreductive' surgery (reducing the numbers of tumour cells present) is *not* failed surgery. The rationale behind cytoreductive surgery is that it is applied in combination with other treatment modalities such as local or systemic chemotherapy, radiotherapy or hyperthermia to try to achieve a cure or improve disease control. In general, radiotherapy is often used as adjunctive therapy to achieve local disease control (soft tissue sarcomas and MCTs) and chemotherapy is used to influence progression of metastatic disease (OSAs and haemangiosarcomas). Cytoreductive surgery improves the efficiency of these adjunctive therapies by reducing the numbers of malignant cells to be treated. Such a multimodal therapy is the optimal form of treatment for limb soft-tissue sarcomas, e.g. the combination of surgical resection and radiotherapy. Another example is the local resection of appendicular OSA and the use of an allograft during a limb-sparing procedure for distal radial OSA in the dog; in this case the tumour resection is regarded as incomplete, the microscopic disease left behind is treated with a slow-release form of cisplatin (Straw *et al.*, 1994; Dawe, 2007; Withrow *et al.*, 2004) and other chemotherapy is used for the systemic metastasis.

Adjunctive therapies such as chemotherapy or radiation therapy are often used postoperatively, when they are more effective due to the small numbers of cells to be sterilized. However, some veterinary oncologists prefer to use such radiation therapy *preoperatively*, because the scattered peripheral cells that they are aiming to kill are best oxygenated at this time and oxygenation of these tissues may be compromised after surgery (see Chapter 8). Postoperative radiation necessitates radiation of the entire surgical scar, which usually results in a larger field than preoperative radiation. This issue has not yet been resolved and presently the use of radiotherapy pre- or postoperatively comes down to personal preference.

Radiation therapy can be used intra-operatively after removal of the tumour when close access to the affected area is required due to problems of damaging surrounding vital structures if postoperative radiation therapy is used. One example of this is intraoperative radiation therapy for bladder carcinomas. Another example is a limb-sparing procedure, where the bone tissue containing OSA is 'flipped' out of the body and irradiated prior to its replacement and fixation in place (Liptak *et al.*, 2004a; Boston *et al.*, 2007). In this way, the tumour cells can be killed and host bone retained, and also the limb 'spared' rather than amputated.

If adjunctive therapies are used preoperatively, the surgical resection should be planned to remove all neoplastic cells, i.e. to be definitive excisional surgery. An example of this would be the 'downstaging' of grade II or III MCTs with chemotherapy prior to definitive surgical excision. The use of chemotherapy to downstage tumours in human medicine is commonplace, e.g. for hepatic tumours.

Palliative surgery

As far as is known, animals have no comprehension of the expected future. Therefore, it is perfectly reasonable to consider performing procedures that markedly improve quality of life, by providing pain relief or relieving poor function, despite the presence of unresolved systemic neoplastic disease. In palliative surgery, the overriding consideration should be the quality of life, not the quantity of life that is expected. There are many situations in which comparatively simple surgical procedures provide the patient with a worthwhile improvement in quality of life despite a poor long-term prognosis. Examples of this include:

- Limb amputation for osteoscaroma causing lameness and pain
- Splenectomy for a bleeding haemangiosarcoma
- Oral resections for a malignant melanoma or haemangiosarcoma causing dysphagia
- Tracheostomy for laryngeal malignancy
- Removal of large ulcerated painful mammary carcinomas
- Placement of a permanent cystostomy catheter to relieve urine outflow obstruction in dogs with transitional cell carcinoma (Smith *et al.*, 1995; Beck *et al.*, 2007).

The risks and benefits must always be weighed and patients selected carefully. Another emerging branch is the increasing use of minimally invasive interventional radiology techniques for placement of palliative vascular, urethral and tracheal stents for management of obstructive disease processes.

Surgical emergencies

Surgical emergencies are relatively common in small animal cancer patients and may include:

- Pericardial effusion and tamponade
- Respiratory distress
- Abdominal haemorrhage
- Urogenital or gastrointestinal obstruction or perforation
- Pathological fracture.

These patients usually require emergency stabilization, and then the ethical question of whether surgical intervention is right and necessary must be addressed. Immediate surgery, prior to definitive diagnosis, may be indicated in some cases but must be followed by appropriate postoperative care. Very often such surgeries are palliative only, such as resection of bleeding splenic haemangiosarcomas, hepatic tumours, resection of ulcerated or obstructive gastrointestinal neoplasms that have already metastasized, or the placement of a permanent cystostomy catheter obviating the need for immediate euthanasia in animals with advanced urethral or bladder cancer. Other surgical procedures include emergency tracheostomy for immediate palliation of life-threatening upper respiratory tract obstructions prior to full evaluation of the extent of the obstructive mass and possible definitive or palliative excision.

Occasionally, surgery is required to deal with complications of radiation or chemotherapy, e.g. treatment of tissue necrosis resulting from extravasated chemotherapeutic agents or radiation-induced tissue necrosis, or fibrosis and subsequent stricture of hollow viscera.

Support surgeries

Support surgeries include the various methods of providing nutritional support (oesophagostomy tubes, gastrostomy tubes, enterostomy tubes) (see also Chapter 10) and the implantation of long-term central catheters or vascular access ports for repeated administration of chemotherapeutic agents or for the repeated administration of anaesthetic agents for hyperfractionated radiotherapy regimens (e.g. radiotherapy three to five times a week). They also include the placement of cystostomy tubes for temporary urinary diversion while local radiation treatment of urethral tumours is carried out.

Surgical treatment of metastatic disease

In human medicine, it has been documented that survival rates for patients where lung metastases have been resected are similar to survival rates for patients who have primary lung tumours resected. Human patients are selected for metastatectomy: when the primary tumour has been controlled; when there is a solitary metastasis or metastases confined to one lobe of the lung; where there has been no local recurrence of the primary tumour following treatment; where there is no extrapulmonary spread; and where there is no circulatory or respiratory insufficiency.

In veterinary medicine, the surgical treatment of metastatic nodules has been suggested in selected patients, although large-scale evaluation is limited (O'Brien *et al.*, 1993; Liptak *et al.*, 2004b). The careful selection of potential patients is important and the basic criteria that have been suggested (Gilson, 1998) are that:

- The primary tumour must be controlled
- The patient must have had a prolonged disease-free interval from the time of treatment of the primary tumour (>300 days)
- The patient must have <3 metastatic nodules
- The metastasis must have a long tumour doubling time (>30 days).

Considerations for oncological surgery

Preoperative preparation

The patient should be generously clipped to facilitate effective preparation and also to allow for changes in the surgical plan during surgery. Gentle cleaning using effective skin preparations (e.g. chlorhexidine/ alcohol mixture) is sufficient; indeed, vigorous scrubbing of skin overlying tumours has been associated with increased metastasis in laboratory mice. Similarly, vigorous palpation of tumours prior to surgery is not advocated, as surface injury, especially to intra-abdominal tumours, may potentiate seeding of neoplastic cells or rupture and haemorrhage.

Oncological surgery often involves operating on patients that have one or more of the patient factors that have been shown to increase the chance of postoperative infection. These include:

- Old age
- Poor nutritional status
- Obesity
- Endocrine disease
- Hypoxaemia
- The presence of remote infection
- Corticosteroid therapy
- Immunocompromise
- Bowel obstruction
- Thrombocytopenia
- Cardiovascular disease
- Poor blood supply to the surgical field.

The infection rates following oncological surgery have been shown to be significantly higher than for other surgical procedures in both the veterinary and human fields. The presence of cancer is not itself a risk factor, but such patients are often at risk of surgical wound infection for the reasons outlined above. Careful planning for pharmacological prevention or treatment of infection will maximize the chances of a successful surgery.

Different classes of antibiotics kill organisms in very different ways and the appropriate dose schedules vary greatly. For example, the beta-lactams and amoxicillin/clavulanate exhibit time-dependent killing and should be given at doses to maintain concentrations above the minimum inhibitory concentration (MIC) for the whole operative period. This may mean repeat dosing (i.e. every 3 hours during surgery). In contrast, the aminoglycosides and quinolones (e.g. enrofloxacin) require a high peak concentration, which determines bacterial killing, and then a period of low concentration to re-establish organism sensitivity. Thus the goal in surgical prophylaxis is for the organisms in the surgical field to encounter just one large dose of the aminoglycoside or quinolone during the operative period.

The timing of antibiotic prophylaxis is crucial. Increased rates of infection are observed if preoperative antibiotic therapy is initiated too early, or continued for too long postoperatively. The best results are seen when antibiotic therapy begins no more than 2 hours before the surgical procedure and continues for no more than 24 hours after the surgical procedure.

Postoperative care

Analgesia

Specific anti-cancer treatments such as surgical resection will often eliminate or reduce very effectively the incidence and severity of the pain associated with a neoplastic disease (see also Chapter

11). However, the surgical procedures are often extensive and can involve reconstructive procedures with the necessity for provision of effective analgesic regimens – at least in the short to medium term. Analgesia can help to prevent secondary adverse effects of postoperative pain, such as increased levels of catabolic hormones, prolonged recovery, and increased skeletal and smooth muscle tone, as well as the suffering caused by the pain itself. Additionally, effective perioperative analgesia in cancer patients may prevent chronic postoperative pain – a phenomenon that is becoming increasingly recognized in human medicine. It is thought to occur due to the superimposition of acute pain on chronic pain.

In line with current thinking, the prevention of postoperative pain should start preoperatively, with effective doses of multiple classes of analgesics (e.g. opioid plus NSAID). If elective surgery for a painful neoplastic lesion is planned, it is probably beneficial to provide effective analgesic therapy for several days prior to surgical intervention in order to minimize central sensitization. This could easily be provided with NSAID therapy. As the surgery planned becomes more extensive, the doses of opioids used (e.g. buprenorphine, morphine) should increase and

pre- (where licensed) or postoperative NSAID therapy should be used.

Local anaesthetics should always be used if possible, as local infiltration, regional blocks or as part of an epidural. If used for local infiltration, care must be exercised not to distort tissue architecture and normal fascial planes in the area of surgery. Figure 6.11 summarizes an analgesic approach to perioperative pain management in oncological patients, an approach that makes the most of pre-emptive analgesia.

Of interest is the recent finding that the provision of analgesics significantly reduces the tumour-promoting effects of undergoing and recovering from surgery (Page *et al.*, 2001). Undergoing surgery is well known to result in the suppression of several immune functions, including natural killer (NK) cell activity in both animals (Sandoval *et al.*, 1996) and humans (Kutza *et al.*, 1997). The reduction in tumour-promoting effects of surgery by analgesics seems to be due to the alleviation of pain-induced reduced NK cell function (Page *et al.*, 2001). So the provision of adequate pain management may be protective against metastatic sequelae in clinical patients.

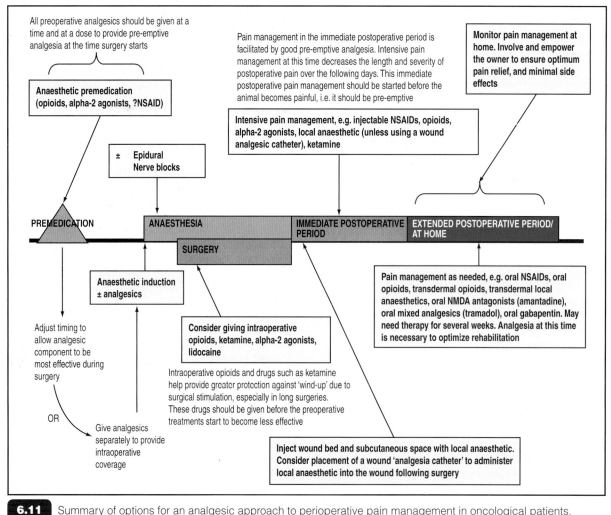

6.11 Summary of options for an analgesic approach to perioperative pain management in oncological patients.

Monitoring and fluid therapy

In the postoperative period, sensible monitoring of cardiopulmonary parameters and major organ function is required to prevent the development of potentially life-threatening complications. The provision of effective fluid therapy in the immediate postoperative period and the instigation of oral or enteral nutrition are particularly important. These factors assume greater importance in many oncological patients who may be older and/or debilitated. Monitoring will be dictated by the types of recognized specific complications that can occur following a given procedure.

Margin evaluation

All tissue resected at surgery *must* be submitted for histopathological analysis for evaluation of the surgical margins, the mitotic index, presence of necrosis, vascular or lymphatic invasion and the grade or degree of differentiation of the tumour (see also Chapter 3). Such information is used to provide the owner with the maximum possible detail regarding prognosis. Following resection, the margins of interest should be clearly identified in order to target the microscopic evaluation of the tissue. It is often difficult for the surgeon to orient a piece of tissue that has just been resected, so one can imagine how difficult it can be for the pathologist, after the tissue has been sitting in formalin for a couple of days. A good plan to follow is:

1. Lay the specimen out in the position it was in the patient.
2. Use sutures to 'reconstruct' the specimen, e.g. to replace displaced muscle in its original *in vivo* position (Figure 6.12).
3. Decide where the resection margin was closest to the gross tumour and mark that margin.
4. Mark other margins that need to be evaluated (e.g. lateral, deep) (Figure 6.13).
5. Draw a picture of the specimen on the histopathological submission form, and also a diagram to indicate where the resection was performed. Also indicate where the tumour was, what margins are inked, and with what colours.

Margins should be tagged or painted with Indian ink or specific tissue dyes immediately after surgery, so that if tumour cells are found in particular margins further surgery or adjunctive therapy such as radiotherapy can be planned optimally. The painting of particular margins of a resected mass with Indian ink is particularly useful, as areas that the surgeon may be suspicious of as being 'dirty' can be assessed accurately by the pathologist, avoiding any misinterpretation (see also Chapter 2). Another way of assessing margins is to submit samples of tissue from aspects of the remaining tissue bed for evaluation of whether or not there are tumour cells present. Such follow-up of cases is a time-consuming but essential part of surgical oncology. [*Editors' note: There are differing opinions on the best way to mark margins; it is best to consult the pathology laboratory as to their preferred method.*]

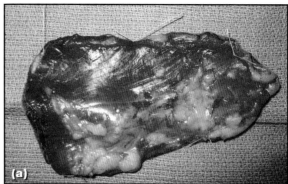
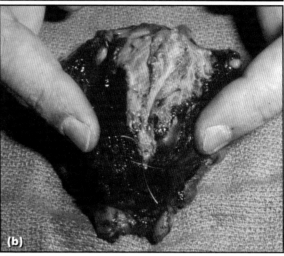

6.12 Prior to submitting any tissue to a pathologist, sutures can be used to 'reconstruct' the specimen (e.g. to replace displaced muscle in its original *in vivo* position). **(a)** The underlying latissimus dorsi muscle tended to 'slip' off the specimen, exposing the ventral part of the mass. **(b)** The muscle was resected as the uninvolved ventral margin to this mass.

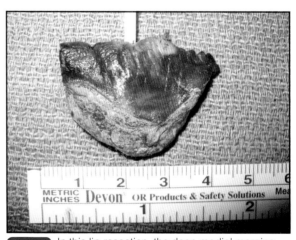

6.13 In this lip resection, the deep medial margins have been inked yellow to allow the pathologist to orient the sections so that he/she can comment on how far away any neoplastic cells are from the inked margins.

There is considerable debate regarding what is considered to be an 'acceptable' clean margin distance from the tissue edge to tumour cells. For example, in humans, the surgical margin status following breast-conserving surgery is considered the strongest predictor for local failure/recurrence. European radiation oncologists require that the clean margin be >5 mm to be considered negative, whereas in many other countries a clean margin is considered to be gained when there are no tumour cells on the inked margin, regardless of how close tumour cells are to the margin (Taghian *et al.*, 2005).

Postoperative appearance

Sometimes surgery can produce a cure in an animal suffering from solid neoplasia, but only with significant alteration of its appearance. Such cosmetic changes can be distressing to look at initially, but it is worth remembering that animals do not appear to be as concerned about their appearance as we are. Potentially, in the right case, if the principles of oncological surgery are adhered to, a cure can be produced, perioperative morbidity can be minimized and the animal can maintain excellent function. Examples of such surgeries are the radical head surgeries (Figure 6.14) and when considering these cases the owners need to be informed of the expected visual outcome. This may be demonstrated using pictures of similar cases and by enlisting the assistance of owners with animals that have undergone such surgeries.

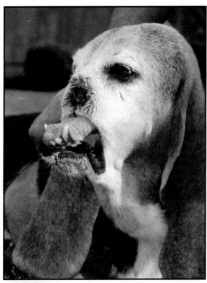

6.14 Owners should be fully informed of the expected appearance of their pet following oncological surgery. The owner of this dog was fully informed of the expected appearance, and was very satisfied with the tumour-curing surgery performed (radical nosectomy for SCC).

Future directions

At present, surgical excision remains the dominant modality of curative therapy. Some of the previously held preconceptions regarding what is possible for patients are evaporating as clients' willingness to pursue more extensive surgery increases, along with their expectations. Increasingly innovative ways are being found to combine currently available treatment modalities such as chemoembolization, receptor-targeted radiotherapy, regional/isolated chemotherapy perfusion and hyperthermia with surgery. There is movement towards more minimally invasive and interventional techniques, with ethanol

and radiofrequency thermal ablation readily available as well as endoscopic surgery and robotic technology. Reconstructive options are increasing, with tissues and organs being engineered in laboratories for transplantation.

References and further reading

Beck AL, Grierson JM, Ogden DM. Hamilton MH and Lipscomb VJ (2007) Outcome of and complications associated with tube cystostomy in dogs and cats: 76 cases (1995–2006). *Journal of the American Veterinary Medical Association* **230**, 1184–1189

Boston SE, Duerr F, Bacon N *et al.* (2007) Intraoperative radiation for limb sparing of the distal aspect of the radius without transcarpal plating in five dogs. *Veterinary Surgery* **36**, 314–323

Britt T, Clifford C, Barger A *et al.* (2007) Diagnosing appendicular osteosarcoma with ultrasound-guided fine-needle aspiration: 36 cases. *Journal of Small Animal Practice* **48**, 145–150

Dawe J (2007) Osteosarcoma in a 6-year-old Newfoundland dog: limb-sparing surgery and cisplatin chemotherapy. *Canadian Veterinary Journal* **48**, 1169–1171

Fulcher RP, Ludwig LL, Bergman PJ *et al.* (2006) Evaluation of a two-centimeter lateral surgical margin for excision of grade I and grade II cutaneous mast cell tumors in dogs. *Journal of the American Veterinary Medical Association* **228**, 210–215

Gilson SD (1998) Principles of surgery for cancer palliation and treatment of metastases. *Clinical Techniques in Small Animal Practice* **13**, 65–69

Halfacree ZJ, Baines SJ, Lipscomb VJ *et al.* (2007) Use of a latissimus dorsi myocutaneous flap for one-stage reconstruction of the thoracic wall after en bloc resection of primary rib chondrosarcoma in five dogs. *Veterinary Surgery* **36**, 587–592

Krag D (2000) Sentinel lymph node biopsy for the detection of metastases. *Cancer Journal* **6** (Suppl. 2), S121–124

Krick EL, Billings AP, Shofer FS, Watanabe S and Sorenmo KU (2009) Cytological lymph node evaluation in dogs with mast cell tumours: association with grade and survival. *Veterinary and Comparative Oncology* **7**, 130–138

Kutza J, Gratz I, Afshar M and Murasko DM (1997) The effects of general anesthesia and surgery on basal and interferon stimulated natural killer cell activity of humans. *Anesthesia and Analgesia* **85**, 918–923

Liptak JM, Dernell WS, Lascelles BD *et al.* (2004a) Intraoperative extracorporeal irradiation for limb sparing in 13 dogs. *Veterinary Surgery* **33**, 446–456

Liptak JM, Dernell WS, Rizzo SA *et al.* (2008) Reconstruction of chest wall defects after rib tumor resection: a comparison of autogenous, prosthetic, and composite techniques in 44 dogs. *Veterinary Surgery* **37**, 479–487

Liptak JM, Monnet E, Dernell WS and Withrow SJ (2004b) Pulmonary metastatectomy in the management of four dogs with hypertrophic osteopathy. *Veterinary and Comparative Oncology* **2**, 1–12

Matthiesen DT, Clark GN, Orsher RJ *et al.* (1992) En bloc resection of primary rib tumors in 40 dogs. *Veterinary Surgery* **21**, 201–204

Moores A and Williams JM (2009) *BSAVA Manual of Canine and Feline Wound Management and Reconstruction, 2nd edn.* BSAVA Publications, Gloucester

O'Brien MG, Straw RC, Withrow SJ *et al.* (1993) Resection of pulmonary metastases in canine osteosarcoma: 36 cases (1983–1992). *Veterinary Surgery* **22**, 105–109

Page GG, Blakely WP and Ben-Eliyahu S (2001) Evidence that postoperative pain is a mediator of the tumor-promoting effects of surgery in rats. *Pain* **90**, 191–199

Pereira CT, Luiz Navarro Marques F, Williams J, Wlademir De Martin B and Primo Bombonato P (2008) 99mTc-labeled dextran for mammary lymphoscintigraphy in dogs. *Veterinary Radiology and Ultrasound* **49**, 487–491

Sandoval BA, Robinson AV, Sulaiman TT, Shenk RR and Stellato TA (1996) Open versus laparoscopic surgery: a comparison of natural antitumoral cellular immunity in a small animal model. *American Journal of Surgery* **62**, 625–630

Schneider R, Dorn CR and Taylor DO (1969) Factors influencing canine mammary cancer development and postsurgical survival. *Journal of the National Cancer Institute* **43**, 1249–1261

Simpson AM, Ludwig LL, Newman SJ *et al.* (2004) Evaluation of surgical margins required for complete excision of cutaneous mast cell tumors in dogs. *Journal of the American Veterinary Medical Associaton* **224**, 236–240

Smith JD, Stone EA and Gilson SD.(1995) Placement of a permanent cystostomy catheter to relieve urine outflow obstruction in dogs with transitional cell carcinoma. *Journal of the American Veterinary Medical Association* **206**, 496–499

Straw RC, Withrow SJ, Douple EB *et al.* (1994) Effects of cisdiammineedichloroplatinum II released from D,L-polylactic acid implanted adjacent to cortical allografts in dogs. *Journal of Orthopaedic Research* **12**, 871–877

Taghian A, Mohiuddin M, Jagsi R *et al.* (2005) Current perceptions regarding surgical margin status after breast-conserving therapy: results of a survey. *Annals of Surgery* **241**, 629–639

Tang J, Li W, Lu F *et al.* (2009) Comparison of gray-scale contrast-enhanced ultrasonography with contrast-enhanced computed tomography in different grading of blunt hepatic and splenic trauma: an animal experiment. *Ultrasound in Medicine and Biology* **35**, 566–575

Virkus WW, Marshall D, Enneking WF and Scarborough MT (2002) The effect of contaminated surgical margins revisited. *Clinical Orthopaedics and Related Research* **397**, 89–94

Wallack ST, Wisner ER, Werner JA *et al.* (2002) Accuracy of magnetic resonance imaging for estimating intramedullary osteosarcoma extent in pre-operative planning of canine limb-salvage procedures. *Veterinary Radiology and Ultrasound* **43**, 432–441

Weisse C, Shofer FS and Sorenmo K (2002) Recurrence rates and sites for grade II canine cutaneous mast cell tumors following complete surgical excision. *Journal of the American Animal Hospital Association* **38**, 71–73

Withrow SJ, Liptak JM, Straw RC *et al.* (2004) Biodegradable cisplatin polymer in limb-sparing surgery for canine osteosarcoma. *Annals of Surgical Oncology* **11**, 705–713

Withrow SJ and Vail DM (2007) *Withrow and MacEwen's Small Animal Clinical Oncology, 4th edn.* Elsevier Saunders, Edinburgh

Zekas LJ, Crawford JT and O'Brien RT (2005) Computed tomography-guided fine-needle aspirate and tissue-core biopsy of intrathoracic lesions in thirty dogs and cats. *Veterinary Radiology and Ultrasound* **46**, 200–204

Zitelli JA, Brown CD and Hanusa BH (1997) Surgical margins for excision of primary cutaneous melanoma. *Journal of the American Academy of Dermatology* **37**, 422–429

7

Principles of chemotherapy

Susan E. Lana and Jane M. Dobson

Introduction

Chemotherapy is a common treatment modality in veterinary cancer medicine. Whether used alone or as an adjunct to surgery or radiation, new drugs, combinations and methods of delivery are constantly being explored. In order to use chemotherapy successfully the clinician must be aware of some basic principles, the potential side effects of the drugs used and the techniques for administering them.

General principles and considerations

Patient factors
Prior to initiation of chemotherapy, several patient factors must be considered.

- Most importantly, an accurate histological diagnosis must be made.
- The biological behaviour of the particular cancer in question must be understood in order to determine whether chemotherapy is appropriate. For some cancer types, such as a low-grade fibrosarcoma of the distal extremity, the disease is confined to the local area and has a very low probability of metastasis; therefore, chemotherapy is not indicated. In other cancer types, such as osteosarcoma (OSA), which displays a highly metastatic behaviour, chemotherapy has been shown to extend the disease-free interval.
- The stage of the disease. (Where in the body is the cancer?)
- The patient's general health status, presence of concurrent disease conditions, and ability to tolerate potential toxicity. Although chemotherapy is generally well tolerated in veterinary patients, there is the potential for side effects. If an animal has underlying renal, hepatic or cardiac dysfunction, the risk of toxicity may be altered, and the chemotherapy protocol may need to be adjusted to serve the needs of the specific patient.

Owner factors
Several owner factors must also be considered prior to initiating chemotherapy.

- Owners should have a thorough understanding of their pet's disease, including expected prognosis and outcome.
- Owners should be made aware of the possible time commitment and costs involved in treatment.
- Owners should be given detailed oral and written information about the cancer treatment recommended for their pet and should be instructed about potential side effects and what to do if toxicity occurs at home. They should also be advised of the potential risks of handling cytotoxic drugs and excreta from animals receiving such agents.

With adequate information and understanding, owners are better able to make treatment choices that are right for their pet and themselves and will be satisfied with those choices regardless of the outcome. The ultimate goal of cancer treatment for the client and veterinary surgeon should be to improve quality of life and overall survival for the patient.

Indications
Chemotherapy is indicated for treatment of tumours known to be chemosensitive, including:

- Haemopoietic malignancies (leukaemia, lymphoma, multiple myeloma)
- Highly metastatic malignancies (such as OSA and haemangiosarcoma).

Chemotherapy is commonly used as a primary treatment for induction, consolidation and, in some cases, maintenance of remission in haemopoietic malignancies. Chemotherapy against solid tumours such as OSA is often used in an adjuvant setting after primary tumour treatment to eradicate occult micrometastatic disease. Neoadjuvant therapy (using chemotherapy prior to definitive treatment) is commonplace in human medicine but has not been widely applied in veterinary medicine. Common terms are explained in Figure 7.1.

Dose and timing
In order for a chemotherapy drug to be effective it must reach the cell in question and must exert a toxic effect within the cell; the cell must be susceptible to the drug of interest and resistance must not have developed. All these pharmacokinetic and pharmacodynamic factors may be influenced by the dose given, the timing of administration and the mechanism of action of a particular chemotherapy agent.

Term	Definition
Remission	Lack of clinical evidence of tumour. A remission may be complete (CR) with no evidence of disease, or partial (PR) with > 50% reduction in tumour volume and no new lesions developing
Induction	A phase of chemotherapy in which the goal is to induce remission. This phase usually involves a more intense therapy (shorter dosing interval/drug combinations)
Consolidation	A phase of treatment in which drugs are administered in order to improve clinical response by reducing microscopic disease that may still be present after the patient is already in remission
Maintenance	The phase of the drug protocol used to keep a patient in remission. Often less intense than previous induction therapy. The indication for maintenance therapy is dependent on the type of cancer being treated
Rescue (salvage) therapy	Treatment used to re-induce remission after a patient fails a previous protocol and the disease returns clinically
Adjuvant	Chemotherapy used *after* surgery or radiation therapy to delay recurrence or distant metastasis
Neoadjuvant	Chemotherapy used to decrease the bulk of the primary tumour *prior to* other treatments such as surgery or radiation

7.1 Common terms used in chemotherapy protocols.

Single *versus* multiple drugs

Chemotherapeutic agents can be used alone or in combination. The advantages and disadvantages of single and multiple protocols are listed in Figure 7.2.

Single agent treatment: As hypothesized by Goldie *et al.* (1982), when tumours become clinically detectable (10^6 cells) they are heterogenous and already contain a population of drug-resistant clones. Single agent therapy has the potential to result in an apparent clinical response but ultimate tumour progression due to survival and proliferation of the drug-resistant clones.

Multiple drug protocols: Several 'rules' should be followed when using multiple drug protocols:

- Each drug should have some efficacy alone against the tumour targeted
- Overlapping toxicities should be avoided or drugs must be scheduled to compensate for this
- Maximum doses should be used when possible
- Drugs with different mechanisms of action against neoplastic cells should be combined to maximize the number of cells killed.

Dosing

The appropriate dose of any drug should be the maximum tolerated dose given at the shortest treatment interval, while still maintaining an acceptable toxicity profile. Chemotherapy drugs are often dosed on the basis of body surface area (BSA) in square metres (m^2). Using this dosage scheme, however, smaller animals (<10 kg) often show increased toxicity to certain drugs, such as doxorubicin. Figures 7.3 and 7.4 show the conversion of weight to BSA for dogs and cats, respectively. Details of specific drug dosages are included later in the chapter, as well as recommendations for those drugs where a dose reduction is indicated for smaller animals.

Single agent treatment		Multiple agent protocols	
Advantages	*Disadvantages*	*Advantages*	*Disadvantages*
Decreased cost Decreased risk of toxicity Decreased time in hospital	Decreased efficacy Lack of tumour control, possibly due to expansion of drug-resistant clones	Greater efficacy Drug resistance slower to develop	Increased cost Increased risk of toxicity Increased time spent at veterinary clinic

7.2 Single *versus* multiple drug protocols.

Weight (kg)	BSA (m^2)	Weight (kg)	BSA (m^2)	Weight (kg)	BSA (m^2)	Weight (kg)	BSA (m^2)	Weight (kg)	BSA (m^2)
		11.0	0.500	21.0	0.769	31.0	0.997	41.0	1.201
2.0	0.160	12.0	0.529	22.0	0.785	32.0	1.018	42.0	1.220
3.0	0.210	13.0	0.553	23.0	0.817	33.0	1.029	43.0	1.240
4.0	0.255	14.0	0.581	24.0	0.840	34.0	1.060	44.0	1.259
5.0	0.295	15.0	0.608	25.0	0.864	35.0	1.081	45.0	1.278
6.0	0.333	16.0	0.641	26.0	0.886	36.0	1.101	46.0	1.297
7.0	0.370	17.0	0.668	27.0	0.909	37.0	1.121	47.0	1.302
8.0	0.404	18.0	0.694	28.0	0.931	38.0	1.142	48.0	1.334
9.0	0.437	19.0	0.719	29.0	0.953	39.0	1.162	49.0	1.352
10.0	0.469	20.0	0.744	30.0	0.975	40.0	1.181	50.0	1.371

7.3 Conversion chart for weight to body surface area (BSA) in dogs.

Weight (kg)	BSA (m²)	Weight (kg)	BSA (m²)	Weight (kg)	BSA (m²)	Weight (kg)	BSA (m²)	Weight (kg)	BSA (m²)
		3.2	0.217	5.2	0.300	7.2	0.373	9.2	0.439
1.4	0.125	3.4	0.226	5.4	0.307	7.4	0.380	9.4	0.445
1.6	0.137	3.6	0.235	5.6	0.315	7.6	0.387	9.6	0.452
1.8	0.148	3.8	0.244	5.8	0.323	7.8	0.393	9.8	0.458
2.0	0.159	4.0	0.252	6.0	0.330	8.0	0.400	10.0	0.464
2.2	0.169	4.2	0.260	6.2	0.337	8.2	0.407		
2.4	0.179	4.4	0.269	6.4	0.345	8.4	0.413		
2.6	0.189	4.6	0.277	6.6	0.352	8.6	0.420		
2.8	0.199	4.8	0.285	6.8	0.360	8.8	0.426		
3.0	0.208	5.0	0.292	7.0	0.366	9.0	0.433		

7.4 Conversion chart for weight to body surface area (BSA) in cats.

The way in which drugs are metabolized and excreted from the body must also be taken into account, as compromised function of the liver or kidneys may lead to increased toxicity or decreased efficacy of certain drugs. An example of this is cyclophosphamide, which must be metabolized in the liver in order to be active. Another example is the potential nephrotoxicity of cisplatin: this drug should be used with caution in animals with renal disease. Dose adjustment guidelines used in humans based on creatinine clearance or bilirubin concentrations are not well standardized in veterinary medicine. A study evaluating the effect of glomerular filtration rate (GFR) on pharmacodynamic endpoints in cats receiving a standardized dose of carboplatin showed that decreases in neutrophil count were directly related to the area under the curve (AUC); clearance of carboplatin and a targeted AUC could be predicted based on GFR (Bailey *et al.*, 2004). The authors proposed that dosing for individualized clearance of the drug could possibly translate into greater dose intensity, acceptable toxicity and ultimately improved outcome. The routine clinical application of such an approach is questionable but it highlights the fact that pharmacokinetic and pharmacodynamic variability between patients can be great.

Timing
The timing of administration of chemotherapy drugs is very important. Ideally, drugs should be given at intervals to allow for maximum tumour cell death but adequate recovery of normal cell populations (e.g. bone marrow, gastrointestinal tract). For this reason, many chemotherapeutic agents are administered in a pulsed fashion. For myelosuppressive drugs such as doxorubicin and cyclophosphamide, the white blood cell count typically reaches a nadir at 7–10 days following administration of maximally tolerated doses and has recovered by day 21, hence the commonly used 3-week cycles of treatment.

Metronomic dosing: A different schedule of treatment currently being investigated is metronomic dosing, or low doses of drugs given continually. These regimes use lower doses of cytotoxic agents (e.g. cyclophosphamide) in a continuous schedule, instead of pulsed maximally tolerated doses. Targeted therapies with specific mechanisms of action are also being studied in combination with low-dose cytotoxic drugs. The exact mechanism of action of this low-dose approach is unknown, though modulation of angiogenic pathways or altering immune effector cells are two of the proposed mechanisms (Gately and Kerbel, 2001). Metronomic dosing regimens have shown promise in animal models and in human clinical trials. Veterinary trials have been reported, but exact drug combinations, doses and efficacy of this approach are not well substantiated at this time (Lana *et al.*, 2007; Elmslie *et al.*, 2008).

Other delivery systems: The *efficacy* of a drug is related to the length of time a cancer cell is exposed to the drug, while the *toxicity* is related to the peak serum concentration. Alternative delivery methods are being devised to increase the time a cell is exposed to a drug and to lessen the peak concentrations. Examples of this include sustained release polymer delivery systems and liposomal encapsulated drugs. Other methods of delivery such as intracavitary or intratumoral administration are designed to give higher concentrations to the tumour cells while decreasing systemic exposure and toxicity.

Drug resistance
Drug resistance is often the ultimate reason for treatment failure and death. Currently there are several known mechanisms of drug resistance (Figure 7.5), including decreased uptake of the drug, altered affinity of the drug for the target, increased inactivation of the drug by the body and increased removal of the drug from the cell.

Mechanism of resistance	Drugs possibly affected
Decreased drug uptake	Methotrexate
Decreased drug activation	Cytarabine, methotrexate
Increased drug target	5-Fluorouracil, methotrexate
Altered drug target	Etoposide, doxorubicin, methotrexate
Increased detoxification (increased glutathione or glutathione transferase)	Alkylating agents
Enhanced DNA repair	Alkylating agents, platinum derivatives, nitrosoureas
Defective recognition of DNA adducts	Cisplatin
Increased drug efflux	Doxorubicin, etoposide, vinca alkaloids, paclitaxel
Defective checkpoint function and/or apoptosis	Most anti-cancer drugs

7.5 Mechanisms of drug resistance.

This last mechanism has been one of the best characterized and involves expression of the *MDR-1* gene, which encodes for P-170 membrane glycoprotein. This glycoprotein works as an efflux pump to remove xenobiotics from the cell. As many cytotoxic drugs are substrates for this pump, development of resistance to one drug through this mechanism can confer resistance to different drugs to which the cell has not been exposed. Other membrane proteins such as MRP (multidrug resistance protein) have also been identified with respect to this phenomenon.

Another reason for drug resistance is the suppression or inactivation of apoptotic or cell-damage control pathways, which occurs during the process of carcinogenesis in many tumours. Apoptosis (programmed cell death) is a common pathway mediating cell death in response to many cytotoxic agents.

Upregulation of *bcl-2* or inactivation of *p53* are examples of genetic changes that could contribute to drug resistance.

As research in this field progresses, it is becoming obvious that drug resistance is often a complex process, involving several mechanisms that may occur in series or in parallel. Because of this, strategies aimed at blocking one specific pathway are often clinically unrewarding. Although work is ongoing with several 'anti-resistance' compounds, definitive results do not yet warrant incorporating these agents into standard protocols.

Preparation and safe handling

With the increasing use of chemotherapy drugs in veterinary practice, more members of the veterinary healthcare team are at risk of exposure to these compounds. This includes veterinary surgeons, nurses, animal technicians, cleaners, and pet owners and their families. Cytotoxic drugs have activity that may cause mutagenic, carcinogenic and teratogenic effects. Studies concerning occupational exposure in the human cancer field have shown changes in the amounts of mutagens in the urine of employees sampled, as well as degrees of work surface contamination in areas of chemotherapy preparation and administration (Conner *et al.*, 1999; Sessink and Bos, 1999).

Exposure can occur in several ways:

- Inhalation of aerosol of drug during mixing or administration
- Absorption through the skin
- Ingestion through contact with contaminated food or other objects (e.g. cigarettes)
- Accidental inoculation.

It is essential that employees are informed of the risks of working with cytotoxic drugs and the safety precautions/procedures that must be taken to minimize exposure. Practices using cytotoxic drugs should develop and implement a set of 'Local Rules' or 'Guidelines' for handling cytotoxic drugs in the practice, as outlined in Figure 7.6. Safety precautions are listed in Figure 7.7.

- All employees must be informed of the risks of working with cytotoxic drugs.
- There must be a procedure for use of personal protective equipment to minimize risk of cytotoxic exposure.
- There must be a procedure and specified equipment for handling (preparation and administration) of cytotoxic drugs to minimize risk of exposure.
- There must be a clear procedure and adequate materials for cleaning spillage of cytotoxic agents.
- All areas where cytotoxic drugs are handled or used must be clearly identified, access to such areas should be restricted during cytotoxic drug usage, and the area should be cleaned before use for other purposes.
- There must be a clear procedure for disposal of all contaminated (and potentially contaminated) materials in accordance with Local Authority Regulations.
- There should be a protocol for cleaning facilities where cytotoxic drugs are used.
- Pregnant women should not handle cytotoxic drugs.

Detailed Guidelines for preventing occupational and environmental exposure to cytotoxic drugs in veterinary medicine have been prepared by the European College of Veterinary Internal Medicine and may be downloaded from their website (www.ecvim-ca.org)

7.6 General guidelines for handling cytotoxic drugs.

- Ideally, drugs should be prepared in a biological safety cabinet or class-II vertical flow containment hood (Figure 7.8a). If this is not possible in the practice setting, drugs should be prepared in a low-traffic area away from doors, windows or draughts. A plastic shield can be used to protect the person preparing the drugs. Preferably a closed-system drug protective device should be used, as discussed below.
- Regardless of where the drugs are prepared, the preparation surface should be covered by a plastic-backed absorbent pad.
- A gown with long sleeves, cuffs and a closed front, made of material with low permeability, should be worn. Specialized cytotoxic protective gloves should be worn and pulled over the cuff of the gown. *Standard surgical gloves are not adequate.*
- If a safety cabinet is not available, the use of a dust-and-mist respirator or a mask with a filter that prevents inhalation of drug aerosols is recommended. A regular surgical mask is not acceptable.
- To prevent formation of aerosols, hydrophobic filters or chemotherapy pins can be used to prevent pressure build-up in a bottle. A filter needle can also be used to prevent aerosol exposure (Figure 7.8b).
- Luer-Lok syringes should also be used to prevent accidental separation of the needle from the syringe or chemo-pin.
- All intravenous lines should be primed prior to addition of cytotoxic agents to the infusion bag.
- After preparation is complete, drugs should be placed in a clearly labelled sealable plastic bag to contain any spills during transport to the area for administration to the patient.
- Materials to be discarded after preparation (e.g. syringes, vials) should be placed in a sealable plastic bag and disposed of as biohazard waste. Needles should be placed in a separate designated 'sharps' container. To prevent accidental inoculation, recapping of needles should be avoided.

7.7 Safety precautions for handling cytotoxic drugs.

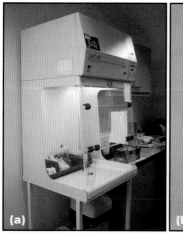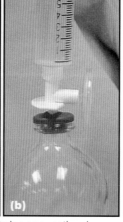

7.8 Equipment used to minimize occupational exposure to chemotherapy agents.
(a) Biological safety cabinet. **(b)** Chemotherapy pin used to prevent aerosolization of any drug.

Closed systems

Closed-system drug transfer devices mechanically prohibit the escape of hazardous drug or vapour concentrations outside the system. The first on the market was the PhaSeal® system (Figure 7.9), which has been shown in numerous studies to reduce exposure to both personnel handling drugs and environmental surfaces (Wick *et al.*, 2003; Jorgensen *et al.*, 2008). The system has two unique qualities. Firstly, when air or liquid is injected into the bottle the pressure is equalized via expansion of the bladder,

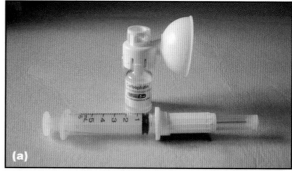

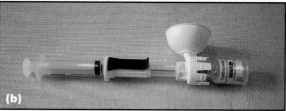

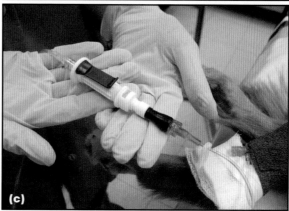

7.9 PhaSeal® system components: **(a)** protective cap, which is fixed to the pharmaceutical bottle; **(b)** injector Luer, which consists of an encapsulated specially ground cannula, used in both preparation and administration. **(c)** Administration to the patient.

which prevents aerosol leakage. Secondly, all components are fitted with sealing membranes that are connected together, and transfer is carried out via a special cannula. When the components are separated the membranes seal completely, preventing any leakage. While this system has reduced exposure dramatically it should not be used as the sole means to prevent contamination: personal protective garments and gloves are still recommended.

Common sense also plays a role in minimizing exposure. Hands should be washed before and after any procedure that involves a chemotherapeutic agent. Another way to decrease chemotherapy exposure is for a local human hospital or drug supplier to prepare the drugs for the veterinary practice.

Spillage and accident procedures

Cytotoxic spill kits (Figure 7.10) should be available in the areas of drug preparation and administration and in the ward where any animal is hospitalized, to prevent and contain contamination in the event of spillage or accidents. The procedures that should be followed in the event of accidental spillage or contamination are outlined in Figure 7.11.

- Disposable protective gown x 2
- Disposable chemotherapy gloves x 2 pairs
- Disposable shoe covers x 2 pairs
- Full face respirator and filters
- pH5 soap tablet
- Sealable plastic bags
- Chemosorb™ pads
- Absorbent disposable towels

7.10 Contents of a spill kit for cytotoxic drugs.

Event	Procedure
Spillage of cytotoxic drugs	1. Call for assistance and warn others. 2. Full personal protective clothing should be worn (including full face respirator and protective shoe coverings). 3. Use dry-absorbent towels to absorb any fluid. 4. Clean contaminated area with 70% alcohol and dry tissue three times. 5. Dispose of all contaminated material as cytotoxic waste.
Contamination of skin	Rinse with large amounts of water and wash with soap
Contamination of eyes	1. Seek help. 2. Remove contact lenses (if worn). 3. Rinse eye(s) with large amounts of water; use eye wash facility if available for at least 20 minutes. 4. Consult a doctor.
All accidents should be reported according to local Health and Safety regulations	

7.11 Procedures in the event of accidental spillage or contamination.

Cytotoxic drug	Period of risk (human data)
5-Fluorouracil	3 days
Carboplatin	5 days
Chlorambucil	2 days
Cisplatin	8 days
Cyclophosphamide	4 days
Cytarabine	3 days
Doxorubicin	7 days
Gemcitabine	7 days
Lomustine	3 days
Mitoxantrone	8 days
Vincristine	3 days
Vinblastine	3 days

7.12 Risk period in human patients after last drug administration. No similar data are available in veterinary medicine.

Drug administration

Oral medication

When administering oral medication, protective gloves should be worn and hands should be washed after administration. Tablets can be given normally, but it is important to ensure that the patient (especially cats) has swallowed the medication. A syringe full of water following administration can be helpful. It may be easier to administer tablets to dogs in a small amount of food, which they can be observed to swallow.

Another important aspect of oral medication is to avoid breaking or splitting pills. Doing so can lead to increased exposure through dust and debris. It may be necessary to alter the dose schedule or have drugs specially compounded by a pharmacy.

Intramuscular, subcutaneous or intralesional administration

Intramuscular and subcutaneous injections are administered in the normal fashion while wearing protective gloves. After insertion of the needle, the syringe must be checked for blood to make sure that a vessel has not been entered inadvertently and that the drug is not given intravenously. Intralesional chemotherapy is often administered in a suspending agent such as oil or another vehicle. Because there is a greater potential for leaking from the injection site, protective gloves, a chemotherapy preparation gown and protective eyewear should be worn. If significant leaking does occur, the areas should be swabbed and cleaned and the materials disposed of as chemotherapy waste.

Intravenous administration

While many chemotherapy drugs are administered intravenously, some of them are vesicants or irritants. Because of this, every attempt must be made

Nursing care of animals that have received cytotoxic drugs

Excreta (saliva, urine, vomit, faeces) of treated animals may contain traces of drugs or their metabolites and are therefore a potential risk. There is very little information available for the period of risk in animals; human data are presented in Figure 7.12.

- Special wards or designated kennels should be used for the hospitalization of animals treated with cytotoxic drugs, with clear identification of the agents used.
- Whilst animals are hospitalized during the period of risk, personal protective clothing should be used by all those taking care of the animal.
- All materials that have been in contact with the animal should be regarded as potentially contaminated.
- All waste should be disposed of as cytotoxic waste.

When animals are discharged from hospital or treated as outpatients, owners should be advised of the potential risk to their own health and environment from contaminated urine and faeces. They should be advised to wear gloves when cleaning up urine or faeces and to avoid being licked by their pet (paying special attention to children).

to ensure that the veins used are cared for and that catheters are placed as cleanly and atraumatically as possible. Peripheral veins should be avoided for routine blood collection in oncology patients, and the jugular vein used instead. Peripheral veins are chosen for intravenous chemotherapy administration because of the ease of monitoring for extravasations. It is good practice to alternate and record the veins being used to allow them to recover between treatments.

Drugs are usually administered with an indwelling catheter when the volume is >3 ml or the infusion is not a bolus injection (Figure 7.13a). For small-volume bolus injections (such as vincristine), a butterfly catheter may be used (Figure 7.13b).

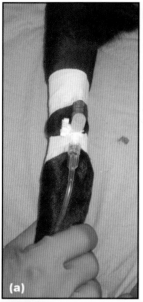

7.13

(a) Most cytotoxic drugs are administered via a cleanly placed intravenous catheter. **(b)** Small volumes of drug given as a bolus can be given through a butterfly catheter. This dog is receiving vincristine into a lateral saphenous vein.

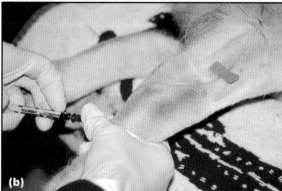

The procedure for intravenous administration of a chemotherapy drug is as follows:

1. Prior to administration, the site is clipped and aseptically prepared.
2. If the venipuncture was not 'clean', a different site should be attempted.
3. After placement, the catheter should be flushed with at least 10 ml of non-heparinized saline to ensure patency. Heparinized saline is avoided as heparin can cause precipitation of some drugs (e.g. doxorubicin).

4. During administration of the drug, the patient is monitored for adverse reaction and extravasation. The site should be visualized and not covered by layers of bandage material.
5. Upon completion of the infusion, the catheter is flushed with at least 10 ml of non-heparinized saline to ensure that the catheter and male adapter or hub have no residual drug present.
6. All materials should be discarded into appropriate chemotherapy waste containers.
7. Accurate record keeping for each treatment is essential, including drug, dose, vein used, administrator and any adverse events or dose reductions required.

Intracavitary administration

It is occasionally indicated that a chemotherapeutic agent (cisplatin, carboplatin) should be administered into a body cavity (thorax or abdomen), especially when a malignant effusion is present.

- For instillation into the chest cavity:
  o The patient is placed in lateral recumbency and the injection site is aseptically prepared. The right side is preferred for injection.
  o A ridged plastic intravenous cannula is inserted between the ribs and flushed with at least 12 ml of saline to ensure patency.
  o If resistance or excessive patient discomfort is noted, the cannula should be removed and a new one inserted.
- For abdominal administration:
  o The patient is placed in dorsal recumbency and a midline site caudal to the umbilicus is prepared. This site is chosen to avoid the spleen. It is advisable to allow the patient to empty the bladder prior to the procedure to reduce risk of bladder puncture.
  o A catheter is placed as described above.
- Once patency is determined, the fluid line is attached and the drug is administered. The maximum volume for the dog is 1 litre/m² in either cavity (Moore *et al.*, 1991). For the cat, maximum volumes of 60 ml for the chest cavity and 250 ml for the abdominal cavity have been recommended (Ogilvie and Moore, 2001b).
- After administration the patient should be allowed to move around in order to distribute the fluid throughout the cavity.
- Because a substantial amount of the drug dose is likely to be absorbed systemically, monitoring and administration guidelines for each drug still apply.

WARNING
Cats are not to receive cisplatin by any route and saline diuresis must still accompany cisplatin administration in dogs.

Toxicity

Many chemotherapy drugs have the potential to cause acute or late treatment-related side effects. Discussed below are some of the more common toxicities that can affect veterinary cancer patients.

Bone marrow suppression

The bone marrow is sensitive to the toxic effects of chemotherapy due to its high growth fraction and mitotic rate. Because the normal bone marrow transit times and circulating half-lives of each cell line are different, neutropenia typically occurs first, followed by thrombocytopenia. Anaemia associated with chemotherapy is rarely manifest clinically in the dog and cat.

Neutropenia: Neutropenia is the dose-limiting toxicity of many frequently used chemotherapeutic agents. Mild neutropenia is common and often not a clinical problem, but severe neutropenia can be complicated by sepsis and may be life-threatening. The neutropenic nadir is usually 7–10 days for most drugs, although each patient will have some variability depending on the drugs being given, dose, route of administration and time since last treatment. Most combination drug protocols are established to account for adequate bone marrow recovery between treatments. Monitoring patients with a complete blood count (CBC) is necessary prior to each chemotherapy treatment. Treatment should be delayed if absolute neutrophil counts are < 2.0–2.5 $\times$ 10^9/l. In most cases of mild neutropenia, the counts will increase in 3–4 days and treatment can then be reinstituted.

Patients with absolute neutrophil counts >1.5 $\times$ 10^9/l are usually non-febrile and asymptomatic. They should be monitored at home for any deterioration in their condition (Figure 7.14). Prophylactic antibiotics with agents such as trimethoprim/sulphonamides (15 mg/kg orally q12h) or fluoroquinolones can be given to guard against infection. When absolute counts drop below 1.0 $\times$ 10^9/l, the risk of developing sepsis rises. If significant neutropenia has developed after chemotherapy, the next dose (once the neutrophil count is sufficiently high) should be reduced by 20–25%.

The neutropenic patient that presents as febrile and possibly septic is a true emergency. The most likely source of infection is bacterial translocation of the patient's own gastrointestinal flora, released when the normal mucosal barrier is damaged by the chemotherapy. Clinically, patients that are severely neutropenic may not have all the signs of infection, due to the lack of cells to produce an inflammatory response. Other signs will include lethargy, collapse, anorexia and general malaise. Gastrointestinal signs may be present or may have preceded the neutropenic episode, and aspiration pneumonia is also possible if vomiting has been occurring. Diagnostic tests, including CBC, platelet count, biochemical profile and urinalysis, should be performed. Other procedures such as chest radiography, urine culture or abdominocentesis, should be carried out if indicated, looking for sites of infection. Blood cultures should be considered, though the likelihood of obtaining a positive result is low. At least two or three blood samples should be taken aseptically, 30 minutes apart. The patient should be carefully evaluated for other sites of infection such as pyoderma, surgical wounds, cellulitis, or radiation treatment sites for acute effects. If a likely area is found, samples should be obtained for culture.

Treatment should consist of supportive care with intravenous fluids and empiric broad-spectrum antibiotic therapy:

- Any electrolyte abnormalities and hydration deficits should be corrected. Strict aseptic technique should be used when placing and handling intravenous catheters
- Appropriate antibiotic choices include a combination of a penicillin or cephalosporin plus an aminoglycoside. Care should be taken when administering aminoglycosides in patients with renal compromise or dehydration. If aminoglycosides are not an appropriate choice for the patient, a second-generation cephalosporin, such as cefoxitin, or a combination of ampicillin and a fluoroquinolone, such as enrofloxacin, can also be used (Figure 7.15)
- Antibiotic therapy should be altered according to sensitivity indicated by any culture results
- Careful monitoring of all body systems and response to therapy is necessary for a successful outcome
- Filgrastim (granulocyte colony stimulating factor, G-CSF) can also be given to increase the neutrophil count. It has a very quick and profound effect of enhancing bone marrow recovery after chemotherapy insult. Only a human recombinant product is available commercially and there is potential for cross-reactive antibody development. Because of this, its routine use is controversial. The author does not recommend its use in afebrile patients or prophylactically. If used in febrile neutropenic patients, the dose is 2.5–10 µg/kg s.c. q24h. One or two doses are often all that is necessary to improve neutrophil counts dramatically.

Absolute neutrophil count (cells/µl)	Is a fever present?	Is the patient showing clinical signs?	Treatment
< 2000	No	No	Delay chemotherapy. No antibiotics needed
< 1000	No	No	Delay chemotherapy. Institute prophylactic antibiotics. Monitor at home for decline in condition
< 2000	Yes	No	Delay chemotherapy. Institute antibiotics. Monitor closely at home
< 1000	Yes	Yes	Delay chemotherapy and hospitalize with intensive monitoring. Give intravenous antibiotics

7.14 Clinical approach to the patient with chemotherapy-induced neutropenia.

Drug	Dose
Trimethoprim/sulphonamide	15 mg/kg orally q12h
Cefalexin	11–22 mg/kg orally q8h
Cefoxitin	22 mg/kg i.v. q8h
Ampicillin	22 mg/kg i.v. q8h
Enrofloxacin	5–10 mg/kg orally or i.v. q12h

7.15 Antibiotics commonly used in veterinary oncology.

With early and aggressive intervention, most febrile neutropenic chemotherapy patients will respond to treatment, but a small proportion will die. Chemotherapy should be withheld until the patient and bone marrow have recovered and then reinstituted at a reduced dose.

Thrombocytopenia: Thrombocytopenia associated with chemotherapy is rarely clinically significant and does not often result in bleeding. If counts are <50 × 10^9/l, administration of bone marrow suppressive drugs can be delayed until counts rise.

Gastrointestinal toxicity

The most common problem observed by pet owners is gastrointestinal toxicity. Vomiting can occur acutely, within 6–12 hours of drug administration, or more commonly is delayed, occurring 24–48 hours after administration, or later. In veterinary medicine, most chemotherapy drugs cause delayed emesis, the most notable exception being cisplatin, which will cause vomiting within the first 6 hours of infusion. In one study of tumour-bearing dogs receiving cisplatin, 27 of 41 dogs (66%) vomited (Knapp et al., 1988).

The mechanism of chemotherapy-induced nausea and vomiting is complex. The emetic centre of the brain is in the medulla and receives input from several sources, including the chemoreceptor trigger zone (CRTZ) in the fourth ventricle, the cerebral cortex, peripheral receptors in the gut and the vestibular system. These areas are influenced by cholinergic, serotonin (5HT-3), histaminergic and adrenergic receptors, which are themselves influenced by certain drugs. The CRTZ is activated by chemical stimuli and is a vital part of chemotherapy-induced nausea and vomiting. Peripheral receptors can be activated directly by chemotherapy or by substances released from cells elsewhere in the gut. Signals from these peripheral receptors ascend to the emetic centre via the vagus nerve and other autonomic afferent pathways. In humans, influence from the cerebral cortex contributes to chemotherapy emesis much more so than in veterinary medicine. Stimuli from these higher centres are likely responsible for 'anticipatory' vomiting and nausea. Input from the vestibular centre probably has minimal influence on chemotherapy-induced emesis.

Clinical signs seen with gastrointestinal toxicity are variable:

- Anorexia alone, occasional vomiting or persistent vomiting accompanied by dehydration, depression and electrolyte abnormalities may be seen

- Stools can be loose, watery or consistent with haemorrhagic colitis, especially after doxorubicin administration
- If severe gastrointestinal toxicity is present, bacterial translocation and sepsis are possible sequelae due to the loss of the normal mucosal integrity
- Nausea and vomiting usually begin 48 hours after drug administration. Diarrhoea will lag behind slightly.

Treatment for chemotherapy-induced gastrointestinal toxicity depends on how severely the patient is affected. Mild signs can usually be managed by withholding food and water if vomiting, and providing an anti-emetic. Offering small amounts of water and a bland diet every 3–4 hours once vomiting has stopped is then indicated.

Significant gastrointestinal toxicity which lasts for >36–48 hours and does not respond to oral anti-emetic therapy should be treated aggressively. Supportive care with intravenous fluids including rehydration and replacing continued losses, along with correction of electrolyte abnormalities, is important. Performing a CBC and biochemical profile is also prudent for severely ill patients, to monitor the possible neutropenia or sepsis that may also occur concurrently. If gastrointestinal effects after chemotherapy administration are severe, instituting prophylactic anti-emetic therapy or a chemotherapy dose reduction may be indicated.

Any nausea or vomiting secondary to chemotherapy should be treated with anti-emetics (Figure 7.16).

Drug	Dose
Metoclopramide	0.2–0.4 mg/kg orally q6–8h or 1–2 mg/kg/day CRI i.v.
Chlorpromazine	0.5 mg/kg i.m. or s.c. q6–8h
Butorphanol	0.1–0.4 mg/kg i.m., i.v. or s.c.
Ondansetron	0.1 mg/kg i.v. or orally q12h
Dolasetron	0.6–3 mg/kg i.v. q24h
Maropitant	1 mg/kg s.c. q24h for 5 days or 2 mg/kg orally q24h for 5 days

7.16 Anti-emetics commonly used in veterinary oncology.

- **Metoclopramide** is one of the most commonly used anti-emetics in veterinary medicine. Its effect is both central, in the CRTZ as a dopamine antagonist, and peripheral, via increasing lower oesophageal sphincter tone and relaxing the pylorus. Metoclopramide is contraindicated in gastrointestinal obstruction.
- **Chlorpromazine** is commonly used for mild nausea. It works centrally in the CRTZ. It can be administered intramuscularly or subcutaneously. A suppository form is also available.
- **Butorphanol** has been used to reduce nausea and vomiting, particularly with cisplatin chemotherapy.

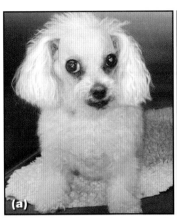
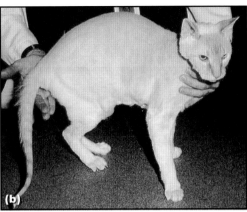
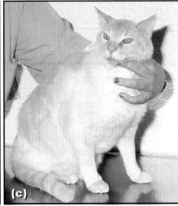

7.17 **(a)** Alopecia in a poodle following treatment with doxorubicin. **(b)** Alopecia, including whisker loss, in a cat with lymphoma treated with cyclophosphamide and vincristine. **(c)** The cat's hair regrew after discontinuation of treatment.

- Serotonin antagonists are very effective anti-emetics currently being used in human and veterinary oncology. They inhibit the 5HT-3 (5hydroxytryptamine) receptor in the CRTZ as well as in the gut afferents. **Ondansetron** is available in an oral or injectable formulation. If given intravenously, it should be given over 2–5 minutes or diluted in 0.9% sodium chloride. **Dolasetron** is also used.
- **Maropitant** is a neurokinin receptor antagonist that blocks the action of substance P in the central nervous system. It is a veterinary product and comes in an oral and injectable (subcutaneous) formulation. Current label indications are to treat acute nausea for use prior to or subsequent to chemotherapy administration for up to 5 consecutive days.

Alopecia

Alopecia or delayed hair growth can occur (Figure 7.17) but is not a universal phenomenon. In the dog, severe alopecia is breed-dependent, typically occurring in breeds with continually growing hair coats such as Poodles, Old English Sheepdogs and some of the terrier breeds. In other breeds, hair may be slow to regrow in areas that have been shaved, or may become sparse. Hair usually grows back after chemotherapy is discontinued and in some cases may return with an altered consistency or colour. Cats rarely develop severe alopecia but will lose their whiskers.

Extravasation

Some chemotherapeutic agents are vesicants and can induce a local tissue irritation or necrosis if they leak out of the vein or are extravasated. In veterinary medicine, the most common agents that cause this reaction are vincristine, vinblastine and doxorubicin (Figure 7.18).

The severity of the reaction is dependent on the agent and the amount that leaks into the tissues. Clinical signs associated with extravasation include pain, erythema, moist dermatitis and necrosis of the area (Figure 7.19). These signs are often not immediate and may occur 1–7 days after administration of vincristine or vinblastine and up to 7–10 days after doxorubicin. If an extravasation reaction occurs, tissue sloughing may follow.

- Cisplatin
- Dactinomycin
- Daunorubicin
- Doxorubicin
- Etoposide
- Mithramycin
- Mitoxantrone
- Vinblastine
- Vincristine

7.18 Chemotherapeutic agents that are vesicants and irritants.

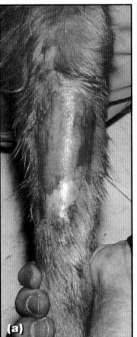
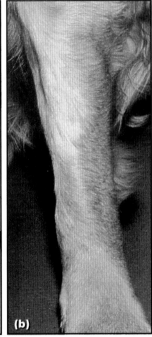

7.19 **(a)** A tissue reaction following vincristine extravasation and **(b)** the healed area several months later.

If an extravasation is suspected, the drug infusion should be stopped and any drug remaining in the catheter should be aspirated back, along with several millilitres of blood if possible.

Standard wound management techniques (dressings, bandaging, pain control) are used to manage mild to moderate reactions, while severe reactions may require surgical debridement and skin grafting.

Anecdotal information exists concerning the use of other agents to treat an immediate extravasation, and minimal clinical information as to their effectiveness exists in veterinary medicine.

- Guidelines borrowed from the human experience for **doxorubicin** include applying cold packs intermittently for up to 12 hours. Dexrazoxane, a free-radical scavenger used to prevent doxorubicin-induced cardiomyopathy, has been reported to reduce extravasation reactions if given shortly after the event (within 3 hours) in people and anecdotally in veterinary patients. Ten times the doxorubicin dose is given intravenously within 3 hours and again at 12 and 24 hours. Topically applied DMSO has also been advocated (Thamm and Vail, 2007).
- For **vinca alkaloid** extravasation, heat is applied for several hours. Infiltrating hyaluronidase (1 ml for every 1 ml extravasated) into the area has been recommended (Spugnini, 2002).

Extravasation is a preventable complication if drugs are administered according to suggested guidelines by appropriately skilled staff. Accurate record keeping of chemotherapy administration, including which vein is used, is also important to help to track extravasation reactions.

Allergic reactions

Agents most commonly associated with hypersensitivity reactions include crisantaspase (L-asparginase) and doxorubicin, while reactions to etoposide and paclitaxel have been linked to the solvents for these compounds (cremophor EL, polysorbate 80).

Careful patient monitoring is recommended during and immediately after drug administration. Clinical signs of hypersensitivity reactions in dogs include urticaria, erythema, restlessness, vomiting, head shaking and oedema of the head, especially the eyelids and lips (Figure 7.20). Severe reactions may lead to hypotension and circulatory collapse. In cats, the signs can be similar but cats may also exhibit respiratory signs such as dyspnoea or open-mouth breathing.

The likelihood of having a reaction in patients receiving crisantaspase increases after repeated doses. Intramuscular administration decreases the chance of reaction when compared with the intra-peritoneal or intravenous route. Doxorubicin administration can induce mast cell degranulation, which will contribute to a hypersensitivity reaction. Slowing the infusion, and/or pretreating with an H-1 blocker (diphenhydramine, 1–2 mg/kg i.m., 30 minutes prior to infusion) and corticosteroid (dexamethasone, 0.5–1 mg/kg i.v.), can eliminate or lessen the effect.

Treatment of anaphylactic or other hypersensitivity reactions to chemotherapy drugs is the same as for any other drug. If a reaction is apparent:

- Discontinue infusion if still in progress
- Administer H-1 blockers (diphenhydramine, 0.2–0.5 mg/kg i.m.) and dexamethasone (0.5–2 mg/kg i.v.)

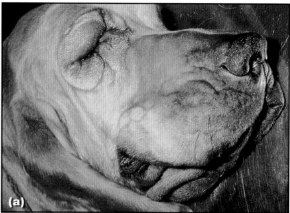
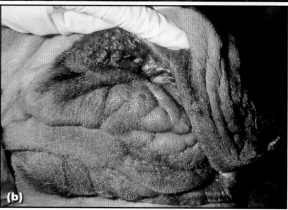

7.20 Hypersensitivity reaction during doxorubicin administration in a Bloodhound. Note **(a)** the oedema around the eyes and **(b)** swelling, redness and induration of the lips.

- If necessary, give intravenous fluids and adrenaline (epinephrine) (0.1–0.3 ml of a 1:1000 solution i.v.)
- Give additional supportive care.

Cardiac toxicity

Cardiotoxicity attributed to chemotherapy administration is usually associated with doxorubicin in the dog. Other drugs, particularly other anthracyclines such as daunorubicin, are associated with cardiac toxicity in humans but are not widely used in veterinary medicine.

There are both acute and chronic forms of doxorubicin cardiotoxicity. The acute form manifests as arrhythmias that occur during or soon after administration of the drug; these are transient. The chronic and more common form of toxicity results in dilated cardiomyopathy and possible congestive heart failure, which is not reversible. In humans, cumulative doses >550 mg/m² have been shown to cause toxicity in up to 30% of the patients studied, while only 1–5% of those who received a cumulative dose <500 mg/m² developed cardiotoxicity. In the dog, cumulative doses between 180 and 240 mg/m² are considered safe, although toxicity has been reported in small numbers of cases at lower doses. In cats, doses of 300 mg/m² given experimentally to non-tumour-bearing cats resulted in no clinical heart disease; however, histopathological changes consistent with damage were present in all hearts examined (O'Keefe et al., 1993).

The mechanism of cardiac damage associated with doxorubicin administration is likely to be due to the formation of free radicals and the oxidative damage that subsequently occurs. Cardiac tissue has relatively low levels of several protective enzymes such as catalase, when compared with other tissues. Histologically, changes consistent with degeneration and atrophy of cardiac myocytes with myofibrillar loss, cytoplasmic vacuolization and cell lysis can be observed, as well as fibrosis.

Diagnosing doxorubicin toxicity prior to clinical signs of congestive heart disease can be difficult due to the lack of sensitivity of tests used. Tachyarrhythmias are often noted first, followed by echocardiographic changes. Nuclear scintigraphy and endomyocardial biopsies are the most sensitive tests used in humans but are not practical in most veterinary clinical settings. Work is being done in both humans and dogs to identify biochemical markers, such as cardiac troponins or atrial natriuretic peptide (ANP), that may provide a more convenient way to monitor and diagnose this toxicity.

Treatment for doxorubicin-induced cardiomyopathy is the same as for any other type of cardiomyopathy.

Prevention of this toxicity can be approached in various ways:

- Use caution in dogs that have risk factors such as a breed predisposition for cardiomyopathy, or previous or concurrent thoracic radiation
- Breeds predisposed to cardiomyopathy should have an echocardiogram prior to beginning therapy. If abnormalities are found, the risk *versus* benefit of doxorubicin therapy must be weighed carefully
- Manipulation of the chemotherapy drug itself is also possible. By increasing infusion time the peak plasma levels are reduced, which can decrease the cardiotoxic effects. Liposomal formulations of doxorubicin have been developed and are less cardiotoxic
- The concurrent use of dexrazoxane has been shown in both humans and dogs to reduce cardiotoxicity significantly. It acts as an iron chelator and ultimately decreases the formation of reactive oxygen species. Other antioxidant drugs studied have not been promising
- If the patient has underlying heart disease, other drugs can be substituted if possible.

Cystitis

Sterile haemorrhagic cystitis is a potential side effect of cyclophosphamide and ifosfamide in the dog and, rarely, in the cat. It usually occurs with chronic use but can happen acutely. This cystitis is due to the toxic effects of acrolein (a metabolite of cyclophosphamide) on the bladder mucosa.

Clinical signs include haematuria, dysuria and pollakiuria. Urine culture should be performed to rule out secondary infections but results are usually negative.

Treatment includes first discontinuing the offending drug. Secondly, prophylactic antibiotics to prevent infection and anti-inflammatory drugs can be given, although symptoms can persist for several weeks.

Improvement has been reported in a small number of dogs when intravesicular DMSO (25–50%) solution has been used (Kisseberth and MacEwan, 2001), but no studies of large numbers of dogs are available.

To decrease the likelihood of sterile haemorrhagic cystitis developing, several strategies can be employed. Treating with furosemide (1 mg/kg) prior to intravenous cyclophosphamide administration has been shown to decrease the incidence of occurrence (Charney *et al.*, 2003). Giving the oral medication first thing in the morning in order to allow for bladder emptying throughout the day is often recommended. Salting food or administering prednisone to promote diuresis have also been advocated. Another preventive strategy used widely in human patients is to give the drug 2-mercaptoethanesulfonate (MESNA) concurrently with cyclophosphamide or ifosfamide. This works by binding acrolein and inactivating its toxic effects on the bladder mucosa, allowing for higher doses of the chemotherapeutic agents. In the dog, administering MESNA with ifosfamide has been shown to mitigate the cystitis normally seen (Rassnick *et al.*, 2000).

Rarely, transitional cell carcinoma of the bladder has been associated with chronic cyclophosphamide use.

Nephrotoxicity

The kidneys are the elimination pathway for many drugs and their metabolites and therefore are potentially susceptible to toxicity. Cisplatin, methotrexate (intermediate and high dose) and, in the cat, doxorubicin are the most commonly used drugs that can lead to nephrotoxicity. Prior to administering these drugs, renal function should be screened using creatinine level, BUN and urinalysis. Pre-existing renal disease is a factor that will predispose a patient to further nephrotoxicity.

In cats, doxorubicin has been reported to cause azotaemia and reduced urine specific gravity in both tumour-bearing and normal animals receiving high cumulative doses of the drug.

In the dog, cisplatin is the most commonly used nephrotoxic drug. Within 48 hours of administration, 80–90% of the drug is excreted in the urine. Cisplatin contains heavy metal and can result in a decreasing glomerular filtration rate as well as damage to the tubules. Because cisplatin is less toxic in a high chloride environment, saline diuresis must accompany cisplatin administration. Several protocols exist for this, ranging in time from 4 to 24 hours. The author currently recommends a 4-hour protocol, involving 3 hours of normal saline at a rate of 25 ml/kg/hour, followed by a 20-minute cisplatin infusion, followed by an additional hour of saline at the previous rate. Other techniques that have been studied include administering hypertonic saline, mannitol, or using drugs such as amiphostine, but their use in a clinical setting remains to be seen.

Neurotoxicity

Neurotoxicity is rare in small animal oncology patients. The drugs most commonly associated with this include the vinca alkaloids, cisplatin and 5-fluorouracil.

Vincristine is reported to cause peripheral neuropathy in the dog, which may manifest as hindlimb weakness. In humans, vincristine can cause peripheral, central or autonomic effects and occurs most often with high, repetitive dose therapy. The most common and initial sign of vincristine neurotoxicity in human patients is depression of deep tendon reflexes and paraesthesia of the distal extremities, which may progress to involve the entire hand or foot. This toxicity is usually clinically reversed once therapy is discontinued. Vincristine is also reported to cause transient ileus and constipation in veterinary patients.

Cisplatin has been reported to cause cortical blindness at high doses in two dogs (Kisseberth and MacEwan, 2001). In humans, ototoxicity and deafness, peripheral neuropathy, cortical blindness and seizures have all been reported. Clinical signs can persist for years after discontinuation of therapy. In veterinary patients, cisplatin neurotoxicity is rare and is not as well characterized.

5-Fluorouracil has been shown to cause rapid, severe neurological signs in cats, including cerebellar ataxia, hyperexcitability, gross dysmetria and death. For this reason, *5-fluorouracil is contraindicated in cats*. Dogs can also develop signs but they are usually less severe.

Acute tumour lysis syndrome

Acute tumour lysis syndrome (ATLS) is an oncological emergency. It is caused by rapid lysis of malignant cells in response to chemotherapy. The resultant release of intracellular products and ions into the circulation exceeds the excretory capacity of the kidneys, resulting in electrolyte abnormalities and metabolic derangements that can be life-threatening. In human medicine, ATLS is often most associated with chemoresponsive diseases such as haematological malignancies (lymphoma, leukaemias) and rarely with solid tumours (Altman, 2001).

In veterinary medicine, ATLS is rare but has been reported in lymphoma patients treated with chemotherapy and/or radiation therapy. Patients at high risk usually have advanced disease, large tumour burdens, are dehydrated, may have underlying renal disease and undergo a rapid response to therapy. Resulting electrolyte abnormalities include hyperkalaemia, hyperphosphataemia, and associated hypocalcaemia and metabolic acidosis due to release of intracellular contents. Additionally, rapidly dividing cancer cells contain high amounts of nucleic acid purines. Normally these purines are catabolized to uric acid and excreted renally. When large amounts are released during massive cell death, the excretory capacity of the renal tubule is exceeded and hyperuricaemia occurs. Ultimately patients may develop acute renal failure, primarily due to uric acid precipitation.

Clinical signs that may occur include acute depression, bradycardia (hyperkalaemia), vomiting, diarrhoea, cardiovascular collapse and shock. Successful management of these patients includes recognition of the syndrome and prompt aggressive fluid therapy with correction of electrolyte and metabolic abnormalities. In humans, treatment with allopurinol to prevent ATLS in high-risk patients is commonplace, and has greatly reduced the incidence and morbidity associated with this syndrome. Allopurinol works by preventing the accumulation of uric acid by blocking xanthine oxidase. Its use for ATLS in veterinary medicine has been infrequent.

Pulmonary toxicity

Bleomycin has been associated with severe pulmonary fibrosis. In cats, even at low doses, cisplatin can induce a severe pulmonary oedema and pleural effusion that is often fatal. Because of this, **cisplatin is contraindicated in cats**. Lomustine (CCNU) is also reported to cause pulmonary toxicity, but it is not commonly reported in veterinary medicine. In humans many drugs have been associated with pulmonary toxicity.

Drugs

General mechanism of action

Chemotherapy drugs cause cell damage in either a cell cycle phase-specific manner or a cell cycle phase non-specific manner. All tissues throughout the body (both normal and tumour tissues) contain cells that are actively dividing as well as cells that are quiescent. The phases of the cell cycle are:

- **G1**: a period of RNA and protein synthesis
- **S**: the period of DNA synthesis
- **G2**: a period of RNA and protein synthesis
- **M**: the period when mitosis occurs
- **G0**: a period of cell rest.

Chemotherapy drugs can damage DNA and prevent cellular replication and/or induce apoptosis, or they can work during a specific phase of the cell cycle, such as mitosis, and prevent the completion of that process.

Listed below according to class are drugs commonly used in veterinary oncology. This is not meant to be an all-inclusive list. Information about specific combination protocols and drugs for specific disease states can be found in other chapters in this book.

Alkylating agents

Alkylating agents all act by cross-linking DNA after insertion of an alkyl group and are considered cell cycle non-specific. There are several classes of alkylating agents, including the nitrogen mustards (cyclophosphamide, chlorambucil, melphalan) and the nitrosoureas (carmustine, lomustine), that are commonly used in veterinary medicine.

Cyclophosphamide

Formulation: Cyclosphosphamide is available as an injectable drug and oral tablets.

Mechanism of action: Cyclosphosphamide works in the same way as the other alkylating agents, but it must be metabolized in the liver to the active form. Excretion is primarily through the renal system.

Dose and administration: Injectable cyclophosphamide is reconstituted with sterile water and used within 24 hours if stored at room temperature or within 6 days if stored in the refrigerator. The tablets must not be split, because of variation in drug distribution throughout the tablet and chemotherapy safe handling guidelines. The dose range is 200–300 mg/m² given every 3 weeks for most applications. When using oral medication, the dose must be adjusted in consideration of the tablet sizes available. In addition, the total dose is typically given over a period of 3–4 days. As an example, a patient requiring 180 mg should receive 175 mg total dose, with a 50 mg tablet given on days 1, 2 and 3, and a 25 mg tablet given on day 4 (the 25 mg tablet is not available in the UK).

Toxicity: Bone marrow suppression (neutropenia, thrombocytopenia) with the nadir around 7 days, gastrointestinal side effects and alopecia are all possible. Sterile haemorrhagic cystitis can occur. If cystitis occurs, the drug should be discontinued and chlorambucil or melphalan may be substituted.

Indications: Cyclophosphamide is a commonly used drug in many multiple drug protocols for lymphoma, leukaemias and various sarcomas and carcinomas.

Chlorambucil

Formulation: Chlorambucil is available as tablets.

Mechanism of action: Chlorambucil works as other alkylating agents and must be metabolized to the active form by the liver. It is excreted as inactive metabolites in the urine and faeces.

Dose and administration: The dose varies depending on the protocol used and disease being treated: 0.1 mg/kg, 2–8 mg/m² q24–48h, or pulsed dosing given in place of cyclophosphamide 1.4 mg/kg orally at once. Tablets must not be broken, so dose may need to be adjusted.

Toxicity: This drug is very well tolerated. Toxicity can include: mild gastrointestinal toxicity; bone marrow suppression, usually late in the course of treatment (2–3 weeks); rare cerebellar toxicity at high doses. Alopecia is rare.

Indications: Chlorambucil is used for the treatment of lymphoma, chronic lymphocytic leukaemia and multiple myeloma.

Melphalan

Formulation: Melphalan is available as an injection and as oral tablets.

Mechanism of action: Melphalan works as the other alkylating agents.

Dose and administration: There are several dosing schemes. For multiple myeloma, for example: 0.1 mg/kg orally q24h for 10 days, then the dose is reduced to 0.05 mg/kg q48h as maintenance therapy. Pulsed therapy is also used at a dose of 7 mg/m² orally q24h for 5 days, repeated every 3 weeks.

Toxicity: Toxicity can include bone marrow toxicity with myelosuppression and, with chronic use, thrombocytopenia. Alopecia is possible.

Indications: Melphalan is most commonly used in multiple myeloma, but its use has been reported in other solid tumours.

Ifosfamide

Formulation: Ifosfamide is available as an injection, packaged with 2-mercaptoethanesulfonate (MESNA), a mandatory uroprotective product.

Mechanism of action: Ifosfamide works as the other alkylating agents.

Dose and administration: 350–375 mg/m² i.v. given every 3 weeks. Fluid diuresis is also recommended, to prevent haemorrhagic cystitis, as well as concurrent administration of the uroprotectant MESNA (at 20% of the ifosfamide dose and given at the same time, and again 2 and 5 hours afterwards).

Toxicity: Toxic reactions include sterile haemorrhagic cystitis (more likely than with cyclophosphamide); 2-mercaptoethanesulfonate should always be given. As with cyclophosphamide, bone marrow suppression is also seen.

Indications: In veterinary medicine, ifosfamide has been used in various tumours with varied response and is currently being investigated.

Busulfan

Formulation: Busulfan is available as tablets.

Mechanism of action: Busulfan works as the other alkylating agents, and is well absorbed orally.

Dose and administration: 2 mg/m² orally q24h.

Toxicity: Bone marrow suppression can occur, both myelosuppression and thrombocytopenia, which may be prolonged. Pulmonary fibrosis has been reported in human patients.

Indications: Busulfan is used in chronic myelogenous or granulocytic leukaemia.

Lomustine (CCNU)

Formulation: Lomustine is available as capsules.

Mechanism of action: Lomustine works as the other alkylating agents. Because it is highly lipophilic, it will penetrate into the central nervous system.

Dose and administration: The dose in dogs is 60–90 mg/m² orally every 3 weeks; in cats, the dose is 50–60 mg/m² every 5–6 weeks.

Toxicity: Bone marrow can be affected, with acute myelosuppression occurring at 7–10 days; this may be severe and can also be delayed and cumulative with additional thrombocytopenia. Hepatotoxicity has also been seen. Pulmonary fibrosis has been reported in the cat.

Indications: Lomustine is used for lymphoma, particularly the cutaneous presentation, and mast cell disease. It is also used for brain tumours due to the ability to cross the blood–brain barrier.

Dacarbazine

Formulation: Dacarbazine is available as an injectable.

Mechanism of action: Dacarbazine works as the other alkylating agents, but may act via other mechanisms.

Dose and administration: 200 mg/m^2 as a slow intravenous bolus given once daily for 5 days, repeated every 3 weeks. It can also be given once as a slow intravenous infusion over 4 hours at a dose of 1000 mg/m^2.

Toxicity: There may be bone marrow suppression, vomiting (occasionally during administration) and alopecia. It is also a vesicant.

Indications: Dacarbazine is primarily used in lymphoma rescue protocols.

Carmustine

Formulation: Carmustine is available as an injection. Drug-impregnated wafers are also available for use in the brain for local therapy.

Mechanism of action: Carmustine works as the other alkylating agents. Like lomustine, this drug also has great penetration into the central nervous system.

Dose and administration: 50 mg/m^2 i.v. over 15–20 minutes, every 6 weeks.

Toxicity: Carmustine may cause severe delayed myelosuppression; nausea and vomiting can also occur. Carmustine is associated with pulmonary fibrosis in human patients.

Indications: Carmustine is primarily used for brain tumours in veterinary medicine.

Plant alkaloids

Plant (vinca) alkaloids are derived from the periwinkle plant. They bind to the microtubule assembly and prevent normal formation and function of the mitotic spindle, resulting in arrest of cell division. These drugs are cell cycle-specific.

Vincristine

Formulation: Vincristine is available for injection.

Mechanism of action: Vincristine inhibits microtubule assembly. It is excreted by the liver into the faeces in a non-active form; severe liver dysfunction may result in decreased metabolism and increased toxicity.

Dose and administration: The dose range is 0.5–0.75 mg/m^2 i.v. weekly or in cycle as part of a combination chemotherapy protocol. The volume administered is typically small (1 ml) and is given as an intravenous bolus. Vincristine is a vesicant and care should be taken with catheter placement.

Toxicity: A tissue reaction will occur if extravasated during administration. Other toxicities include alopecia, gastrointestinal toxicity (including constipation) and peripheral neuropathy (rare). Myelosuppression is considered minimal, although it can occur if vincristine is used in some drug combinations.

Indications: Vincristine is used in multiple drug combination protocols for lymphoma, leukaemias, sarcomas and mast cell tumours (MCTs). Vincristine will cure 90% of transmissible venereal tumours in an average of 3.3 doses. This drug will also cause premature release of platelets from megakaryocytes and may be used in the management of thrombocytopenia.

Vinblastine

Formulation: Vinblastine is available as an injection.

Mechanism of action: The drug binds to the mitotic spindle and prevents assembly. Vinblastine is metabolized in the liver and excreted in the bile/faeces. Significant liver dysfunction can result in increased toxicity.

Dose and administration: 2 mg/m^2 i.v. weekly, or as directed by the specific protocol.

Toxicity: Vinblastine causes myelosuppression (nadir at 4–9 days), alopecia, mild gastrointestinal toxicity, and is a vesicant that will cause a tissue reaction if administered perivascularly. Neurotoxicity is reported but is usually mild and less common that that seen with vincristine.

Indications: Vinblastine is used for mast cell disease and lymphoma.

Anti-metabolites

Anti-metabolites work by interfering with the biosynthesis of nucleic acids by substituting for normal metabolites and inhibiting normal enzymatic reactions. They are typically cell cycle-specific.

Methotrexate

Formulation: Methotrexate is available as tablets and an injection.

Mechanism of action: Methotrexate inhibits the conversion of folic acid to tetrahydrofolic acid by binding to the enzyme dihydrofolate reductase. This inhibits thymidine and purine synthesis, which are essential for DNA replication. Methotrexate is partially metabolized by gastrointestinal flora after oral administration. After absorption, it is metabolized in the liver and excreted in the urine.

Dose and administration: 0.6–0.8 mg/kg i.v. or orally; 2.5 mg/m² orally i.v., i.m. or s.c., q24h, or as part of a combination chemotherapy protocol. High-dose methotrexate with leucovorin rescue is used in human patients but is rarely used in veterinary medicine due to the expense and intensive monitoring required.

Toxicity: Gastrointestinal toxicity (vomiting, anorexia, diarrhoea), myelosuppression (nadir 6–9 days), alopecia, renal toxicity and hepatotoxicity may be seen.

Indications: Methotrexate is used in combination protocols to treat lymphoma, Sertoli cell tumours and OSA.

5-Fluorouracil

Formulation: 5-Fluorouracil is available as an injection and 1% or 2% topical creams/ointments.

Mechanism of action: 5-Fluorouracil is metabolized into a nucleotide which is incorporated into RNA; this subsequently alters DNA synthesis.

Dose and administration: 5-Fluorouracil is applied topically with minimal systemic absorption. Intravenous use has been reported at a dose of 150 mg/m² once weekly. This drug also penetrates the central nervous system.

Toxicity: **Severe fatal toxicity occurs in cats; 5-fluorouracil should never be used in cats.** Other effects include gastrointestinal toxicity, myelosuppression and milder neurotoxicity in dogs.

Indications: 5-Fluorouracil has been used for various sarcomas and carcinomas with variable success.

Cytarabine (cytosine arabinoside)

Formulation: Cytarabine is available as an injection.

Mechanism of action: Cytarabine is a pyrimidine analogue that inhibits DNA synthesis, possibly inhibiting DNA polymerase. This drug is cell cycle-specific (killing cells undergoing DNA synthesis (S phase)). It reaches therapeutic concentrations in the cerebrospinal fluid. The circulating half-life in the dog is very short.

Dose and administration: Dosing ranges from a constant rate infusion of 100 mg/m² i.v. q24h for 3–4 days, to higher pulsed dosing, 150 mg/m² s.c. twice daily for 2 days or 600 mg/m² i.v. or s.c. once weekly. Constant-rate infusion is ideal but not always clinically practical.

Toxicity: Cytarabine may cause gastrointestinal symptoms, alopecia and myelosuppression.

Indications: Cytarabine is used in lymphoma (especially with CNS involvement) and some leukaemias (myelogenous).

Gemcitabine

Formulation: Gemcitabine is available as an injection.

Mechanism of action: Gemcitabine is a deoxycytidine analogue, the active metabolite of which is incorporated into DNA, resulting in inhibition of synthesis.

Dose and administration: The maximally tolerated dose (MTD) in dogs and the appropriate dose interval have yet to be determined. 300 mg/m² i.v. given once weekly for 3 or 4 weeks has been safely used in the dog. Other dosing regimens reported include 675 mg/m² given every 2 weeks. It can be used in cats, but most reports evaluate concurrent radiation treatment so the MTD has not been established.

Toxicity: Myelosuppression is the dose-limiting toxicity, and gastrointestinal toxicity can occur.

Indications: In humans, gemcitabine has been used successfully in lung cancer, pancreatic cancer and bladder cancer, as well as several other carcinomas. Its spectrum of activity has not been determined in veterinary medicine.

Anti-tumour antibiotics

Anti-tumour antibiotics form stable complexes and intercalate with DNA, preventing DNA and RNA synthesis. This class of drugs is cell cycle non-specific.

Doxorubicin

Formulation: Doxorubicin is available as an injection.

Mechanism of action: This anthracycline antibiotic has several mechanisms of action. It intercalates DNA, promotes free-radical formation and inhibits topoisomerase enzymes required for DNA replication.

Dose and administration: In the dog, the dose is 30 mg/m² i.v. given every 2–3 weeks, depending on the disease being treated and other drugs being used. In smaller dogs (< 10 kg) the dose is reduced to 1 mg/kg due to an increase in toxicity when dosed on a body surface area basis. Cats are also dosed at 1 mg/kg. The drug is diluted in saline to a volume of 35–150 ml, depending on the size of the patient. Doxorubicin is administered through an intravenous catheter placed without traumatizing the vein, because the drug is a vesicant. A 20–30 minute infusion is recommended.

Toxicity: Myelosuppression (nadir at 7–10 days), alopecia, gastrointestinal toxicity (particularly haemorrhagic colitis), allergic reaction, tissue reaction if given perivascularly and a unique cumulative cardiac toxicity are all possible. Renal toxicity has been reported (especially in cats) and is thought to be cumulative.

Indications: This drug has a wide range of reported anti-tumour activity. It is commonly used to treat lymphoma, leukaemias, OSA, haemangiosarcoma, mammary adenocarcinoma and a variety of other tumour types.

Comment: Dexrazoxane can be used as a cardioprotectant with doxorubicin administration. It is available in 250 mg and 500 mg vials. The dose is based on the amount of doxorubicin given. The recommended ratio is 10:1, for example if 30 mg of doxorubicin is given, then 300 mg of dexrazoxane is needed. The drug is given by slow intravenous bolus, 30 minutes prior to doxorubicin administration.

Epirubicin

Formulation: Epirubicin is available as an injection.

Mechanism of action: This is similar to the action of doxorubicin, including intercalating DNA and inhibiting topoisomerase enzymes required for DNA replication.

Dose and administration: In the dog, the dose is 30 mg/m^2 i.v. given every 3 weeks. In smaller dogs (<10 kg) the dose is reduced to 1 mg/kg due to an increase in toxicity when dosed on a body surface area basis. Cats are also dosed at 1 mg/kg. The drug is diluted in saline to a volume of 35–150 ml, depending on the size of the patient.

Toxicity: Myelosuppression (nadir at 7–10 days), alopecia, gastrointestinal toxicity, allergic reaction and a tissue reaction if given perivascularly are all possible. Although cardiac toxicity is less of a problem than with doxorubicin, it has been reported and so caution must be exercised if epirubicin is used in patients with pre-existing heart disease.

Indications: Epirubicin has the same clinical indications as doxorubicin; however, it is most frequently used for treatment of lymphoma and leukaemias.

Mitoxantrone

Formulation: Mitoxantrone is available as an injection.

Mechanism of action: This is a synthetic anti-tumour antibiotic whose mechanism of action is by inhibition of topoisomerase II enzymes.

Dose and administration: In the dog, it is given at a dose of 5.5 mg/m^2 i.v. once every 3 weeks. In the cat, the dose is 6.5 mg/m^2 i.v. once every 3 weeks. The drug is diluted in 35 ml of saline and administered over 15–20 minutes through a catheter placed without traumatizing the vein.

Toxicity: Myelosuppression (nadir at 7–10 days) is the dose-limiting toxicity. Gastrointestinal toxicity may occur but is usually mild. Also seen are alopecia and tissue irritation (mild) if extravasation occurs. Cardiotoxicity and allergic reactions are not common.

Indications: Mitoxantrone has been used for lymphoma as a rescue or as a substitute for doxorubicin, as well as for transitional cell carcinoma and squamous cell carcinoma (SCC).

Dactinomycin (Actinomycin D)

Formulation: Dactinomycin is available as a 0.5 mg vial of powder for reconstitution.

Mechanism of action: Dactinomycin works by intercalation of DNA, which prevents protein synthesis. Excretion is through urine and faeces.

Dose and administration: The dose range is 0.5–0.9 mg/m^2 i.v. given every 2–3 weeks. It is diluted in 25–150 ml of 0.9% saline and given over 20–30 minutes. A clean stick catheter should be used.

Toxicity: Toxicity may cause gastrointestinal signs (infrequent), alopecia, myelosuppression (nadir 7–10 days) and tissue reaction if given perivascularly.

Indications: Dactinomycin is used in place of doxorubicin in multiple drug protocols for lymphoma, as a rescue agent for lymphoma, and reported in a variety of other cancers with variable success.

Miscellaneous agents

Cisplatin

Formulation: Cisplatin is available as an injection.

Mechanism of action: Cisplatin is a heavy metal that binds to DNA, causing intra- and interstrand cross-links, preventing protein synthesis. This drug is excreted by the kidneys.

Dose and administration: The dose range is 50–70 mg/m^2 i.v. every 3 weeks. Saline diuresis must be given concurrently. The author recommends a 4-hour protocol using a fluid rate of 25 ml/kg/hour for 3 hours, followed by a 20-minute drug infusion, followed by an additional hour of saline diuresis at the previous fluid rate. Anti-emetics should be considered to combat acute nausea and vomiting that will occur. Cisplatin can also be used intracavitarily.

Toxicity: Nephrotoxicity is the reason for diuresis during administration. Gastrointestinal toxicity manifested by acute emesis is common. Myelosuppression with both neutropenia and thrombocytopenia is also possible, with a bimodal nadir at 6 and 15 days. Alopecia can occur. Cisplatin causes fatal pulmonary oedema and pleural effusion in cats. **The use of cisplatin is contraindicated in cats by any route!**

Indications: Cisplatin has shown efficacy for OSA, SCC, mesothelioma, bladder tumours and other carcinomas.

Carboplatin

Formulation: Carboplatin is available as an injection.

Mechanism of action: This drug is a heavy metal that works, like cisplatin, by binding between and within DNA strands. It is excreted by the kidneys.

Dose and administration: The dose for dogs is 300 mg/m^2 i.v., over 5–10 minutes, given every 3 weeks. Its use is safe in the cat and the dose range is 200–250 mg/m^2 i.v. given every 3 weeks.

Toxicity: Carboplatin is not as nephrotoxic as cisplatin and diuresis is not required. It is excreted in the kidneys and caution should be used in patients with renal compromise. Gastrointestinal toxicity is possible but acute emesis is rare. Myelosuppression is common, with the nadir being reported in the dog at 11–14 days, and 14–21 days in the cat.

Indications: Carboplatin has been used successfully for OSA in dogs and is presumed to have a similar spectrum of action as cisplatin.

Paclitaxel

Formulation: Paclitaxel is available as an injection.

Mechanism of action: The taxanes bind to the microtubular assembly and prevent its disassembly, thereby inhibiting the completion of mitosis. These drugs are cell cycle-specific.

Dose and administration: In the dog, a dose of 135 mg/m^2 i.v. by slow infusion given every 3 weeks has been shown to be tolerated. The dose in the cat, which is under investigation, is 5 mg/kg i.v. every 3 weeks.

Toxicity: Paclitaxel is dissolved in cremophor EL, which causes significant hypersensitivity reactions in dogs. Premedication with diphenhydramine (4 mg/kg i.m.), cimetidine (4 mg/kg i.v.), and dexamethasone SP (2 mg/kg i.v.) given 30 minutes prior to infusion will help to prevent this reaction. Other toxicities include myelosuppression (nadir at 3–5 days) and rare gastrointestinal toxicity.

Indications: Paclitaxel has been used to treat mammary carcinoma and some sarcomas with variable success.

Hydroxycarbamide (Hydroxyurea)

Formulation: Hydroxycarbamide is available as capsules.

Mechanism of action: Hydroxycarbamide inhibits the conversion of ribonucleotides to deoxyribonucleotides through the destruction of ribonucleoside diphosphate reductase.

Dose and administration: In dogs, the dose is 50 mg/kg orally daily, decreasing to every other day as the disease responds to treatment. Cats should be given 10 mg/kg orally daily, decreasing to every other day as disease responds.

Toxicity: Side effects include myelosuppression and gastrointestinal toxicity. Sloughing of toenails has been reported in the dog.

Indications: Hydroxycarbamide is used for polycythaemia vera and myelogenous or basophilic leukaemia.

Piroxicam

Formulation: Piroxicam is available as capsules.

Mechanism of action: Piroxicam is a non-steroidal anti-inflammatory drug (NSAID). In addition to having anti-inflammatory effects, it is thought to have anti-tumour effects through possible cyclo-oxygenase-2 (COX-2) inhibition.

Dose and administration: The dose in dogs is 0.3 mg/kg orally daily or every other day. The same dose has been used in cats, but usually on an every-other-day schedule. Piroxicam can cause significant gastrointestinal bleeding, and the newer COX-2 specific NSAIDs may be a safer choice. Accurate dosing is important to avoid toxicity and capsules can be readily formulated. Liquid preparations have questionable stability (particularly aqueous preparations).

Toxicity: The spectrum of toxicity mirrors that of other NSAIDs. Gastrointestinal toxicities including ulceration are possible, as well as renal toxicity. Gastrointestinal protectants can be used concurrently but are not usually needed routinely in dogs. Combining piroxicam with other renal toxins or ulcer-promoting drugs should be avoided.

Indications: Piroxicam is used for transitional cell carcinoma of the bladder, SCC and as an anti-inflammatory for pain control.

Prednisone or prednisolone

Formulation: These are available as tablets and injections.

Mechanism of action: Prednisone and prednisolone act as a hormone that binds to receptors in the nucleus and inhibits DNA synthesis.

Dose and administration: The dose is variable depending on the protocol used and disease being treated. A general anti-tumour dose is 1–2 mg/kg daily.

Toxicity: Side effects include iatrogenic hyperadrenocorticism, polyuria and polydypsia, hepatomegaly, hair loss, muscle wasting, gastrointestinal ulceration and panting.

Indications: Prednisone and prednisolone have anti-tumour activity against lymphoma, MCTs, leukaemias and plasma cell tumours. Other indications include symptomatic treatment of oedema and hyperinsulinism associated with insulinoma.

Crisantaspase (ʟ-Asparginase)

Formulation: This is available as a 10,000 IU vial for reconstitution.

Mechanism of action: Crisantaspase is an enzyme derived from a bacterium. It inhibits the enzyme asparagine synthetase and depletes the tumour cell of asparagine. It is a foreign protein and antibodies will form to it, leading to resistance.

Dose and administration: 400 IU/kg i.m. or s.c.; or 10,000 IU/m² i.m. or s.c.. Intramuscular administration has been shown to cause less anaphylaxis than intraperitoneal dosing. After drug administration, patients should be observed for 20–30 minutes for possible anaphylaxis.

Toxicity: Anaphylaxis is reported with repeated dosing. Rare toxicities include myelosuppression, pancreatitis and disseminated intravascular coagulation.

Indications: Crisantaspase is used in multiple drug protocols for the treatment of lymphoma.

New frontiers

Pharmacogenetics

Inter-individual variability in pharmacokinetic and pharmacodynamic parameters is a result of several influences, including genetic polymorphisms in drug metabolizing enzymes, transporters, or drug targets. This variability leads to the differences in efficacy and toxicity that are seen between patients treated with the same drugs for the same disease. Pharmacogenetics is the study of the genetic polymorphisms that determine an individual's response to drugs. Anticancer drugs often undergo biotransformation or detoxification by enzyme systems that are known in humans to be areas of genetic polymorphism, potentially leading to increased toxicity or decreased efficacy (Nagasubramanian *et al.*, 2003). In veterinary medicine less is known about specific genetic differences, although breed differences with respect to sensitivity to different drugs are well documented. In order to improve the ability to address this issue the Animal Pharmaceutics and Technology Focus Group of the American Association of Pharmaceutical Scientists (AAPS) developed a working group to examine breed-specific differences in metabolism that could alter drug disposition. A recent review article summarizes their findings (Fleischer *et al.*, 2008).

MDR1 mutations and breed predisposition to toxicity

A clinically applicable pharmacogenetics example in veterinary oncology is a mutation in the *ABCB-1* (formerly *MDR1*) gene which encodes for the drug transport protein, P-glycoprotein (P-gp). P-gp effectively acts as a drug barrier for certain tissues such as the brain, testis and placenta. When this protein is not functional, drugs that are substrates for P-gp are not excreted normally, leading to increased drug exposure and increased clinical toxicity. Chemotherapeutic drugs that are substrates for P-gp include the vinca alkaloids, doxorubicin, dactinomycin and the taxanes (Mealey, 2004). Dogs that are homozygous or have the mutation in two alleles are 100 times as susceptible as wild-type dogs to developing ivermectin-induced neurological toxicity. This mutation occurs most commonly in herding breeds and several studies have been reported looking at the incidence of mutation amongst various breeds originating from various countries. A recent study looking at breed distribution of the polymorphism in over 5000 dogs that had samples submitted for testing found collies and Australian Shepherd Dogs to be affected most commonly. In the collies the frequency of *mut/mut* allelic status was 35% with *mut/wt* frequency of 42%. Australian Shepherd Dogs were 10% *mut/mut* and 37% *mut/wt*. This study also identified German Shepherd Dogs with the mutation; and a surprising number of mixed-breed dogs that did not appear to be of herding dog mix also had the mutation (Mealey and Meurs, 2008). Where a patient is scheduled to undergo chemotherapy with P-gp substrate drugs, testing should be considered if the patient is of a breed that has been reported to have a high frequency of mutation in this gene. If the patient is homozygous, these drugs should be avoided or used with extreme caution to prevent unacceptable toxicity.

Targeted therapy

Targeted therapy is another expanding treatment area (see Chapter 9). Identification of signal transduction pathways that drive cellular proliferation has led to the discovery of many potential 'drugable' targets.

One such group of molecules is the tyrosine kinases which, when activated by mutation, result in aberrant cell growth (Griffin, 2001). A disease in human medicine in which this type of mutation is important is chronic myelogenous leukaemia, where the reciprocal translocation of chromosomes 9 and 22 results in the *bcr–abl* oncogenic product. One of the first targeted agents successfully developed, imatinib mesylate, disrupts this important pathway. Clinical trials with this agent in humans showed unexpected and exciting responses with refractory disease. This agent is now part of the standard of care for this disease.

In veterinary medicine an excellent example of targeted therapy having a clinical impact on how disease will be treated lies with canine mast cell tumours (MCTs). Studies have shown that 20–30% of canine MCTs express a mutated form of the receptor tyrosine kinase KIT, which is involved in cell growth and differentiation. Several *in vitro* and *in vivo* proof-of-concept studies have been published showing activity of targeted tyrosine kinase-inhibiting compounds (London *et al.* 2003; Gleixner *et al.*, 2007). Results of a double-blind randomized placebo-controlled phase III clinical trial were reported by Hahn *et al.* (2008), who evaluated the efficacy of the drug masitinib, a selective inhibitor of KIT. The treatment was well tolerated and resulted in an overall increase in time to progression, an effect that was more pronounced in patients who were given masitinib as a front-line therapy. They concluded that this targeted therapy was safe and effective at delaying tumour progression in dogs with recurrent or non-resectable grade II or III non-metastatic MCTs. Masitinib (Masivet, AB Science) and toceranib phosphate (Palladia, Pfizer) have both recently been authorized for treatment of canine mast cell tumours and may yet find application in treatment of other tumour types.

Based on results in human trials, it is clear that targeted therapies are susceptible to the development of resistance. It is unlikely that these agents will replace standard chemotherapy, but they are likely to be used in combination with other drugs to achieve better tumour control.

References and further reading

Altman A (2001) Acute tumor lysis syndrome. *Seminars in Oncology* **28** (suppl. 5), 3–8

Bailey DB, Rassnick KM, Erb HN *et al.* (2004) Effects of glomerular filtration rate on clearance and mylotoxicity of carboplatin in cats with tumors. *American Journal of Veterinary Research* **65**, 1502–1507

Charney SC, Bergman PJ, Hohenhaus AE and McKnight JA (2003) Risk factors for sterile hemorrhagic cystitis in dogs with lymphoma receiving cyclophosphamide with or without concurrent administration of furosemide: 216 cases (1990–1996). *Journal of the American Veterinary Medicine Association* **222**, 1388–1393

Chu E and DeVita VT (2001) Principles of cancer management: chemotherapy. In: *Cancer Principles and Practice of Oncology, 6th edn*, ed. VT DeVita *et al.*, pp. 289–306. Lippincott, Philadelphia

Chun R, Garrett LD and Vail DM (2001) Cancer chemotherapy. In: *Small Animal Clinical Oncology, 3rd edn*, ed. SJ Withrow *et al.*, pp. 92–118. WB Saunders, Philadelphia

Clifford CA and Sorenmo K (1999) Doxorubicin cardiotoxicity: current concepts in pathogenesis, cardioprotection and screening. *Veterinary Cancer Society Newsletter* **23**, 1–5

Conner TH, Anderson RW, Sessink PJ, Broadfield L and Power LA (1999) Surface contamination with antineoplastic agents in six cancer treatment centers in Canada and the United States. *American Journal of Health System – Pharmacy* **56**, 1427–1432

Dickinson KL and Ogilvie GK (1995) Safe handling and administration of chemotherapeutic agents in veterinary medicine. In: *Current Veterinary Therapy XII. Small Animal Practice*, ed. RW Kirk *et al.*, pp. 475–478. WB Saunders, Philadelphia

Elmslie RE and Dow SW (2000) Gene therapy for cancer. In: *Current Veterinary Therapy XIII Small Animal Practice*, ed. J Bonagura, pp. 493–498. WB Saunders, Philadelphia

Elmslie RE, Glawe P and Dow SW (2008) Metronomic therapy with cyclophosphamide and proxicam effectively delays tumor recurrence in dogs with incompletely resected soft tissue sarcomas. *Journal of Veterinary Internal Medicine* **22**, 1373–1379

Fleischer S, Sharkey M, Mealey K, Ostrander EA and Martinez M (2008) Pharmacogenetic and metabolic differences between dog breeds: their impact on canine medicine and the use of the dog as a preclinical animal model. *The AAPS Journal* **10**, 110–119

Folkman J. (1997) Antiangiogenic therapy. In: *Cancer: Principles and Practice of Oncology, 5th edn*, ed. VT Devita *et al.*, pp. 3075–3085. Lippincott, Philadelphia

Gately S and Kerbel R (2001) Antiangiogenic scheduling of lower dose cancer chemotherapy. *Cancer Journal* **7**, 427–436

Gleixner KV, Rebuzzi L, Mayerhofer M *et al.* (2007) Synergistic antiproliferative effects of KIT tyrosine kinase inhibitors on neoplastic canine mast cells. *Experimental Hematology* **24**, 1510–1521

Goldie JH, Coldman AJ and Gudauskas GA (1982) Rationale for the use of alternating non-cross-resistant chemotherapy. *Cancer Treatment Reports* **66**, 439–449

Griffin J (2001) The biology of signal transduction inhibition: basic science to novel therapies. *Seminars in Oncology* **28** (suppl. 17), 3–8

Hahn KA, Ogilvie G, Rusk T *et al.* (2008) Masitinib is safe and effective for the treatment of canine mast cell tumors. *Journal of Veterinary Internal Medicine* **22**, 1301–1309

Jones A and Hunter AL (1998) New developments in angiogenesis: a major mechanism for tumor growth and target for therapy. *The Cancer Journal from Scientific American* **4**, 209–217

Jorgenson JA, Spivey SM, Au C *et al.* (2008) Contamination comparison of transfer devices intended for handling hazardous drugs. *Hospital Pharmacy* **43**, 732–727

Kaufman DC and Chabner BA (2001) Clinical strategies for cancer treatment: the role of drugs. In: *Cancer Chemotherapy and Biotherapy, Principles and Practice, 3rd edn*, ed. BA Chabner *et al.*, pp. 1–16. Lippincott, Philadelphia

Keefe DL (2001) Anthracycline induced cardiomyopathy. *Seminars in Oncology* **28** (suppl. 12), 2–7

Kisseberth WC and MacEwen EG (2001) Complications of cancer and its treatment. In: *Small Animal Clinical Oncology, 3rd edn*, ed. SJ Withrow *et al.*, pp. 198–219. WB Saunders, Philadelphia

Knapp DW, Richardson RC, Bonney PL *et al.* (1988) Cisplatin therapy in 41 dogs with malignant tumors. *Journal of Veterinary Internal Medicine* **2**, 41–46

Kosarek CE, Kisseberth WC, Gallant SL and Couto CG (2005) Clinical evaluation of gemciabine in dogs with spontaneously occurring malignancies. *Journal of Veterinary Internal Medicine* **19**, 81–86

Lana SE, U'ren L, Plaza S *et al.* (2007) Comparison of continuous low dose oral chemotherapy with conventional doxorubicin chemotherapy for adjuvant therapy of hemangiosarcoma in dogs. *Journal of Veterinary Internal Medicine* **21**, 764–769

London CA, Hannah AL, Zadovoskaya R *et al.* (2003) Phase I dose escalating study of SU11654, a small molecule receptor tyrosine kinase inhibitor in dogs with spontaneous malignancies. *Clinical Cancer Research* **9**, 2755–2768

Mauldin GE, Fox PR, Patnaik AK *et al.* (1992) Doxorubicin-induced cardiotoxicosis: clinical features in 32 dogs. *Journal of Veterinary Internal Medicine* **6**, 82–88

Mealey KL (2004) Therapeutic implications of the MDR-1 gene. *Journal of Veterinary Pharmacology and Therapeutics* **27**, 257–264

Mealey KL and Meurs KM (2008) Breed distribution of the ABCB1-1delta polymorphism (multidrug sensitivity) among dogs undergoing ABCB1 phenotyping. *Journal of the American Veterinary Medical Association* **233**, 921–924

Moore AS, Kirk C and Cardona A (1991) Intracavitary cisplatin chemotherapy experience in six dogs. *Journal of Veterinary Internal Medicine* **5**, 227–231

Nagasubramanian R, Innocenti F and Ratain MJ (2003) Pharmacogenetics in cancer treatment *Annual Review of Medicine* **54**, 437–452

Ogilvie GK and Moore AS (2001a) Chemotherapy – properties, uses and patient management. In: *Feline Oncology*, ed. GK Ogilvie *et al.*, pp. 62–76. Veterinary Learning Systems, Trenton, New Jersey

Ogilvie GK and Moore AS (2001b) Drug handling and administration. In: *Feline Oncology*, ed. GK Ogilvie *et al.*, pp. 53–61. Veterinary Learning Systems, Trenton, New Jersey

O'Keefe DA, Sisson DD, Gelberg HB, Shaeffer DJ and Krawiec DR (1993) Systemic toxicity associated with doxorubicin administration in cats. *Journal of Veterinary Internal Medicine* **7**, 309–317

Rassnick KM, Frimberger AE, Wood CA *et al.* (2000) Evaluation of ifosfamide for treatment of various canine neoplasms. *Journal of Veterinary Internal Medicine* **14**, 271–276

Sessink PJ and Bos RP (1999) Drugs hazardous to healthcare workers. Evaluation of methods for monitoring occupational exposure to cytostatic drugs. *Drug Safety* **20**, 347–359

Spugnini EP (2002) Use of hyaluronase for the treatment of extravasation of chemotherapeutic agents in six dogs. *Journal of the American Veterinary Medical Association* **221**, 1437–1440

Tannock IF and Goldenberg GJ (1998) Drug resistance and experimental chemotherapy. In: *The Basic Science of Oncology, 3rd edn*, ed. IF Tannock *et al.*, pp. 392–419. McGraw-Hill, New York

Thamm DM and Vail DM (2007) Aftershocks of cancer chemotherapy: managing adverse effects. *Journal of the American Animal Hospital Association* **43**, 1–7

Wick C, Slawson MH, Jorgenson JA and Tyler LS (2003) Using a closed system protective device to reduce personnel exposure to antineoplastic agents. *American Journal of Health-System Pharmacy* **60**, 2314–2320

8

Principles of radiation therapy

Amy F. Pruitt and Donald E. Thrall

Introduction

When considering treatment options for a solid tumour, often the first choice is to use a single modality, commonly surgery. Although many solid tumours can be cured with surgery, in others it is impossible to obtain tumour-free margins. In these patients, disease-free interval or survival can often be extended with a combination of surgery and radiation therapy.

The best chance of achieving tumour cure is always with a logical, preplanned approach, particularly when dual or multimodal treatment therapy is indicated as the first treatment. Any concern that surgery may not achieve complete excision warrants consultation with both a surgeon and radiation oncologist before initiating treatment. The combination of surgery to reduce the tumour volume (preferably to microscopic levels) followed by radiation therapy to treat remaining disease is a very effective treatment option and can provide long-term control in situations where neither modality alone is sufficient to accomplish that goal. For optimal outcome when combining surgery and radiation therapy, thorough preplanning and communication are required among all involved as well as adherence to good oncological surgical principles.

Radiation therapy may be administered preoperatively or postoperatively, and the decision on which sequence to use depends on tumour type, size and/or location. For tumours where compartmental resection is theoretically possible, preoperative radiation is favoured as the radiation field is typically smaller and the tumour may become easier to excise. When using postoperative irradiation, careful presurgical planning will decrease the chance of radiation therapy complications. Poorly thought out surgery may leave large scars or scar orientations and locations that can prevent or hinder the ability to administer a subsequent course of radiation therapy safely and effectively if surgical excision is incomplete. This emphasizes the need for meaningful pretreatment communication between the surgeon and radiation oncologist.

Permanent or long-term local control of various solid tumours may be achieved with the combination of surgery and radiation. Common tumours where this approach is applicable include grade II canine mast cell tumours and canine and feline soft tissue sarcomas.

The ability to achieve tumour control or cure for a recurrent tumour may be compromised or prohibited by previously administered therapy. A tumour recurring after surgery may be more difficult to return surgically to microscopic disease. Often recurrent tumours will require a second excision, resulting in radiation fields that are larger than they would have been had margins been assessed and postoperative radiation used initially. Also, recurrent tumours are often more aggressive in behaviour than the initial tumour, giving rise to cells capable of metastasis and acquiring resistance to drugs and radiation. For these reasons, it is critical that the first therapy applied to a solid tumour be the optimal therapy.

Indications for radiation therapy

Generally, radiation therapy has the best chance of leading to cure or long-term remission when used for localized microscopic disease. For tumours having a high metastatic potential, adjuvant chemotherapy should also be considered. Volume is the biggest factor negatively affecting tumour response to radiation therapy and, as described above, for most solid tumours the best approach is a combination of surgery and radiation. However, there are some indications where the tumour is not amenable to surgical resection due to the anatomical site. These include intranasal tumours, fixed thyroid carcinomas and brain tumours. In these instances, there is usually a small chance that radiation will lead to long-term tumour control. Definitive treatment of these tumours is acceptable provided that the expectations are clear. Rarely, radiation therapy alone will be effective for macroscopic tumours that are fairly radiosensitive and not amenable to complete or partial resection; examples include acanthomatous epulis (also referred to as basal cell carcinoma and acanthomatous ameloblastoma), small (1–2 cm) oral carcinomas, small grade II mast cell tumours and transmissible venereal tumours.

Definitive and palliative intent
Radiation therapy can be delivered with either curative (definitive) or palliative intent:

- **Definitive cancer therapy:** Can also be referred to as 'curative intent' therapy. It is a treatment plan designed potentially to cure cancer, using one or a combination of treatment modalities

- **Palliative cancer therapy:** Treatment specifically directed to help to improve the clinical signs associated with an incurable cancer. The primary objective of palliative care is to improve the patient's quality of life.

Curative radiation therapy

With definitive intent, the goal is to deliver the maximally tolerated radiation dose and to achieve permanent tumour control, or the longest remission possible. This requires prescribing a more aggressive course of therapy and expecting the development of acute side effects.

Palliative radiation therapy

Palliative radiation therapy has a role in veterinary medicine for the purpose of relieving pain or clinical signs of an incurable tumour. The goal of palliative radiation therapy for an incurable cancer is not long-term control but to improve the quality of life of the patient by decreasing any distressing clinical symptoms associated with the tumour.

Palliative radiation therapy often involves using the simplest radiation schedule that will give the maximum relief with the least morbidity and cost. Thus, most palliative protocols use lower total doses and a higher dose per fraction to avoid acute radiation side effects and prolonged hospitalization. Palliative prescriptions are not intended for the sake of convenience, or to address financial limitations.

It is important to establish and communicate the goal of palliative radiation therapy to the owner. Although prolongation of life is not a goal of true palliative radiation therapy, successful palliation can lead to increased survival. As such, the choice of radiation prescription for palliative treatments is not trivial and the use of large doses per fraction for palliative radiation therapy does have some drawbacks. The risk for development of serious late side effects in patients receiving large doses per fraction is increased if they live longer than expected. Also, if the tumour responds more favourably than expected to the palliative treatment, the administration of additional radiation is complicated by the large doses per fraction used in the initial prescription.

Principles of radiation therapy

Ionizing radiation kills cells by producing chemical damage in DNA, which eventually leads to cell death. The lesions in DNA prevent normal replication but do not lead to immediate cell death. Radiation damage is manifested when the irradiated cells attempt to divide. Tissue responses to radiation therapy are classified as acute and late effects:

- Acute effects occur in both the tumour and proliferating normal tissues
- Late effects occur in slowly proliferating or non-proliferating normal tissues.

Fractionation

The goal of radiation therapy is to destroy the reproductive capacity of the tumour without excessive damage to the surrounding normal tissues. To achieve this goal, the total dose of radiation is divided into multiple, smaller fractions, with total doses of 48–60 Gy usually delivered using 16–25 separate daily fractions of 2.5–3 Gy.

Radiation therapy is administered in this way because higher total doses can be given with less risk of late effects when divided into smaller dose fractions, and higher total doses are associated with improved tumour control. Fractionating the dose also allows for proliferative recovery of normal tissue in the radiation field as the radiation therapy progresses.

In contemporary radiation therapy practices, daily fractionation using relatively small doses per fraction (≤3 Gy) is standard practice and it is difficult to justify deviating from this prescription. Large doses per fraction will preferentially damage slowly proliferating normal tissues with no benefit to tumour control. While slowly dividing cells appear to be somewhat less sensitive to small doses of radiation than the more rapidly dividing cells, they sustain more relative damage if radiation is delivered in larger doses per fraction. Thus, the chance that a serious normal tissue complication will develop is not only a direct function of the total radiation dose, but also of the size of each of the fractions wherein the total dose is administered.

Dose distribution

When administering radiation therapy, tumour volumes are defined to include all known gross disease plus a margin of adjacent normal tissue that is at risk for suspected microscopic tumour extension. It is the response of the adjacent normal tissue that limits the amount of radiation that can be administered safely.

Most contemporary radiation treatments are planned based on computer modelling of dose distribution in computed tomography (CT) images of the tumour region (Shiran *et al.*, 2006). A variety of proprietary programs are available for this purpose. This highly detailed anatomical basis of radiation planning allows optimization of the radiation dose distribution in the tumour, and sparing of normal tissue (Figure 8.1). Due to the importance of patient positioning for radiation therapy administration, it is important that a radiation oncologist be intimately involved with acquisition of the CT images used for radiation planning.

Equipment

Though a detailed discussion of the physics of radiation therapy is beyond the scope of this chapter, some preliminary information is provided. Modern veterinary radiation therapy is based around the use of a **linear accelerator** that can generate high-energy X-rays suitable for treatment of tumours lying deep to the surface, and generation of electrons for treatment of very superficial tumours in the skin. This equipment has replaced the use of cobalt machines and orthovoltage X-ray machines.

Cobalt machines used the photons arising from radioactive decay of ^{60}Co for treatment. Although these photons were of relatively high energy, cobalt

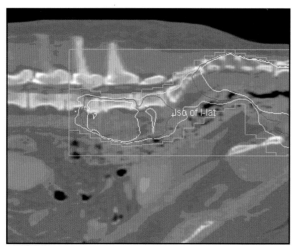

8.1 Sagittal CT image of the caudal abdomen of a dog with an incompletely resected anal sac tumour (no gross tumour is present) and regional lymph node metastasis. The green stepped lines represent a radiation field configured using a multileaf collimator (see text). Computer software enables radiation doses to be estimated once a treatment configuration is chosen. In this image the white, purple and yellow lines represent the periphery of areas receiving at least 49, 48 and 47 Gy, respectively. By assessing radiation dose in the tumour and adjacent normal tissue, the treatment configuration can be optimized.

sources required periodic replacement and the dose fall-off at the edge of the treatment field was quite broad, leading to irradiation of more normal tissue than necessary and uncertainties in treatment planning. Unfortunately, the rise of terrorism in the world resulted in greatly increased regulatory control of these large radiation sources, which complicated maintaining such equipment.

Orthovoltage machines are nearly obsolete in veterinary radiation therapy. These machines operate much like a diagnostic X-ray machine, producing relatively high-energy X-rays, but not nearly as energetic as the radiation coming from a cobalt unit or a linear accelerator. Therefore, they were suited mainly for treatment of superficial lesions. The complications associated with orthovoltage use were more frequent and more severe than encountered when using a linear accelerator. The electron-generating capability of linear accelerators replaces the need to use orthovoltage X-ray machines to treat very superficial tumours.

Acute and late radiation effects

Figure 8.2 is a compilation of potential acute and late radiation-induced tissue/organ side effects.

Acute effects

Regularly dividing tissues, such as skin and mucosa, are referred to as acutely responding normal tissues. Acute effects that develop in these tissues as a result of radiation therapy are observed during or shortly after completion of radiation therapy. Manifestation of radiation injury in acutely responding normal tissues is due to depletion of stem cells, with failure to maintain the functional cell compartment that is the population of differentiated cells that provide function of the tissue at risk. Radiation dose intensity (the amount of radiation delivered per unit of time) is directly associated with the development and severity of acute radiation effects.

Acute effects in proliferating tissues may cause discomfort and require supportive therapy. However, acute damage is repaired rapidly, rarely has significant consequences and rarely limits administration of the prescribed dose. Attempting to avoid acute reactions by altering the radiation schedule should be discouraged, because it will result in the decreased efficacy of the treatment. Giving less radiation dose or irradiating over a protracted period of time to decrease acute reactions will also spare the tumour, leading to decreased tumour control.

Tissue/organ/region	Acute effects	Late effects
Skin	Epidermis: erythema, dry desquamation, moist desquamation (see Figure 8.3ab)	Dermis: fibrosis, contracture, non-healing ulcer, telangiectasia, alopecia, leucotrichia, hyperpigmentation (see Figure 8.3c)
Oral cavity	Mucositis (see Figure 8.4)	Ulceration, osteoradionecrosis, periodontal disease
Salivary gland		Xerostomia
Nasal cavity	Mucositis, nasal discharge	Osteoradionecrosis, chronic nasal discharge
Eye	Conjunctivitis, corneal ulcer, uveitis	Cataract, keratoconjunctivitis sicca, retinal blindness
Ear	Otitis media	
Brain and spinal cord		Infarction, necrosis
Cervical region	Oesophagitis, tracheitis	Oesophageal ulceration and stricture, hypothyroidism
Thoracic region		Chronic pneumonitis, pericarditis, pancarditis
Kidney		Chronic nephrosclerosis
Pelvic region	Colitis, cystitis, urethritis, prostatitis	Bladder constricture, colon/rectal ulcer, stenosis, fistula, perforation, chronic colitis

8.2 Potential acute and late radiation-induced tissue/organ side effects.

Skin

Acute radiation side effects to the skin are common in dogs but less common in cats. Radiation-induced skin side effects manifest initially as slight erythema and can progress to dry desquamation or moist desquamation (Figure 8.3). Acute skin side effects are usually worse if the treated site includes skin that is subject to friction, such as the axilla or groin regions. Its occurrence is also worse in particularly sensitive areas, including the perianal region and paws.

Skin side effects can persist for several weeks following completion of therapy, with the treated area usually healed 3–6 weeks after treatment completion. Treatment is mainly supportive with gentle cleansing/soaking of the area with mild soap (dilute nolvasan or chlorhexidine solution) and prescription of anti-inflammatory (NSAIDs or corticosteroids), analgesic and antibiotic medications. After cleansing, the radiation site should be gently blotted dry (not rubbed) with a soft, clean towel. The prevention of self-trauma by the use of Elizabethan collars or other devices used to prevent access to the site is of utmost importance.

A large number of ointments and creams have been used for the prevention and management of acute radiation skin side effects in human and veterinary medicine. There is a lack of well designed studies in both human and veterinary medicine to evaluate the effectiveness of these topical therapies. In a recent review of 54 private and university teaching veterinary hospitals (Flynn and Lurie, 2007), the most common options out of 25 different topical therapies reported included aloe vera-based lotions or silver sulfadiazine cream.

Irradiation of the paw results in painful sloughing of pads and loss of nails. Oral analgesics alone may not be sufficient for adequate pain control and often the patient will benefit from local nerve blocks.

Mucosa

If areas of mucosa are included in the radiation field, the most significant acute side effect is mucositis (Figure 8.4), which often develops midway through therapy. Mucositis can be patchy in its distribution or can progresses to a confluent mucositis.

Treatment consists of supportive care with gentle cleansing/rinsing of the area and prescription of anti-inflammatory, antibiotic and analgesic medications. Topical analgesics include 2% lidocaine gel and 'miracle' mouthwash formulations that typically include some combination of lidocaine, benzocaine, diphenhydramine, kaolin, milk of magnesia and/or sucralfate,

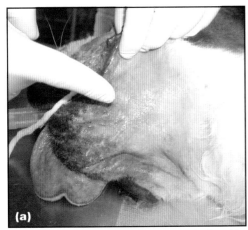 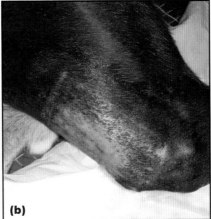 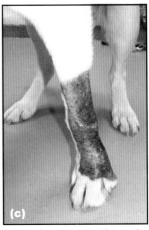

8.3 Radiation side effects seen in the skin. **(a)** Marked confluent moist desquamation of the skin seen near the end of radiation therapy. **(b)** Mild patchy desquamation of the skin seen at the end of radiation therapy. **(c)** Permanent alopecia and hyperpigmentation of the skin after definitive radiation therapy.

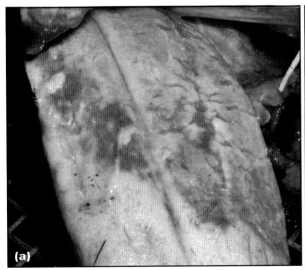 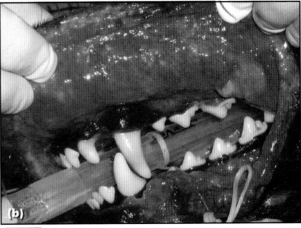

8.4 Acute radiation side effects seen in the oral cavity. **(a)** Oral mucositis of the caudal tongue. **(b)** Oral mucositis of the buccal mucosa.

compounded by the pharmacy as directed (Treister and Sonis, 2007). At North Carolina State University, a formulation of diphenhydramine 2.5 mg/ml, Maalox suspension and lidocaine 2% gel compounded in equal amounts is used to coat the areas of oral mucositis. Also, if the oral cavity is involved, it is important to maintain adequate hydration and nutrition, which may necessitate the placement of a temporary gastrostomy or oesophagostomy tube.

If the perianal region is in the radiation field, mucositis can make defecation very painful and may require the placement of a lumbosacral epidural catheter for constant rate infusion of analgesics.

Late effects

Tissues such as brain, spinal cord and bone that do not divide regularly are referred to as late-responding normal tissues. These tissues will not express radiation injury until many months or years after being irradiated. In tissues where cells divide only rarely, cellular damage remains latent for a long period of time and is revealed slowly.

In late-responding normal tissues, the development and severity of late radiation effects are not related to the time over which the radiation is given, but rather are a function of the individual fraction size and the total dose. The larger the fraction size, the lower is the total dose required to produce serious complications. Radiation injury in late-responding tissues may manifest as fibrosis, vascular damage, demyelination or necrosis.

Late radiation effects limit the dose that can be given safely because they are progressive, often not treatable and adversely affect the animal's quality of life. Late-responding normal tissues are therefore referred to as the dose-limiting tissues. Necrosis or fibrosis of critical non-proliferating tissues such as the brain, spinal cord or heart can be life-threatening and should be avoided if at all possible.

In general, radiation doses are selected that offer the greatest chance of tumour control with some acceptable finite but small (<5%) probability of serious normal tissue complication.

Implications for wound healing

Radiation creates both acute and delayed effects to the skin and subcutaneous tissues within the radiation field and these effects have implications for surgical wound healing.

Acute effects

Acutely, radiation produces degenerative changes in basement membranes, increases vascular permeability, can result in vasculature stasis or thrombosis and may reduce neovascularization. Radiation decreases the ability of fibroblasts to multiply and decreases their production of collagen, or results in production of collagen that does not mature as quickly as needed for wound healing (Tibbs, 1997). The force required to break apart a healing linear surgical incision can be directly measured by the wound bursting strength (WBS), which has been shown to be reduced after radiation therapy (Bernstein et al., 1993).

Delayed effects

A wound produced in tissue that was irradiated months or even years prior also exhibits altered wound healing capacity, though less pronounced. Delayed effects to the skin and subcutaneous tissues due to fibroblast injury include atrophy, contraction and fibrosis. The skin and subcutaneous tissues become atrophic and less pliable than normal, while reduced vascularity and tissue hypoxia can impair normal wound healing response and predispose to bacterial infection (Tibbs, 1997).

Surgical complications

Occasionally, the need to perform a surgical procedure in previously irradiated tissue arises. The safety of such a procedure depends on a number of factors, including the size of the original treatment field, the total dose delivered, the fraction size used, the time between completion of radiation therapy and the planned surgery, and the inherent tissue repair characteristics of the individual patient. There are no hard and fast rules governing whether surgery will be tolerated. Negative risk factors are a large radiation field, a high total dose, a large fraction size and a short time between radiation and surgery. In general, surgery can be tolerated in tissue that has been irradiated to 48 Gy in 3 Gy fractions, even when the surgery and radiation are in close proximity.

When considering the effect of radiation on wound healing, another issue is the type of surgery itself. Large, extensive surgery requires healing of a larger wound. Also, scars under increased tension in irradiated tissue are likely to be at a higher risk of having wound healing complications than if in non-irradiated tissue.

Tumour radiation responsiveness

Tumour response to radiation therapy can vary depending on species, tumour histology, tumour location, volume and histopathological grade. Figures 8.5 and 8.6 show some of the reported results for tumours commonly irradiated in dogs and cats, respectively.

Tumour type	Number of patients	Treatments	Results	Reference
Mast cell tumour (MCT) Grade II Stage 0	32	Surgery and megavoltage radiation	94% 1 year disease-free interval. 86% 2–5 years disease-free interval	Al-Sarraf et al. (1996)
	37	Surgery and orthovoltage or megavoltage radiation	97% 1 year disease-free interval. 93% 3 years disease-free interval	Frimberger et al. (1997)

8.5 Some of the reported results for tumours commonly irradiated in dogs. (continues) ▶

Tumour type	Number of patients	Treatments	Results	Reference
MCT Grade I–III (mostly grade II) Stage 1	56	35/56 surgery and megavoltage radiation 21/56 megavoltage radiation	32.7 months overall median disease-free interval: 12 months if measurable disease, 54 months if microscopic	LaDue *et al.* (1998)
MCT Grade I–III (mostly grade II) Stage 2	19	Surgery and megavoltage radiation to primary tumour and metastatic lymph node. Prednisone 18/19	40.7 months median disease-free survival	Chaffin and Thrall (2002)
MCT Grade III Stage 0	31	Surgery and megavoltage radiation	Median duration of control and survival 27.7 months and 28 months, respectively	Hahn *et al.* (2004)
Soft tissue sarcomas	48	Surgery and megavoltage radiation	35.5 months median disease-free interval	McKnight *et al.* (2000)
	37	Surgery and megavoltage radiation	61 months median survival. Median time to local recurrence > 2 years	Forrest *et al.* (2000)
	29	Megavoltage radiation and local hyperthermia	14.5 months median time to local failure	Thrall *et al.* (1996)
	122	Megavoltage radiation and local hyperthermia (low dose and high dose hyperthermia)	Median duration of local control 1.9 years in high hyperthermia dose group; 1.2 years in low hyperthermia dose group	Thrall *et al.* (2005)
Infiltrative lipoma	13 (4 microscopic; 9 macroscopic disease)	Megavoltage radiation	40 months median survival. Macroscopic disease: 2/9 complete response, 2/9 partial response, 4/9 stable disease	McEntee *et al.* (2000)
Osteosarcoma	14	Definitive megavoltage radiation, median total dose 57 Gy, and chemotherapy	6.9 months median survival	Walter *et al.* (2005)
	95	Palliative megavoltage radiation, 16 or 30 Gy, ± chemotherapy	4 months median survival. 74 % pain relief response – 2.5–4 months reported duration	Ramirez *et al.* (1999)
Nasal cavity tumours	77 and 130	Definitive megavoltage radiation, most total doses 48–57 Gy	9–13 months median survival	Theon *et al.* (1993); LaDue *et al.* (1999)
	56 and 48	Palliative megavoltage radiation, total dose 24–36 Gy	4.9–7 months median survival	Mellanby *et al.* (2002b); Gieger *et al.* (2008)
	51	Megavoltage radiation and slow-release cisplatin	15.6 months median survival	Lana *et al.* (2004
Nasal planum squamous cell carcinoma	8	Orthovoltage radiation	6 months median survival. 2.9 months mean time to failure	Thrall and Adams (1982)
	3	Surgery and megavoltage radiation	2 months stable disease, then progressive disease	Rogers *et al.* (1995)
	11	Surgery and hypofractionated radiation; 7/11 or hypofractionated radiation alone; 4/11	9 weeks median time to recurrence, whatever treatment	Lascelles *et al.* (2000)
Oral tumours: acanthomatous epulis	39	Orthovoltage radiation	37–47.5 months median survival	Thrall (1984)
	57	Megavoltage radiation	39.8 months median time to first event	McEntee *et al.* (2004)
Oral tumours: melanoma	38	Megavoltage radiation	8 months median survival	Theon *et al.* (1997)
	140	Megavoltage radiation: 3 different protocols 30–57 Gy	5 months median time to first event, 7 months median survival. Risk factors (RFs) identified: 1-0 RF median survival 11–21 months; 3-2 RFs median survival 3–5 months	Proulx *et al.* (2003)

8.5 (continued) Some of the reported results for tumours commonly irradiated in dogs. (continues) ▶

Tumour type	Number of patients	Treatments	Results	Reference
Oral tumours: squamous cell carcinoma (SCC)	14	Megavoltage radiation	12 and 15 months median disease-free interval and survival, respectively	LaDue-Miller *et al.* (1996)
	39	Megavoltage radiation	36 months median progression-free survival	Theon *et al.* (1997)
Oral tumours: SCC – tonsillar	8	Surgery + megavoltage radiation or surgery, megavoltage radiation + chemotherapy	75% local disease control but 5 months median survival	MacMillan *et al.* (1982)
	6		9 months median survival	Brooks *et al.* (1988)
Oral tumours: SCC – tongue	11	Orthovoltage radiation and local hyperthermia	4 months median survival	Beck *et al.* (1986)
Oral tumours: fibrosarcoma	8	Megavoltage radiation	18 months median survival	Ciekot *et al.* (1994)
	28	Megavoltage radiation	26 months median disease-free interval	Theon *et al.* (1997)
Thyroid carcinoma	25	Megavoltage radiation	45 months mean progression-free survival; median not reached Time to max tumour size reduction ≥ 8 months	Theon *et al.* (2000)
Salivary gland carcinoma	6	Surgery and megavoltage radiation	18 months median survival	Hammer *et al.* (2001)
Apocrine gland anal sac adenocarcinoma	15–27	Megavoltage radiation ± surgery ±chemotherapy	18–31.5 months median survival	Turek *el al.* (2003) Williams *et al.* (2003)
Intracranial tumours: pituitary macroadenoma	13–19	Megavoltage radiation	13–46 months median survival	Theon and Feldman (1998) Kent *et al.* (2007)
Intracranial tumours: meningioma	20–31	Surgery and megavoltage radiation	16.5–30 months median survival	Theon *et al.* (2000) Axlund *et al.* (2002)
Intracranial tumours: mixed (no histopathology)	29–46	Megavoltage radiation	8–23 months median survival	Spugnini *et al.* (2000) Bley *et al.* (2005)
Spinal cord tumours: mostly meningiomas	6–9	Surgery and megavoltage radiation	17 to ~36 months median survival	Siegel *et al.* (1996) Petersen *et al.* (2008)
Transitional cell carcinoma (TCC), bladder	10	Palliative radiation and mitoxantrone and piroxicam	10.7 months median survival; 22% partial response and 90% clinical improvement	Poirier *et al.* (2004)
Bladder TCC and prostatic Ca/TCC	10	Definitive radiation alone	7–8 months median survival	Authors' experience
Thymoma	17	Megavoltage radiation	8.2 months median survival	Smith *et al.* (2001)
Transmissible venereal tumour	Variable	Variable, but orthovoltage or megavoltage radiation the most common method	24–25 months median disease-free interval and survival	Thrall and Adams (1982) Rogers *et al.* (1998)

8.5 (continued) Some of the reported results for tumours commonly irradiated in dogs.

Tumour type	Patient number	Treatments	Results	Reference
Injection site sarcomas	92	Megavoltage radiation followed by surgery ± chemotherapy	19.2 months median time to first event (recurrence, metastasis, or death). 32.4 months if complete excision versus 9.7 months if incomplete	Kobayashi et al. (2002)
	18	Surgery followed by megavoltage radiation and chemotherapy	21.7 months median disease-free interval	Bregazzi et al. (2001)
	76		13.3 months median disease-free interval	Cohen et al. (2001)
Oral squamous cell carcinoma (SCC)	Variable	Radiation: orthovoltage or megavoltage, palliative or definitive ± surgery ± chemotherapy	2–6 months median survival	Postorino et al. (1993); Jones et al. (2003); Fidel et al. (2007)
Nasal planum SCC	90	Orthovoltage radiation	16.5 months median progression-free survival	Theon et al. (1995)
	12	Orthovoltage radiation	13.6 months disease-free interval	Melzer et al. (2006)
Nasal cavity tumours, non-lymphoid	8–16	Megavoltage radiation	11–13 months median survival	Theon et al. (1994); Mellanby et al. (2002a)
Salivary gland tumour	30	Surgery and megavoltage radiation	17 months median survival	Hammer et al. (2001)
Thymoma	7	Megavoltage radiation	23.6 months median survival	Smith et al. (2001)
Pituitary macroadenoma	8	Megavoltage radiation	17.4 months median survival. Endocrine disorder improved within 1–5 months	Mayer et al. (2006)

8.6 Some of the reported results for tumours commonly irradiated in cats.

Future directions

Although considerable progress has been made in optimizing the response of tumours in animals to radiation treatment, many solid tumours still recur following radiation therapy. This may be due to insufficient killing of tumour clonogens due to inadequate radiation dose, or to biological characteristics of the tumour that render it radioresistant. New directions in veterinary oncology are aimed at each of these problems.

Conformal radiation dose delivery

With regard to inadequate tumour radiation dose, effort is being directed towards making the radiation dose delivery more conformal. This implies tailoring the shape of the radiation dose distribution to the shape of the tumour, to allow higher tumour doses to be given with no increased risk, or perhaps even a decreased risk, of normal tissue complications.

A key component of conformal radiation dose delivery is the **multileaf collimator**. Whereas until now the collimator of a therapeutic photon beam has essentially been identical to that of a diagnostic X-ray machine, with X and Y leaves that can be adjusted to create rectangular treatment fields, new collimators are composed of multiple leaflets – up to 60 on each of two sides – that allow creation of irregularly shaped photon beams that tailor the shape of the radiation dose more closely to the shape of the tumour (Figure 8.7).

Also, software used for radiation planning is undergoing extensive modification. Rather than

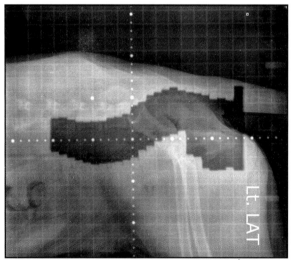

8.7 Portal radiograph of a dog being treated for an anal sac carcinoma. The treatment field, configured by a multileaf collimator, is shown superimposed on a digitally reconstructed radiograph of the caudal abdomen. The field is relatively large in the region of the primary tumour, but then becomes more conformal for treatment of regional lymph nodes, sparing the ventral colon wall and the cauda equina. Shaping a field this extensively is essentially impossible without use of a multileaf collimator. This is the same field shown in Figure 8.1.

computing the radiation dose that results from preselected radiation field shapes and sizes, as illustrated in Figure 8.1, software can now prescribe the size and shape of multiple photon beams, all configured with a multileaf collimator, and the dose to be delivered from each beam, to optimize tumour radiation dose. Thus, software has gone from a reporting tool to a prescribing tool. This type of radiation dose prescription, based on computerized iterations of treatment delivery, is called **intensity-modulated radiation therapy**. IMRT can ultimately lead to an increase in the dose delivered to the tumour with no increase, or possibly even a decrease, in the dose delivered to the normal tissue. Dose escalation using this method may lead to improved tumour control and various studies are under way testing this new dose delivery method in a variety of canine and feline tumours.

Tumour biology

Modulating the biology of the tumour to augment radiation therapy is an exciting new direction for veterinary oncology. Full discussion of this topic is beyond the scope of this chapter, but the following is a brief description of some selected approaches to sensitize tumour cells with novel anticancer therapies directed at specific molecular targets. The rapid advances in molecular oncology have offered remarkable insights into the molecular basis of biological factors that influence the response of tumour cells to radiation and can guide the modern molecular radiation oncologist to identify novel agents that can modulate tumour response to irradiation.

EGF/VEGF inhibition

A great deal of work has been directed at developing inhibitors of different components of cell signal transduction pathways and angiogenesis. Epidermal growth factor (EGF) and vascular endothelial growth factor (VEGF) signalling pathways are upregulated in many tumour types. Inhibition of EGF receptor and VEGF has been shown to be effective in increasing the radiation responsiveness of neoplastic cells both *in vitro* and in human trials. Integrating targeted therapies against the EGF receptor and angiogenesis pathways into standard radiation treatment paradigms may be beneficial for treating canine patients with tumours shown to over-express EGF receptor and VEGF.

Dose painting

There is a mounting interest in integrating biological information (factors that influence treatment outcome such as tumour proliferation and hypoxia) into radiation treatment planning for the purpose of targeting radiation-resistant regions inside the tumour. One strategy is biological image-guided dose escalation with a procedure called dose painting. Dose painting relies on non-invasive biological imaging such as positron emission tomography, functional magnetic resonance imaging and magnetic resonance spectroscopy to obtain a three-dimensional distribution of tumour factors that may influence radiation response. This is then used to guide focal dose escalation to radioresistant regions within the tumour. Image-guided biological dose escalation may significantly increase the probability of tumour control and decrease normal tissue toxicity.

Nuclear radiation therapy

Brachytherapy

Brachytherapy is the implantation of radioactive sources directly into the tissue. These sources may remain in place permanently, or be removed after a certain dose is delivered.

Brachytherapy is not discussed here in detail, as it really has no application for companion animal radiation therapy. It is only useful for treatment of small localized tumours, as the dose fall-off at the edge of the implant is very rapid. There are no sites in dogs or cats where brachytherapy is the preferred modality. This is in contrast to humans, where highly localized tumours of the prostate gland and cervix can be effectively treated using brachytherapy.

In large animals where access to a linear accelerator is problematic, and daily anaesthesia is not possible, small superficial tumours, such as incompletely resected periocular carcinomas, can be effectively treated with brachytherapy.

Internal radiotherapy

In addition to brachytherapy, internal radiotherapy can be achieved by injection of a small radioactive source that seeks out the target area.

Iodine-131

[131]Iodine is commonly used to treat thyroid cancer in people and has been successfully used for the treatment of hyperthyroidism in cats. Treatment with iodine-131 can be particularly useful for cats when there is bilateral thyroid involvement or ectopic thyroid tissue, or with the rare case of thyroid carcinoma. In one retrospective study with 524 hyperthyroid cats treated with iodine-131, overall response to treatment was considered good in 94.2% of the cats and median survival time in the cats was 2.0 years. The percentage of cats alive 1, 2, and 3 years after treatment was 89, 72, and 52%, respectively (Peterson and Becker, 1995).

Less is known about the use of iodine-131 in dogs with thyroid tumours. Results from one retrospective study suggested that iodine-131 therapy may result in prolonged survival times in dogs with non-resectable thyroid tumours, regardless of serum thyroxine concentration prior to treatment (54% of the dogs were hyperthyroid) (Turrel et al., 2006b).

Samarium-153

[153]Samarium is another isotope used in internal radiotherapy as a palliative therapy. It is effective in relieving the pain of metastatic cancer lesions to the bone in human medicine. Results from a recent study evaluating its use in 35 dogs with primary bone tumours suggest that samarium-153 lexidronam may be useful in veterinary medicine for the palliation of bone pain (Barnard et al., 2007).

Plesiotherapy

Plesiotherapy involves the direct therapeutic application of a radiation source on to an area of pathology. The use of strontium-90 (^{90}Sr) in this way has been successfully employed for treatment of superficial

feline nasal planum squamous cell carcinoma. One retrospective study evaluating 49 cats that underwent ^{90}Sr plesiotherapy reported that 98% had a response to treatment and 88% had a complete response. Reported median progression free survival time was 1,710 days (Hammond *et al.*, 2007).

Irradiation with ^{90}Sr has also been evaluated in the treatment of 54 cutaneous mast cell tumours in 35 cats. Treatment resulted in local tumour control in 53 of 54 (98%) tumours with a median follow-up time of 783 days after treatment (Turrel *et al.*, 2006a).

Lesions treated with ^{90}Sr plesiotherapy should be very superficial, since its effective treatment depth is only a couple of millimetres.

References and further reading

Al-Sarraf R, Mauldin GN, Patnaik AK *et al.* (1996) A prospective study of radiation therapy for the treatment of grade 2 mast cell tumours in 32 dogs. *Journal of Veterinary Internal Medicine* **10**, 376–378

Axlund TW, McGlasson ML and Smith AN (2002) Surgery alone or in combination with radiation therapy for treatment of intracranial meningiomas in dogs: 31 cases (1989–2002). *Journal of the American Veterinary Medical Association* **221**, 1597–1600

Barnard SM, Zuber RM and Moore AS (2007) Samarium Sm 153 lexidronam for the palliative treatment of dogs with primary bone tumours: 35 cases (1999–2005). *Journal of the American Veterinary Medical Association* **230**, 1877–1881

Beck ER, Withrow SJ, McChesney AE *et al.* (1986) Canine tongue tumours: a retrospective review of 57 cases. *Journal of the American Animal Hospital Association* **22**, 525–532

Bernstein EF, Salomon GD, Harisiadis L *et al.* (1993) Collagen gene expression and wound strength in normal and radiation-impaired wounds. *Journal of Dermatology, Surgery and Oncology* **19**, 564–570

Bley CR, Sumova A, Roos M *et al.* (2005) Irradiation of brain tumours in dogs with neurologic disease. *Journal of Veterinary Internal Medicine* **19**, 849–854

Bregazzi VS, LaRue SM, McNiel E *et al.* (2001) Treatment with a combination of doxorubicin, surgery, and radiation versus surgery and radiation alone for cats with vaccine-associated sarcomas: 25 cases (1995–2000). *Journal of the American Veterinary Medical Association* **218**, 547–550

Brooks MB, Matus RE, Leifer CE *et al.* (1988) Chemotherapy versus chemotherapy plus radiotherapy in the treatment of tonsillar squamous cell carcinoma in the dog. *Journal of Veterinary Internal Medicine* **2**, 206–211

Chaffin K and Thrall DE (2002) Results of radiation therapy in 19 dogs with cutaneous mast cell tumour and regional lymph node metastasis. *Veterinary Radiology and Ultrasound* **43**, 392–395

Ciekot PA, Powers BE, Withrow SJ *et al.* (1994) Histologically low-grade, yet biologically high-grade, fibrosarcomas of the mandible and maxilla in dogs: 25 cases (1982–1991). *Journal of the American Veterinary Medical Association* **204**, 610–615

Cohen M, Wright JC, Brawner WR *et al.* (2001) Use of surgery and electron beam irradiation, with or without chemotherapy, for treatment of vaccine-associated sarcomas in cats: 78 cases (1996–2000). *Journal of the American Veterinary Medical Association* **219**, 1582–1589

Fidel JL, Sellon RK, Houston RK *et al.* (2007) A nine-day accelerated radiation protocol for feline squamous cell carcinoma. *Veterinary Radiology and Ultrasound* **48**, 482–485

Flynn AK and Lurie DM (2007) Canine acute radiation dermatitis, a survey of current management practices in North America. *Veterinary and Comparative Oncology* **5**, 197–207

Forrest LJ, Chun R, Adams WM *et al.* (2000) Postoperative radiotherapy for canine soft tissue sarcoma. *Journal of Veterinary Internal Medicine* **14**, 578–582

Frimberger AE, Moore AS, LaRue SM *et al.* (1997) Radiotherapy of incompletely resected, moderately differentiated mast cell tumours in the dog: 37 cases (1989–1993). *Journal of the American Animal Hospital Association* **33**, 320–324

Gieger T, Rassnick K, Siegel S *et al.* (2008) Palliation of clinical signs in 48 dogs with nasal carcinomas treated with coarse-fraction radiation therapy. *Journal of the American Animal Hospital Association* **44**, 116–123

Hahn KA, King GK and Carreras JK (2004) Efficacy of radiation therapy for incompletely resected grade-III mast cell tumours in dogs: 31 cases (1987–1998). *Journal of the American Veterinary Medical Association* **224**, 79–82

Hammer A, Getzy D, Ogilvie G *et al.* (2001) Salivary gland neoplasia in the dog and cat: survival times and prognostic factors. *Journal of the American Animal Hospital Association* **37**, 478–482

Hammond GM, Gordon IK, Theon AP *et al.* (2007) Evaluation of strontium Sr 90 for the treatment of superficial squamous cell carcinoma of the nasal planum in cats: 49 cases (1990–2006). *Journal of the American Veterinary Medical Association* **231**, 736–741

Head KW, Else RW and Dubielzig RR (2002) Tumours of the alimentary tract. In: *Tumours in Domestic Animals, 4th edn*, ed. DJ Meuten, pp. 401–481. Iowa State University Press, Iowa

Jones PD, de Lorimier LP, Kitchell BE *et al.* (2003) Gemcitabine as a radiosensitizer for nonresectable feline oral squamous cell carcinoma. *Journal of the American Animal Hospital Association* **39**, 463–467

Kent MS, Bommarito D, Feldman E *et al.* (2007) Survival, neurologic response, and prognostic factors in dogs with pituitary masses treated with radiation therapy and untreated dogs. *Journal of Veterinary Internal Medicine* **21**, 1027–1033

Kobayashi T, Hauck ML, Dodge R *et al.* (2002) Preoperative radiotherapy for vaccine associated sarcoma in 92 cats. *Veterinary Radiology and Ultrasound* **43**, 473–479

LaDue TA, Dodge R, Page RL *et al.* (1999) Factors influencing survival after radiotherapy of nasal tumours in 130 dogs. *Veterinary Radiology and Ultrasound* **40**, 312–317

LaDue T, Price GS, Dodge R *et al.* (1998) Radiation therapy for incompletely resected canine mast cell tumours. *Veterinary Radiology and Ultrasound* **39**, 57–62

LaDue-Miller T, Price GS, Page RL *et al.* (1996) Radiotherapy of canine non-tonsillar squamous cell carcinoma. *Veterinary Radiology and Ultrasound* **37**, 74–77

Lana SE, Dernell WS, Lafferty MH *et al.* (2004) Use of radiation and a slow-release cisplatin formulation for treatment of canine nasal tumours. *Veterinary Radiology and Ultrasound* **45**, 577–581

Lascelles BD, Parry AT, Stidworthy MF *et al.* (2000) Squamous cell carcinoma of the nasal planum in 17 dogs. *Veterinary Record* **147**, 473–476

MacMillan R, Withrow SJ and Gillette EL (1982) Surgery and regional irradiation for treatment of canine tonsillar squamous cell carcinoma: a retrospective review of eight cases. *Journal of the American Animal Hospital Association* **18**, 311–314

Mayer MN, Greco DS and LaRue SM (2006) Outcomes of pituitary tumour irradiation in cats. *Journal of Veterinary Internal Medicine* **20**, 1151–1154

McEntee MC, Page RL, Mauldin GN *et al.* (2000) Results of irradiation of infiltrative lipoma in 13 dogs. *Veterinary Radiology and Ultrasound* **41**, 554–556

McEntee MC, Page RL, Theon AP *et al.* (2004) Malignant tumour formation in dogs previously irradiated for acanthomatous epulis. *Veterinary Radiology and Ultrasound* **45**, 357–361

McKnight JA, Mauldin GN, McEntee MC *et al.* (2000) Radiation treatment for incompletely resected soft-tissue sarcomas in dogs. *Journal of the American Veterinary Medical Association* **217**, 205–210

McLeod DA and Thrall DE (1989) The combination of surgery and radiation in the treatment of cancer. A review. *Veterinary Surgery* **18**, 1–6

Mellanby RJ, Herrtage ME and Dobson JM (2002a) Long-term outcome of eight cats with non-lymphoproliferative nasal tumours treated by megavoltage radiotherapy. *Journal of Feline Medicine and Surgery* **4**, 77–81

Mellanby RJ, Stevenson RK, Herrtage ME *et al.* (2002b) Long-term outcome of 56 dogs with nasal tumours treated with four doses of radiation at intervals of seven days. *Veterinary Record* **151**, 253–257

Melzer K, Guscetti F, Rohrer Bley C *et al.* (2006) Ki67 reactivity in nasal and periocular squamous cell carcinomas in cats treated with electron beam radiation therapy. *Journal of Veterinary Internal Medicine* **20**, 676–681

Petersen SA, Sturges BK, Dickkenson PJ *et al.* (2008) Canine intraspinal meningiomas: imaging features, histopathologic classification, and long-term outcome in 34 dogs. *Journal of Veterinary Internal Medicine* **22**, 946–953

Peterson ME and Becker DV (1995) Radioiodine treatment of 524 cats with hyperthyroidism. *Journal of the American Veterinary Medical Association* **207**, 1422–1428

Poirier VJ, Forrest LJ, Adams WM *et al.* (2004) Piroxicam, mitoxantrone, and coarse fraction radiotherapy for the treatment of transitional cell carcinoma of the bladder in 10 dogs: a pilot study. *Journal of the American Animal Hospital Association* **40**, 131–136

Postorino NC, Turrel JM and Withrow SJ (1993) Oral squamous cell carcinoma in the cat. *Journal of the American Animal Hospital Association* **29**, 438–441

Proulx DR, Ruslander DM, Dodge R *et al.* (2003) A retrospective analysis of 140 dogs with oral melanoma treated with external beam radiation. *Veterinary Radiology and Ultrasound* **44**, 352–359

Ramirez O, Dodge RK, Page RL *et al.* (1999) Palliative radiotherapy of appendicular osteosarcoma in 95 dogs. *Veterinary Radiology and Ultrasound* **40**, 517–522

Rogers KS, Helman RG and Walker MA (1995) Squamous cell carcinoma of the canine nasal planum: eight cases (1988–1994). *Journal of the American Animal Hospital Association* **31**, 373–378

Rogers KS, Walker MA and Dillon HB (1998) Transmissible venereal tumour: a retrospective study of 29 cases. *Journal of the American Animal Hospital Association* **34**, 463–470

Shiran MR, Proctor NJ, Howgate EM *et al.* (2006) Prediction of metabolic drug clearance in humans: in vitro–in vivo extrapolation vs allometric scaling. *Xenobiotica* **36**, 567–580

Siegel S, Kornegay JN and Thrall DE (1996) Postoperative irradiation of spinal cord tumours in 9 dogs. *Veterinary Radiology and Ultrasound* **37**, 150–153

Smith AN, Wright JC, Brawner WR *et al.* (2001) Radiation therapy in the treatment of canine and feline thymomas: a retrospective study (1985–1999). *Journal of the American Animal Hospital Association* **37**, 489–496

Spugnini EP, Thrall DE, Price GS *et al.* (2000) Primary irradiation of canine intracranial masses. *Veterinary Radiology and Ultrasound* **41**, 377–380

Theon AP and Feldman EC (1998) Megavoltage irradiation of pituitary macrotumours in dogs with neurologic signs. *Journal of the American Veterinary Medical Association* **213**, 225–231

Theon AP, Lecouteur RA, Carr EA *et al.* (2000) Influence of tumour cell proliferation and sex-hormone receptors on effectiveness of radiation therapy for dogs with incompletely resected meningiomas. *Journal of the American Veterinary Medical Association* **216**, 701–707

Theon AP, Madewell BR, Harb MF *et al.* (1993) Megavoltage irradiation of neoplasms of the nasal and paranasal cavities in 77 dogs. *Journal of the American Veterinary Medical Association* **202**, 1469–1475

Theon AP, Madewell BR, Shearn VI *et al.* (1995) Prognostic factors associated with radiotherapy of squamous cell carcinoma of the nasal planum in cats. *Journal of the American Veterinary Medical Association* **206**, 991–996

Theon AP, Marks SL, Feldman ES *et al.* (2000) Prognostic factors and patterns of treatment failure in dogs with unresectable differentiated thyroid carcinomas treated with megavoltage irradiation. *Journal of the American Veterinary Medical Association* **216**, 1775–1779

Theon AP, Peaston AE, Madewell BR *et al.* (1994) Irradiation of nonlymphoproliferative neoplasms of the nasal cavity and paranasal sinuses in 16 cats. *Journal of the American Veterinary Medical Association* **204**, 78–83

Theon AP, Rodriguez C, Griffy S *et al.* (1997) Analysis of prognostic factors and patterns of failure in dogs with malignant oral tumours treated with megavoltage irradiation. *Journal of the American Veterinary Medical Association* **210**, 778–784

Thrall DE (1982) Orthovoltage radiotherapy of canine transmissible venereal tumours. *Veterinary Radiology* **23**, 217–219

Thrall DE (1984) Orthovoltage radiotherapy of acanthomatous epulides in 39 dogs. *Journal of the American Veterinary Medical Association* **184**, 826–829

Thrall DE and Adams WM (1982) Radiotherapy of squamous cell carcinoma of the canine nasal plane. *Veterinary Radiology* **23**, 193–195

Thrall DE, LaRue SM, Yu D *et al.* (2005) Thermal dose is related to duration of local control in canine sarcomas treated with thermoradiotherapy. *Clinical Cancer Research* **11**, 5206–5214

Thrall DE, Prescott DM, Samulski TV *et al.* (1996) Radiation plus local hyperthermia versus radiation plus the combination of local and whole-body hyperthermia in canine sarcomas. *International Journal of Radiation Oncology, Biology and Physics* **34**, 1087–1096

Tibbs DE (1997) Wound healing following radiation therapy: a review. *Radiotherapy and Oncology* **42**, 99–106

Treister N and Sonis S (2007) Mucositis: biology and management. *Current Opinion in Otolaryngology and Head and Neck Surgery* **15**, 123–129

Turek MM, Forrest LJ, Adams WM *et al.* (2003) Postoperative radiotherapy and mitoxantrone for anal sac adenocarcinoma in the dog: 15 cases (1991–2001). *Veterinary and Comparative Oncology* **1**, 94–104

Turrel JM, Farrelly J, Page RL *et al.* (2006a) Evaluation of strontium 90 irradiation in treatment of cutaneous mast cell tumours in cats: 35 cases (1992–2002). *Journal of the American Veterinary Medical Association* **226**, 898–901

Turrel JM, McEntee MC, Burke BP *et al.* (2006b) Sodium iodide I131 treatment of dogs with nonresectable thyroid tumours: 39 cases (1990–2003). *Journal of the American Veterinary Medical Association* **229**, 542–548

Walter CU, Dernell WS, LaRue SM *et al.* (2005) Curative-intent radiation therapy as a treatment modality for appendicular and axial osteosarcoma: a preliminary retrospective evaluation of 14 dogs with the disease. *Veterinary and Comparative Oncology* **3**, 1–7

Williams LE, Gliatto JM, Dodge RK *et al.* (2003) Carcinoma of the apocrine glands of the anal sac in dogs: 113 cases (1985–1995). *Journal of the American Veterinary Medical Association* **223**, 825–831

9

Therapies of the future

Stuart C. Helfand

Introduction

Advances in molecular biology, immunology and cell biology have greatly expanded our understanding of abnormalities underlying malignancy. A clearer understanding of the subcellular and genetic derangements that lead to malignant transformation, coupled with increased awareness of the role of the tumour microenvironment, have gradually revealed an array of potential targets within cancer cells that may offer opportunities for therapeutic intervention. In contrast to the 'slash and burn' effects associated with traditional chemotherapy that interfere with DNA synthesis, mitosis, DNA integrity and protein synthesis indiscriminately, the new anticancer agents in the therapeutic pipeline are designed to exploit specific and potentially vulnerable targets within the tumour cell or microenvironment.

The discovery of proteins that mediate cellular cross-talk and intracellular signalling has helped to explain cancer cell proliferation, microenvironment interactions, metastasis, apoptosis and angiogenesis. Membrane receptors acting as switches turned on by extracellular ligands initiate complex intracellular signalling cascades that affect expression of various cellular proteins, promoting proliferation, apoptosis, or stress responses. Development of drugs that can interrupt growth signals or activate apoptotic pathways is of high priority. Some drugs have made their way to the human oncology clinic and have been highly successful, such as tyrosine kinase inhibitors (e.g. imatinib, dasatinib). Still other new approaches seek to regulate epigenetic events, such as modulating gene transcription by histone deacetylase inhibitors.

The major paradigm switch towards agents that target antigens, receptors and signalling kinases holds enormous promise. Redundant and overlapping signalling cascades offer many pivotal and hub-like targets common to multiple pathways (Figure 9.1). A

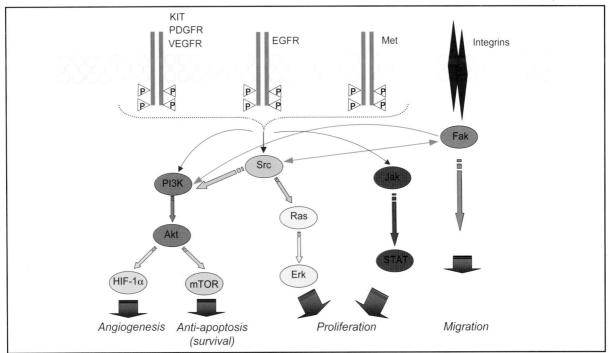

9.1 Cell signalling pathways associated with features of malignancy. This is a simplified schematic of some of the pathways used by cells that promote cell proliferation, survival, angiogenesis and migration. Receptor tyrosine kinases and membrane adhesion molecules (integrins) interact with extracellular ligands that trigger propagation of signals within the cell. Dependent downstream signalling partners ultimately activate transcription factors that affect DNA transcription and cell function. In addition to various stimulatory cascades, there are numerous inhibitors of signal transduction (not shown) that normally help to control and regulate cell function.

number of targeting strategies have been pursued. These include: small molecules that selectively bind to and block function of signalling molecules intracellularly; and monoclonal antibodies that accomplish a similar result by binding to growth factor receptors on the cell surface and compete with stimulatory ligands for access to the receptor (see Figure 9.2). Antibodies can also mediate a number of immunological functions toxic to the cancer cell (Weiner *et al.*, 2009).

A seemingly endless array of potential cancer targets has emerged, stimulating a multitude of preclinical studies examining novel targeting strategies. Universal antigens, such as telomerase (a protein that confers immortality to many types of tumour cells), can serve as an immunological target using a vaccine strategy (Beatty and Vonderheide, 2008). Other innovations have been proposed such as targeting non-neoplastic proteins within the tumour microenvironment of most malignancies. For example, targeting adhesion molecules expressed on endothelial cells of the new blood vessels within the tumour milieu, such as $\alpha_v\beta_3$ integrin (Dickerson *et al.*, 2004; Cai and Chen, 2006; Tucker, 2006; Sun *et al.*, 2009), can be anti-angiogenic as well as being a more stable target in contrast to mutating targets expressed by unstable tumour cells. Hopes for cancer immunotherapy, the ultimate form of targeting, continue to be high as a better understanding and mastery of the complexities of the immune response are revealed (Mohebtash *et al.*, 2009). Indeed, veterinary medicine was the first to bring a commercial cancer vaccine to the oncology clinic (Bergman *et al.*, 2003, 2006).

Ultimately, it is likely that truly successful cancer therapy will employ combinations of strategies that maximize synergistic effects. Learning what they may look like will require a rigorous methodical process as the practice of veterinary oncology gains a solid understanding of how individual drugs work, what can be expected from them, and what are the clinically relevant toxicities.

The challenge to veterinary oncology

There is great enthusiasm for developing targeted therapy for the treatment of human cancer patients and excitement also runs high in veterinary oncology. However, veterinary oncology faces unique challenges that may ultimately limit the use of new strategies in veterinary cancer patients.

Not the least of these is the high cost associated with new drug development. Development costs ultimately passed on to consumers may be prohibitive for pet owners. This problem is complicated by the relative paucity of biotechnology companies dedicated to development of new oncology drugs for the veterinary market. Given their likely expense, new agents must meet expectations to maintain enthusiasm for continued development. Thus, a modicum of caution is warranted as we embark on a new era of cancer treatment.

Furthermore, there has always been a tendency to extrapolate new developments for human health directly into veterinary practice. While chemotherapeutic agents have for the most part been amenable to this way of thinking, targeted agents need to be subjected to rigorous confirmation that comparable targets are present in animal cancers and drugs bind to targets that are effective at clinically achievable concentrations. It may not be appropriate to prescribe new, expensive and potentially toxic agents for pet animals until preclinical validation is confirmed. For example, rituximab, a monoclonal antibody of tremendous benefit for the treatment of human B-cell lymphoma, has no role in veterinary clinical oncology because it does not recognize a comparable epitope of the CD20 target in canine lymphoma (Jubala *et al.*, 2005; Impellizeri *et al.*, 2006).

However, veterinary oncology may benefit from a 'coat tails' effect due to an overflow of novel ideas associated with robust development efforts in human oncology. The development of agents that block signal transduction mediated by tyrosine kinases is the best example and the introduction of tyrosine kinase inhibitors to veterinary oncology signals the dawn of a new day in cancer therapeutics for pet animals.

Tyrosine kinase inhibitors

Nearly 100 tyrosine kinases have been identified in the human kinome. It is likely that a similar number exists in veterinary species. These proteins are responsible for transmitting signals from the extracellular environment, starting with the activation of receptor tyrosine kinases that span the cell membrane (Figure 9.2). These in turn transduce signals intracellularly to trigger activation of cytoplasmic tyrosine kinases along vertical and horizontal axes within the cell. Signals are purposeful and control gene expression that promotes growth, survival, angiogenesis and motility (see Figure 9.1).

Activation confers conformational change associated with phosphorylation of tyrosine residues in the kinase domain that activate downstream signalling partners in a cascading chain reaction. In health, ligands bind specifically to their unique receptors and initiate the signalling cascade.

Activating mutations imparting gain-of-function to tyrosine kinases have now been recognized in numerous malignancies and comprise a steadily expanding group of dysregulated kinases regarded as the 'cancer kinome' that can be targeted individually and collectively. The prototypical cancer tyrosine kinase is the illegitimate bcr-abl fusion protein associated with chronic myelogenous leukaemia in humans (Ben-Neriah *et al.*, 1986). This kinase is constantly activated and is responsible for uncontrolled triggering of proliferation signals.

Canine mast cell tumours: c-kit mutations and KIT targeting

Targeting tyrosine kinases

Imatinib, developed and validated as an effective drug for human chronic myelogenous leukaemia patients (Druker *et al.*, 2006), was the first tyrosine kinase inhibitor to enter clinical practice and represented a milestone in cancer therapy. This drug competes with adenosine triphosphate (ATP) for the phosphorylation-binding pocket in the bcr-abl kinase

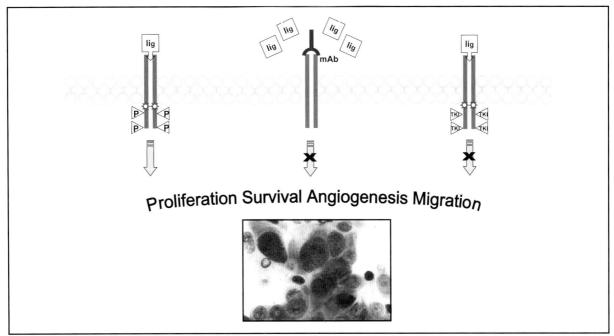

9.2 Targeting tyrosine kinases in malignancy. Over-expression of receptor tyrosine kinases on the cell surface can result in excessive stimulation when ligand (lig) in the extracellular environment binds and activates (i.e. phosphorylates, P) large numbers of receptors that in turn promote cell growth and malignant behaviour (left). Alternatively, activating mutations in the regulatory juxtamembrane domain (red/white star, left) account for autophosphorylation of the receptor's cytoplasmic kinase domain (P), independent of external ligand binding, resulting in continuous intracellular signalling stimulatory to growth. Monoclonal antibody (mAb) that specifically binds to the receptor's extracellular domain can block ligand binding by competitive inhibition and extinguish generation of stimulatory signals (centre). Small molecules (tyrosine kinase inhibitors, TKI) that compete for the ATP binding pocket in the receptor's cytoplasmic domain suppress downstream signalling by preventing receptor phosphorylation (right).

domain, thereby interrupting constitutive signals originating from this kinase. Imatinib also proved to be effective in suppressing several other mutated tyrosine kinases in human cancer, including in gastrointestinal stromal tumours (GIST) (Dematteo *et al.*, 2009). A mutation in canine chronic myelogenous leukaemia comparable to bcr-abl in human leukaemia has been recognized in veterinary medicine, suggesting that similar opportunities with tyrosine kinase inhibitors are of emerging importance in veterinary oncology (Breen and Modiano, 2008).

To this end, activating mutations in the receptor tyrosine kinase c-kit have been extensively investigated in malignant canine mast cells. Since expression of c-kit by malignant canine mast cells was first reported (London *et al.*, 1996), a repeatable pattern of mutations in exons 11 and 12 of canine c-kit in malignant mast cells has been demonstrated (London *et al.*, 1999). Mutations comprising repeats of small stretches of DNA (internal tandem duplications) within the negative regulatory coding region of the c-kit juxtamembrane domain have been most commonly reported. c-kit juxtamembrane mutations confer gain-of-function activity resulting in constitutive KIT phosphorylation in the absence of ligand binding. Additional sites of KIT mutation associated with gain-of-function have been described in exons 8 and 9 in canine mast cell tumours (MCTs) (Letard *et al.*, 2008). KIT activation (i.e. phosphorylation) is an early event in the propagation of intracellular signalling that culminates in DNA replication and cell division.

The revelation of ligand-independent KIT autophosphorylation in canine mast cell c-kit mutants has not only shed light on the pathogenesis of canine mast cell cancer, but has also laid the foundation for rationally designed targeted drug therapy with tyrosine kinase inhibitors that specifically block KIT phosphorylation.

Toceranib

The attractiveness of targeting c-kit in canine MCTs was further substantiated by demonstration of activated KIT *in vivo* in canine MCTs and the capacity of a novel tyrosine kinase inhibitor, SU11654, to inhibit KIT phosphorylation *in vivo* in the tumour-bearing dogs (Pryer *et al.*, 2003).

Coincident with this study, a phase I trial was conducted in dogs with various malignancies with SU11654 (London *et al.*, 2003), which is an indolinone purported to inhibit activation of a group of structurally related receptor tyrosine kinases, including KIT, platelet-derived growth factor receptor (PDGFR), vascular endothelial growth factor receptor (VEGFR) and fibroblast growth factor receptor (FGFR), by competitive inhibition of ATP binding to each receptor's catalytic domain within the cytoplasm.

This trial provided useful clues that tyrosine kinase inhibitor treatment of dogs with MCTs, especially those bearing the juxtamembrane KIT mutation, can arrest tumour growth and induce clinically meaningful remission (i.e. 9 of 11 dogs) at clinically achievable doses with only modest toxicity. Dogs with MCTs lacking c-kit mutations showed a lower response rate (2 of 11 dogs). In addition, responses of metastatic carcinoma and sarcoma were documented in a small number of treated dogs, notably complete resolution of pulmonary metastases.

The preclinical studies of SU11654 culminated in 2009 following a large field trial of the drug (London *et al.*, 2009), with the launch of Palladia® (toceranib phosphate, formerly known as SU11654, Pfizer Animal Health). This product heralded a new era in veterinary oncology and represents another milestone in how (mast cell) cancer will be treated in veterinary oncology.

Responses of c-kit mutant negative tumours, though not as robust as mutants, has been attributed to drug effects on the tumour microenvironment, specifically suppression of angiogenesis through interruption of VEGFR-2 and PDGFR-β signalling by angiogenic endothelial cells recruited in response to tumour stimuli. Alternative explanations could be direct inhibition of signalling triggered by activating mutations in exons 8 or 9 (Letard *et al.*, 2008) that were not reported as part of the study. The overall biological response rate (i.e. complete responders, partial responders, stable disease) was 60%.

With more clinical experience, it will be interesting to see the role for toceranib in the management of canine cancer as it will likely have value in a variety of tumours. For example, toceranib appears active against canine GIST when juxtamembrane domain c-kit mutations are present (CA London, 2009, personal communication) and the results of the phase I trial support continued investigation of efficacy in canine soft tissue sarcoma and mammary carcinoma.

Masitinib

Masitinib mesylate, another newly available competitive inhibitor of KIT, has shown efficacy in mediating biological effects that slowed growth of canine MCTs and improved survival time of dogs with grade II and III tumours (Hahn *et al.*, 2008). Its benefit to dogs with non-resectable tumours has been documented: dogs with MCTs expressing KIT mutations lived more than twice as long as did placebo-treated dogs bearing MCTs with KIT mutations (417 vs. 242 days) when masitinib was administered as first-line therapy. There was a significant prolongation in the time to tumour progression compared with placebo when masitinib was given to dogs with MCTs as the initial treatment (175 vs. 78 days) (Hahn *et al.*, 2008). This benefit was observed independently of the mutational status of KIT amongst MCTs, suggesting, as observed with toceranib, that masitinib impacts on the tumour's extracellular microenvironment.

Masitinib has received approval in Europe (by the European Medicines Agency, Masivet, AB Science). At the time of this writing, it is nearing approval in the United States (Kinavet, AB Science) for use in dogs with grade II and III MCTs. The same drug is under development for various human cancers as well. For example, masitinib exhibited greater *in vitro* activity and selectivity than imatinib for human wild-type GIST as well as GIST with KIT mutations in the juxtamembrane region (Bui *et al.*, 2007).

Masitinib should provide veterinary oncology with a unique perspective in that it is one of few (perhaps the only) tyrosine kinase inhibitors to date to be marketed both for human and canine cancer patients. Given the improvement in tumour control in dogs with MCTs treated with masitinib as first-line therapy, veterinary oncology is fortunate to acquire two new tyrosine kinase inhibitors with which to treat canine MCTs that are not curable with surgery alone. Furthermore, although masitinib's patent claim is as a KIT inhibitor, developers of this drug have presented data supporting activity of masitinib against several other tyrosine kinases, including PDGFR.

Future use of KIT inhibitors

Another study documented a benefit of imatinib in the treatment of canine MCTs (Isotani *et al.*, 2008); and its potential to control mastocytosis in human patients has been described (Droogendijk *et al.*, 2006). As was seen with masitinib and toceranib, responses were greater in dogs with KIT mutations in exon 11, though the authors observed objective responses to imatinib by tumours lacking KIT mutations in exon 11 (Isotani *et al.*, 2008). Taken together, a benefit of KIT inhibitors for the treatment of canine MCTs has clearly been established, making future use of these drugs a welcome addition to the therapeutic toolbox for mast cell cancer in dogs. Hopefully, these agents will live up to expectations as more experience is gained with them either singly or in combination with chemotherapeutic agents.

Feline mast cell tumours

Compared with canine mast cell cancer, there are far fewer studies documenting KIT juxtamembrane mutations in feline MCTs. An earlier study did not find activating c-kit mutations in malignant feline mast cells comprising the neoplastic infiltrates of excised spleens from cats with splenic mastocytosis (Dank *et al.*, 2002). Nevertheless, a role for tyrosine kinase inhibitors in treating feline cancer is likely and a c-kit internal tandem duplication associated with systemic mast cell cancer in a cat has been described (Isotani *et al.*, 2006). Seemingly this mutation, located within the fifth immunoglobulin-like domain of c-kit, induced cellular activation (and proliferation) as the affected cat reportedly experienced complete resolution of clinically detectable tumour in response to treatment with imatinib (Isotani *et al.*, 2006). Results of a small phase I trial of imatinib in cats with various malignancies reported low toxicity, but the one cat with mast cell cancer in this report did not respond to treatment (Lachowicz *et al.*, 2005). The role of KIT inhibition in management of feline MCTs awaits further clarification but, given the report by Isotani *et al.* (2006), it seems likely that some cats will benefit from KIT inhibitors.

Platelet-derived growth factor receptor-beta (PDGFR-β)

PDGFR-β, another receptor tyrosine kinase, structurally related to KIT, appears to be involved in the malignant transformation of feline injection site sarcoma (feline ISS). Inhibition of PDGFR-β signalling by tyrosine kinase inhibitors may represent a novel treatment option for this malignancy. Specifically, drugs such as imatinib, toceranib and masitinib are competitive inhibitors of ATP binding to the activation sites of the split receptor tyrosine kinase family, which includes KIT, PDGFR-β, and VEGFR-2.

As mentioned earlier, one proposed explanation for clinical improvement of MCTs negative for activating KIT mutations is suppression of PDGFR-β signalling in angiogenic endothelial cells within the tumour microenvironment by tyrosine kinase inhibitors. PDGFR-β is a signalling molecule widely expressed by mesenchymal cells (Heldin and Westermark, 1999) and, not unexpectedly, it is highly expressed by the malignant fibroblasts comprising the sarcoma (Hendrick, 1999). The anti-PDGFR-β activity of imatinib appears to inhibit the constitutive phosphorylation of PDGFR-β in cultured feline ISS cell lines (Katayama *et al.*, 2004). Furthermore, imatinib was capable of suppressing *in vitro* growth of feline ISS, presumably due to interruption of mitogenic PDGFR-β signal transduction; the effect was best demonstrated when imatinib was combined with traditional chemotherapeutic agents (i.e. doxorubicin, carboplatin) (Katayama *et al.*, 2004) giving clues to its optimal usage in clinically affected cats.

Epidermal growth factor receptor (EGFR)

Opportunities abound for developing tyrosine kinase inhibitors for veterinary patients. Targeting signal transduction pathways is a unifying strategy for many cancers; and as more abnormalities are identified in these proteins in cancer cells, expanded interest in use of specifically targeted tyrosine kinase inhibitors can be expected.

As an example, feline oral squamous cell carcinoma, the most common oral malignancy in the cat, remains a highly aggressive infiltrative neoplasm that is not easily eradicated despite radical surgical intervention and radiation therapy (Northrup *et al.*, 2006; Fidel *et al.*, 2007). The identification of EGFR, another receptor tyrosine kinase, on feline oral squamous cell carcinoma (SCC) biopsy samples (Looper *et al.*, 2006), provides a compelling rationale to evaluate inhibitors of EGFR signalling in this tumour. In humans with head and neck squamous cell carcinoma, the tyrosine kinase inhibitor erlotinib (Tarceva®, Genentech/OSI in the US, Roche elsewhere) has shown efficacy in preclinical studies (Chinnaiyan *et al.*, 2005; Ahmed and Cohen, 2007; Thomas *et al.*, 2007).

Because it has been difficult to demonstrate EGFR activating mutations in these patients (Lemos-González *et al.*, 2007), the role of tyrosine kinase inhibitors in the management of this cancer is uncertain since the greatest effect of these drugs is usually seen in tumours with constitutive kinase activation secondary to mutation. However, overexpression of EGFR in human head and neck SCC also leads to oncogenesis due to ligand hyperstimulation of receptors that trigger mitogenic responses (Sun *et al.*, 2009). As shown in Figure 9.2, monoclonal antibodies that compete with ligand for binding to the extracellular domain of receptor tyrosine kinases provide an alternative strategy to inhibit signalling.

Cetuximab

Cetuximab (Erbitux®, ImClone Systems Incorporated, also known as C225) is a humanized murine IgG1 monoclonal antibody that binds to the extracellular domain of human EGFR. It has been approved for treatment of human head and neck SCC in combination with radiotherapy for advanced tumours and as a single agent for incurable recurrent/metastatic disease (Mehra *et al.*, 2008; Harari *et al.*, 2009). Importantly, its effectiveness is independent of mutational status of EGFR. This may be due in part to an antibody-dependent cellular cytotoxicity (ADCC) mechanism mediated by natural killer cells binding to antibody attached to the EGFR (López-Albaitero *et al.*, 2009).

The author and colleagues examined binding of cetuximab to archived feline oral SCC biopsy samples. Immunohistochemical staining revealed strong binding of cetuximab to three of three separate feline oral SCC biopsy samples (Figure 9.3), indicating the

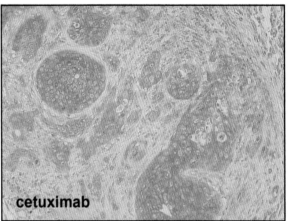
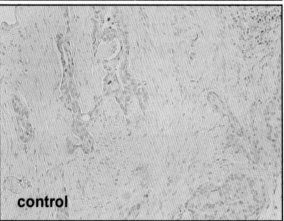

9.3 Feline oral SCCs express EGFR. Positively staining feline SCC cells from the oral cavity appear brown (left) after binding cetuximab, a monoclonal antibody that recognizes EFGR. An irrelevant antibody was used on the control tissue (right), followed by the reagents needed to generate the brown colour (immunoperoxidase methodology). Control tissues were counterstained with haematoxylin. Widespread EGFR expression by feline oral SCC, demonstrated by strong cetuximab binding, suggests a possible role for cetuximab in the treatment of cats with this malignancy. Humans with oral SCC are routinely treated with the combination of cetuximab and radiation therapy. (Immunohistochemistry kindly provided by Eric Armstrong in the laboratory of Dr Paul Harari, University of Wisconsin-Madison, Madison, Wisconsin)

potential to use this antibody in cats. Whether antibody binding is sufficient to block EGF binding is unknown and the ability of feline Fc receptors to trigger cytotoxic responses in natural killer cells by binding a human Fc end present in cetuximab awaits clarification. Canine natural killer cells mediate potent ADCC with a chimerized antibody (i.e. human Fc end) (Helfand *et al.*, 1994) and so perhaps feline cells can too.

Hepatocyte growth factor (HGF) and c-Met

It is likely that tyrosine kinase inhibitors will be used for other tumours in veterinary oncology as more of the intricacies of signal transduction and the proto-oncogenes that encode signalling molecules are revealed. In the future, there will likely be efforts to inhibit signalling through c-Met, a receptor tyrosine kinase activated by hepatocyte growth factor (HGF) binding ligand that has been implicated in human head and neck SCC (Seiwert *et al.*, 2009) and various other carcinomas. A functional germ line mutation in canine Met that has been described in Rottweilers may contribute to tumorigenesis in this breed (Liao *et al.*, 2006), providing a rationale to explore Met targeting in this breed. The potential for a Met/HGF autophosphorylation loop has been shown for a number of cultured canine cancer cell lines and a tyrosine kinase inhibitor partially blocked phosphorylation of key signalling molecules, function and proliferation of osteosarcoma and melanoma cells *in vitro* (Liao *et al.*, 2005). The author's laboratory has been interested in the role of tyrosine kinase abnormalities in canine haemangiosarcoma; preliminary data suggest that there will be an opportunity to impact on this cancer with tyrosine kinase inhibitors.

A note of caution

Compared with human oncology, veterinary oncology has yet to gain extensive experience with tyrosine kinase inhibitor therapeutics. While the promise of this approach is obvious, the other part of the story deals with development of resistance. Though stunning improvements with tyrosine kinase inhibitor strategies have been reported in humans with leukaemia, head and neck SCC and breast cancer, to name a few, drug resistance is often seen with chronic treatment. This reflects the addiction of cancer cells to utilize alternative kinase signalling pathways in promoting cell growth and survival (Benavente *et al.*, 2009). Overcoming resistance to tyrosine kinase inhibitors will be one of the biggest challenges for these agents to meet their full potential.

Immunotherapy

The dream of enlisting the patient's immune system to help to fight cancer has never gone away. Harnessing the body's own immune defences for cancer cell surveillance and annihilation is the most targeted form of therapy. In addition to being highly selective for their targets, immune cells circulate and are long-lived; thus the sustained interest in focusing these responses against cancer cells. There remains a common belief that 'the immune system can be trained to recognize cancer as being something foreign and dangerous' (Wolchok, 2007).

The overriding challenge in 'training' the immune system to recognize and mount anti-tumour responses is the need to break immune tolerance. Furthermore, it is not enough for the immune system merely to recognize tumour cells; the immune response needs to trigger cytotoxicity of clinical significance to be of value to cancer patients.

During the ontogeny of the T-cell repertoire, primitive T lymphocytes that exhibit the capacity to recognize self antigens are carefully deleted to prevent autoimmune tissue destruction. With the exception of some viral-induced tumours, cancer cells are usually immunologically indistinguishable from normal tissue and so effective cancer immunotherapy seemingly goes against the natural order of immune function. Malignant cells, however, may over-express antigens compared with normal counterparts, providing a potential therapeutic window for immune intervention.

The immune system is basically composed of immune cells, antibodies, antigens and regulators and so strategies to manipulate immune responses need to work through these compartments. Just what are the most effective approaches is still an unanswered question. No simple means for identification of antigens that can be targeted in cancer cells has emerged. Which immune cells should be stimulated, how to provide stimulatory signals, and how immunostimulatory factors are best delivered remain some of the major questions in cancer immunotherapy. Despite the challenges, continually expanding knowledge of the workings of the immune system present novel opportunities for immune intervention. While the immune system can mediate powerful responses to cancer, responses are limited by the finite nature of the immune system – implying that immunotherapy may be most effective in the minimal residual disease setting.

Cancer vaccines

Whereas earlier immunotherapy approaches focused on providing more T-cell help in the form of exogenously administered cytokines or non-specific activators of tumoricidal macrophages, there is now more emphasis on developing cancer 'vaccines' that help the immune system to recognize tumour cells in the face of disease. Traditional vaccines used in veterinary medicine are intended to prevent infectious disease by stimulating immune responses to immunizing antigens associated with a pathogen prior to infection. Cancer vaccines differ in that they are given after a cancer diagnosis, but they are similar in regard to the goal of eliciting a specific immune response.

Antigen presentation

Antigen presentation initiates the immune response and a number of novel approaches designed to isolate, activate and prime antigen-presenting cells (APCs) (e.g. dendritic cells, B-cells) with tumour antigen have been described in the veterinary literature (Figure 9.4).

Strategy	Goal	Method	References
Vaccine	Provide tumour antigen	Allotumour cell vaccine	U'Ren et al. (2007)
		Xenotumour vaccine (melanoma, cDNA)	Bergman et al. (2003)
Cell therapy	Antigen-presenting cells (dendritic cells (DCs), B-lymphocytes)	Adeno-DC melanoma (xenoantigen-loaded antigen-presenting cells)	Gyorffy et al. (2005)
		Ex vivo DC culture	Catchpole et al. (2002); Wang et al. (2007)
		DC–allotumour fusion	Bird et al. (2008)
		Tumour RNA-transfected CD40-activated B-cells	Mason et al. (2008)
Humoral	Target immunodominant tumour antigens	Single-chain fragment variable targeting systems (haemangiosarcoma)	Mason (2009, personal communication)
Reverse endogenous suppressed anti-tumour immunity	Deplete regulatory T-lymphocytes (Tregs)	Metronomic chemotherapy	Elmslie et al. (2008)
		CD25$^+$CD4$^+$FoxP3$^+$ T-lymphocyte depletion	Biller et al. (2007); O'Neill et al. (2009)

9.4 Immunotherapy approaches of interest in veterinary oncology.

Immune responses triggered by APCs offer the potential of a holistic, physiological immune response that can engage a variety of effector mechanisms. Recruiting APCs as a means to induce anti-tumour response offers promise and is an area of great interest in human cancer immunotherapy.

One distinct drawback to this type of cell therapy is the need to generate large numbers of autologous dendritic or other APCs in the laboratory, which can be laborious, time consuming and expensive. The approaches of Bird et al. (2008) and Mason et al. (2008) are noteworthy for their use of allogeneic established cell lines derived from malignant APCs so that the problem of autologous cell expansion was avoided. Mason et al. actually used a genetically modified xenogeneic (human) B-cell line to present antigen. Both studies documented in vivo generation of tumour antigen-specific T-cell immune responses in dogs (normal and tumour-bearing) following immunization with the respective APCs that had been modified to present tumour antigen. While these results are encouraging, demonstration of in vivo anti-tumour activity or improved survival time in tumour-bearing dogs given APC therapy has yet to be reported.

Melanoma vaccine
In 2007, the commercial release of a cDNA melanoma vaccine for dogs marked a new era in veterinary immuno-oncology. This is a milestone because it was the first licensed cancer vaccine for any species and employs a cutting-edge gene transfer strategy to stimulate an immune response. This is a xeno-vaccine, because it contains cDNA that codes for human tyrosinase, an enzyme present in pigmented cells that is needed for melanin synthesis. Expression of human tyrosinase by dog cells produces a protein foreign to the canine immune system that can stimulate anti-tyrosinase immunoreactivity. Immune responses to the foreign (xenogeneic) tyrosinase have the potential to elicit a bystander effect against endogenous canine tyrosinase associated with the dog's melanoma cells. The vaccine can be effective against metastasis when given to appropriate-stage dogs with oral melanoma; complete local control of oral malignant melanoma is recommended before vaccine administration.

This is a sophisticated approach to melanoma immunotherapy in the dog, but it is only a beginning because not all dogs benefit from it (even those with the appropriate clinical stage melanoma) and the need to obtain local control first significantly adds to cost and morbidity. Perhaps future modifications of the approach may also contain immunostimulatory genes that can provide additional help to responding dendritic cells and T-cells, enhancing the anti-melanoma immune response.

Regulatory T-cells (Tregs)
The recent report of increased numbers of regulatory T-cells (Tregs) in canine cancer patients (O'Neill et al., 2009) promises to be a discovery that will likely impact on immunotherapy in dogs. Tregs are immunomodulatory, ostensibly promoting self-tolerance by acting as negative regulators of immune responses and inflammation (Lu and Rudensky, 2009). Increased numbers of Tregs in the tumour microenvironment can be deleterious by hindering development of an effective anti-tumour immune response (Beyer and Schultze 2009).

Therapeutic targeting of Tregs provides an opportunity to significantly improve the effectiveness of anti-tumour immune responses (Banham and Pulford, 2009; Zhang et al., 2009). This effect was shown in several animal models that demonstrated enhancement of the Th1 cell-mediated anti-tumour immune response and improved survival time in tumour-bearing animals when Tregs were targeted (Nair et al., 2007; Banham and Pulford, 2009). As more information about Tregs in animals becomes available, strategies to deplete these cells in veterinary cancer patients seem likely, as this is a novel and promising idea.

Photodynamic therapy

Photodynamic therapy has been on the fringes of veterinary oncology for 20 years. It is a very specialized form of cancer treatment that employs both physical (i.e. laser energy) and chemical means (i.e. photosensitizing drugs) to elicit tumoricidal effects. The specialized nature of this modality has likely contributed to its limited accessibility and intermittent advances in veterinary medicine. Yet, in the right situations, results can be dramatic for superficial tumours that are readily accessible to laser irradiation.

In photodynamic therapy, a photosensitizing chemical (e.g. porphyrin precursor or other photosensitizer) is administered (intravenously, orally, or topically) and laser light of an appropriate wavelength that is excitatory to the photosensitizer is directed on to the tumour. Growing neoplastic cells accumulate more porphyrins than normal tissue, providing a therapeutic window. Porphyrin excitation by laser light generates reactive oxygen species and free radicals that damage intracellular organelles and triggers apoptosis. It also induces anti-angiogenic and immunomodulatory effects (Ortner, 2009). Issues pertaining to optimizing photosensitization agents, route of photosensitizer administration, depth of penetration of laser energy, timing of laser excitation and access to tissue present the important challenges to development of this modality.

Superficial tumours, especially those of the skin, obviously lend themselves more readily to photodynamic therapy, given the easy access for laser irradiation. In cats with solar-induced SCC of the nasal planum, for example, responses have been impressive although relapses are common, probably due to inadequacy of exposure of deeply seated tumour cells to surface laser treatment. One report indicated a remarkable 96% response rate of cats with nasal planum SCC to photodynamic therapy and most were considered complete clinical remissions (Bexfield et al., 2008). Early relapses were a problem, however, as the median remission time was reported to be 157 days. Highly invasive tumours are reportedly far less responsive (Ferreira et al., 2009). Newer photosensitizing agents may provide better results (Buchholz et al., 2007).

There is increasing interest in the use of photodynamic therapy for tumours that may require surgical access for directing the laser light on to the tumour. For example, several recent reports support the use of intraoperative photodynamic therapy for treatment of the canine prostate (Lucroy et al., 2003a; Huang et al., 2005; Moore et al., 2008), and the potential for treatment of canine bladder cancer has also attracted attention (Lucroy et al., 2003b). Several investigators reported positive results using photodynamic therapy for the treatment of canine nasal tumours (Lucroy et al., 2003c; Osaki et al., 2009).

As the veterinary profession gains more experience with photodynamic therapy, it is a niche modality that may evolve into a valuable adjunct to traditional therapy. It is particularly appealing for non-resectable tumours that cannot be irradiated or managed effectively by other means. Although the costs of laser instrumentation and photosensitizers are not inconsequential, photodynamic therapy may one day find a role as an alternative for radiotherapy for some cancers in veterinary oncology.

Other novel approaches

There are many other interesting novel approaches under investigation, too many to elaborate here but some are attracting attention for veterinary oncology and several are mentioned here for completeness. They represent a broad range of strategies, each intended to take advantage of a potentially vulnerable target in cancer cells or to correct a known oncogenic transformation.

Mammalian target of rapamycin (mTOR)

Figure 9.1 (see earlier) is a greatly simplified schematic of some signalling pathways used by cells for survival, growth, and proliferation. Of considerable interest as a target is the PI3kinase/Akt/mTOR axis. This is a complex pathway that interacts with other signalling cascades and is important for cellular regulation of growth and metabolism. The pathway is activated in a variety of cancers. Inhibitors of mTOR (mammalian target of rapamycin) are in various phase I/II trials for various human cancers. Several reports in the veterinary literature suggest that targeting mTOR may be important in some canine cancers (Gordon et al., 2008; Kent et al., 2009). Given the association of the PI3kinase/Akt/mTOR pathway with so many human cancers and its apparent involvement in canine cancer, mTOR targeting (as well as PI3 kinase and Akt targeting) appears to offer an important opportunity for development of new effective therapies in veterinary oncology and bears following.

Histone deacetylase

Interest in histone deacetylase (HDAC) inhibitors in veterinary medicine was sparked following a case report of long-term survival of a dog with splenic haemangiosarcoma treated with the HDAC inhibitor suberoylanilide hydroxamic acid (SAHA, also known as vorinostat, Zolinza) (Cohen et al., 2004). Histones are integral to the supercoiling of DNA and acetyl groups on histones help the DNA wrapped around them to be accessible to transcription factors and DNA reading enzymes; decreased acetylation results in DNA that is overly wound and cannot uncoil to be read. Excessive, unregulated histone deacetylation in cancer cells hinders transcription of important regulatory genes, some of which are thought to code for proteins that inhibit cell growth (i.e. tumour suppressor genes). Development of HDAC inhibitors continues to be a priority in human oncology, especially since vorinostat was approved for treatment of human cutaneous T-cell lymphoma in 2007 (Mann et al., 2007). Preclinical studies in the dog suggest that HDAC inhibitors may be useful in various cancers (Kisseberth et al., 2008).

Angiogenesis

Angiogenesis is the formation of new blood vessels from existing ones and its inhibition is a goal of contemporary cancer therapy. Tumour cells play an active role in providing the stimuli that mature endothelial cells require to become mitogenically active and generate tumour neovasculature. While some drugs are specifically developed to inhibit angiogenesis as their primary function, others mediate anti-angiogenic effects in combination with additional activities. For example, HDAC inhibitors have shown anti-angiogenic activity by altering patterns of gene expression to favour an anti-angiogenic effect (Liang et al., 2006). Likewise, receptor tyrosine kinase inhibitors reportedly mediate anti-angiogenic effects by suppressing PDGFR and VEGFR signal transduction that is stimulatory to angiogenesis. There are also beginning to be studies in veterinary medicine of agents specifically developed for anti-angiogenic activity, such as thrombospondin analogues (Rusk et al., 2006a,b).

Transcriptional gene silencing

Transcriptional gene silencing due to DNA hypermethylation has emerged as an important target in oncology and has become of interest in veterinary oncology (Bryan et al., 2008). Structural changes to certain DNA nucleotides, e.g. methylation of cytosines, that are otherwise present in an unmutated DNA sequence can result in gene silencing and can be an important cause of cancer. As more is learned about this, correcting transforming epigenetic events in cancer, such as that documented in canine lymphoma (Bryan et al., 2008) will likely become an important focus of future therapy.

Heat shock proteins

Heat shock proteins (molecular chaperones that protect and shuttle various cellular proteins within the cell) have been recognized as vulnerable targets in malignancy. Incapacitating heat shock proteins can have a ripple effect and can be a means to suppress function of transported client proteins important in cancer. For example, some oncogenic mutant forms of KIT in malignant canine mast cells that are resistant to tyrosine kinase inhibitors can be suppressed by targeting a KIT-associated heat shock protein, Hsp90, that results in proteasomal degradation of the oncogenic KIT client protein, causing cell growth inhibition and apoptosis (Lin et al., 2008). Recent in vitro studies of canine osteosarcoma demonstrated effectiveness of a heat shock protein inhibitor against canine osteosarcoma growth and it was highly effective in causing tumour regression in a canine osteosarcoma xenograft model (McCleese et al., 2009). This field is rapidly growing in human oncology and is likely to take on more importance in veterinary oncology.

Apoptosis

One final interesting idea worth mentioning is the development of approaches that directly serve as apoptotic cell triggers. While apoptosis is a terminal event in many cancer strategies, several are being examined for the capacity to directly activate cellular death domains such as that triggered by the interaction of Fas ligand (FasL) with endogenous Fas.

Impressive results were reported in dogs with oral melanoma given FasL by intratumoral injection (Bianco et al., 2003). The convenience of direct injection into accessible tumours is attractive, but novel delivery methods, such as use of adenovirus, could extend utility of the concept. Kolluri et al. (2008) described the potential to use a derivative of the anti-apoptotic protein, Bcl-2, to turn Bcl-2 into a proapoptotic trigger. Converting a powerful anti-apoptotic protein such as Bcl-2, considered the 'antidote to apoptosis' (Hockenbery et al., 1991), into a cellular death trigger is a highly innovative concept, given that many tumours ensure their longevity by upregulation of Bcl-2.

Conclusion

Advances in molecular biology, immunology and cellular techniques have resulted in rapid proliferation of potential targets for cancer therapy. The willingness of pharmaceutical companies to develop some novel drug concepts into clinically available medicines for the treatment of cancer in pet animals is a giant step forward for veterinary oncology. Despite exciting preclinical data, validation of new agents must come from thoughtfully designed clinical trials in veterinary cancer patients. In the future, we can expect to witness availability of not only more drugs against validated targets but also drugs that are the result of discoveries that today can only be imagined.

References and further reading

Ahmed SM and Cohen EE (2007) Treatment of squamous cell carcinoma of the head and neck in the metastatic and refractory settings: advances in chemotherapy and the emergence of small molecule epidermal growth factor receptor kinase inhibitors. Current Cancer Drug Targets **7**, 666–673

Banham AH and Pulford K (2009) Therapeutic targeting of FOXP3-positive regulatory T cells using a FOXP3 peptide vaccine WO2008081581. Expert Opinion on Therapeutic Patents **19**, 1023–1028

Beatty GL and Vonderheide RH (2008) Telomerase as a universal tumor antigen for cancer vaccines Expert Review of Vaccines **7**, 881–887

Ben-Neriah Y, Daley GQ, Mes-Masson AM et al. (1986) The chronic myelogenous leukemia-specific P210 protein is the product of the bcr/abl hybrid gene. Science **233**, 212–214

Benavente S, Huang S, Armstrong EA et al. (2009) Establishment and characterization of a model of acquired resistance to epidermal growth factor receptor targeting agents in human cancer cells. Clinical Cancer Research **15**, 1585–1592

Bergman PJ, Camps-Palau MA, McKnight, JA et al. (2006) Development of a xenogeneic DNA vaccine program for canine malignant melanoma at the Animal Medical Center. Vaccine **24**, 4582–4585

Bergman PJ, McKnight J, Novosad A et al. (2003) Long-term survival of dogs with advanced malignant melanoma after DNA vaccination with xenogeneic human tyrosinase: a phase I trial. Clinical Cancer Research **9**, 1284–1290

Bexfield NH, Stell AJ, Gear RN et al. (2008) Photodynamic therapy of superficial nasal planum squamous cell carcinomas in cats: 55 cases. Journal of Veterinary Internal Medicine **22**, 1385–1389

Beyer M and Schultze JL (2009) Regulatory T cells: major players in the tumor microenvironment. Current Pharmaceutical Design **15**, 1879–1892

Bianco SR, Sun J, Fosmire SP et al. (2003) Enhancing antimelanoma immune responses through apoptosis. Cancer Gene Therapy **10**, 726–736

Biller BJ, Elmslie RE, Burnett RC et al. (2007) Use of FoxP3 expression to identify regulatory T cells in healthy dogs and dogs with cancer. Veterinary Immunology and Immunopathology **116**, 68–78

Bird RC, Deinnocentes P, Lenz S et al. (2008) An allogeneic hybrid-cell fusion vaccine against canine mammary cancer Veterinary

Immunology and Immunopathology **123**, 289–304

Breen M and Modiano JF (2008) Evolutionarily conserved cytogenetic changes in hematological malignancies of dogs and humans – man and his best friend share more than companionship. *Chromosome Research* **16**, 145–154

Bryan JN, Taylor KH, Henry CJ et al. (2008) DNA methylation in cancer: techniques and preliminary evidence of hypermethylation in canine lymphoma. *Cancer Therapy* **6(A–2)**, 137–148

Buchholz J, Wergin M, Walt H et al. (2007) Photodynamic therapy of feline cutaneous squamous cell carcinoma using a newly developed liposomal photosensitizer: preliminary results concerning drug safety and efficacy. *Journal of Veterinary Internal Medicine* **21**, 770–775

Bui BN, Blay J, Duffaud F et al. (2007) Preliminary efficacy and safety results of Masitinib administered, front line in patients with advanced GIST. A phase II study. *Journal of Clinical Oncology* **25(18S)**, 10025

Cai W and Chen X (2006) Anti-angiogenic cancer therapy based on integrin alpha-v beta-3 antagonism. *Anticancer Agents in Medicinal Chemistry* **6**, 407–428

Catchpole B, Stell AJ, and Dobson JM (2002) Generation of blood-derived dendritic cells in dogs with oral malignant melanoma. *Journal of Comparative Pathology* **126**, 238–241

Chinnaiyan P, Huang S, Vallabhaneni G et al. (2005) Mechanisms of enhanced radiation response following epidermal growth factor receptor signaling inhibition by erlotinib (Tarceva). *Cancer Research* **65**, 3328–3335

Cohen LA, Powers B, Amin S et al. (2004) Treatment of canine haemangiosarcoma with suberoylanilide hydroxamic acid, a histone deacetylase inhibitor. *Veterinary and Comparative Oncology* **2**, 243–248

Dank G, Chien MB, and London CA (2002) Activating mutations in the catalytic or juxtamembrane domain of c-kit in splenic mast cell tumors of cats. *American Journal of Veterinary Research* **63**, 1129–1133

Dematteo RP, Ballman KV, Antonescu CR et al. (2009) Adjuvant imatinib mesylate after resection of localised, primary gastrointestinal stromal tumour: a randomised, double-blind, placebo–controlled trial. *Lancet* **373**, 1097–1104

Dickerson EB, Akhtar N, Steinberg H et al. (2004) Enhancement of the antiangiogenic activity of interleukin-12 by peptide targeted delivery of the cytokine to alpha-v beta-3 integrin. *Molecular Cancer Research* **2**, 663–673

Droogendijk HJ, Kluin-Nelemans HJ, van Doormaal JJ et al. (2006) Imatinib mesylate in the treatment of systemic mastocytosis: a phase II trial. *Cancer* **107**, 345–351

Druker BJ, Guilhot F, O'Brien SG et al. (2006) Five-year follow-up of patients receiving imatinib for chronic myeloid leukemia. *New England Journal of Medicine* **355**, 2408–2417

Elmslie RE, Glawe P and Dow SW (2008) Metronomic therapy with cyclophosphamide and piroxicam effectively delays tumor recurrence in dogs with incompletely resected soft tissue sarcomas. *Journal of Veterinary Internal Medicine* **22**, 1373–1379

Ferreira I, Rahal SC, Rocha NS et al. (2009) Hematoporphyrin-based photodynamic therapy for cutaneous squamous cell carcinoma in cats. *Veterinary Dermatology* **20**, 174–178

Fidel JL, Sellon RK, Houston RK et al. (2007) A nine-day accelerated radiation protocol for feline squamous cell carcinoma. *Veterinary Radiology and Ultrasound* **48**, 482–485

Gordon IK, Ye F, and Kent MS (2008) Evaluation of the mammalian target of rapamycin pathway and the effect of rapamycin on target expression and cellular proliferation in osteosarcoma cells from dogs. *American Journal of Veterinary Research* **69**, 1079–1084

Gyorffy S, Rodriguez-Lecompte JC, Woods JP et al. (2005) Bone marrow-derived dendritic cell vaccination of dogs with naturally occurring melanoma by using human gp100 antigen. *Journal of Veterinary Internal Medicine* **19**, 56–63

Hahn KA, Ogilvie G, Rusk T et al. (2008) Masitinib is safe and effective for the treatment of canine mast cell tumors. *Journal of Veterinary Internal Medicine* **22**, 1301–1309

Harari PM, Wheeler DL and Grandis JR (2009) Molecular target approaches in head and neck cancer: epidermal growth factor receptor and beyond. *Seminars in Radiation Oncology* **19**, 63–68

Heldin CH and Westermark B (1999) Mechanism of action and in vivo role of platelet-derived growth factor. *Physiological Reviews* **79**, 1283–1316

Helfand SC, Soergel SA, Donner RL et al. (1994) Potential to involve multiple effector cells with human recombinant interleukin-2 and antiganglioside monoclonal antibodies in a canine malignant melanoma immunotherapy model. *Journal of Immunotherapy with Emphasis on Tumor Immunology* **16**, 188–197

Hendrick MJ (1999) Feline vaccine-associated sarcomas. *Cancer Investigation* **17**, 273–277

Hockenbery DM, Zutter M, Hickey W et al. (1991) BCL2 protein is topographically restricted in tissues characterized by apoptotic cell death. *Proceedings of the National Academy of Science of the United States of America* **88**, 6961–6965

Huang Z, Chen Q, Luck D et al. (2005) Studies of a vascular-acting photosensitizer, Pd-bacteriopheophorbide (Tookad), in normal canine prostate and spontaneous canine prostate cancer. *Lasers in Surgery and Medicine* **36**, 390–397

Impellizeri JA, Howell K, McKeever KP et al. (2006) The role of rituximab in the treatment of canine lymphoma: an *ex vivo* evaluation. *Veterinary Journal* **171**, 556–558

Isotani M, Ishida N, Tominaga M et al. (2008) Effect of tyrosine kinase inhibition by imatinib mesylate on mast cell tumors in dogs. *Journal of Veterinary Internal Medicine* **22**, 985–988

Isotani M, Tamura K, Yagihara H et al. (2006) Identification of a c-kit exon 8 internal tandem duplication in a feline mast cell tumor case and its favorable response to the tyrosine kinase inhibitor imatinib mesylate. *Veterinary Immunology and Immunopathology* **114**, 168–172

Jubala CM, Wojcieszyn JW, Valli VE et al. (2005) CD20 expression in normal canine B cells and in canine non-Hodgkin lymphoma. *Veterinary Pathology* **42**, 468–476

Katayama R, Huelsmeyer MK, Marr AK et al. (2004) Imatinib mesylate inhibits platelet-derived growth factor activity and increases chemosensitivity in feline vaccine-associated sarcoma. *Cancer Chemotherapy and Pharmacology* **54**, 25–33

Kent MS, Collins CJ and Ye F (2009) Activation of the AKT and mammalian target of rapamycin pathways and the inhibitory effects of rapamycin on those pathways in canine malignant melanoma cell lines. *American Journal of Veterinary Research* **70**, 263–269

Kisseberth WC, Murahari S, London CA et al. (2008) Evaluation of the effects of histone deacetylase inhibitors on cells from canine cancer cell lines. *American Journal of Veterinary Research* **69**, 938–945

Kolluri SK, Zhu X, Zhou X et al. (2008) A short Nur77-derived peptide converts Bcl-2 from a protector to a killer. *Cancer Cell* **14**, 285–298

Lachowicz JL, Post GS, and Brodsky E (2005) A phase I clinical trial evaluating imatinib mesylate (Gleevec) in tumor-bearing cats. *Journal of Veterinary Internal Medicine* **19**, 860–864

Lemos-González Y, Páez de la Cadena M, Rodríguez-Berrocal FJ et al. (2007) Absence of activating mutations in the EGFR kinase domain in Spanish head and neck cancer patients. *Tumour Biology* **28**, 273–279

Letard S, Yang Y, Hanssens K et al. (2008) Gain-of-function mutations in the extracellular domain of KIT are common in canine mast cell tumors. *Molecular Cancer Research* **6**, 1137–1145

Liang D, Kong X and Sang N (2006) Effects of histone deacetylase inhibitors on HIF-1. *Cell Cycle* **5**, 2430–2435

Liao AT, McMahon M and London C (2005) Characterization, expression and function of c-Met in canine spontaneous cancers. *Veterinary and Comparative Oncology* **3**, 61–72

Liao AT, McMahon M and London CA (2006) Identification of a novel germline MET mutation in dogs. *Animal Genetics* **37**, 248–252

Lin TY, Bear M, Du Z et al. (2008) The novel HSP90 inhibitor STA-9090 exhibits activity against Kit-dependent and -independent malignant mast cell tumors. *Experimental Hematology* **36**, 1266–1277

London CA, Galli SJ, Yuuki T et al. (1999) Spontaneous canine mast cell tumors express tandem duplications in the proto-oncogene c-kit. *Experimental Hematology* **27**, 689–697

London CA, Hannah AL, Zadovoskaya R et al. (2003) Phase I dose-escalating study of SU11654, a small molecule receptor tyrosine kinase inhibitor, in dogs with spontaneous malignancies. *Clinical Cancer Research* **9**, 2755–2768

London CA, Kisseberth WC, Galli SJ et al. (1996) Expression of stem cell factor receptor (c-kit) by the malignant mast cells from spontaneous canine mast cell tumours. *Journal of Comparative Pathology* **115**, 399–414

London C, Malpas PB, Wood-Follis SL et al. (2009) Multi-center, placebo-controlled, double-blind, randomized study of oral toceranib phosphate (SU11654), a receptor tyrosine kinase inhibitor, for the treatment of dogs with recurrent (either local or distant) mast cell tumor following surgical excision. *Clinical Cancer Research* **15**, 3856–3865

Looper JS, Malarkey DE, Ruslander D et al. (2006) Epidermal growth factor receptor expression in feline oral squamous cell carcinomas. *Veterinary and Comparative Oncology* **4**, 33–40

López-Albaitero A, Lee SC, Morgan S et al. (2009) Role of polymorphic Fc gamma receptor IIIa and EGFR expression level in cetuximab mediated, NK cell dependent in vitro cytotoxicity of head and neck squamous cell carcinoma cells. *Cancer Immunology Immunotherapy* **58**, 1853–1862

Lu LF and Rudensky A (2009) Molecular orchestration of differentiation and function of regulatory T cells. *Genes and Development* **23**, 1270–1282

Lucroy MD, Bowles MH, Higbee RG et al. (2003a) Photodynamic therapy for prostatic carcinoma in a dog. *Journal of Veterinary Internal Medicine* **17**, 235–237

Lucroy MD, Ridgway TD, Peavy GM et al. (2003b) Preclinical evaluation of 5–aminolevulinic acid–based photodynamic therapy for canine transitional cell carcinoma. *Veterinary and Comparative Oncology* **1**, 76–85

Lucroy, MD, Long KR, Blaik MA et al. (2003c) Photodynamic therapy for the treatment of intranasal tumors in 3 dogs and 1 cat. *Journal of Veterinary Internal Medicine* **17**, 727–729

Mann BS, Johnson JR, Cohen MS *et al.* (2007) FDA approval summary: vorinostat for treatment of advanced primary cutaneous T-cell lymphoma. *Oncologist* **12**, 1247–1252

Mason NJ, Coughlin CM, Overley B *et al.* (2008) RNA-loaded CD40-activated B cells stimulate antigen-specific T-cell responses in dogs with spontaneous lymphoma. *Gene Therapy* **15**, 955–965

McCleese JK, Bear MD, Fossey SL *et al.* (2009) The novel HSP90 inhibitor STA-1474 exhibits biologic activity against osteosarcoma cell lines. *International Journal of Cancer* Epub June 19, 2009

Mehra R, Cohen RB and Burtness BA (2008) The role of cetuximab for the treatment of squamous cell carcinoma of the head and neck. *Clinical Advances in Hematology and Oncology* **6**, 742–750

Mohebtash M, Gulley JL, Madan RA *et al.* (2009) Cancer vaccines: current directions and perspectives in prostate cancer. *Current Opinion in Molecular Therapeutics* **11**, 31–36.

Moore RB, Xiao Z, Owen RJ *et al.* (2008) Photodynamic therapy of the canine prostate: intra-arterial drug delivery. *Cardiovascular and Interventional Radiology* **31**, 164–176

Nair S, Boczkowski D, Fassnacht M *et al.* (2007) Vaccination against the forkhead family transcription factor Foxp3 enhances tumor immunity. *Cancer Research* **67**, 371–380

Northrup NC, Selting KA, Rassnick KM *et al.* (2006). Outcomes of cats with oral tumors treated with mandibulectomy: 42 cases. *Journal of the American Animal Hospital Association* **42**, 350–369.

O'Neill K, Guth A, Biller B *et al.* (2009) Changes in regulatory T cells in dogs with cancer and associations with tumor type. *Journal of Veterinary Internal Medicine* **23**, 875–881

Ortner MA (2009) Photodynamic therapy for cholangiocarcinoma: overview and new developments. *Current Opinion in Gastroenterology* **25**(5), 466–471

Osaki T, Takagi S, Hoshino Y *et al.* (2009) Efficacy of antivascular photodynamic therapy using benzoporphyrin derivative monoacid ring A (BPD-MA) in 14 dogs with oral and nasal tumors. *Journal of Veterinary Medical Science* **71**, 125–132

Pryer NK, Lee LB, Zadovaskaya R *et al.* (2003) Proof of target for SU11654: inhibition of KIT phosphorylation in canine mast cell tumors. *Clinical Cancer Research* **9**, 5729–5734

Rusk A, Cozzi E, Stebbins M *et al.* (2006a) Cooperative activity of cytotoxic chemotherapy with antiangiogenic thrombospondin-I peptides, ABT-526 in pet dogs with relapsed lymphoma. *Clinical Cancer Research* **12**, 7456–7464

Rusk A, McKeegan E, Haviv F *et al.* (2006b) Preclinical evaluation of antiangiogenic thrombospondin-1 peptide mimetics, ABT-526 and ABT-510, in companion dogs with naturally occurring cancers. *Clinical Cancer Research* **12**, 7444–7455

Seiwert TY, Jagadeeswaran R, Faoro L *et al.* (2009) The MET receptor tyrosine kinase is a potential novel therapeutic target for head and neck squamous cell carcinoma. *Cancer Research* **69**, 3021–3031

Sun Q, Ming L, Thomas SM *et al.* (2009) PUMA mediates EGFR tyrosine kinase inhibitor-induced apoptosis in head and neck cancer cells. *Oncogene* **28**, 2348–2357

Thomas F, Rochaix P, Benlyazid A *et al.* (2007) Pilot study of neoadjuvant treatment with erlotinib in nonmetastatic head and neck squamous cell carcinoma. *Clinical Cancer Research* **13**, 7086–7092

Tucker GC (2006) Integrins: molecular targets in cancer therapy. *Current Oncology Reports* **8**, 96–103

U'Ren LW, Biller BJ, Elmslie RE *et al.* (2007) Evaluation of a novel tumor vaccine in dogs with hemangiosarcoma. *Journal of Veterinary Internal Medicine* **21**, 113–120

Wang YS, Chi KH, Liao KW *et al.* (2007) Characterization of canine monocyte-derived dendritic cells with phenotypic and functional differentiation. *Canadian Journal of Veterinary Research* **71**, 165–174

Weiner LM, Dhodapkar MV and Ferrone S (2009) Monoclonal antibodies for cancer immunotherapy. *Lancet* **373**, 1033–1040

Wolchok JD (2007) Dogs shed new light on cancer genes in humans. *Lehrer News Hour* (www.pbs.org/newshour/bb/science/jan–june07/cancer_03–15.html)

Zhang Y, Wang L, Li D *et al.* (2009) Taming regulatory T cells by autologous T cell immunization: a potential new strategy for cancer immune therapy. *International Immunopharmacology* **9**, 593–595

10

Principles of nutrition for the cancer patient

Korinn E. Saker

Introduction

Tumours, not unlike a parasite, live in or on a host and obtain their nourishment from the host organism. The unfortunate host suffers from consequences of malnutrition and organ malfunction associated with tumour growth and metastasis. Tumour–host competition for energy substrates is ongoing, with survival the endpoint. An overview of nutrient utilization by both tumour and host will help to elucidate the rationale behind nutritional support strategies for the cancer patient to prolong survival and maximize quality of life.

To date, the majority of investigations into tumour–host nutrient interactions in veterinary patients have been focused on the metabolic effects of multicentric lymphoma, tumours of the gastrointestinal tract and solid nasal tumours. The mechanism of nutrient utilization by many solid tumours in canine and feline companions is not as well documented as in human patients with widespread disease. Therefore, not unlike other medical scenarios, it is necessary to combine the documented knowledge base from human and veterinary oncology research to devise nutritional support plans for patients with a variety of neoplastic diseases. As the knowledge base in veterinary medicine develops, nutritional management of cancer patients will become more refined.

Metabolism of energy substrates by the tumour cell

Glucose metabolism

Energy production starts in the cytoplasm of the cell with anaerobic glycolysis and ends in the mitochondria of the cell with electron transport chain (ETC) production of adenosine triphosphate (ATP) under aerobic conditions. Under normal circumstances, glucose is metabolized to pyruvate, which is shuffled into the Krebs (tricarboxylic acid, TCA) cycle for metabolism. TCA cycle substrates are then utilized in the ETC for respiratory metabolism (oxidative phosphorylation) to ATP (energy).

When compared with an untransformed (normal) cell, the tumour cell has a distinctive, altered metabolism that allows it to exhibit increased glycolysis and pentose phosphate cycle activity, while demonstrating reduced rates of respiration. This dysregulation between glycolytic metabolism and respiration

results in cell death in normal cells, but the tumour cell has acquired the ability to escape this fate. The mechanisms that tumour cells have acquired for survival are varied (Argiles and Azcon, 1988; Spitz et al., 2000) and include:

- An accelerated rate of glycolysis enabled by unhampered glucose uptake into transformed cells
- Promotion of metabolic inefficiency in the host via lactate conversion to glucose by way of the Cori cycle
- Reduction of mitochondrial number in tumour cells, forcing/promoting anaerobic glycolysis as the predominant energy pathway
- Detoxification of intracellular oxidants (i.e. hydroperoxides), rendering tumour cells resistant to oxidant-induced cytotoxicity.

This glucose-dependent state of most tumour cells suggests a potential target for inhibiting tumour cell growth.

Protein (amino acid) metabolism

Tumours have the ability to act as a nitrogen sink, whereby amino acids are retained and used for oxidation and protein synthesis in transformed cells. The synthesis of extracellular protein (i.e. hormones) is reduced while enzymes catalysing synthesis of purines and pyrimidines to promote cell proliferation are increased. Additionally, the tumour can modify protein synthesis and/or degradation in normal cells, which results in an altered protein status of the host (i.e. clinical hypoalbuminaemia) and increased production of ectopic hormones (i.e. ACTH, parathyroid hormone and growth factors) (Argiles and Azcon, 1988).

Although all amino acids are involved in protein synthesis in both normal and transformed cells, specific amino acids have been identified as essential for tumour growth in certain cancer-bearing states (Mackenzie and Baracos, 2004; Muscaritoli et al., 2004). Glutamine, a conditionally essential amino acid for healthy cats and dogs and the primary fuel source for intestinal mucosal cells, is considered, along with glucose, to be a major compound contributing to the energy needs of most tumour cells. An understanding of the select amino acid utilization by transformed cells (Figure 10.1) can help to elucidate dietary protein strategies that promote host survival.

Function	Amino acid(s)
Protein synthesis	All
ATP production	Glutamine
Glucose production	Alanine, threonine, serine, glycine
Nucleotide synthesis	Glutamine
Polyamine synthesis	Arginine, ornithine
Nitric oxide synthesis	Arginine
Methyl group transfer	Methionine
Serotonin synthesis	Tryptophan

10.1 Functions of amino acids in tumour cells.

Lipid metabolism

The role of lipids as an energy substrate for tumour cells is not as well defined as the role of glucose and amino acids. Fatty acids are presented to, taken up by and utilized by the tumour cell, in varying degrees, to support metabolic needs. At least one reported mechanism to promote lipid utilization is an up-regulation of lipoprotein lipase (LPL) production. This is a key enzyme in promoting entry of fatty acids into the tumour cell for metabolism. These findings, along with earlier reported studies indicating *de novo* synthesis (lipogenesis) of fatty acids in specific tumour cell types (Herber *et al.*, 1985; Argiles and Azcon, 1988), support the implication of lipid utilization as a metabolic substrate in certain tumour cells.

In regard to normal cell energy metabolism, ketone bodies produced from fatty acid oxidation provide an alternative fuel source in scenarios of inadequate glucose, such as in the case of simple starvation. Information elucidating the role of ketone bodies (acetoacetate and β-hydroxybutyrate) by the cancer cell is limited.

Metabolic substrate needs and tumour type

Depending on the particular tumour growth pattern, cancer cells preferentially utilize glucose, amino acids or lipids as their primary fuel source to meet their energy or biosynthetic needs. Lipids are most efficiently utilized by very slow-growing tumours, relying almost entirely on mitochondrial ATP as an energy source for growth. In contrast, the energy requirement of rapidly growing tumour types is preferentially met by glucose oxidation. Tumour growth does affect the plasma amino acid profile of patients based on tumour type, the stage of disease progression and concurrent physiological state (Muscaritoli *et al.*, 2004). The nutritional relevance of altered amino acid profiles in the cancer patient is under investigation. Original studies based on patients with cancer of varying origins reported a consistent reduction in gluconeogenic amino acids (GAAs) and normal or increased concentration of branched-chain amino acids (BCAAs). More recent studies have identified that specific amino acids are preferentially utilized by solid *versus* haematological malignancies;

within the solid tumour category, amino acid profiles vary with specificity/location of the tumour (i.e. lung, breast, hepatocelllular, squamous cell). Clearly, matching amino acid profiles to specific tumours and malignancies, along with differentiating whether the amino acid imbalance primarily impacts tumour metabolism or systemic metabolic changes in the host, requires further investigation to enable practical feeding application.

Tumour *versus* host survival

General tumour–host interaction

The presence of a tumour results in alterations of metabolism in the host. These alterations can be appreciated at two levels.

- The tumour successfully drains the host's dietary supply of metabolites and trophic factors, causing the host to shift into the 'starvation' and 'anoxia' mode, utilizing body stores of fat and protein for needed energy. As body reserves continue to diminish, a cachexic condition ensues, which can rapidly progress to severe malnutrition, multiple organ failure and death.
- The tumour can decrease differentiation of certain host cells. This altered differentiation can result in a change in enzyme sensitivity to hormone signals, disturbing the feedback systems that coordinate endocrine gland activity in the host, therefore adversely influencing energy homeostasis.

Effects of tumours on the host: cancer cachexia

Tumours appear to have a two-pronged survival mechanism:

- The tumour cell must obtain nutrients to provide it with the necessary fuel for growth, as described above
- Tumours secrete a variety of cachexia-promoting compounds, which hasten a malnourished state in the host (patient), eventually resulting in death.

Studies in human and animal models, as well as observations in clinical veterinary cases, suggest that the depletion of body fat can be disproportionate to protein loss and may account for the majority of *initial* weight loss seen in cancer-bearing patients (Kalantar-Zadeh *et al.*, 2007; Skipworth *et al.*, 2007). In the first stages of tumour growth, a lipolytic factor is secreted by the tumour, which is associated with lipid mobilization from adipose stores and some degree of thymic involution. The resultant hyperlipidaemia in the host, in conjunction with the tumour-induced hypoglycaemic environment, triggers the metabolic machinery responsible for oxidation of fatty acids as an alternative energy source for the host in place of glucose metabolism. While mobilized free fatty acids are oxidized to ketone bodies via beta oxidation in the liver, the glycerol component of the mobilized triglyceride is utilized as a glucogenic substrate within hepatocytes. These energy-requiring processes help to explain the fat depletion, enhanced gluconeogenesis and overall negative energy balance in cancer patients.

Whether the cachexia is fully accounted for by inadequate energy intake and increased energy expenditure is still unclear; but the increased uncoupling of oxidative phosphorylation associated with this imbalance of energy homeostasis in the host supports the cachexic state. Likewise, up-regulation of the ubiquitin–proteosome pathway (UPP) in cancer patients promotes cachexia. The UPP is the major non-lysosomal process responsible for the breakdown of most short- and long-lived proteins in mammalian cells. The ubiquination process associated with cancer cachexia is controlled by sulphated glycoproteins produced by cachexia-inducing tumours (Ciechanover et al., 2000). An example is proteolysis-inducing factor (PIF), which has been found in the urine of weight-losing patients with gastrointestinal tumours (Cabal-Manzano et al., 2001). PIF is also thought to be involved in the inflammatory response of cachexia, leading to increased tumour production and secretion of interleukins (IL-6, IL-8) and C-reactive protein (Cabal-Manzano et al., 2001; McMillan, 2009). Ultimately, the increased rate of protein catabolism, increased requirement for mediator production, increased urinary and gastrointestinal losses, and protein loss to tumour cells promotes a negative nitrogen (protein) balance in the patient. This protein-deficient state adversely influences immune cell function, wound healing and overall strength of the patient.

Anti-cancer treatment effects on the host

Multimodal therapy (combinations of surgery, chemotherapy, radiation therapy, immunotherapy, hyperthermia, etc.) for veterinary cancer patients is considered the current standard of care. Each treatment modality presents systemic and/or site-specific biological alterations that affect the patient's recovery and quality of life.

- Acute and chronic effects of *radiation therapy* associated with the head/neck region can be appreciated as mucositis (Ogilvie, 2006; Keefe *et al.*, 2007; Saker and Selting, 2009), dry mouth, dental disease, or altered smell and taste (see Chapter 8). Radiation treatment of the abdominal region can result in nausea, vomiting and diarrhoea as acute effects. In chronic situations, intestinal obstruction, fistula formation or chronic enteritis may be observed.
- Although *chemotherapy* is utilized as a treatment for numerous tumour types and locations, common sequelae of chemotherapy include gastrointestinal side effects (see Chapter 7). Effects that may have nutritional implications include decreased appetite, alterations in smell/taste, food aversions, nausea, vomiting, diarrhoea, constipation and inflammation of the oropharyngeal region (Saker and Selting, 2009).
- The effects of *surgical* intervention on cancer patients, although site-specific, can influence overall nutrient utilization and metabolic disease state of the patient (Bozzetti *et al.*, 2007; Saker and Selting, 2009). For example, some oral

therapies will diminish a patient's ability to prehend, chew or swallow food, whereas a pancreatectomy may result in the onset of diabetes mellitus.

Individually the treatment modalities are reported to adversely influence metabolic and functional aspects of the patient. When utilizing a multimodality approach, the adverse sequelae often become magnified, putting the patient at higher risk for malnutrition and its consequences if not addressed in an appropriate and timely manner.

Nutritional support for the host

Goals of nutritional support

In the cancer patient, the goals of nutritional support and the feeding plan will be dynamic and therefore subject to revision based on sequential patient assessments. General goals for every patient should target:

- Optimizing quality of life
- Maintaining a reasonably optimal body condition
- Preventing metabolic complications from feeding
- Feeding via the gastrointestinal tract whenever possible
- Slowing the onset and progression of cachexia
- Replacing nutrient losses associated with the disease process and/or anti-cancer treatments.

Assessment of each patient will allow for these general goals to be tailored to focus on the specific needs of the patient and determine the appropriate nutritional support options. As in the case of any terminal disease state, treatment and associated management options range from choosing no intervention to choosing every possible intervention modality currently available. Nutritional support guidelines can be provided across this continuum of disease management scenarios.

A caregiver may choose to take no specific action (**NA**) in regard to nutritional support for a pet diagnosed with cancer, and this would be considered a feeding approach. Basically this means they have decided to let the pet eat whatever it will eat, whenever it has the interest in eating. In this scenario, reasonable recommendations would be to avoid offering foods that contain noxious or harmful ingredients and ensure that there is plenty of fresh water available at all times. The next feeding approach for nutritional support focuses efforts on optimizing voluntary intake (**VI**) so as to provide the pet's daily energy requirement and address specific *nutrients of concern* based on the pet's clinical condition. The last feeding approach for nutritional support is assisted feeding (**AF**), a more aggressive approach to nutrient delivery. The AF approach ranges from the very simple technique of hand or syringe feeding to the more complex technique of parenteral feeding. Both VI and AF are most successful when a nutritional assessment of the patient is performed prior to developing a comprehensive feeding plan. Figure 10.2 summarizes these feeding approaches.

Feeding approach	Requirements	Practical recommendations
No specific action (**NA**)	Allow the patient to eat whatever it will eat, whenever it will eat	Avoid offering foods that contain noxious or harmful ingredients. Ensure plenty of fresh water is available
Optimize voluntary intake (**VI**)	Ensure the patient's daily energy requirements are met and address specific nutrients of concern	Calculate daily energy/nutrient requirements. Identify and feed appropriate diet type/ amount. Monitor daily intake
Assisted feeding (**AF**)	Ensure the patient's daily energy requirements are met and address specific nutrients of concern	Hand or syringe feeding, tube feeding, or parenteral feeding

10.2 Options for nutritional support of the cancer patient: feeding approaches.

Nutritional assessment

The American College of Veterinary Nutrition suggests an integrated approach to patient nutritional assessment referred to as the **iterative process** (Thatcher et al., 2004), which includes assessment of:

- The patient
- The food (diet)
- The feeding method.

This approach helps to ensure a complete and accurate nutritional assessment of each patient.

Patient assessment

In the iterative approach, assessment of the patient is based on:

- Physical examination
- Clinical history
- Dietary history
- Routine diagnostics (CBC, chemistry profile, urinalysis)
- Other pertinent diagnostics.

Translating the patient assessment data into a useful information base for developing an appropriate feeding plan can be quite daunting for practitioners not trained in clinical nutrition. To simplify this process, a modification of the **subjective global assessment** (SGA) technique common to human medicine can be used. The SGA technique is based on using clinical history and physical examination parameters to identify patients at

risk for complications, and assumes the 'at risk' patient will benefit from appropriate nutritional support (Detsky et al., 1987). SGA involves identifying the cause of the malnourished state and the categories include:

- Maldigestion of food
- Malabsorption of the ingesta
- Decreased intake of food (calories).

This assessment technique includes correlations between malnutrition with specific organ function and alterations in bodyweight/composition, as well as identifying how the disease process influences the patient's nutrient requirements.

SGA can be adapted to the cancer patient by focusing more specifically on:

- Body condition and weight changes
- Voluntary diet intake
- Signs of GI intolerance associated with the cancer or the treatment
- Functional capacity of the patient.

The findings of clinical, historical and physical assessment can be translated into one of three nutritional status categories (Figure 10.3):

- Well nourished
- Borderline, or at risk of becoming malnourished
- Significantly malnourished.

Category standing is used to indicate which feeding approach will most benefit the patient.

Category	Definition	Criteria	Suggested feeding approach
1	Well nourished	Consistent intake of daily energy needs Weight maintenance Maintain optimal (or near optimal) BCS Muscle mass score 2–3 Normal serum albumin No change in BW No nutrient losses	VI
2	Borderline malnourished	Inconsistent intake of daily energy needs Weight loss of <10% BCS variable Muscle mass score 1–2 Normal to mild hypoalbuminaemia Undesired weight loss Moderate, but controlled nutrient losses (i.e. diarrhoea, vomiting, regurgitation, urinary)	VI and/or AF

10.3 Nutritional status categories. BCS, body condition score; RER, resting energy requirement. (continues) ▶

Category	Definition	Criteria		Suggested feeding approach
3	Significantly malnourished	Daily energy intake ≤66% RER Weight loss ≥10% Poor BCS (≤2.5/5 or 3/9) Moderate to severe hypoalbuminaemia Muscle mass score 0–1 Undesired/uncontrolled weight loss Ongoing, uncontrolled nutrient losses		AF

10.3 (continued) Nutritional status categories. BCS, body condition score; RER, resting energy requirement.

Body condition and weight changes: Current *bodyweight* is easily determined, but just as important is the history and time frame of *weight change*. Accurate reporting of weight using the same scales and a scale of appropriate sensitivity is ideal. The more rapid the weight loss, the more likely it is to be associated with loss of lean muscle mass (LMM) *versus* fat tissue, although both are documented in the cancer cachexia syndrome. Close physical examination will reveal the presence of ascites or oedema, both of which will obscure true bodyweight, as well as composition of LMM *versus* fat tissue. The rate of lean tissue catabolism (breakdown) is inversely correlated with survival.

During the physical examination, an assessment of body condition and assignment of a **body condition score** (BCS) (on a 5-point or 9-point scale) is useful for current and future assessment. Current BCS systems are based on subjective evaluation of fat tissue covering ribs, tail-base, backbone, and other obvious bony prominences (Thatcher *et al.*, 2004). Assignment of a BCS equal to 1 indicates an emaciated condition, using either the 5 or 9 scoring scale. Conversely, a BCS assignment of 5/5 or 9/9 indicates extreme obesity. An optimal body condition would be scored 3/5 or 4.5–5/9. With practice, assigning a BCS to a dog or cat can be done with high accuracy. Cancer patients, especially cats, have a very high incidence of muscle wasting in the face of adequate or excessive fat stores. Therefore, it is imperative to evaluate *muscle mass* subjectively along with the traditional BCS systems (Figure 10.4).

Score	Criteria
0	Severe pronounced muscle wasting over scapulae, skull or wings of the ilium
1	Moderate muscle wasting over these areas
2	Mild muscle wasting
3	Normal muscle mass over these areas

10.4 The muscle mass scoring system.

Voluntary dietary intake: The voluntary dietary intake must be evaluated against a daily caloric goal calculated as resting energy requirement (RER) of the patient while hospitalized and daily energy requirement (DER) when managed at home.

RER is based on bodyweight (BW) and is calculated as:

$$70 \times BW(kg)^{0.75}\ kcal/day$$

or

$$[BW(kg) \times 30] + 70\ kcal/day$$

This is an *interspecies* equation, making it relevant for both canine and feline patients. Depending on the patient's clinical condition at the time of diagnosis and the plan for treatment (general, chemotherapy, radiation), hospitalized cancer patients should be receiving a *minimum* of 66% of RER calories, and in some instances a determined percentage greater than RER calories.

Accurate determination of DER for the veterinary cancer patient is still a challenge. The following DER calculation should be used as a starting point, but since bedside calorimetry is not feasible in pets, reassessment of the patient at regular intervals will help to determine whether adjustments to DER are necessary.

For dogs:
$$DER_{canine} = RER_{\text{at optimal BW}} \times (1.6\ to\ 3.0)\ kcal/day$$

For cats:
$$DER_{feline} = RER_{\text{at optimal BW}} \times (1.2\ to\ 2.5)\ kcal/day$$

DER accounts for daily calorie needs that are associated with food digestion, activity, thermoregulation and maintenance of lean body mass. It should be remembered that the cachexic patient has a much higher daily energy expenditure than may be appreciated, due to rapidly ongoing catabolism, increased respiratory efforts, excessive production of cytokines and the influence of drug metabolism on liver and cardiac function.

To simplify the DER calculations for a cancer patient, while using the above equations as a starting point it should be realized that adjustments will probably be necessary to optimize calorie intake for each patient. In the author's experience of feeding the cachexic cancer patient, many cases benefit from an increase in DER of up to two-fold in order to match their daily calorie expenditure adequately. DER factors for dogs are consistently higher than for cats, based on the more sedentary lifestyle of cats compared to most dogs.

Signs of intolerance and functional capacity: Assessment of the patient with regard to the two remaining SGA focus areas – signs of GI intolerance associated with the cancer or the cancer treatment; and the functional capacity of the patient – can further help to clarify which nutrition support category best describes each patient. This categorization, along with consideration of the patient's cancer diagnosis, stage, treatment protocol and prognosis, will aid in identifying the most beneficial feeding approach.

Although the 'golden rule' in nutritional support for any species is to 'feed the gut whenever possible', gut function and tolerance level, patient metabolic status and nutritional status category may limit the total calories either provided or tolerated via the enteral route, in which case a combination of nutrient delivery methods, also utilizing the parenteral route, is indicated.

Diet

Diet assessment is the next component of the iterative process approach to a comprehensive nutritional assessment. Choosing appropriate diet options involves matching the specific nutrient and diet characteristic needs of the patient with what the diet provides. In general, diet options that help to minimize gastric/intestinal complications and maximize nutrient digestion and absorption in the presence of either ongoing tumour cell development or destruction of tumour cells via chemotherapy and/or radiation would be preferred.

Despite the current understanding of nutrient accretion and metabolism of macronutrients by tumour cells, there is limited scientifically founded information available regarding cancer diets for pets. To date, the focus for nutritional recommendations appears to be based on research using the canine GI lymphoma model (Saker and Selting, 2009) and extrapolation from nutritional intervention studies for human cancer patients, resulting in little consensus of appropriate dietary recommendations for veterinary cancer patients. Diet choices should be made based on a desired anti-tumour growth nutrient profile and the nutrients needed to address anti-cancer treatment sequelae experienced by the patient.

Carbohydrate: From a strictly tumour-growth perspective, dietary carbohydrate restriction and omega-3 fatty acid supplementation are nutritional management foci supported by multiple *in vitro* and *in vivo* animal studies. Glucose deprivation causes cytotoxicity in multiple human tumour cell lines, including fibroblasts, aorta, colon and breast cells, and studies indicate that transformed cells appear to be more susceptible to glucose deprivation-induced cytotoxicity than matched untransformed cells (Spitz *et al.*, 2000). Based on studies utilizing the canine GI lymphoma model, dietary carbohydrate calories should be restricted and fat calories increased, but it should be borne in mind that this dietary recommendation may not be universal for all cancers. The rapidly growing, poorly differentiated tumour types utilize glucose oxidation, which suggests that a carbohydrate-restricted diet will slow or minimize tumour growth. Conversely, slower-growing well differentiated tumours rely on mitochondrial ATP, which suggests that dietary fat restriction would adversely influence tumour growth.

Fat and fatty acids: Omega-3 fatty acid (*n*-3 FA) metabolites, eicosapentaenoic acid (EPA) and docosahexaenoic acid (DHA) have been reported as having anti-tumorigenic and anti-cachexic functions. Several mechanisms of *n*-3 FA and tumour growth suppression have been identified. Omega-3 FA can competitively down-regulate the *n*-6 metabolites and up-regulate EPA and DHA, minimizing the angiogenesis-promoting effects of pro-inflammatory eicosanoids (Cowing and Saker, 2001; Saker, 2006; Grimble, 2007). EPA and DHA have been shown to stimulate programmed cell death, induce differentiation and inhibit cell proliferation by down-regulating NFκB, Bcl-2 and MAPK mechanisms in specific tumour cells (Cowing and Saker, 2001; Saker, 2006). Canine and feline studies indicate that both the essential fatty acid ratio (*n*-6:*n*-3) and the total *n*-3 FA concentration in the diet influences the tumour cell. Dietary recommendations based on research associated with the commercial canine cancer diet and feline nutrition cancer studies suggest 337 mg EPA/DHA per 100 kcal and an *n*-6:*n*-3 ratio of 1:1 to 2.5:1 as effective feeding guidelines.

Protein: It is the experience-based opinion of this author that dietary protein levels should be based on the following considerations (in this order):

1. Protein tolerance of the patient
2. Current protein status, immunocompetence and body condition
3. Tumour type.

Ongoing kidney or liver dysfunction with associated clinical consequences should take precedence over altered protein requirements due to tumour–patient competition. Accordingly, excessive protein losses due to related or unrelated malabsorptive/maldigestive disorders will increase patient protein requirements above cancer needs alone.

Canine lymphoma studies suggest increased arginine and/or glutamine as beneficial for wound healing, enhanced immune function and GI enterocyte nourishment associated with anti-cancer treatment protocols. Conversely, these amino acids are reported to be instrumental for energy production and synthesis of nucleotides, nitric oxide and polyamines in tumour cells (Muscaritoli *et al.*, 2004). Supplementation to the patient may simultaneously promote tumour growth. This is where timing is important: delivery of therapeutic levels of arginine and/or glutamine immediately following a chemotherapy, radiation or surgical procedure would seemingly benefit the patient by minimizing complications associated with anti-cancer treatment, yet provide little or no benefit to the dead or dying tumour.

Antioxidants: A similar rationale may apply to dietary antioxidants and cancer. Studies have shown that glucose metabolism is related to the metabolic detoxification of intracellular hydroperoxides formed as a consequence of cellular oxidative metabolism; therefore, glucose deprivation to tumour cells from dietary carbohydrate restriction in the host limits hydroperoxide detoxification in tumour cells, rendering them more susceptible to oxidant-induced cytotoxicity (Spitz *et al.*, 2000). Dietary antioxidant supplementation can 'detoxify' damaging oxidant species in both normal and transformed cells, preventing tumour cell devitalization and destruction. Targeted antioxidant delivery following an anticancer treatment would specifically provide protection to normal cells against secretory substances from tumour cells and from damaging reactive oxidant species derived from treatment protocols and damaged or dying cells. Numerous antioxidant products are readily available. Vitamin E protects lipid cell membranes through free-radical scavenging and the succinate and α-tocopherol acetate forms have been reported as having anti-proliferative activity. Additionally, both vitamins E and C reportedly inhibit nitrozation reactions that can induce cancers (Saker and Selting, 2009). Specific trace minerals, flavonoids and other vitamins are described as having anti-cancer activity, but evidence-based research for veterinary cancer patients is not available.

The feeding method
Assessment of feeding method is the final component of a comprehensive nutritional assessment approach.

Voluntary intake: The least invasive, most physiological feeding approach is VI. The diet should be offered, primarily, in a meal-feeding manner, with calculated RER or DER divided between multiple meals each day. This allows for more accurate monitoring of calculated *versus* actual food intake. In the case where body condition is poor, appetite is still good and VI is tolerated, a combination of meal and free-choice feeding can optimize maintenance of desired body condition.

Assisted feeding: If a patient cannot or will not consume desired calories voluntarily and in a consistent manner, then AF is indicated. Enteral assisted feeding methods range from hand or syringe feeding to diet delivery via a feeding tube. Feeding tube placement is recommended for the cancer patient when hand or syringe feeding is no longer tolerated or feasible. The decision regarding tube type and location of placement will depend on:

- Amount of functional GI tract
- Length of time AF is required
- Whether at-home or hospitalized feeding
- Availability of resources (i.e. equipment, technical experience).

During short-term hospitalization, hand feeding, syringe feeding and/or supplemental diet delivery via naso-oesophageal tube are appropriate options. If an inconsistent appetite is expected at home, placement of an oesophagostomy or gastrostomy tube should be considered prior to hospital discharge for ease of at-home supplemental assisted feeding. Detailed guidelines for tube placement and management can be found in the *BSAVA Manual of Canine and Feline Rehabilitation, Supportive and Palliative Care*. Figure 10.5 summarizes tube types, recommended feeding method, and diet form(s) for enteral assisted feeding.

Parenteral feeding is reserved for hospitalized patients that require either temporary avoidance of the enteral feeding route or supplemental nutrient delivery. The feeding approach does not have to be an either/or approach. In many situations a combination of VI and AF or combining enteral with parenteral AF is indicated and extremely beneficial for the patient.

Feeding plan
Basic steps to developing a feeding plan based on nutritional status category (see Figure 10.3) are as follows.

Category 1: well nourished patient
1. Calculate required kcal/day as RER $_{current\ BW}$, then DER using RER × 1.6 (canine) or RER × 1.2 (feline).

Tube type and size	Use	Sedation/anaesthesia requirements	Feeding method	Diet type
Orogastric 16–20 Fr	Ultra-short term (1–2 days) In-hospital use	± Sedation	B	L, CB
Naso-oesophageal 5–10 Fr	Short term (3–7 days) In-hospital or at-home use	± Sedation. Topical anaesthetic required	CRI, B	L
Oesophagostomy 14–19 Fr	Weeks to several months In-hospital or at-home use	General anaesthesia required	CRI, B	L, CB
Gastrostomy 18–28 Fr	Weeks to years In-hospital or at-home use	General anaesthesia required for surgical, endoscopic or non-endoscopic placement	CRI, B	L, CB
Enterostomy 5–8 Fr	Short term In-hospital use	General anaesthesia required – surgical placement	CRI	L

10.5 Feeding tubes for canine and feline patients. The enterostomy tube is commonly referred to as a J-tube, as placement is in the jejunum. A J-tube can also be placed as a 'J-thru-G' tube to access both the upper small intestine and stomach as needed for feeding and/or residual monitoring. B, bolus feeding; CB, canned diet blended with a liquid (water or liquid diet); CRI, constant-rate infusion; L, commercial liquid diet.

2. Identify low-carbohydrate (<8 g CHO/100 kcal), increased-fat diet (>4.5 g fat/100 kcal) enriched in omega-3 fatty acids and highly digestible (low crude fibre content). Consider diet categories as:
   i. Commercial cancer management diet
   ii. Growth diets, kitten or puppy
   iii. Canine performance diets (for dogs only)
   iv. Fish-based diets, canine or feline.
3. Minimize dietary and supplemental antioxidant intake during anti-cancer treatment.
4. Feed twice to three times per day.
5. Monitor appetite, bodyweight and condition and nutrient losses, daily.

Category 2: borderline malnourished patient

1. Calculate RER $_{optimal\ BW}$, then DER using RER × (1.6 to 3.0) (canine) or RER × (1.2 to 2.5) (feline).
2. Identify appropriate diet nutrient profile (see *Category 1*). Consider diet categories as:
   i. Commercial cancer management diet
   ii. Feline diabetes management diet (for dog or cat)
   iii. Kitten growth diet (for dog or cat)
   iv. Canine performance diets (for dogs only)
   v. Fish-based diets, canine or feline
   vi. Veterinary and human liquid diets.
3. Avoid dietary and supplemental antioxidant intake during anti-cancer treatment.
4. Feed two to four times per day.
5. If daily voluntary calorie intake is less than calculated RER$_{optimal\ BW}$, initiate assisted feeding (i.e. hand, syringe, or tube feeding) to ensure delivery of RER (minimally) and DER (optimally) to cover daily caloric deficit.
6. Monitor appetite, bodyweight changes/condition and nutrient losses, daily. Protein and electrolyte status as indicated by clinical picture.

Note that limited veterinary liquid diets are available that match desired nutrient profile and that human liquid diets may require supplementation with select amino acids and linoleic acid based on essential nutrients of the patient.

Category 3: malnourished patient

1. Calculate RER$_{current\ BW}$ for in-hospital feeding; RER$_{optimal\ BW}$ for at-home feeding.
2. Calculate DER using RER × (1.6 to 3.0) (canine) or RER × (1.2 to 2.5) (feline) for home feeding.
3. Choose assisted feeding method (i.e. syringe, tube, parenteral or combination):
   i. Enteral feeding contraindicated if patient exhibiting chronic vomiting or regurgitation; utilize parenteral option
   ii. Parenteral admixtures formulated to match patient's specific nutrient needs.
4. Identify enteral diet based on nutrient profile (see Categories 1 and 2) and feeding tube size/ location (see Figure 10.5).
5. Avoid dietary and supplemental antioxidant intake during anti-cancer treatment.
6. Feeding frequency as constant-rate infusion or bolus schedule: follow appropriate tube feeding and tube maintenance protocols.

7. Offer fresh diet prior to a scheduled tube feeding if not vomiting.
8. Monitor attitude, appetite, bodyweight changes/ condition and nutrient losses, daily; monitor protein and electrolyte status as indicated by clinical picture.

Roadblocks to adequate nutritional support

Food aversions are not an uncommon sequel to anti-cancer treatments and to a progressing disease state in general. The veterinary patient may associate nausea, pain, or overall discomfort with the act of eating, or simply with the sight or scent of food (Michel and Sorenmo, 2008). Clinical signs associated with food aversion include: initial interest in food followed by refusal after smelling or tasting the food; salivation; repeated swallowing or turning away from food when offered; and distancing from the feeding bowl.

- Altering the flavour/scent, texture and temperature of the food may entice the patient to eat.
- Presentation of some unique food stuff may interest the patient and jump-start voluntary food intake.
- The use of appetite-stimulating drugs in conjunction with diet change and palliative medications to decrease nausea may promote and sustain appropriate caloric intake.
- If food aversion behaviour persists with resultant weight loss, an assisted feeding approach should be initiated.

Non-compliance with dietary and feeding guidelines can be a multifactorial issue, involving the patient, caregiver and/or attending veterinary surgeon:

- Is the recommended diet unavailable?
- Is the caregiver unable to adhere to the recommended feeding schedule?
- Does the caregiver have reservations about diet options?
- Is there poor diet acceptance and/or tolerance by the patient?
- Are the nutrition support recommendations unclear?

Identification of these issues can help to rectify any non-compliance.

Summary

The principles of nutritional support for the veterinary cancer patient can be summarized as follows.

- Evaluation of growth characteristics of the tumour helps to target specific nutrient utilization by tumour cells, allowing for efficacious anti-tumour nutritional support.
- A comprehensive nutritional assessment identifies specific nutrient needs and DER for each patient.

- Use nutritional status category criteria to direct the approach to feeding.
- Minimize the calorie contribution from soluble carbohydrates; target an *n*-6:*n*-3 FA ratio (2.5:1 to 1:1) by increasing EPA/DHA sources such as menhaden fish oil.
- Dietary protein intake calculations should reflect patient needs and tolerance level.
- Time antioxidant supplementation with anti-cancer treatments.
- Utilize assisted feeding alone or in combination with voluntary intake as needed.
- Despite best intentions to feed an anti-tumour diet, the biggest nutritional impact on survival is consistent intake of adequate calories.

Although feeding protocols targeted to prevent or cure cancer would be ideal, the present state of veterinary nutritional oncology realistically is focused on development of feeding protocols to complement anti-cancer treatment modalities. As studies continue to reveal the mechanisms of tumour cell metabolism and varied host responses to tumour cell growth, feeding protocols can make the transition from management to prevention and possibly cure.

References and further reading

Argiles JM and Azcon J (1988) The metabolic environment of cancer. *Molecular and Cellular Biochemistry* **81**, 3–17

Bing C and Trayhurn P (2008) Regulation of adipose tissue metabolism in cancer cachexia. *Current Opinion in Clinical Nutrition and Metabolic Care* **11**, 201–207

Bozzetti F, Gianotti L, Braga M *et al.* (2007) Postoperative complications in gastrointestinal cancer patients: the joint role of the nutritional status and the nutritional support. *Clinical Nutrition* **6**, 698–709

Cabal-Manzano R, Bhargava P, Torres-Durate A *et al.* (2001) Proteolysis inducing factor is expressed in tumours of patients with gastrointestinal cancers and correlates with weight loss. *British Journal of Cancer* **94**, 1599–1601

Ciechanover A, Orian A and Schwartz AL (2000) Ubiquitin-mediated proteolysis: biological regulation via destruction. *Bioessays* **22**, 442–451

Cowing BE and Saker KE (2001) Polyunsaturated fatty acids and EGFR-MAPK signaling in mammary cancer. *Journal of Nutrition* **131**, 1125–1128

Detsky AS, McLaughlin JR, Baker JP *et al.* (1987) What is subjective global assessment of nutritional support? *Journal of Parenteral and Enteral Nutrition* **11**, 8–13

Grimble RF (2007) Immunomodulatory impact of dietary lipids. *Clinical Nutrition Highlights* **3**, 2–7

Herber D, Byerly LO and Chlebowski RT (1985) Metabolic abnormalities in the cancer patient. *Cancer* **55**, 225–232

Johnen H, Lin S, Kuffner T *et al.* (2007) Tumour-induced anorexia and weight loss are mediated by the TGF-beta superfamily cytokine MIC-1. *Nature Medicine* **13**, 1333–1340

Kalantar-Zadeh K, Horwich TB, Oeropoulos A *et al.* (2007) Risk factor paradox in wasting diseases. *Current Opinion in Clinical Nutrition and Metabolic Care* **10**, 433–442

Keefe DM, Rassias G, O'Neil L *et al.* (2007) Severe mucositis: how can nutrition help? *Current Opinion in Clinical Nutrition and Metabolic Care* **5**, 627–631

Mackenzie M and Baracos VE (2004) Cancer-associated cachexia: altered metabolism of protein and amino acids. In: *Metabolic and Therapeutic Aspects of Amino Acids in Clinical Nutrition, 2nd edn,* ed. LC Cynober, pp. 339–354. CRC Press, Boca Raton, Florida

Marks DL, Ling N and Cone RD (2001) Role of the central melancortin system in cachexia. *Cancer Research* **61**, 1432–1438

McMillan DC (2009) Systemic inflammation, nutritional status and survival in patients with cancer. *Current Opinion in Clinical Nutrition and Metabolic Care* **12**, 223–226

Michel KE and Sorenmo KU (2008) Nutritional status of cats with cancer: nutritional evaluation and recommendations. In: *Encyclopedia of Feline Clinical Nutrition, 1st edn,* ed. P Pibot *et al.,* pp. 385–402. Royal Canin/Aniwa SAS, Aimargues, France

Muscaritoli M, Fanelli FR, Meguid MM *et al.* (2004) Amino acid requirement in cancer. In: *Metabolic and Therapeutic Aspects of Amino Acids in Clinical Nutrition, 2nd edn,* ed. LC Cynober, pp. 689–704. CRC Press, Boca Raton, Florida

Ogilvie GK (2006) Amazing advances in veterinary oncology today. *Veterinary Forum* July, 39–46

Saker KE (2006) Clinical value of fatty acids for our feline friends. *Proceedings of Hill's Global Symposium on Feline Care,* pp. 28–34

Saker KE and Selting KA (2009) Cancer. In: *Small Animal Clinical Nutrition, 5th edn,* ed. M Hand *et al.,* pp. 587–607. Mark Morris Institute, Topeka, Kansas

Skipworth RJC, Stewart GD, Dejong CHC *et al.* (2007) Pathophysiology of cancer cachexia: much more than host–tumour interaction? *Clinical Nutrition* **83**, 667–676

Spitz DR, Sim JE, Ridnour LA *et al.* (2000) Glucose deprivation-induced oxidative stress in human tumour cells. A fundamental defect in metabolism? *Annals of the New York Academy of Sciences* **899**, 349–362

Thatcher CD, Hand MS and Remillard RL (2004) Small animal clinical nutrition: an iterative process. In: *Small Animal Clinical Nutrition, 4th edn,* ed. M Hand *et al.,* pp. 1–19. Mark Morris Institute, Topeka, Kansas

Watson P and Chan DL (2010) Principles of clinical nutrition. In: *BSAVA Manual of Canine and Feline Rehabilitation, Supportive and Palliative Care: Case Studies in Patient Management,* ed. S Lindley and P Watson, pp. 42–59. BSAVA Publications, Gloucester

11

Relief of chronic cancer pain

Brian J. Trumpatori and B. Duncan X. Lascelles

Introduction

In human medicine there is a significant amount of interest in cancer pain, both in its neurobiology and in novel methods to alleviate it. However, little is known about the relationship between pain and cancer in animals. Yoxall (1978) stated: 'It is surprising, for instance, how much a dog's quality of life, observed by the owner, may be improved by the administration of a simple analgesic if the dog is suffering from a tumour, which although painless on palpation, may be causing considerable chronic pain.' Despite this statement, and the fact that obvious pain associated with specific tumours such as osteosarcoma has been emphasized for a long time as a diagnostic criterion, there is a complete absence of controlled studies specifically investigating the occurrence of cancer pain in companion animals and a relative lack of studies specifically investigating the alleviation of pain in animals suffering from cancer.

Given the lack of animal clinical studies, the information in this chapter cannot be based on peer-reviewed investigations. Rather, it is a combination of the authors' experience and the experience of others who are heavily involved in the treatment of animal cancer patients. It is also based on considered extrapolations from human medicine and from veterinary research in other chronically painful conditions, such as osteoarthritis.

It is estimated that cancer pain could be managed effectively in up to 90% of human patients with currently available drugs and techniques, but that problems related to healthcare professionals, patients and healthcare systems lead to frequent undertreating of cancer pain. The same drugs and techniques recommended for use in humans can probably be used to good effect in animals.

There are no estimates for the numbers of animals with cancer pain that receive analgesic therapy, nor for how effective that therapy is. At the time the previous edition of this manual was published, surveys into the use of analgesics in the perioperative setting found that significant numbers of animals were not receiving analgesic drugs. Since that time, significant improvements have been made with regard to the identification and management of pain. As a result, preventing and managing pain has become a fundamental part of how veterinary patients are cared for. In spite of this, there is still room for further improvement. The most recent AAHA/AAFP Pain Management Guidelines list oncological pain as a frequently overlooked source of pain.

Barriers to effective cancer pain control in animals probably include:

- Lack of appreciation that many cancers are associated with significant pain
- Overly focusing on treating the cancer and not 'present-moment' quality of life of the patient
- Inability to assess pain in cancer patients
- Lack of knowledge of drugs, drug therapy combination and other pain-relieving techniques
- Lack of communication with clients and lack of involvement of clients in the assessment and treatment phases
- Underuse of nursing staff for assessment and re-evaluation of pain in cancer patients.

This chapter deals with the assessment and treatment of chronic cancer pain in dogs and cats. The control of perioperative pain in cancer patients is very important (see 'Relationship between cancer and pain') and readers are encouraged to refer to appropriate texts for information on perioperative pain control and also to Chapter 6, which outlines the principles of perioperative analgesia.

How common is cancer pain in dogs and cats?

As discussed in Chapter 1, the available information indicates that cancer has a significant prevalence within the pet population. The next question that has to be asked is: 'How painful is cancer?' Not all tumours are painful, and the amount of pain is likely to vary considerably from one animal to another, even with similar tumour types. The authors' experience, and the experience of others, would suggest that, using a conservative estimate, 30% of tumours are associated with some degree of pain. Tumours most likely to be associated with pain include those at the following sites: oral cavity; bone; urogenital tract; eyes; nose; liver; gastrointestinal tract; and skin (Figure 11.1). That the figure of 30% is conservative is suggested by looking at the figures from human medicine: pain is experienced by 20–50% of patients when the lesion is diagnosed, by nearly half of all patients in active treatment, and by up to 90% of

Tumour category	Notes
Tumours involving bone	Primary bone tumours (both of the appendicular and axial skeleton) and metastasis to bone are painful. Just as in humans, sometimes metastasis to bone can be relatively non-painful, but this should be considered to be the exception
Central nervous system tumours	Extradural tumours that expand and put pressure on neural tissue are often associated with pain, but tumours originating from within the neural tissue are often not associated with pain until later on in the course of disease. In humans with primary brain tumours or metastases to brain, 60–90% suffer from headaches; it can be presumed that animals also suffer such headaches
Gastrointestinal tumours	Especially oesophagus, stomach, colon and rectum. Colonic and rectal pain is often manifest as perineal discomfort
Inflammatory mammary carcinoma	This form of mammary cancer is very painful in humans. Dogs with this form of mammary cancer appear to exhibit obvious signs of pain
Genitourinary tract tumours	Stretching of the renal capsule appears to produce significant pain. Bladder tumours appear to be predictably associated with pain. Tumours of the distal genitourinary tract are often manifest as perineal pain
Prostate tumours	Prostatic tumours appear to be particularly painful, especially if local metastasis to bone is present
Oral and pharangeal tumours	Soft tissue tumours that are growing by projecting from the surface (e.g. from the gingival surface) appear to be relatively non-painful. Tumours involving bone, or that are growing within the tissues of the maxilla or mandible, appear to be significantly more painful. Soft tissue tumours of the pharynx and caudal oral cavity are particularly painful
Intranasal tumours	Pain probably results both from the destruction of turbinates and from the destruction of bone of the nasal cavity
Invasive soft tissue sarcomas	The aggressive 'injection site sarcomas' (ISSs) in cats are particularly painful, the apparent size of the lesion not correlating with the degree of pain. Other invasive sarcomas in both species are painful. In both cats and dogs, non-invasive soft tissue sarcomas that are pressing on nerves and other sensitive structures will be painful. One form of soft tissue sarcoma, the peripheral nerve sheath tumour (PNST), is sometimes reported to be painful if touched
Invasive cutaneous tumours	Especially those that are ulcerative
Liver and biliary tumours	Especially those that are expansile, stretching the liver capsule. Expansile liver tumours are reported to be painful in humans
Disseminated intrathoracic and intra-abdominal tumours, e.g. mesothelioma, malignant histiocytosis	The signs associated with such tumours are particularly vague, but often intracavitary analgesia (such as intra-abdominal local anaesthetic) can markedly improve the animal's demeanour, and thus, just as in humans, it appears that disseminated neoplasia of these cavities is associated with significant pain
Lung tumours	Although significant pain is reported in humans with lung cancer, often animals appear to show few signs of pain. However, even in those animals, the provision of an analgesic can often improve demeanour
Pain following surgical removal of a tumour	Pain well beyond the postoperative period occurs in animals that have undergone surgery. Most often it is associated with tumour recurrence, but true phantom pain (such as phantom limb pain) that is not associated with tumour recurrence does appear to exist in animals

11.1 Tumours that are probably associated with pain in veterinary patients. In many of these it is difficult for the veterinary surgeon to appreciate that pain may be present. However, the administration of an analgesic to animals suffering from these conditions is reported by owners to result in an improvement in demeanour. In the face of lack of evidence to the contrary, it is suggested that this improvement in demeanour is due to the alleviation of pain.

patients with far advanced or terminal cancer. In humans an overall average of about 70% of patients with advanced cancer suffer pain. Much of this is due to metastasis of breast and prostate cancer to bone. In addition to pain caused by the tumour itself, pain in cancer patients can also be caused by chemotherapy, radiation therapy or surgery (perioperative pain, postoperative pain, and conditions such as 'phantom limb' pain) and by concurrent non-cancerous disease, most notably osteoarthritis.

The importance of alleviating pain

The alleviation of pain is important from physiological and biological standpoints, as well as from an ethical point of view. The role of the veterinary surgeon is to alleviate suffering and maintain the welfare of the animals in their care.

In terms of animal welfare, five freedoms, initially proposed by the Brambell Committee in reference to farmed animals, may equally be applied to the context of companion animals. They are:

- Freedom from hunger and thirst
- Freedom from physical and thermal discomfort
- Freedom from pain, injury, and disease
- Freedom to express normal behaviour
- Freedom from fear and distress.

Thus, pain is one aspect that is considered to compromise welfare. Superimposed on this should be a consideration of the severity and duration of the pain for the individual patient. The greater the duration of pain, such as in longstanding painful cancers, the greater is the compromise of welfare. However, it must also be remembered that animals, as far as we know, have no ability to judge the future and so unrelieved pain at a moment in time may be a significant welfare compromise, even if the pain is going to subside over the subsequent several days.

The approach to the cancer patient should be one that considers all aspects of welfare. In many cases, cancer pain is removed with treatment of the cancer. In cases where owners do not want definitive treatment, or where definitive treatment is not possible and owners do not want to elect for euthanasia, pain control is important. With the increasing demand for 'hospice' type care for pets, pain control is an aspect every veterinary surgeon should become familiar with.

The majority of veterinary surgeons probably agree that it is 'right' to alleviate the pain associated with cancer, and most of the lack of treatment or under-treatment of cancer pain probably stems from a lack of knowledge, lack of recognition of pain and lack of re-evaluation of patients. It does not usually stem from a lack of concern.

Additional effects of analgesics

Physiologically, pain can induce a stress response, with elevations in 'stress hormones' (aldosterone, angiotensin II, antidiuretic hormone, adrenocorticotropic hormone, catecholamines, cortisol and renin) and decreases in other hormones (insulin and testosterone). These changes result in a catabolic state, with muscle protein catabolism. A stress response can result in decreased healing and can also adversely affect the cardiopulmonary and gastrointestinal systems. Such systems are stressed already by the presence of cancer. Of interest is the finding that the provision of analgesics significantly reduces the tumour-promoting effects of undergoing and recovering from surgery. Undergoing surgery is known to result in the suppression of several immune functions, including natural killer (NK) cell activity, probably as a result of released substances such as catecholamines and prostaglandins. This suppression of NK cell activity can enhance metastasis. The reduction of the tumour-promoting effects of surgery by analgesics seems to be due to the alleviation of pain-induced reduced NK cell function, but it is likely that hitherto unrecognized factors other than immune cells also play a role (Page *et al.*, 2001). Thus, the provision of adequate perioperative pain management in oncological surgery may be protective against metastatic sequelae in clinical patients (Bar-Yosef *et al.*, 2001; Benish *et al.*, 2008). It may also be that the treatment of chronic pain, often associated with cancer, is somewhat protective against metastasis and possibly the local extension of cancer.

Classification of cancer pain

Pain is a multifactorial experience with sensory (the sensation), affective/emotional (how it makes the subject feel) and functional (can the subject still perform particular functions?) components. It can result from obvious causes (e.g. ulcerated skin tumour) and last an expected time period. However, in many cases (e.g. post-amputation pain), the pain persists after the original painful cancer has been removed or surgical wound appears to be healed.

In the past, pain has often been categorized as 'acute' or 'chronic' based solely on duration – the latter arbitrarily being pain that lasts more than 3–6 months – but it is now accepted that this may not be a helpful classification. It has been suggested that the terms adaptive and maladaptive be adopted.

- **Adaptive pain** refers to a normal response to tissue damage and involves an inflammatory component (e.g. a surgical incision). It is reversible over an expected, relatively short, time period.
- **Maladaptive pain** results from changes in the spinal cord and brain that result in abnormal sensory processing, and is usually persistent.

Maladaptive pain can result from poorly treated adaptive pain and can occur quickly in some circumstances. Until proven otherwise, cancer pain should be considered maladaptive, with both peripheral and central changes in the pain processing system contributing to the pain, in addition to noxious input from the cancer or pathological area.

Ideally, pain would be classified by the underlying mechanism: for example, inflammatory or neuropathic. However, many diseases are associated with overlapping 'forms' of pain. Taken one step further, pain occurring in different diseases or conditions would be further classified by the underlying mechanisms in that particular disease, and even patient. This could be referred to as the neurobiological signature of pain in a particular disease or patient. Knowing this would better guide the practitioner in the choice of treatment. For example, a diagnosis of 'cancer' pain is not very helpful, since the cause could be mechanical compression of a nerve, inflammation from tissue necrosis, mechanical distension of an organ or neuropathic pain, or a combination of these. A diagnosis of 'osteosarcoma bone pain' with the associated knowledge of the upregulation of peripheral TRPV1 and ASIC receptors, and central COX-2 enzyme, is far more informative in terms of guiding clinical treatment. Without this information, treatment is empirical – perhaps better termed 'hit or miss'.

A key feature of maladaptive pain is central sensitization – changes in the central nervous system (anywhere from the dorsal root ganglion rostrally) that are likely initiated by cellular 'wind-up' and result in amplification and facilitation of nociceptive signal generation and transmission (Figure 11.2). A cancer that is associated with pain (such as an osteosarcoma) results in a barrage of sensory information going into the spinal cord in the area of the dorsal horn. As the problem progresses, peripheral sensitization develops and increases the amount of noxious stimuli going into the spinal cord and CNS.

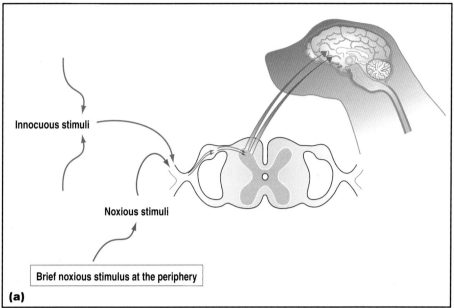

(a)

Innocuous stimuli

Noxious stimuli

Brief noxious stimulus at the periphery

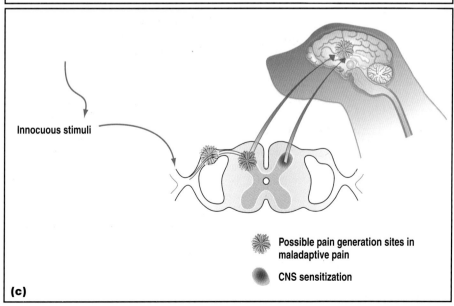

(b)

Innocuous stimuli

Noxious stimuli

Tumour

● CNS sensitization

(c)

Innocuous stimuli

✳ Possible pain generation sites in maladaptive pain

● CNS sensitization

11.2 Peripheral and central sensitization and cancer pain. **(a)** In the normal animal, noxious stimuli (red arrows) are transmitted via the spinal cord to the brain and perceived by the brain as painful. Non-noxious stimuli (blue arrows) travel through the system and are perceived by the brain as non-painful stimuli. **(b)** A cancer that is associated with pain results in a barrage of sensory information going into the spinal cord in the area of the dorsal horn. Peripheral sensitization develops (see text for details), making it easier for a signal to get through and be perceived as painful (hyperalgesia). Also, usually innocuous stimuli are felt as painful (blue arrow into spinal cord becomes a red arrow to the brain). These changes are known as *central hypersensitivity*. **(c)** Occasionally, after resolution of the initiating problem (e.g. amputation for limb osteosarcoma), behaviour indicative of pain remains or recurs. This may be due to the establishment of 'pain generator' centres.

From this point a number of processes take place, including: rostral transmission of the noxious stimulus (perceived as 'pain'); activation of receptors on dorsal horn neurons (e.g. NMDA receptors); and the induction of longer-term changes within the primary afferent fibre and the CNS (e.g. sodium channel, opioid receptor, serotinergic and noradrenergic changes). These result in modulation of nociceptive information processing within the spinal cord. The end result of these changes is a heightened activity and responsiveness of the spinal cord, making it easier for a signal to get through and be perceived as painful (*hyperalgesia*). In addition, stimuli that would not normally have been felt as painful (both from the site of surgery and from other areas) are perceived as painful (*allodynia*). These changes are known as *central hypersensitivity*. In patients experiencing long-lasting persistent pain, as is the case with many types of cancer, peripheral or central sensitization may contribute to the further development of pain, separate from the initial inciting cause, and should be considered in patients with pain that is unresponsive to first-line or conventional analgesics.

Occasionally, after resolution of the initiating problem (e.g. amputation for limb osteosarcoma), behaviour indicative of pain remains or recurs. This may be due to the establishment of 'pain generator' centres (Figure 11.2c), probably resulting from changes similar to those described for central sensitization. There is much debate as to where these 'generators' are, and indeed they may exist at multiple levels. These 'generators' are thought to be responsible for syndromes such as 'phantom limb' pain.

Early intervention is recommended to limit cellular wind-up and prevent central sensitization.

Assessment of cancer pain

It is likely that the tolerance of pain in veterinary patients varies greatly from individual to individual, as it does in humans. Coupled with the innate ability of dogs and, particularly, cats to mask significant disease and probably pain, this makes it very difficult to assess pain. Because there is no obvious external injury, it is often difficult for some clinicians and owners to appreciate that many cancers are associated with pain. Failure of the practitioner to assess pain adequately, both initially and throughout cancer treatment, is likely a major contributor to under-treatment, as it is difficult to assess behaviour and efficacy of treatment if a baseline is not established early on. Unfortunately, little work has been carried out on the assessment of cancer pain in cats or dogs.

Physiological parameters
Physiological variables such as heart rate, respiratory rate, temperature and pupil size have been shown to be unreliable measures of acute perioperative pain in dogs and they are therefore unlikely to be useful in chronic pain states. These variables are affected by psychological factors, disease states and drugs, and thus cannot be relied upon to determine whether an animal is in pain.

Behavioural changes
The mainstay of pain assessment in cats and dogs suffering from cancer is likely to be changes in behaviour. Figure 11.3 outlines behaviours that are probably indicative, in certain situations, of pain. The main point to remember is that any change in behaviour can be associated with pain.

Behaviour	Notes
Vocalization	Although often thought of as associated with pain, vocalization is rare in response to chronic pain in dogs and cats. Occasionally there may be hissing, plaintive miaowing or purring in cats, or whining in dogs. Owners are more likely to report these behaviours, as they are seldom seen in the clinic
Facial expression	Head hung low, squinted eyes in cats with the eyes drawn together by a 'furrowed forehead'. 'Sad' expression in dogs, head carried low
Activity	Less activity than normal; decreased jumping; less playing; less venturing outside; less willing to go on walks (dogs); stiff gait, altered gait or lameness can be associated with generalized pain, but more often associated with limb or joint pain; slow to rise and get moving after rest (osteoarthritis – which is often concurrently present)
Respiration	May be elevated with cancer pain
Attitude	Any change in behaviour can be associated with pain, such as hitherto unseen aggressiveness, dullness, shyness, 'clinginess'
Appetite	Often decreased with chronic pain; tartar build-up on one side of dental arcade relative to other can indicate chronic oral pain; dropping of food can be indicative of intra-oral pain
Urinary and bowel habits	Failure to use litter box (cats); urinating and defecating inside (dogs)
Grooming	Failure to groom, especially with chronic pain – can be due to either painful oral lesion or generalized pain
Response to palpation	One of the best ways to diagnose and monitor pain. Pain can be elicited by palpation of affected area, or manipulation of affected area, which exacerbates low-grade pain to produce transient severe pain, manifested as aversion response from animal, i.e. animal attempts to escape procedure, or yowls, cries, hisses or bites. Pain is inferred when this occurs
Posture	Unusual posture can be an early indicator of the presence of pain
Self-traumatization	Licking at an area (e.g. joint with osteoarthritis, bone with primary bone cancer, abdomen with intra-abdominal cancer) can indicate pain; scratching can indicate pain (e.g. scratching at cutaneous tumours, scratching and biting at flank with prostatic or colonic neoplasia; scratching at area that has received radiation therapy). Pulling out of hair or fur can indicate pain in that area of the body at or below the surface (e.g. hair pulling at flank in cats with renal tumours). Licking at an area can also be indicative of neuropathic pain or neurogenic pain; e.g. after radiation therapy of a limb, constant licking at the area or more distal parts of limb may indicate neuropathic pain

11.3 Behaviours that may be seen in cancer-associated or cancer therapy-associated pain and other chronic pain in cats and dogs.

To be able to assess pain, the veterinary surgeon needs to have a basic understanding of normal behaviour in the species. Ideally, they should have knowledge of the individual animal's normal behaviour. This is not possible in most cases and so the best people to assess the animal's behaviour are the owners. The veterinary surgeon must work closely with the owner to assess the level of pain present at the initial evaluation and also during the re-evaluations that must take place throughout treatment. Owners may not be able to assess the level of pain itself but they are usually able to assess 'quality of life'.

Spontaneous behaviours

It is important to assess spontaneous behaviours.

- Animals that are in pain, especially pain associated with the musculoskeletal system, do not move around as much as they did prior to the pain. Because cats self-regulate exercise and are not generally taken for walks as dogs are, this is more difficult to assess in cats.
- Jumping, climbing and playing are all activities that can be decreased when pain is present, either localized musculoskeletal pain, localized pain not associated with the musculoskeletal system, or more generalized pain.
- In cats, grooming is often decreased. This can be evaluated by examining the condition of the coat.
- In dogs, in particular, attention is paid to painful areas, indicated by licking at such areas.
- Both cats and dogs in pain have decreased appetites, but drinking is usually unaffected unless the pain is severe.

Localized pain can result in specific signs:

- Localized joint, bone or soft tissue pain will result in lameness, muscle wastage or altered gait
- Oral pain can result in an uneven appearance to tartar build-up on teeth, with more tartar being found on the painful side, and can also result in problems with eating or anorexia.

These are examples of clues to the possible presence of pain, which may be detected on clinical examination.

The problem with assessing spontaneous behaviours is that there are many factors released by the tumour itself that can result in depression and lethargy and so altered behaviours are not always associated with pain. For example, lymphoma also often results in anorexia, but probably does not often have a significant pain component. The anorexia in this case is possibly due to many factors, including substances produced by the tumour itself. Also, many diseases alter behaviour, but probably do not produce pain (e.g. hyperthyroidism).

Induced or reactive behaviours

During clinical examination it is routine to use elicitation of pain as a marker of pathology. The same approach should be used to assess pain associated with a tumour. Pain may be elicited by palpation of a tumour, which exacerbates low-grade pain to produce transient severe pain. This is manifested as an aversion response from the animal, i.e. the cat or dog attempts to escape the procedure, or yowls, cries, hisses or bites. Pain is inferred when this occurs and it can therefore be assumed that the tumour is painful. While it is impossible to be sure that the intensity of the reaction to manipulation is truly representative of the severity of the pain felt by the animal in the absence of stimulation, it should be assumed that pain is present and steps should be taken to alleviate it.

The efficacy of analgesic treatments, whether drugs or adjunctive therapies such as acupuncture, should be monitored using palpation and manipulation. Also, it is important to assess cancer patients for non-cancerous related painful conditions, such as osteoarthritis, and to monitor the pain associated with these.

Response to analgesic therapy

Another very good way to determine whether a cat or dog is in pain is to examine its response to analgesic therapy. Both spontaneous and induced or reactive behaviours are assessed. The owner's input here is vital, and assessing the response to analgesic therapy is a central part of tailoring effective treatment to the individual animal.

Health-related quality of life assessment

Over the past two decades, there has been considerable focus on assessment of quality of life (QoL) in human medicine. In humans, cancer pain has been shown to interfere significantly with many aspects of daily life, thus altering overall QoL. A variety of tools have been developed and validated which have proved useful in assessing the impact that specific diseases, including cancer, have on a patient's QoL. Quality of life is most often measured on the basis of a patient's responses to questions in the form of a structured questionnaire.

Though still in its relative infancy, there is a growing interest in developing similar tools for assessing the impact of certain diseases on the QoL of animals. An additional challenge encountered in veterinary medicine is that assessments of QoL must be provided by a proxy informant, typically the owner or primary caregiver – a situation similar to assessment of QoL in human neonates, mentally disabled patients or those who are severely ill.

The impact of cancer pain on QoL in dogs has been investigated using a specifically designed questionnaire, demonstrating a significantly lower QoL in animals with signs of pain from cancer when compared with healthy animals or those with chronic skin disease (Yazbek and Fantoni, 2005). Other authors have reported the use of questionnaires to assess the impact of chronic diseases, including osteoarthritis (Hudson et al., 2004; Wiseman-Orr et al., 2004, 2006; Brown et al., 2007, 2009; Hielm-Bjorkman et al., 2009), spinal cord injuries (Budke et al., 2008) and heart disease (Freeman et al., 2005), on the quality of life in animals. While these tools are unlikely to replace clinical evaluation, they represent yet another option for assessment of patients with chronically painful conditions – maladaptive pain. These instruments can serve both a discriminative and evaluative function: they can identify an absolute QoL score at a particular point in time, as well as determine any changes that occur as a result of disease progression or treatment. Though not yet evaluated in animals, it has been demonstrated in humans that QoL scores can independently predict survival time for patients with a variety of types of cancer.

An approach to cancer pain management

Although drug treatment is the mainstay of cancer pain treatment (see below), adjunctive non-drug therapies such as acupuncture play an important role in pain management of the cancer patient. It must also be remembered that surgery (see Chapter 6) and radiation therapy (see Chapter 8) have very important roles in the management of cancer pain through treatment or palliation of the disease.

A basic approach to cancer pain management could be summarized as follows.

1. Assess the pain. Ask for the owner's perceptions of the pain present or of any compromise of the animal's quality of life.
2. Believe the owner. The owner sees the pet every day in its own environment and knows when alterations in behaviour occur. The owner can rarely suggest diagnoses, but they do know when something is wrong and when their pet is in pain, just as a mother knows when something is wrong with her child.
3. Choose appropriate therapy depending on the stage of the disease. Anything other than mild pain should be treated with more than one class of analgesic, or an analgesic drug combined with non-drug adjunctive therapy. Also consider concurrent problems and drug therapy; be aware of potential drug interactions.
4. Deliver the therapy in a logical coordinated manner and explain carefully to the owner about any possible side effects.
5. Empower clients to participate actively in their pet's treatment; ask for feedback and updates on how the therapy is working.

Principles of drug therapy

Drugs are the mainstay of cancer pain management, although non-drug adjunctive therapies are becoming recognized as increasingly important. It is currently unknown which of the approaches outlined below is most appropriate; indeed, one approach may be best at one stage of the disease, and the other later on.

The 'analgesic ladder'

The World Health Organization has outlined a general approach to the management of cancer pain based on the use of the following 'groups' of analgesics:

- Non-opioid analgesics (e.g. non-steroidal anti-inflammatory drugs (NSAIDs), acetaminophen)
- Weak opioid drugs (e.g. codeine)
- Strong opioid drugs (e.g. morphine)
- Adjuvant drugs (e.g. corticosteroids, tricyclic antidepressants, anticonvulsants, N-methyl D-aspartate (NMDA) antagonists).

This 'analgesic ladder' (Figure 11.4) was developed on the premise that healthcare professionals should learn how to use a few drugs well. It is based on three stepped levels of treatment intensity:

- Some types of pain respond to non-opioid therapy alone
- Pain of a greater intensity can be relieved with the combination of a non-opioid and a 'weak' opioid
- More severe pain requires the addition of a higher dose of opioid, and the use of a 'strong' opioid that is titrated to the pain present.

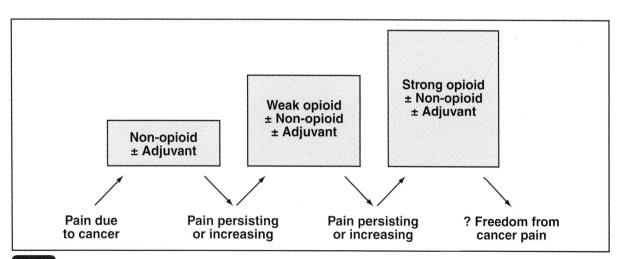

11.4   The WHO 'analgesic ladder' for the treatment of cancer pain.

At any of these three levels, adjunctive analgesics can be used to augment analgesia. This approach is a sound one where the pain is initially at a relatively low level and gradually becomes more severe. However, there are two problems with the use of the WHO analgesic ladder in veterinary medicine. The first is that there is very little information from human medicine, and virtually none from veterinary medicine, on which drugs are most effective for which particular types of cancer pain (see later). It may well be that so-called 'fourth tier' drugs might be most effective for a particular condition and therefore best used up front. This comment relates back to the discussion of the 'neurobiological signature' of different cancer pains. The second problem is that such an approach is not so suited to patients that present initially with significant to severe pain.

The multimodal approach

Many veterinary cancer patients present at an advanced stage of disease and thus are already in pain. Once pain has been present for a period of time, changes have taken place in the central nervous system that alter the way pain signals are processed: maladaptive pain (see above). As a result, the CNS of patients experiencing maladaptive pain may be more sensitive to additional painful stimuli. The clinical implications of this central hypersensitivity are that, once 'pain' is established, analgesic drugs, for a given dose, are much less effective (i.e. pain is more difficult to control); and the 'pain' felt by the animal is greater. Clinical cancer pain is a combination of central hypersensitivity and peripheral hypersensitivity and can be considered maladaptive pain in most cases. Both peripheral and central hypersensitivity are probably well established in most veterinary patients with painful cancers. The implication of this is that the pain is more difficult to treat (due to the established changes at the periphery and in the central nervous system) and thus a *multimodal drug therapy* approach should be employed (using drugs from several different classes). Once the pain is minimized, and central changes are partially reversed, the amounts of drugs

being administered, and the number of classes of analgesic drugs being used, can be decreased. This approach is termed (by this author and others) the *analgesic reverse pyramid* approach.

The most important aspect to remember in the treatment of cancer pain is that, for the majority of situations, multimodal therapy (i.e. concurrent use of more than one class of drug) is required for successful alleviation of the pain. The theory behind a multimodal approach to the management of cancer pain stems from the understanding that pain transmission involves a variety of different pathways, mechanisms and transmitter systems and it is unlikely that a single class of analgesic will provide complete pain control. Multimodal approaches combine several drugs with differing mechanisms of action to affect the perception, transmission and modulation of pain.

In addition to providing more complete pain control, another major advantage of this approach is the ability to reduce the dose, and therefore the potential for the occurrence of side effects associated with each individual drug. This is especially important when considering the risk of adverse events with certain medications (e.g. NSAIDs) or the perception of owners to the untoward effects of others (opioids).

Choice of drugs

As we begin to embrace a mechanistic approach to pain, we understand that different mechanisms might underlie pain associated with different tumours, or different tumours *versus* other long-term pain conditions, such as osteoarthritis. The result is the need for treatments geared toward the individual patient's specific needs and the use of a single class of analgesic for every patient would be inappropriate. However, multimodal therapy can have negative side effects associated with it and these have not been defined in veterinary medicine. Drugs that can be used for chronic cancer pain management are outlined in Figures 11.5 and 11.6. The following notes are not a comprehensive appraisal of each class of drug, but are pointers to their use for cancer pain. Figure 11.7 outlines a decision-making tree for the process of treating cancer pain in dogs and cats.

Drug	Dose in dogs	Comments
Paracetamol	10–15 mg/kg orally q8h for 5 days Long-term therapy: up to 10 mg/kg q12h	Seems to be associated with fewer GI side effects than 'regular' NSAIDs. Not noted to be associated with renal toxicity. Toxicity not evaluated clinically in dogs. Can be combined with regular NSAIDs in severe cancer pain, but combination not evaluated for toxicity
Paracetamol + codeine	Dose based on 10–15 mg/kg of paracetamol – correspond to codeine at 2 mg/kg	Sedation can be seen as side effect
Amantadine	4.0–5.0 mg/kg orally q24h	Loose stools and excess GI gas can be seen at higher doses for a few days. *Should not be combined with drugs such as selegiline or sertraline until more is known about drug interactions*
Amitriptyline	0.5–2.0 mg/kg orally q24h	Not evaluated for clinical toxicity in the dog, but suggested should not be administered concurrently with tramadol or other drugs with 'serotinergic' actions
Aspirin	10 mg/kg orally q12h	Causes significantly more GI ulceration than approved NSAIDs. *Do not use near time of surgery, due to inhibition of platelet function*
Butorphanol	0.2–0.5 mg/kg orally up to q8h	May produce sedation at higher doses. Not a very predictable analgesic, and best when used in combination (e.g. with NSAIDs)

11.5 Analgesics that may be considered for alleviation of chronic cancer pain in dogs. Note that *none* of the drugs is authorized for this use. (continues) ▶

Drug	Dose in dogs	Comments
Codeine	0.5–2.0 mg/kg orally q12h	Sedation can be seen at higher doses
Carprofen	2 mg/kg orally q12h or 4 mg/kg orally q24h	
Deracoxib	1–2 mg/kg orally q24h	(Only available in the US)
Etodolac	5–15 mg/kg orally q24h	(Only available in the US)
Fentanyl, transdermal	2–5 μg/kg/h	Can be very useful short term. Usefulness limited due to need to change patch every 4–5 days and expense involved
Firocoxib	5 mg/kg q24h	
Gabapentin	10 mg/kg orally q12h	Not evaluated for analgesic effects but appears to be useful for certain neuropathic pain (e.g. after limb amputation, nerve root tumour pain, other cancer pain involving nerve damage). Best effects seen when used in combination (e.g. with NSAIDs or paracetamol)
Glucosamine and chondroitin sulphate	13–15 mg/kg chondroitin sulphate orally q24h	Often not considered for cancer pain. Mild anti-inflammatory and analgesic effects. Preparations with avocado–soya unsaponifiables may be more effective as mild analgesics
Meloxicam	0.2 mg/kg orally day 1, then 0.1 mg/kg q24h	
Morphine, liquid	0.2–0.5 mg/kg orally q6–8h	Can be useful for dosing smaller dogs where tablets not suitable. Sedation and (particularly) constipation are side effects as dose is increased, but see text on first-pass effects
Morphine, sustained release	0.5–3.0 mg/kg orally q8–12h	Doses >0.5–1.0 mg/kg are often associated with unacceptable constipation according to owners, so suggest 0.5 mg/kg several times a day. See text on first-pass effects
Pamidronate	1–1.5 mg/kg slowly i.v. q3–5wks	Inhibits osteoclast activity and provides analgesia in cases suffering from primary or metastatic bone tumour causing osteolysis
Piroxicam	0.3 mg/kg orally q24–48h	
Polysulphated glycosaminoglycan	5 mg/kg i.m. twice weekly, then once a month	Has not been evaluated for cancer pain, but may provide mild analgesic effects. *Suggested not used in cancer patients with haemostatic disorders*
Prednisolone	0.25–1 mg/kg orally q12–24h; taper to q48h if possible after 14 days	*Do not use concurrently with NSAIDs.* Can be particularly useful in providing analgesia when there is significant inflammatory component associated with tumour
Robenacoxib	1 mg/kg	
Tepoxalin	10 mg/kg q24h	
Tramadol	4–5 mg/kg orally q8–12h	Not evaluated for efficacy or toxicity in dogs but appears to be useful adjunctive analgesic (when combined e.g. acetaminophen or NSAIDs). Note comments in text about GI ulceration
Vedaprofen	0.5 mg/kg q24h	

11.5 (continued) Analgesics that may be considered for alleviation of chronic cancer pain in dogs. Note that *none* of the drugs is authorized for this use.

Drug	Cat dose	Notes
Paracetamol (acetaminophen)	**Contraindicated**	**Contraindicated – small doses cause death in cats**
Amantadine	3.0–5.0 mg/kg orally q24h	Not evaluated for toxicity but well tolerated in dogs and humans, with occasional side effects of agitation and GI irritation. May be useful addition to NSAIDs in treatment of chronic cancer pain conditions. The 100 mg capsules need to be re-compounded for cats (can be done using amantadine powder)
Amitriptyline	0.5–2.0 mg/kg orally q24h	Appears to be well tolerated for up to 12 months of daily administration. Has been used for interstitial cystitis; somnolence (<10%), weight gain, decreased grooming and transient cystic calculi were observed during treatment in some cats. May be useful addition to NSAIDs for treatment of cancer pain conditions
Aspirin	10 mg/kg orally q48h	Can cause significant gastrointestinal ulceration
Buprenorphine	0.02 mg/kg sublingual q8–12h	Sublingual route not resented by cats; may be good way to provide postoperative analgesia at home. Feedback from owners indicates anorexia develops after 2–3 days at this dose. Smaller doses (5–10 *micrograms* per kg) may be more appropriate for 'long-term' administration, especially in combination with other drugs

11.6 Suggested dosages of analgesics that might be considered for the alleviation of cancer pain in cats. Note that *none* of these is authorized in any country for the treatment of cancer pain in the cat; some are approved for inflammatory or painful conditions in the cat in certain countries, and doses for the control of cancer pain are extrapolated from these. The dosages given come from the authors' experience and that of others working in the area of clinical cancer pain control. (continues) ▶

Drug	Cat dose	Notes
Butorphanol	0.2–1.0 mg/kg orally q6h	One study suggests oral butorphanol after surgery may be beneficial. Generally considered to be poor analgesic in cats except for visceral pain, but author has found it useful as part of multimodal approach to cancer pain therapy
Carprofen	Not enough data to enable recommendations for long-term administration	
Etodolac	Not enough data to enable recommendations	
Fentanyl, transdermal	2–5 µg/kg/h	Patches may provide 5–7 days analgesia in some cases. Following removal at 3 days, decay in plasma levels is slow
Firocoxib	Not enough data to enable recommendations	Not been used in clinical cases. Has half-life 8–12 hours in cat. At 3 mg/kg provided anti-pyrexia effects in pyrexia model
Flunixin meglumine	1 mg/kg orally q24h for 7 days	Daily dosing for 7 days results in increased rate of metabolism of drug. Rise in liver enzymes suggests liver toxicity *may* be problem with prolonged dosing
Gabapentin	10 mg/kg q12h	Appears to be particularly effective in chronic pain in cats where increase in sensitivity has occurred, or where pain appears to be excessive in comparison with lesion present
Glucosamine/chondroitin sulphate combinations	Approx 15 mg/kg chondroitin sulphate orally q12–24h	Appear to produce mild anti-inflammatory and analgesic effects in cats more predictably than in dogs
Glucosamine/chondroitin sulphate combination with avocado–soya extracts	Labelled dose	This preparation has only just become available, but addition of ASU (Dasuquin®) appears to boost analgesic effects of Glu/Cho4
Ketoprofen	1.0 mg/kg orally q24h; maximum 5 days	Probably well tolerated as pulse therapy for cancer pain, with a few days 'rest' between treatments. Has also been used at 1 mg/kg q3d long term. Another approach has been 0.5 mg/kg q24h for 5 days (weekdays) followed by no drug over weekend, and this is repeated
Meloxicam	0.1 mg/kg orally on day 1, followed by 0.05 mg/kg orally q24h for 4 days, then 0.05 mg/kg q48h thereafter, *or* 0.025 mg/kg q24h	Particularly well received by cats due to formulation as honey syrup. Drop formulation makes it very easy to decrease dose gradually and accurately. Meloxicam should be dosed accurately using syringes – drop size dispensed from the bottle varies significantly. Suggested dosing regimen not evaluated for clinical toxicity. Approval gained in Europe (June 2007) for long-term (unlimited) use of meloxicam in cat at 0.1 mg/kg on day 1, followed by 0.05 mg/kg q24h for musculoskeletal pain
Morphine, oral liquid	0.2–0.5 mg/kg orally q6–8h	Best compounded into palatable flavoured syrup but cats usually strongly resent this medication. Morphine may not be as effective in cats as in dogs
Morphine, oral sustained release	Tablets too large for dosing cats	
Piroxicam	0.2–0.3 mg/cat orally q24h	Daily dosing for 7 days results in slight increase in half-life. Recent work suggests daily piroxicam tolerated well in cats with cancer, with main side effects GI signs
Polysulphated glycosaminoglycans	5 mg/kg s.c. twice weekly for 4 weeks; then once weekly for 4 weeks; then once monthly (other suggested regimens call for once weekly injections for 4 weeks, then once monthly)	No evidence-based medicine that it provides any effect, but anecdotal information suggests efficacy in some cancer pain
Prednisolone	0.5–1.0 mg/kg orally q24h	Can be very effective for some cancer pain. *NOT to be combined with concurrent NSAID administration*
Robenacoxib	1–2 mg/kg q24h for up to 6 days	Short half-life (1–2 hours) in cat. Demonstrates tissue selectivity
Tepoxalin	Not enough data to enable recommendations	
Tolfenamic acid	4 mg/kg orally q24h for 3 days max	Recent objective measurements demonstrate analgesia in cat when administered perioperatively
Tramadol	1–2 mg/kg q12–24h	Recent studies indicate metabolism of tramadol slower in cat than dog, and production of M1 metabolite very much greater, leading to greater tendency to see 'opioid'-like side effects
Vedaprofen	0.5 mg/kg q24h for 3 days	Evaluated for controlling pyrexia in upper respiratory infection and for controlling postoperative pain following ovariohysterectomy

11.6 (continued) Suggested dosages of analgesics that might be considered for the alleviation of cancer pain in cats. Note that *none* of these is authorized in any country for the treatment of cancer pain in the cat; some are approved for inflammatory or painful conditions in the cat in certain countries, and doses for the control of cancer pain are extrapolated from these. The dosages given come from the authors' experience and that of others working in the area of clinical cancer pain control.

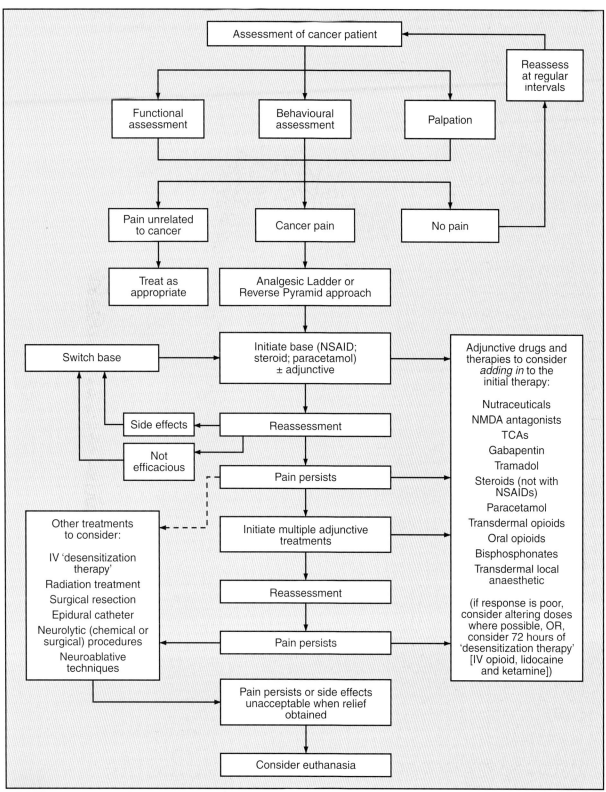

11.7 Decision-making tree for the treatment of cancer pain in cats and dogs. This should be considered as a guide only; approaches in individual patients will vary. For example, it may be most appropriate to initiate treatment of pain associated with osteosarcoma with an NSAID and palliative radiation before moving to other adjunctive drugs.

Non-steroidal anti-inflammatory drugs

New impetus to the fields of analgesia and inflammation research was provided by the finding that the cyclo-oxygenase enzyme (COX) exists in (at least) two different forms. It was found that COX activity was stimulated by bacterial endotoxin and that this increase in activity was due to the *de novo* synthesis of new COX protein. Shortly after this, the inducible COX protein was characterized as a distinct isoform of cyclo-oxygenase, COX-2, and was shown to be encoded by a different gene from that producing the constitutive enzyme, renamed COX-1. Thus, there are now known to be two types of cyclo-oxygenase enzyme, one producing 'essential prostaglandins' (e.g. prostaglandins that are involved in maintaining mucosal integrity of the stomach) on a minute-to-minute basis, and avnother that is activated by tissue trauma and results in the production of 'inflammatory' or 'pain-mediating' prostaglandins. However, it is not as simple as COX-1 being 'good' and COX-2 'bad', as COX-2 has been shown to be expressed constitutively in certain tissues, such as the canine kidney and canine gastrointestinal tract (Wooten *et al.*, 2008) and may play a role in protection and healing of gastric and duodenal mucosa (Goodman *et al.*, 2009). So, although theory would suggest that selective or specific COX-2 inhibitors might be associated with fewer gastrointestinal side effects than a non-selective drug, this has not yet been proved in veterinary medicine. Additionally, if gastroduodenal ulceration is present, selective or specific COX-2 inhibitors may interfere with healing. The clinical significance of this has not been defined. Theory would also suggest that COX-2 selective drugs are *not* any safer to the kidney than are the non-selective drugs. Again, widespread clinical experience in dogs is required to substantiate this, though the COX-2 selective drugs used in humans have been found to be associated with a similar incidence of renal toxicity as traditional NSAIDs.

NSAIDs are the most widely used analgesic drugs in human and veterinary medicine and the mainstay for treatment of long-standing pain, especially in osteoarthritis. They have both central analgesic and peripheral anti-inflammatory effects. When combined with other medications, such as opioids, they exhibit a synergistic effect, allowing for the reduction in dose, and in theory the potential for the development of adverse effects associated. They should be considered as a component of a multimodal pain management plan in patients for which there is not a specific contraindication to administration (e.g. renal, hepatic or gastrointestinal disease; concurrent steroid administration).

Apart from the concern over side effects produced by NSAIDs, discussion of COX enzymes has further relevance to cancer pain therapy. Of particular interest in cancer pain management is the finding that NSAIDs that inhibit COX-2 may not only produce pain alleviation in cancer pain states but also demonstrate anti-tumour effects. In recent years, there has been a considerable amount of research published regarding the expression of COX-2 and/or PGE_2 by a variety of epithelial and non-epithelial tumours, including canine transitional cell, prostatic and renal carcinoma, osteosarcoma, oral and cutaneous squamous cell carcinomas, oral melanoma and colorectal adenocarcinoma. In cats, both oral squamous cell carcinoma and transitional cell carcinomas have been reported to express the COX-2 enzyme (Spugnini *et al.*, 2005; Hayes, 2007). These findings have resulted in interest in the clinical use of NSAIDs as a component of treatment for these tumours, particularly now with the widespread availability of COX-2 selective or specific inhibitors.

The choice of NSAIDs available can be bewildering, and continues to increase, but there are a few key points to note.

- On a population basis, all NSAIDs are equally efficacious in relieving pain associated with osteoarthritis, but for a given patient one drug is often more effective than another drug. This is probably even more true for cancer pain, where the mechanisms of pain may be very different from one patient to another.
- Gastrointestinal side effects associated with NSAID use may be more common with drugs that preferentially block COX-1 over COX-2, but COX-2 selective drugs may delay or inhibit the healing of gastric erosions and ulcers.
- There is no difference in renal toxicity between COX-1 selective drugs and COX-2 selective drugs. Both COX-1 and COX-2 are constitutively expressed in the kidney.
- Liver toxicity with NSAIDs is an idiosyncratic event that can happen with any NSAID.
- The total level of side effects seen with the different NSAIDs is probably the same, but the type of side effects seen with different NSAIDs appears to differ.

Thus, veterinary surgeons should start treatment using an NSAID with which they are comfortable, and possibly consider the aspect of COX-2 inhibition or published work demonstrating an anti-cancer effect of a particular NSAID.

Monitoring: If the drug is effective, it should be continued. If not, therapy should be switched to another NSAID. The patient should be monitored for toxicity. This consists of two aspects:

- Informing the owner of potential toxicity and what signs to watch for (lethargy, depression, vomiting, melaena, increased water ingestion)
- Regular blood work (and urinalysis) to evaluate renal function (urea, creatinine, urine specific gravity) and liver function (alkaline phosphatase and alanine aminotransferase and, if these enzymes are raised, bile acids). A baseline should be obtained when therapy is initiated and parameters monitored on a regular basis thereafter. There are no guidelines on this, but the author repeats the evaluation after 2–4 weeks, and then at 2–4-monthly intervals as dictated by the individual patient and client. This re-evaluation is done more frequently if multiple drugs are used, as there is no information on clinical toxicity associated with combinations of analgesics administered chronically. Caution should be used when administering any NSAID to dogs with renal disease; paracetamol may be a good alternative in these cases.

NSAIDS in cats: NSAIDs are considered potentially more toxic to cats than to dogs or humans. Interestingly, there seems to be significant variation among individual cats in the metabolism of NSAIDs and also inconsistent variation in the rate of metabolism of different NSAIDS compared with other species. The use of NSAIDs in cats has been comprehensively reviewed (Lascelles *et al.*, 2007) and pertinent developments since that publication are the approval in Europe and other countries (including Australia) of meloxicam to treat chronic musculoskeletal pain. An additional development is that the first coxib class of NSAIDs, robenacoxib, has been granted approval in Europe for use in cats.

Cats are more sensitive to NSAIDs than are dogs and so monitoring should probably be carried out more frequently than in dogs. There are no guidelines for monitoring cats receiving chronic NSAID administration. The authors consider it very important to monitor these patients closely, and suggest the following:

- A biochemistry panel, packed cell volume, total protein assay and urinalysis measurements prior to starting the NSAID
- Re-evaluation at 1 week, 4 weeks and every 4–6 weeks thereafter.

This should be done in conjunction with continual reassessment of the patient so that the dose can be tapered down to the smallest effective amount as soon as possible. Although decreasing specific gravity is not an early indicator of renal disease in cats as it is in the dog, but is rather a late phenomenon, urinalysis should still be performed on a regular basis. Decreasing the drug dose to the lowest effective amount is probably a very important factor in limiting clinical toxicity of NSAIDs in the cat. These suggestions are based on very limited information that the authors have gathered on the toxicity of NSAIDs in cats. Owners should be informed about the possibility of toxicity and given the signs to look for.

Additional drugs for use with NSAIDs: If pain relief with NSAIDs is inadequate, other drugs can be administered in conjunction with them. Agents that can be used include: paracetamol; fentanyl patches; amantadine (an NMDA antagonist); anticonvulsants/ calcium channel modulators, such as gabapentin; and tricyclic antidepressants, such as amitriptyline. Transdermal lidocaine patches can be used to treat localized pain and it is believed that they may provide relief in some maladaptive pain states. These can all be combined with NSAIDs. However, the toxicity related to such polypharmacy has not been defined and clinicians are advised to monitor carefully for side effects.

Paracetamol

Paracetamol (acetaminophen) is a non-acid NSAID; many authorities do not consider it an NSAID as it probably acts through different mechanisms. Although its mechanism of action is poorly understood, it is likely that it acts through several central mechanisms, possibly including inhibition of the activity of a splice variant of COX-1 and by acting through the endogenous cannabinoid system. With any maladaptive pain, there are always CNS changes, so for what seems a 'peripheral' problem, such as many cancers, centrally acting analgesics can be very effective. *Although highly toxic in the cat (even in small quantities)* it can be effectively used in dogs for pain control. No studies of toxicity in dogs have been done, but if toxicity is seen it will probably affect the gastrointestinal system and, in larger doses, the liver. It can be used on its own or in a preparation combined with codeine and is initially dosed at about 10–15 mg/kg q12h. The author often uses it as the first line of analgesic therapy in dogs with renal compromise where NSAIDs cannot be used, or in dogs that appear to be otherwise intolerant to NSAIDs (e.g. vomiting or gastrointestinal ulceration).

Opioids

In humans, opioids represent the primary class of analgesics for management of moderate to severe cancer pain. Many veterinary surgeons, however, may be unfamiliar with the use of opioids outside the perioperative period. Opioids act at all levels of the pain pathway – peripherally, and centrally at the spinal cord and brain. Opioid receptors interact positively with other analgesic systems such as the NMDA and alpha-2 receptors and therefore can be a very effective part of the management of cancer pain as part of a multimodal approach.

Opioids may be classified as pure μ-agonists (e.g. morphine, hydromorphone, oxymorphone, fentanyl, codeine, meperidine), partial agonists or κ-agonist/ μ-antagonists. Pure μ-agonists are thought to produce the most complete analgesia. Buprenorphine is a commonly used partial μ-agonist. Butorphanol is an example of a κ-agonist/μ-antagonist and is generally regarded as a weak analgesic drug; as such, its use in treating cancer pain is limited.

Most commonly, pure μ-agonists are given by injection, but oral, epidural and transdermal routes of administration may also be used.

Oral route: Oral opioid medications such as codeine, codeine-combination drugs (such as paracetamol plus codeine), morphine, methadone or butorphanol can be administered to dogs, but very little is known about their efficacy by this route. When given orally, opioids are subject to a high 'first pass' effect in the liver; published studies have demonstrated that oral morphine and methadone are not well absorbed in the dog, which may limit their effectiveness clinically (Kukanich *et al.*, 2005ab). However, unpublished data suggest that other oral opioids (such as codeine) may be absorbed into the systemic circulation and thus have the opportunity of being effective.

Transdermal route: Transdermal delivery of opioids has become an increasingly popular method for managing both acute and chronic pain in humans. In animals, transdermal delivery of opioids avoids the hepatic first-pass metabolism associated with oral opioids. The primary use of transdermal opioids has been for the treatment of acute postoperative pain. Fentanyl is the only opioid medication for which studies have demonstrated effective transdermal delivery and resulting analgesia in animals. Fentanyl patches require 12–24 hours to take effect and last as long as 4 days. Analgesia achieved following fentanyl patch placement alone is generally mild to moderate, but in cases of more severe pain it may allow for reduction in the doses of adjuvant medications.

More recently, transdermal buprenorphine patches have been introduced in humans for use in a variety of chronic pain conditions, including cancer pain and chronic neuropathic pain. There are currently no data to support the use of these patches for dogs.

It is of note that none of these drugs has been fully evaluated for clinical toxicity when administered in the long term, nor for efficacy against cancer pain in the dog or cat. It is important to realize that dosing must be done on an individual basis, and adjustment of the dose to produce analgesia without undesirable side effects requires excellent interaction and communication with clients.

Epidural route: In addition to the routes listed above, opioids may be administered via the epidural route, either as a single perioperative injection, or following the placement of an epidural catheter for continuous infusion following surgery or as a component of hospice-type care.

Side effects: Side effects of opioids can include diarrhoea, vomiting, constipation with long-term use and occasionally sedation. It is very often the constipation, and occasionally the sedation seen, that owners seem to object to most, especially with the administration of oral opioids.

Opioids in cats: There is currently no information on the long-term use of opioids for pain in the cat. Interestingly, there seems to be significant individual variation in the level of analgesia obtained with certain opioids, especially morphine and butorphanol, in the acute setting. Buprenorphine appears to produce predictable analgesia when given sublingually in the cat (Robertson *et al.,* 2005). Compared with humans, the sublingual route appears more effective in cats; this may be a result of differences in ionization in the alkaline environment (pH 8–9) of the cat's mouth compared with that of humans (pH 6.5–7). Sublingual administration of buprenorphine is well accepted by cats, with no resentment or salivation, and so there is no need to compound the injectable solution. Based on clinical feedback from owners, this is a very acceptable technique for them to perform at home and the authors have found it useful to use sublingual buprenorphine in the management of certain types of cancer pain in the cat. However, some owners do not like the behavioural changes it can induce in cats (euphoria) nor the dilated pupils. In addition, inappetence can occur after several days of treatment. Sometimes slightly lower doses can overcome these problems.

The pharmacodynamics and kinetics of transdermal fentanyl have been evaluated in the cat and this method of delivery has proven efficacy for routine perioperative analgesia. Significant variations in plasma concentrations of fentanyl have been reported, however, and it should not be presumed that the placement of a fentanyl patch provides sufficient analgesia. Animals with fentanyl patches should be regularly assessed and supplemental analgesics should be provided if necessary. Recently published data evaluating the analgesic effect of transdermal buprenorphine in cats failed to demonstrate a significant anti-nociceptive benefit (Murrell *et al.*, 2007).

NMDA antagonists

The *N*-methyl D-aspartate receptor appears to be central to the induction and maintenance of central sensitization, and the use of NMDA receptor antagonists would appear to offer benefit in the treatment of pain where central sensitization has become established (i.e. especially maladaptive pain).

Ketamine, tiletamine, dextromethorphan, memantadine and amantadine possess NMDA antagonist properties, among other actions. Dogs may not make the active metabolite after administration of dextromethorphan, which probably negates its use in dogs for chronic pain (Kukanich and Papich, 2004b). Studies have suggested a benefit of using ketamine perioperatively in low doses.

Amantadine has been used for the treatment of neuropathic pain in humans. It does not have the undesirable side effects associated with ketamine administration. The authors have been using amantadine over the past few years as an adjunctive drug (usually together with an NSAID) for the alleviation of cancer pain. Recent data suggest that it appears to augment pain relief in dogs with osteoarthritis, with a low incidence of side effects (mainly agitation and diarrhoea over the first few days of administration) (Lascelles *et al.*, 2008). This work suggested that it may take up to 2 weeks to see the full effect and so it may be a drug to start earlier rather than later in cancer pain treatment. Amantadine should probably not be used in patients with congestive heart failure, nor in patients on selegiline, sertraline or tricyclic antidepressants.

The development of more specific NMDA antagonists is an exciting area of research, but the development of clinically useful and targeted antagonists is hampered by the fact that the NMDA receptor is known to exist in numerous forms which may change rapidly following nociceptive input. Additionally, the form and quantity of the specific NMDA receptor may differ significantly from one painful condition to the next.

Combination analgesics

Tramadol is a centrally acting analgesic with complex interactions between opiate, adrenergic and serotonergic receptors. Opioid receptors are well known to be involved in pain states, and the descending serotonergic system is known to be one of the body's endogenous 'analgesic' mechanisms. In humans, clinical response to tramadol is determined by its metabolism, primarily due to the analgesic effects of its metabolites. Hepatic demethylation of tramadol produces the major active metabolite, O-desmethyltramadol (M1), which is reported to be 200 times more potent at the μ-receptor than the parent drug, which has a weak affinity for the opioid receptors. Both the parent drug and metabolite exist as a racemic mixture, and different metabolites interact differently with the target receptors (Kukanich and Papich, 2004a).

Pharmacokinetic studies have been performed in both dogs and cats (Kukanich and Papich, 2004a; Pypendop and Ilkiw, 2008) and have suggested sufficient absorption of the oral form and plasma levels that are similar to those achieved in humans, with a significantly shorter elimination half-life. Plasma elimination half-life of the M1 metabolite is longer in cats than in dogs, possibly due to cats' poor ability to glucuronidate compounds. More recent pharmacokinetic data call into question the amount of the M1 metabolite that is formed in dogs following intravenous (McMillan et al., 2008) and oral (Giorgi et al., 2009b) administration and, as a result, calls into question the effectiveness of tramadol as an analgesic in animals. Very few studies have been performed assessing the analgesic effect of tramadol in the dog or cat and none have evaluated its use in treating musculoskeletal or cancer pain. In veterinary medicine, the standard oral formulation is most commonly prescribed; and based on recent pharmacokinetic data, it appears that the extended-release formulation does not allow for once-daily dosing, as in humans (Giorgi et al., 2009ab).

Tramadol has not been evaluated for toxicity in the dog or cat and almost nothing is known about the side effects when tramadol is combined with other drugs in human or veterinary patients. A recent study in humans found that, for patients hospitalized for peptic ulcer treatment, tramadol use prior to admission was associated with a greater risk of mortality than was NSAID use prior to admission. Additionally, mortality was 2.02- and 1.41-fold higher in these groups of patients, respectively, than in patients who used neither tramadol nor NSAIDs (Torring et al., 2008). The authors of that study suggested that this may be due to the ability of tramadol to mask visceral pain associated with gastrointestinal irritation and perforation. However, a recent study evaluating the analgesic effects of various doses of rofecoxib and tramadol, both alone and in combination, found that the most analgesic combination of tramadol and rofecoxib produced gastric injury in rats that was more severe than with either drug alone (Garcia-Hernandez et al., 2007). The cause of this injury is unknown but these data do suggest that, under certain circumstances, caution may need to be exercised when combining NSAIDs and tramadol. However, there are no data from dogs or cats, and other data on tramadol suggest protective effects on the gastrointestinal tract.

α2-Agonists

This class of drugs exerts analgesic and sedative effects by interaction with the α_2-adrenergic receptors in the dorsal horn of the spinal cord and within the brain stem. Though not commonly used as first-line analgesics, drugs such as medetomidine, detomidine and dexmedetomidine have the potential to provide excellent analgesia when used as an adjunct to other medications. These drugs are most commonly administered intravenously and are generally used as a component of a multimodal perioperative pain management plan. In addition to the intravenous route, α_2-agonist may be administered via epidural injection (in combination with morphine and/or a local anaesthetic), intra-articularly, or as a component of a peripheral nerve block. Their use perioperatively may help to prevent long-term postoperative pain or neuropathic pain.

Anticonvulsant drugs

In humans many anticonvulsants, such as carbamazepine, phenytoin, baclofen and, more recently, gabapentin, have been used to treat chronic pain, including neuropathic pain and chemotherapy-induced peripheral neuropathies. Gabapentin and the more recently introduced pregabalin appear to be among the most effective drugs available for neuropathic pain, but have also been demonstrated to be effective when used to treat acute postoperative pain. While the exact mechanism of action of these drugs is unclear, one potential mode by which they exert their analgesic effect is by binding to the alpha-2-delta protein subunit of voltage-gated calcium channels, thereby reducing excitatory neurotransmitter release through channel modulation or channel trafficking.

In dogs, although there is considerable information on gabapentin disposition (Vollmer et al., 1986; Radulovic et al., 1995) and some information on its use as an anticonvulsant (Platt et al., 2006), there is as yet no information on its use for pain control. Very recently, information on the kinetics of gabapentin in cats has become available (unpublished) but there are no scientific publications demonstrating its efficacy for long-term pain in this species. While the indications for gabapentin (and pregabalin) are at present unclear in veterinary patients, they do appear to be useful for cancer pain in some patients and are probably particularly effective in cancers that have some neurogenic or nerve destruction component. The authors start at 10 mg/kg twice daily.

Tricyclic antidepressants

Tricyclic antidepressants have been used for many years for the treatment of chronic pain syndromes in humans and are becoming widely used for the modulation of behavioural disorders in animals. Within the central nervous system, there are descending inhibitory serotonergic and noradrenergic pathways that reduce pain transmission in the spinal cord. Tricyclic antidepressants, such as amitriptyline, clomipramine, fluoxetine, imipramine, maprotiline and paroxetine, primarily inhibit the reuptake of various monoamines (serotonin for clomipramine, fluoxetine and paroxetine; noradrenaline for imipramine, amitriptyline and maprotiline). Tricyclic antidepressants can also interact directly with 5HT and peripheral noradrenergic receptors and may also contribute other actions such as voltage-gated sodium channel blockade and reduction in peripheral PGE_2-like activity or tumour necrosis factor (TNF) production.

These drugs have been used in humans for the treatment of chronic and neuropathic pain at doses considerably lower than those used to treat depression. Several recent systematic reviews of the human literature confirm the efficacy of antidepressant medications (specifically tricyclic antidepressants) in treating certain chronic pain conditions such as neuropathic pain, fibromyalgia, lower back pain and headaches. The authors of these studies identify that, even in human medicine, there is a relative lack of controlled clinical trials specifically evaluating the efficacy of antidepressants in treating cancer pain, with the exception of two studies demonstrating a lack of efficacy in the treatment of chemotherapy-induced peripheral neuropathy.

Given the possibility that many behavioural disorders are in fact due to chronic pain, tricyclic antidepressants may not be directly affecting behaviour but rather pain itself, resulting in behavioural modification. The opposite argument could also be made. It is not unrealistic to assume that, although more difficult to appreciate or evaluate, chronic painful conditions may also affect mood or behaviour in veterinary patients, and the symptomatic treatment of behavioural alterations may, in turn, give the appearance of a decrease in pain as perceived by the owner.

The tricyclic antidepressant amitriptyline appears to be effective in the cat for pain alleviation in interstitial cystitis and many practitioners are reporting efficacy in other chronically painful conditions in the cat, including osteoarthritis. Amitriptyline has been used daily for periods up to 1 year for interstitial cystitis and few side effects have been reported. The author has used amitriptyline in the cat for cancer pain with some encouraging results. It should probably not be used concurrently with other drugs that modify the serotonergic system, such as amantadine or tramadol, until more is known about drug interactions.

Sodium channel blockade
Alterations in the level of expression, cellular localization and distribution of sodium channels are seen in many pain states. These aberrantly expressed sodium channels result in hyperexcitability and ectopic activity in peripheral and central nerves that encode nociceptive information. Low doses of lidocaine and other sodium-channel blockers readily block these aberrantly expressed sodium channels, producing pain relief.

Sodium channel blockers may be administered orally, intravenously, intrathecally or as a component of a peripheral nerve or plexus block. Although not a convenient mode of delivery for veterinary patients unless hospitalized, low-dose intravenous lidocaine has proved as effective as other commonly used medications for treatment of neuropathic pain in humans and the authors use such an approach to 'down-regulate' central sensitization in veterinary cancer patients.

There is increasing interest in the use of transdermal lidocaine patches for treatment of chronic neurological and osteoarthritic pain in humans. Although most recommendations suggest that the patches be placed close to the site of the painful stimulus, it is possible they may have analgesic actions due to the systemic absorption of lidocaine. Human patients do not report a loss of sensitivity or numbness. While the mechanism of this differential blockade is not completely understood, it has been suggested that the lidocaine patch delivers adequate amounts of drug to block small, injured or dysfunctional pain fibres, while large myelinated A-β sensory fibres are unaffected. Studies have been performed evaluating the kinetics of lidocaine absorbed from patches applied to dogs and cats (Weiland et al., 2006; Ko et al., 2007, 2008; Weil et al., 2007). Peak plasma concentrations of lidocaine were obtained 10–24 hours after application in dogs and at 65 hours after application in cats. The results of these studies indicate that, as in humans, systemic absorption of lidocaine from the patch is minimal. Peak plasma concentrations were over 100 times below the level reported to induce neurological signs and 10 times below the level reported to result in myocardial depression in dogs, and 25 times lower than that observed following an intravenous injection of lidocaine (2 mg/kg) in cats (Weiland et al., 2006; Ko et al., 2007, 2008). Potential systemic toxicity associated with lidocaine administration including bradycardia, hypotension, cardiac arrest, muscle or facial twitching, tremors, seizures, nausea and vomiting were not noted in any study.

While dosing guidelines have been suggested (Weil et al., 2007), there have been no published reports evaluating the analgesic efficacy of lidocaine patches in veterinary patients. Based on the authors' experience, cats appear to be particularly sensitive to the effects of lidocaine and care should be exercised if lidocaine patches are utilized.

Steroids
Steroids have a mild analgesic action and can also produce a state of euphoria; they are often used for these reasons to palliate cancer and cancer pain in cats and dogs. They should not be used concurrently with NSAIDs, because the risk of side effects is increased dramatically.

Bisphosphonates and other targeted therapies for skeletal neoplasia
Malignant bone disease creates a unique pain state, with a neurobiological signature distinct from that of inflammatory and neuropathic pain. Bone pain induced by primary or metastatic bone tumours is thought to be initiated and perpetuated by dysregulated osteoclast activity and activation of nociceptors by prostaglandins, cytokines and hydrogen ions. Therapies that block osteoclast activity and aim to prevent bone resorption not only have the potential to reduce bone pain markedly, but may also mitigate other skeletal complications associated with neoplastic conditions, including pathological fractures and hypercalcaemia of malignancy (Fan et al., 2007).

Bisphosphonates are synthetic analogues of pyrophosphate whose primary effect is to inhibit osteoclast activity. After administration, bisphosphonates accumulate in areas of bone that are more metabolically active, such as trabecular bone, growing bone, and areas of osteolysis and repair. Following osteoclast-mediated bone resorption, bisphosphonates are released from hydroxyapatite and then disrupt cellular functions, resulting in osteoclast death. Oral absorption of bisphosphonates tends to be poor and intravenous dosing is the preferred route of administration.

While most reports suggest that these drugs are relatively non-toxic, adverse effects have been reported and include oesophageal and gastrointestinal tract irritation (following oral dosing), nephrotoxicity (following intravenous administration), electrolyte abnormalities and acute-phase reactions (Milner et al., 2004).

In addition to the inhibitory effects of bisphosphonates on osteoclasts, reports suggest that they may also exert direct effects on cancer cells, including canine osteosarcoma and fibrosarcoma lines, through a variety of different mechanisms. Several studies have demonstrated beneficial effects of intravenous pamidronate for the treatment of malignant osteolysis and pain associated with primary and secondary bone neoplasms (Fan et al., 2005, 2007, 2008, 2009). These studies have collectively demonstrated a reduction in focal bone lysis and an improvement in both subjective and objective measures of pain and lameness in dogs with a variety of tumours. As is the case in humans, however, the addition of pamidronate to standard palliative therapies (radiation, chemotherapy) does not appear to improve the duration of pain control in dogs with osteosarcoma, though there is evidence that the degree of pain alleviation may be greater (Fan et al., 2009). Pamidronate may be administered at a dose of 1–2 mg/kg as a 2–4-hour infusion (diluted in saline) and repeated at intervals of 3–5 weeks.

Other examples of bisphosphonates that can be used in dogs are clodronate, aledronate and zoledronate (Tomlin et al., 2000; de Lorimier and Fan, 2005; Martin-Jimenez et al., 2007; Fan et al., 2008; Wypij et al., 2008).

Samarium-153 is a radioisotope that has been evaluated for use in both humans and dogs (Milner et al., 1998). When administered as [153]Sm-lexidronam, the compound concentrates in areas of increased osteoblastic activity and binds to hydroxyapatite crystals, which allows for targeted therapy of bone tumours. Beta decay of the isotope is reported to result in both tissue-destructive and therapeutic effects. The most common adverse effect reported in both humans and dogs is myelosupression resulting in thrombocytopenia and leucopenia. While the use of [153]Sm-lexidronam in veterinary medicine is still limited, results of a recent study demonstrated an improvement in lameness scores in 63% of dogs, suggesting that this therapy may be useful in the palliation of pain in dogs with bone tumours in which curative-intent treatment is not pursued (Barnard et al., 2007). Further research is needed to determine the ultimate role that this therapy may play.

Nutraceuticals

These are often used in osteoarthritis and there is evidence that they provide a mild anti-inflammatory effect and an analgesic effect. The authors have found them to be of benefit in the alleviation of cancer pain but only when used as part of a multimodal approach. The analgesic effect appears to be more predictable in cats than in dogs, and the authors prefer combinations of glucosamine and chondroitin sulphate with avocado–soya unsaponifiables.

Radiation therapy

Radiation therapy is a useful tool in the palliation of certain cancer pain. However, radiation pain is a recognized side effect of radiation treatment of tumours in animals, and the pain associated with this is extremely difficult to control. Chapter 8 gives detailed information on topical mixtures that can be useful in decreasing radiation-associated pain. The authors recommend an aggressive multimodal analgesic drug approach that is instigated early in patients undergoing radiation therapy.

Acupuncture

There are no published studies on the use of non-drug therapy (apart from surgery and radiation) for the alleviation of cancer pain. From veterinary clinical experience, one of the most useful adjuncts to drug therapy appears to be acupuncture. Placement of needles at specific acupuncture points can relieve pain through several mechanisms.

- Acupuncture may decrease muscle spasms when needles are inserted into pressure points. Lack of spasms considerably increases patient comfort. Muscle spasms are often present in cancer patients with pain, due to altered gait from a painful limb, or altered gait from concurrent osteoarthritis.
- Acupuncture can also induce the release of a variety of neurotransmitters, which can affect the processing of the pain impulse.

Acupuncture can be provided through simple needle placement, or by needle placement combined with electrical stimulation (of high or low frequency, though most types of pain respond to low-frequency stimulation). Results of a study by Culp et al. (2005) demonstrated a weak analgesic effect of electroacupuncture in anaesthetized patients as evaluated by a reduction in the MAC of inhaled anaesthetic agent. More recent data utilizing a rodent model suggested that electroacupuncture may have beneficial effects in treatment of pain associated with bone cancer (Zhang et al., 2007, 2008). In contrast, Kapatkin et al. (2006) found no benefit of electroacupuncture on the severity of lameness in a group of dogs with osteoarthritis. It is likely that the benefits of acupuncture are variable and specific to the type and degree of pain that is experienced.

A recent systematic review of the use of acupuncture in veterinary medicine concluded that the evidence for the effectiveness in domestic animals was 'generally weak and not sufficiently compelling to recommend or reject its use in treating any condition' (Habacher et al., 2006). The authors did suggest that the data regarding the alleviation of cutaneous pain were encouraging and warranted further investigation utilizing more rigorous investigative methods.

In addition to potential analgesic effects, acupuncture may also help to increase appetite and alleviate nausea induced by the administration of certain chemotherapeutic or analgesic drugs.

The future: towards a mechanistic understanding of cancer pain

Over the past few years, it has become evident that the pain transmission system is plastic, i.e. it alters in response to inputs. It is also becoming understood that this plasticity results in a unique neurobiological signature within the peripheral and central nervous system for each painful disease. Reading and understanding the individual neurobiological signatures for different disease processes should allow novel, targeted and more effective treatments to be established. This approach should also allow for a more informed choice to be made regarding which of the currently available drugs might be most effective.

It may surprise readers that only in the past 10 years has the first relevant model of cancer pain been established in rats: an osteosarcoma model. Prior to this, evaluation of mechanisms and treatments was undertaken in various chronic pain models such as sciatic nerve ligation, or injection of chronic irritants – models that did not involve cancer. The establishment of more recent models, such as the osteosarcoma pain model, have shown that the neurobiological signature of pain in clinically relevant models is very different from that in the older models of chronic pain.

The new approach of using clinically relevant models has allowed targeted pain treatments to be developed. Such models will also allow for the screening of the potential efficacy of other novel treatments, such as selective neuroablation techniques. Recently published research has demonstrated very promising results utilizing such novel approaches as substance P-saporin and resiniferatoxin for the treatment of chronic pain. These substances, when administered intrathecally, induce selective destruction or inactivation of neurons involved in pain transmission, resulting in prolonged analgesia in patients in which conventional analgesics are ineffective. The effectiveness of such approaches has been demonstrated in dogs with osteosarcoma of the limbs (Brown *et al.*, 2005).

References and further reading

Bar-Yosef S, Melamed R, Page GG *et al.* (2001) Attenuation of the tumor-promoting effect of surgery by spinal blockade in rats. *Anesthesiology* **94**, 1066–1073

Barnard SM, Zuber RM and Moore AS (2007) Samarium Sm 153 lexidronam for the palliative treatment of dogs with primary bone tumors: 35 cases (1999–2005). *Journal of the American Veterinary Medical Association* **230**, 1877–1881

Benish M, Bartal I, Goldfarb Y *et al.* (2008) Perioperative use of beta-blockers and COX-2 inhibitors may improve immune competence and reduce the risk of tumor metastasis. *Annals of Surgical Oncology* **15**, 2042–2052

Brown DC, Boston RC, Coyne JC and Farrar JT (2007) Development and psychometric testing of an instrument designed to measure chronic pain in dogs with osteoarthritis. *American Journal of Veterinary Research* **68**, 631–637

Brown DC, Boston R, Coyne JC and Farrar JT (2009) A novel approach to the use of animals in studies of pain: validation of the canine brief pain inventory in canine bone cancer. *Pain Medicine* **10**, 133–142

Brown DC, Iadarola MJ, Perkowski SZ *et al.* (2005) Physiologic and antinociceptive effects of intrathecal resiniferatoxin in a canine bone cancer model. *Anesthesiology* **103**, 1052–1059

Budke CM, Levine JM, Kerwin SC *et al.* (2008) Evaluation of a questionnaire for obtaining owner-perceived, weighted quality-of-life assessments for dogs with spinal cord injuries. *Journal of the American Veterinary Medical Association* **233**, 925–930

Culp LB, Skarda RT and Muir WW (2005) Comparisons of the effects of acupuncture, electroacupuncture, and transcutaneous cranial electrical stimulation on the minimum alveolar concentration of isoflurane in dogs. *American Journal of Veterinary Research* **66**, 1364–1370

de Lorimier LP and Fan TM (2005) Bone metabolic effects of single-dose zoledronate in healthy dogs. *Journal of Veterinary Internal Medicine* **19**, 924–927

Fan TM, Charney SC, de Lorimier LP *et al.* (2009) Double-blind placebo-controlled trial of adjuvant pamidronate with palliative radiotherapy and intravenous doxorubicin for canine appendicular osteosarcoma bone pain. *Journal of Veterinary Internal Medicine* **23**, 152–160

Fan TM, de Lorimier LP, Charney SC and Hintermeister JG (2005) Evaluation of intravenous pamidronate administration in 33 cancer-bearing dogs with primary or secondary bone involvement. *Journal of Veterinary Internal Medicine* **19**, 74–80

Fan TM, de Lorimier LP, Garrett LD and Lacoste HI (2008) The bone biologic effects of zoledronate in healthy dogs and dogs with malignant osteolysis. *Journal of Veterinary Internal Medicine* **22**, 380–387

Fan TM, de Lorimier LP, O'Dell-Anderson K, Lacoste HI and Charney SC (2007) Single-agent pamidronate for palliative therapy of canine appendicular osteosarcoma bone pain. *Journal of Veterinary Internal Medicine* **21**, 431–439

Freeman LM, Rush JE, Farabaugh AE and Must A (2005) Development and evaluation of a questionnaire for assessing health-related quality of life in dogs with cardiac disease. *Journal of the American Veterinary Medical Association* **226**, 1864–1868

Garcia-Hernandez L, Deciga-Campos M, Guevara-Lopez U and Lopez-Munoz FJ (2007) Co-administration of rofecoxib and tramadol results in additive or sub-additive interaction during arthritic nociception in rat. *Pharmacology Biochemistry and Behaviour* **87**, 331–340

Giorgi M, Del Carlo S, Saccomanni G *et al.* (2009a) Biopharmaceutical profile of tramadol in the dog. *Veterinary Research Communications* **33**(Suppl.1), 189–192

Giorgi M, Saccomanni G, Lebkowska-Wieruszewska B and Kowalski C (2009b) Pharmacokinetic evaluation of tramadol and its major metabolites after single oral sustained tablet administration in the dog: a pilot study. *Veterinary Journal* **180**, 253–255

Goodman L, Torres B, Punke J *et al.* (2009) Effects of firocoxib and tepoxalin on healing in a canine gastric mucosal injury model. *Journal of Veterinary Internal Medicine* **23**, 56–62

Habacher G, Pittler MH and Ernst E (2006) Effectiveness of acupuncture in veterinary medicine: systematic review. *Journal of Veterinary Internal Medicine* **20**, 480–488

Hayes A (2007) Cancer, cyclo-oxygenase and nonsteroidal anti-inflammatory drugs; can we combine all three? *Veterinary and Comparative Oncology* **5**, 1–13

Hielm-Bjorkman AK, Rita H and Tulamo RM (2009) Psychometric testing of the Helsinki chronic pain index by completion of a questionnaire in Finnish by owners of dogs with chronic signs of pain caused by osteoarthritis. *American Journal of Veterinary Research* **70**, 727–734

Hudson JT, Slater MR. Taylor L, Scott HM and Kerwin SC (2004) Assessing repeatability and validity of a visual analogue scale questionnaire for use in assessing pain and lameness in dogs. *American Journal of Veterinary Research* **65**, 1634–1643

Kapatkin AS, Tomasic M, Beech J *et al.* (2006) Effects of electrostimulated acupuncture on ground reaction forces and pain scores in dogs with chronic elbow joint arthritis. *Journal of American Veterinary Medical Association* **228**, 1350–1354

Ko J, Weil A, Maxwell L, Kitao T and Haydon T (2007) Plasma concentrations of lidocaine in dogs following lidocaine patch application. *Journal of the American Animal Hospital Association* **43**, 280–283

Ko JC, Maxwell LK, Abbo LA and Weil AB (2008) Pharmacokinetics of lidocaine following the application of 5% lidocaine patches to cats. *Journal of Veterinary Pharmacology and Therapeutics* **31**, 359–367

Kukanich B, Lascelles BD, Aman AM, Mealey KL and Papich MG (2005a) The effects of inhibiting cytochrome P450 3A, p-glycoprotein, and gastric acid secretion on the oral bioavailability of methadone in dogs. *Journal of Veterinary Pharmacology and Therapeutics* **28**, 461–466

Kukanich B, Lascelles BD and Papich MG (2005) Pharmacokinetics of morphine and plasma concentrations of morphine-6-glucuronide following morphine administration to dogs. *Journal of Veterinary Pharmacology and Therapeutics* **28**, 371–376

Kukanich B and Papich MG (2004a) Pharmacokinetics of tramadol and the metabolite O-desmethyltramadol in dogs. *Journal of Veterinary Pharmacology and Therapeutics* **27**, 239–246

Kukanich B and Papich MG (2004b) Plasma profile and pharmacokinetics of dextromethorphan after intravenous and oral administration in healthy dogs. *Journal of Veterinary Pharmacology and Therapeutics* **27**, 337–341

Lascelles BD, Court MH, Hardie EM and Robertson SA (2007) Nonsteroidal anti-inflammatory drugs in cats: a review. *Veterinary Anesthesia and Analgesia* **34**, 228–250

Lascelles BD, Gaynor JS, Smith ES *et al.* (2008) Amantadine in a multimodal analgesic regimen for alleviation of refractory osteoarthritis pain in dogs. *Journal of Veterinary Internal Medicine* **22**, 53–59

Lindley S and Taylor P (2010) Chronic pain. In: *BSAVA Manual of Canine and Feline Rehabilitation, Supportive and Palliative Care: Case Studies in Patient Management*, ed. S Lindley and P Watson, pp. 42–59. BSAVA Publications, Gloucester

Martin-Jimenez T, De Lorimier LP, Fan TM and Freise KJ (2007) Pharmacokinetics and pharmacodynamics of a single dose of zoledronate in healthy dogs. *Journal of Veterinary Pharmacology and Therapeutics* **30**, 492–495

McMillan CJ, Livingston A, Clark CR *et al.* (2008) Pharmacokinetics of intravenous tramadol in dogs. *Canadian Journal of Veterinary Research* **72**, 325–331

Milner RJ, Dormehl I, Louw WK and Croft S (1998) Targeted radiotherapy with Sm-153-EDTMP in nine cases of canine primary bone tumours. *Journal of the South African Veterinary Association* **69**, 12–17

Milner RJ, Farese J, Henry CJ *et al.* (2004) Bisphosphonates and cancer. *Journal of Veterinary Internal Medicine* **18**, 597–604

Murrell JC, Robertson SA, Taylor PM *et al.* (2007) Use of a transdermal matrix patch of buprenorphine in cats: preliminary pharmacokinetic and pharmacodynamic data. *Veterinary Record* **160**, 578–583

Page GG, Blakely WP and Ben-Eliyahu S (2001) Evidence that postoperative pain is a mediator of the tumor-promoting effects of surgery in rats. *Pain* **90**, 191–199

Platt SR, Adams V, Garosi LS *et al.* (2006) Treatment with gabapentin of 11 dogs with refractory idiopathic epilepsy. *Veterinary Record* **159**, 881–884

Pypendop BH and Ilkiw JE (2008) Pharmacokinetics of tramadol, and its metabolite O-desmethyl-tramadol, in cats. *Journal of Veterinary Pharmacology and Therapeutics* **31**, 52–59

Radulovic LL, Turck D, von Hodenberg A *et al.* (1995) Disposition of gabapentin (neurontin) in mice, rats, dogs, and monkeys. *Drug Metabolism and Disposition* **23**, 441–448

Robertson SA, Lascelles BD, Taylor PM and Sear JW (2005) PK-PD modeling of buprenorphine in cats: intravenous and oral transmucosal administration. *Journal of Veterinary Pharmacology and Therapeutics* **28**, 453–460

Spugnini EP, Porrello A, Citro G and Baldi A (2005) COX-2 overexpression in canine tumors: potential therapeutic targets in oncology. *Histology and Histopathology* **20**, 1309–1312

Tomlin JL, Sturgeon C, Pead MJ and Muir P (2000) Use of the bisphosphonate drug alendronate for palliative management of osteosarcoma in two dogs. *Veterinary Record* **147**, 129–132

Torring ML, Riis A, Christensen S *et al.* (2008) Perforated peptic ulcer and short-term mortality among tramadol users. *British Journal of Clinical Pharmacology* **65**, 565–572

Vollmer KO, von Hodenberg A and Kolle EU (1986) Pharmacokinetics and metabolism of gabapentin in rat, dog and man. *Arzneimittelforschung* **36**, 830–839

Weil AB, Ko J and Inoue T (2007) The use of lidocaine patches. *Compendium Continuing Education for Veterinarians* **29**, 208–210, 212, 214–216

Weiland L, Croubels S, Baert K *et al.* (2006) Pharmacokinetics of a lidocaine patch 5% in dogs. *Journal of Veterinary Medicine. A, Physiology, Pathology, Clinical Medicine* **53**, 34–39

Wiseman-Orr ML, Nolan AM, Reid J and Scott EM (2004) Development of a questionnaire to measure the effects of chronic pain on health-related quality of life in dogs. *American Journal of Veterinary Research* **65**, 1077–1084

Wiseman-Orr ML, Scott EM, Reid J and Nolan AM (2006) Validation of a structured questionnaire as an instrument to measure chronic pain in dogs on the basis of effects on health-related quality of life. *American Journal of Veterinary Research* **67**, 1826–1836

Wooten JG, Blikslager AT, Ryan KA *et al.* (2008) Cyclooxygenase expression and prostanoid production in pyloric and duodenal mucosae in dogs after administration of nonsteroidal anti-inflammatory drugs. *American Journal of Veterinary Research* **69**, 457–464

Wypij JM, Fan TM, Fredrickson RL *et al.* (2008) In vivo and in vitro efficacy of zoledronate for treating oral squamous cell carcinoma in cats. *Journal of Veterinary Internal Medicine* **22**, 158–163

Yazbek KV and Fantoni DT (2005) Validity of a health-related quality-of-life scale for dogs with signs of pain secondary to cancer. *Journal of the American Veterinary Medical Association* **226**, 1354–1358

Yoxall AT (1978) Pain in small animals – its recognition and control. *Journal of Small Animal Practice* **19**, 423–438

Zhang RX, Li A, Liu B *et al.* (2007) Electroacupuncture attenuates bone cancer pain and inhibits spinal interleukin-1 beta expression in a rat model. *Anesthesia and Analgesia* **105**, 1482–1488

Zhang RX, Li A, Liu B *et al.* (2008) Electroacupuncture attenuates bone-cancer-induced hyperalgesia and inhibits spinal preprodynorphin expression in a rat model. *European Journal of Pain* **12**, 870–878

12

Tumours of the skin and subcutaneous tissues

Laura Blackwood

Introduction

Tumours of the skin and subcutaneous tissues account for approximately one-third of tumours in dogs and one-quarter of tumours in cats. Most skin and subcutaneous tumours in the dog are benign (70–80%), but the majority of feline tumours (50–65%) are malignant. Most tumours are primary and metastatic lesions are uncommon.

Based on pathological submissions, mast cell tumours (MCTs) are the commonest skin tumours in dogs, but benign lesions are also common (lipomas, benign epithelial tumours, papillomas). In cats, basal cell tumours, squamous cell carcinomas, MCTs and fibrosarcomas are commonest, though historically basal cell tumours have probably been over-diagnosed.

Many non-neoplastic skin lesions can mimic tumours, especially if proliferative or ulcerated. Examples include:

* Eosinophilic granuloma complex
* Flea allergic dermatitis
* Mycoses
* Poxvirus
* Dermatophytoses
* Autoimmune disease.

Approach to the patient

Clinical and historical features help to refine differential diagnoses for skin lesions, particularly when there are non-neoplastic differentials. Clinical features typical of a malignant tumour include rapid growth, fixation, invasion into deep tissues or overlying skin, ulceration, or poorly defined margins. Clinical criteria can suggest that a lesion is malignant, but apparently less aggressive behaviour should not result in the lesion being assumed to be benign. Aggressive mesenchymal tumours may appear well demarcated due to pseudocapsule formation, and MCTs can mimic many benign lesions, including lipomas.

Tumours of the skin and subcutis are seldom imaged, but magnetic resonance imaging or computed tomography can inform surgical planning for sarcomas. Ultrasonography can help to confirm that a lesion is a lipoma (because of the distinct echogenicity of fat), or guide aspiration or biopsy.

Neither cytology nor histopathology is 100% sensitive or specific in the diagnosis of skin tumours, though histopathology remains the gold standard. Cytology will usually differentiate between neoplastic and inflammatory lesions, and determine whether tumours are malignant or benign. It will broadly ascertain tumour type (epithelial, mesenchymal, round cell or melanocytic tumour) but not exact histogenesis; for example, sarcoma may be diagnosed, but histology will be required to determine type. Cytological samples contain fewer cells than biopsy samples and these may not be representative of the whole lesion; furthermore, tissue architecture cannot be appreciated. There are other pitfalls: dysplastic epithelial or mesenchymal cells may mimic neoplastic change and this is particularly problematic where there is inflammation. However, aspirates are easy to perform, of low cost and yield rapid results.

Histopathology can also be limited by small or non-representative samples. When harvesting incisional biopsies:

* Avoid ulcerated and necrotic areas
* Do not increase the surgical field by sampling at the junction of normal and neoplastic tissue
* Plan the biopsy site so that the entire biopsy tract can be resected at definitive surgery.

Excisional biopsy

Excisional biopsy is widely used in the management of skin tumours. Often this is appropriate and successful, particularly in dogs, where many skin tumours are benign. It is less successful in the management of subcutaneous tumours. In a minority of cases, this intervention can have disastrous consequences for the future management of the case and the opportunity for curative treatment can be lost forever. This most often occurs where there is incomplete excision of soft tissue sarcomas or MCTs. The difficulty in achieving a complete excision at second surgery is compounded where large surgeries have been performed and/or complex closure methods used.

Excisional biopsy is appropriate where adequate excision is likely to be achieved by simple surgery. This decision is best made in the light of a diagnosis based on fine-needle aspiration (FNA) rather than on clinical criteria alone. The owner should understand that further surgery may be recommended on the basis of biopsy results after excisional biopsy. The whole specimen must be submitted to the pathologist for diagnosis and assessment of margins of excision. Benign proliferative epithelial tumours have a relatively distinctive appearance and excisional biopsy is justifiable in these cases, as there is a high likelihood that the clinical diagnosis is correct, but care should be taken where squamous cell carcinoma is a differential diagnosis.

Clinical features that suggest excisional biopsy of a cutaneous or subcutaneous mass would be inappropriate include:

* Rapidly growing mass
* Ill-defined or poorly demarcated lesion (Figure 12.1)
* Peritumoral oedema or erythema
* Ulceration of overlying skin
* Injection site masses in cats
* FNA suspicion of soft tissue sarcoma or MCT
* Non-diagnostic FNA:
  o No cells harvested (common in sarcomas)
  o Very bloody sample, or haemorrhage only (may be seen in MCTs and some sarcomas)
  o Haemorrhage and eosiniphils (suspicious for MCT)

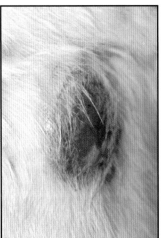

12.1 An ulcerated rapidly growing and poorly demarcated skin mass on a middle-aged crossbred dog. Aspiration of this lesion to achieve a diagnosis prior to surgery is recommended.

Staging for metastases
Local and regional lymph nodes should be evaluated by palpation. Nodes that are abnormal in size or texture should be aspirated; and apparently normal nodes should also be aspirated in patients known or suspected to have highly malignant tumours and in all cases of MCT. Metastases may be found in nodes that are palpably normal.

Further tumour staging, to assess for distant metastatic spread, is appropriate for malignant lesions and investigations are dictated by tumour type.

Solitary skin tumours

Dermatopathologists are keen to classify tumours accurately, but the cell of origin of some dermal tumours has been difficult to determine. Terminology has changed as histochemistry and immunohistochemistry have allowed determination of the true cell of origin of tumours. A large number of different terms are used, particularly for epithelial tumours, as the epithelium has many different cells and complex adnexal structures.

Hamartomas and naevi also cause confusion. **Hamartomas** are benign nodules created by disorganized overgrowth of mature cells and tissues normally found in the affected area. Hamartoma is the preferred term for these tumour-like malformations, whether congenital or acquired. **Naevus** implies congenital origin.

Most solitary skin tumours in dogs arise from the epithelial tissues, including the adnexae, but tumours may arise from mesenchymal tissues, neural tissue, melanocytes, histiocytes, mast cells and lymphoid cells.

Epithelial tumours

The common epithelial tumours (and pseudonyms) are summarized in Figures 12.2, 12.6, 12.9 and 12.10. Epithelial tumours include epidermal, follicular, sebaceous and sweat gland tumours. Non-neoplastic mass lesions that may mimic tumours are included where relevant.

Epidermal tumours
Epidermal tumours are summarized in Figure 12.2. Oncologically, the squamous cell carcinoma group is most important.

Lesions (and pseudonyms)	Signalment/predisposition	Predilection site	Clinical features	Possible treatment/ comments
Dermoid cyst	Rhodesian Ridgeback	Dorsal midline	Congenital lesions where there is a focal reduplication of the entire skin structure. Dermal or s.c. mass, central pore, hair may protrude. May be multiple	Surgical excision (if required)
Squamous papilloma (misnomer fibrous papilloma)	None	Face, eyelids, feet, conjunctiva	Delicate fimbriated pedunculated mass	Surgical excision (if required)

12.2 Epidermal tumours and tumour-like lesions in dogs and cats. (continues) ▶

Lesions (and pseudonyms)	Signalment/predisposition	Predilection site	Clinical features	Possible treatment/ comments
Viral papilloma	Dogs <3 years old. Whippet, Bernese Mountain Dog, Irish Setter, Beagle, Great Dane, Cocker Spaniel, Kerry Blue Terrier	Haired skin or mucosa (oral, eyelids, nasal planum)	Mainly exophytic wart-like fimbriated hyperkeratotic lesions. Rarely inverted	Usually regress
Viral plaque (canine pigmented viral plaque, verruca plana, epidermodysplasia verruciformis)	Young adults. Pug, Miniature Schnauzer, Boston Terrier, French Bulldog	Ventral abdomen, thorax, medial legs (dogs only)	Flat wart, may be pigmented	May progress to malignancy, especially in cats (may precede SCC)
Actinic keratosis (actinic carcinoma *in situ*, solar keratosis, keratinocytic intradermal neoplasia)	Sunny climate, high altitude, lower latitude, arid environment. White cats, dogs with thin/white haircoat	Pinna, nose and eyelids of cats. Ventral abdomen and medial thigh in dogs	Plaque-like or papillated lesion. Scaly, crusty	See text
Multifocal SCC *in situ* (Bowenoid carcinoma *in situ*, Bowen's disease, multicentric papillomavirus induced SCC *in situ*)	Older animals	Any site	Multifocal, heavily crusted plaques and verricose lesions. May be pigmented.	May progress to squamous cell carcinoma or basal cell carcinoma. See text: Bowenoid should not be used to refer to multicentric disease
Squamous cell carcinoma	Sunny climate, high altitude, lower latitude, arid environment. White cats, dogs with thin/white haircoat	Pinna, nose and eyelids of cats. Ventral abdomen and medial thigh in dogs	Plaque-like or papillated, scaly, crusty. Crateriform or ulcerated mass, papillary or fungiform mass. Often indurated	Surgical excision, radiotherapy, photodynamic therapy (see text)
Basal cell carcinoma (basal cell epithelioma)	UV exposure a risk factor for BCC in humans but not proven in dogs and cats. Mean age of cats with BCC is 10 years. Older dogs	Nose, face and ears of cat. Trunk of dogs	Indurated plaques, umbilicated nodules, alopecia, crusting, pigmentation	Surgical excision

12.2 (continued) Epidermal tumours and tumour-like lesions in dogs and cats.

Feline actinic keratosis

It is proposed that actinic keratosis (AK) is renamed keratinocytic intradermal neoplasia or actinic carcinoma *in situ*, as it is an early form of squamous cell carcinoma (SCC) *in situ* (i.e. non-invasive). Many of the molecular and genetic lesions found in SCC are also found in AK, and many AK lesions progress to SCC, so both basic science and clinical experience support this.

Aetiology, pathogenesis and predispositions: The aetiology and risk factors for AK in cats are the same as for SCC, and the lesions occur at the same sites (see below).

Clinical presentation: Clinically, these lesions are scaly, crusty, scabby plaque-like or papillated lesions (Figure 12.3).

Treatment: Surgical excision is generally curative. Alternative treatments include photodynamic therapy or imiquimod (see below).

Prognosis: The prognosis for AK is variable. Although the disease course is often very long, lesions can progress through SCC *in situ* to full-blown SCC, and earlier intervention is more likely to achieve cure. Active monitoring is only appropriate if

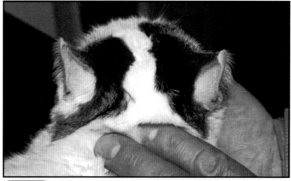

12.3 Actinic dermatosis affecting the pinnae of a middle-aged female neutered DSH cat. (Courtesy of T Nuttall)

there is intervention before the lesion ceases to be surgically curable.

Squamous cell carcinoma

Squamous cell carcinoma is the commonest malignant skin tumour in cats (up to 50% of skin tumours) and the second commonest in dogs (up to 20% of skin tumours).

Aetiology, pathogenesis and predispositions: The wide variation in reported incidence of SCC is largely dependent on geographical factors reflecting ultraviolet (UV) exposure (arid climate, lower latitude and higher altitude will increase risk). UV-related p53 mutations have been identified in feline tumours. Patient risk factors are white hair coat in cats and short or white/piebald ventral hair coat in dogs. White cats have 13 times the risk of developing SCC than cats with any other coat colour. Papillomavirus may have an aetiological role, and SCC has been reported after thermal injury. Tumours of the nasal planum in dogs are thought to be associated with chronic inflammation rather than UV exposure. Canine nail-bed SCC is commonest in large dogs with dark/black hair coats. Nail-bed SCC is uncommon in cats.

Older cats (median 11 years) and dogs (median 10 years) tend to be affected.

Presentation and clinical signs: In cats, tumours tend to arise on the nasal planum, pinnae (Figure 12.4) and eyelids. In dogs, the ventral abdomen, flanks and medial thighs are most commonly affected. SCCs are often plaque-like, or may form ulcerated, crateriform or fungiform masses. Crusting and ulceration are common and there may be associated fibrous tissue so that the lesion is indurated (thickened or hardened), especially where there has been chronic AK.

Dogs with SCC of the nail bed usually present with a single swollen deformed digit with or without loss of the nail. Although lesions are usually solitary, multiple digits can be affected synchronously or metachronously (e.g. in Giant Schnauzers). Metastasis to regional lymph nodes is common and distant metastasis occurs in up to 30% of cases. Tumours of the nasal planum in dogs are ulcerated lesions (Figure 12.5) and are aggressively locally invasive, often with nodal metastases.

Multifocal SCC may occur in both dogs and cats. In dogs, multiple lesions have been reported affecting relatively thin-haired areas of pale-skinned dogs chronically exposed to sunlight. In cats, multiple lesions are common, affecting ear and nose, synchronously or sequentially; and SCC, SCC *in situ* and AK may coexist. Multifocal lesions of SCC *in situ* may histologically resemble Bowen's disease in

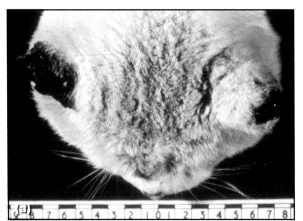

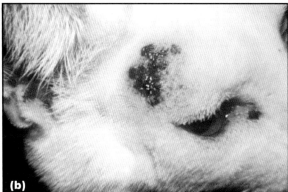

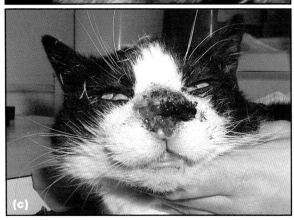

12.4 SCC in three light-coated DSH cats. Invasive erosive lesions are seen affecting **(a)** pinnae, **(b)** forehead and **(c)** the rhinarium. The rhinarial tumour is a postsurgical recurrence. (Photograph (b) courtesy of C Gaskell)

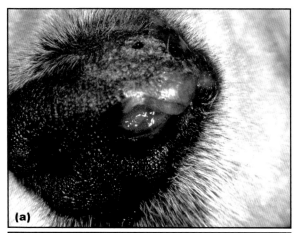

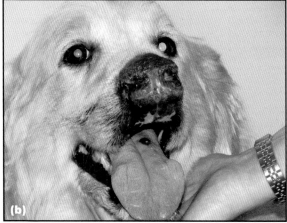

12.5 Rhinarial SCC in dogs. **(a)** Untreated lesion in a 7-year-old male Golden Retriever. **(b)** Recurrent tumour in a 10-year-old neutered male Golden Retriever 4 months after surgery and radiotherapy.

humans, but this is most often a solitary tumour, associated with sunlight exposure, which rarely progresses to invasion. The use of Bowen's disease as a term for multicentric SCC *in situ* is discouraged.

Clinical approach and management: Biopsy is required for diagnosis and local lymph nodes should be evaluated. For both SCC *in situ* and invasive SCC, even in multiple sites, treatment options are surgical excision, radiotherapy (strontium plesiotherapy, or electron beam or orthovoltage external beam therapy) and photodynamic therapy (PDT). Radiation therapy and PDT are most appropriate for early disease, and invasive or extensive disease usually requires surgical management.

Early feline rhinarial (or ear tip or eyelid) SCC generally responds well to radiation therapy. PDT may also be appropriate for superficial lesions, but recurrence is common. Either radiotherapy or PDT may achieve long-term control after a single treatment in very superficial lesions. Topical imiquimod has also been reported to produce clinical remission. For invasive tumours, surgical excision is the treatment of choice (see Chapter 18).

Canine rhinarial SCC has a rapidly progressive clinical course characterized by local infiltration, rapid recurrence after surgery and/or radiotherapy, and local/regional metastatic disease.

Local failure rather than metastatic disease is the most common cause of death in patients with SCC. There is no proven role for systemic chemotherapy. Intra-lesional chemotherapy (5-fluorouracil and cisplatin, neither of which can be used systemically in cats) has been described with 30–64% response rates. Intra-lesional chemotherapy requires special formulation to avoid systemic toxicity and is rarely used.

Prognosis: The prognosis for feline SCC is variable, but for SCC *in situ* the disease course may be long. For invasive SCC, the prognosis is largely dictated by the efficacy of local treatment. Where surgery is used, this depends upon the ability to achieve complete excision. Histological degree of differentiation is also associated with prognosis in cats: poorly differentiated SCC is associated with short survival times (median 3 months) whereas median survival times (MSTs) may be >1 year with well differentiated tumours. Rhinarial SCC in dogs carries a poor prognosis.

SCC of the oral cavity is discussed in Chapter 15a.

Basal cell carcinoma
Before it was possible to confirm the diagnosis with cytokeratin immunostaining, basal cell carcinomas (BCCs) were over-diagnosed. Many tumours previously classified as BCC were trichoblastomas or sweat gland tumours. In the cat, the majority of tumours diagnosed as BCC were benign sweat gland adenomas, with few carcinomas or true BCCs. True BCCs are uncommon, and of low malignancy. They are described in Figure 12.2, above.

Follicular tumours
Follicular tumours are summarized in Figure 12.6. As there is a relatively large number of follicular tissues and tumours are compound, i.e. originate from more than one tissue (supposedly due to the close ontogeny of tissues), there is a very complex histological classification system for these common tumours and Figure 12.6 includes notes on origin. Many of these behave clinically in a similar manner. Although each individual subtype is not very common, overall follicular tumours are relatively common in dogs.

Lesions (and pseudonyms)	Tissue of origin	Signalment/ predispositions	Predilection site	Clinical features	Possible treatment
Follicular hamartoma (follicular naevus)	Hair follicle (non-neoplastic malformation)			Single nodule or multiple grouped plaques or small nodules, 'orange peel skin', thick brush-like hairs	Surgical excision if required
Fibroadnexal hamartoma (fibroadnexal dysplasia/focal adnexal dysplasia)	Possible malformations of folliculosebaceous units and/or dermal collagen	Possible association with trauma/scarring Large breed dogs	Pressure points, interdigital space (or any site)	Solitary firm mass, polypoid or dome-shaped, may be alopecic	Surgical excision if required
Follicular cyst		Boxer, Shih-Tzu, Miniature Schnauzer, Old English Sheepdog	May occur at pressure points or in scars because of follicular entrapment	Solitary, firm, intradermal or s.c. nodule. Alopecic. Often appear black/white/yellow. May have central pore (± protruding keratin)	Surgical excision if required
Dilated pore (pore of Winer)	Proliferative variant of follicular cyst	Older cats	Head and neck	Solitary firm mass, central keratin protrusion	Surgical excision if required
Trichofolliculoma	Probably a form of hamartoma, resembling entire follicular/folliculosebaceous unit			Solitary or dome-shaped nodule with a central pore/depression	Surgical excision if required

12.6 Follicular tumours and tumour-like lesions in cats and dogs. (continues) ▶

Lesions (and pseudonyms)	Tissue of origin	Signalment/ predispositions	Predilection site	Clinical features	Possible treatment
Trichoepithelioma	Benign neoplasm that differentiates towards all three segments of the hair follicle	Common in dogs, uncommon in cats. Bassett, Bull Mastiff, English Springer Spaniel, Golden Retriever, Gordon Setter, Standard Poodle	Tail in cat	Round to oval dermal nodules to subcutaneous masses. Alopecia or ulceration if large. (Occasionally multiple)	Surgical excision if required *NB: infiltrative trichoepithelioma should be considered malignant (see text)*
Infundibular keratinizing acanthoma (intracutaneous cornifying epithelioma)	Not really an epithelioma; benign follicular lesion	Norwegian Elkhound, Lhasa Apso, Pekingese, Yorkshire Terrier, German Shepherd Dog		Solitary or multiple partially alopecic dermal nodules. May have central pore with protruding keratin. May be multiple in Norwegian Elkhound, Lhasa Apso	Surgical excision if required
Tricholemmoma	Benign tumour of the outer root sheath of hair follicle	Rare. Older animals		Firm circumscribed solitary nodule	Surgical excision if required
Pilomatrixoma (pilomatrixoma, calcifying epithelioma)	Benign tumour arising from follicular matrix or hair bulb	Uncommon in dogs (but seen in Poodle, Kerry Blue, Old English Sheepdog, Soft-coated Wheaten Terrier, Bouvier de Flandres, Bichon Frise, Schnauzer, Basset). Continuously growing coat may predispose. Rare in cats	Legs and trunk	Solitary firm well circumscribed dome to plaque-like mass	Surgical excision if required
Trichoblastoma (basal cell tumour)	Benign tumour derived follicular stem cells	Common in dogs (Poodle, Cocker Spaniel), reasonably common in cats	Base of ear in dogs, head/cranial half of body in cats	Solitary firm dome or polypoid nodules, alopecia or ulceration (if large)	Surgical excision if required
Malignant trichoepithelioma (matrical carcinoma, infiltrative epithelioma, follicular carcinoma)	Malignant tumour with matrical and inner root sheath features			Large, poorly circumscribed often plaque-like masses. Alopecia or ulceration common	Surgical excision
Malignant pilomatrixoma (matrical carcinoma, pilomatrix carcinoma)	May arise from pilomatrixoma (not proven in animals)	Rare, dog only		Large, poorly circumscribed often plaque-like masses. Alopecia or ulceration if large	Surgical excision

12.6 (continued) Follicular tumours and tumour-like lesions in cats and dogs.

Most follicular tumours are solitary, firm, well circumscribed cutaneous nodules, which may be alopecic. The majority are benign and can be cured by excisional biopsy. However, histologically infiltrative behaviour suggests a more malignant variant. In particular, invasive trichoepitheliomas are malignant rather than benign. Malignant lesions require more aggressive investigation, treatment and active monitoring. For malignant follicular tumours (or benign tumours causing a clinical problem), surgical excision is the treatment of choice. Radiation therapy may be of benefit for non-resectable or residual malignant disease, but there are few data. There is no proven role for systemic chemotherapy.

Sebaceous tumours

Like follicular tumours, there is a complex classification system for sebaceous tumours, but most are benign and simple to manage. Nodular sebaceous hyperplasia (senile sebaceous hyperplasia) (Figure 12.7) accounts for 25% of non-malignant skin masses in dogs and up to 11% of non-malignant skin lesions in cats. Sebaceous adenomas (Figure 12.8) (benign neoplasms of combined glandular and ductal origin) are also relatively common, accounting for about 6–7% of skin tumours in dogs and 2–4% in cats. However, this group includes perianal gland tumours, which may be aggressively malignant. Features of these lesions and sebaceous tumours are summarized in Figure 12.9.

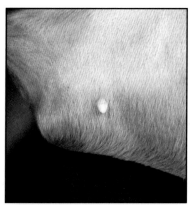

12.7
Nodular sebaceous hyperplasia on the medial aspect of the elbow of an 8-year-old male Weimaraner.

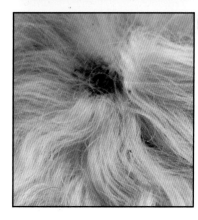

12.8
Sebaceous adenoma on the dorsum of the head of an 11-year-old neutered female Standard Poodle.

True sebaceous cysts are rare in dogs and very rare in cats. Follicular cysts are often erroneously called sebaceous cysts because of their grumous keratinaceous contents, but sebum is a white milky liquid.

Sebaceous epitheliomas

These controversial tumours may possess low malignant potential, and have a tendency to recur after incomplete/marginal excision. Histologically, it is difficult to differentiate a true epithelioma from its malignant variant. If the tumour appears clinically malignant (large mass, infiltrative margins, rapid proliferation) it should be treated as malignant in spite of the apparently benign histological diagnosis. Treatment is by surgical excision.

Sebaceous carcinomas

These are locally aggressive tumours that show local/regional metastatic behaviour but rarely distant metastases. Treatment is surgical excision: radiotherapy can be used to treat residual disease or nodal metastases, but there are few data on outcome.

Perianal gland tumours

Perianal (hepatoid) gland tumours arise from the hepatoid glands, which are modified sebaceous glands found in the skin of the perianal area,

Lesions (and pseudonyms)	Signalment or other predisposition	Predilection site	Clinical features	Possible treatment/comments
Sebaceous duct cyst	Rare in dogs, very rare in cats	Eyelid: meibomian cyst	Small nodules	Surgical excision if required
Nodular sebaceous hyperplasia (senile sebaceous hyperplasia)	Poodle, Cocker Spaniel, Manchester Terrier, Wheaten Terrier	Dorsal head, ears, face, neck	Warty with a waxy or pearly alopecic surface. Dome-shaped or papillated, pale or yellowy-white	Aspiration can be difficult as masses often very small. No treatment usually required
Sebaceous hamartoma			Solitary alopecic nodule	Variant of fibroadnexal hamartoma
Sebaceous adenoma	Cocker Spaniel, Siberian Husky, Miniature Poodle, Coonhound, Samoyed, Beagle, Dachshund, Persian cats	Head, any site	Dome-shaped or papillated nodule, yellow opalescent or pigmented, may be alopecic or ulcerated	Surgical excision if required
Sebaceous epithelioma	Common in dogs (Cocker Spaniel and others predisposed to sebaceous adenoma), rare in cats	Head, ears, dorsum	Firm nodular plaque or fungiform masses, often ulcerated, may be pigmented	Surgical excision if required
Sebaceous carcinoma	Cocker Spaniel, Cavalier King Charles Spaniel, Scottish Terrier, Siberian Husky	Head	Often large, alopecic and ulcerated	Surgical excision (see text)
Perianal gland adenoma (hepatoid gland adenoma, perianal gland adenoma)	Dogs only, older (8 years plus), mostly male (male to female ratio at least 3:1, and neutered female to entire female ratio 3:1). Cocker Spaniel, Samoyed, Siberian Husky, English Bulldog, Beagle, crossbreeds	Perianal skin, tail, prepuce, thigh	Nodular, polypoid or anular masses. Rubbery firm texture, may ulcerate	Hormonal (castration, or delmadinone acetate). Surgical excision may be indicated, but may be facilitated by prior hormonal therapy
Perianal gland epithelioma			As adenomas	As adenomas
Perianal gland carcinoma	German Shepherd Dog, Arctic Circle breeds	Mainly perianal, occasionally tail or prepuce	Nodular, polypoid or anular masses. Rubbery firm texture. Often poorly demarcated, may ulcerate	See text

12.9 Sebaceous tumours in dogs and cats.

proximal third of the tail, dorsal lumbosacral area, and lateral to the prepuce. In dogs, these androgen-dependent glands are larger and more extensive in adult males than in females. There are no hepatoid glands in cats.

- **Perianal gland adenomas** account for up to 18% of canine skin tumours (perianal gland epitheliomas are sometimes reported by pathologists and should be approached as adenomas). Features are summarized in Figure 12.9.
- **Perianal gland carcinomas** are relatively uncommon, representing 0.25–2.6% of skin tumour submissions. Their features are summarized in Figure 12.9.

Well differentiated tumours are managed in the same way as adenomas. Poorly differentiated tumours tend to show aggressive behaviour, presenting as large poorly circumscribed lesions, which metastasize early in the disease course. Aggressive carcinomas are often androgen-independent.

Surgical excision is the treatment of choice but complete excision may not be feasible: adjunctive radiotherapy may be used in these cases. There are limited data on chemotherapy, but there are anecdotal reports of long-term survival after chemotherapy (using the VAC regime) for individual patients. Histopathological grade is predictive of behaviour.

Sweat gland tumours

Sweat gland tumours are summarized in Figure 12.10. Over recent years pathologists have introduced more precise classification of these tumours and found that many tumours previously classified as basal cell carcinomas in cats are in fact apocrine ductular adenomas (60%) or trichoblastomas (40%). Both these tumours are benign.

Apocrine carcinomas account for 0.6–2.2% of canine skin tumours and 2.5–3.6% of cat skin tumours. They can be classified into different histological subtypes, but the clinical value of this is unclear. The degree of malignancy may correlate with the degree of differentiation. These tumours are locally invasive, with variable metastatic potential. Overall, the metastatic rate is low and so treatment is usually focused on the primary tumour. Surgery is the mainstay of therapy, with adjunctive radiotherapy used for residual disease.

Mesenchymal tumours

Mesenchymal tumours are summarized in Figure 12.11 and discussed in detail in Chapter 14.

Canine nodular dermatofibrosis is a benign skin lesion, but is associated with renal epithelial tumours (including cystadenocarcinoma, cystadenoma) or cysts, or less commonly uterine leiomyoma. The renal lesions are often multicentric and bilateral and

Lesions (and pseudonyms)	Signalment or other predisposition	Predilection site	Clinical features	Possible treatment/comments
Apocrine cyst (sweat gland cyst, epitrichial sweat gland cyst)	Old English Sheepdog, Weimaraner, Persian cat	Head, neck, legs, dorsal trunk in dogs. Ear canal in cats	Bullous nodules with bluish or reddish contents visible through alopecic skin. Well defined, tense or fluctuant	Surgical excision if required
Apocrine cystomatosis	Rare in dogs, uncommon in cats	Head and neck in dogs. Ear canal or pinna in cats	Multiple clusters of dilated sweat glands, often look blue/black on cats	Surgical excision if required
Apocrine cystadenoma (sweat gland cystadenoma, apocrine hidrocystoma)	Great Pyrenean, Chow Chow, Malamute, Old English Sheepdog, Persian cat	Head, neck, dorsum in dogs. Head in cats	As apocrine cyst	Surgical excision if required
Apocrine secretory adenoma (sweat gland adenoma/epitrichial sweat gland adenoma)	Great Pyrenean, Chow Chow, Malamute, Old English sheepdog	Head, neck, dorsum in dogs. Head in cats	Well circumscribed firm or fluctuant dermal nodules	Surgical excision if required
Apocrine ductal adenoma (ductular sweat gland adenoma, basaloid sweat gland adenoma, nodular hidroadenoma)	Rare in dogs, more common in cats. Pitbull Terrier, Old English Sheepdog, English Springer Spaniel	Head and neck	Circumscribed dermal or s.c. nodules; may be alopecic and blue-black-brown; can be ulcerated	Surgical excision if required
Apocrine secretory adenocarcinoma	Older cats and dogs. Coonhound, Norwegian Elkhound, Siamese cat	Legs of dogs or cats; head, abdomen and chin of cats	Solitary, fluctuant or firm, may be poorly demarcated, alopecic, ulcerated	Surgical excision
Apocrine ductular carcinoma (ductular sweat gland adenocarcioma, malignant nodular hidradenoma, hidradenocarcinoma)	Incidence unclear. Older cats and dogs. Coonhound, Norwegian Elkhound and Siamese cat	Legs of dogs or cats, head and abdomen of cats	Solitary, fluctuant or firm, may be poorly demarcated, alopecic, ulcerated	Surgical excision

12.10 Sweat gland tumours in dogs and cats.

Lesions (and pseudonyms)	Signalment/ predispositions	Predilection site	Clinical features	Possible treatment/ comments
Collagenous hamartoma	Relatively common in dogs	Head, neck, proximal limbs	Small solitary dome-shaped firm nodule. May be alopecic, hyperpigmented	May be diagnosed as fibroma. Management is the same: surgical excision
Canine nodular dermatofibrosis	German Shepherd Dog (rare inherited autosomal recessive disorder), middle aged and older	Legs, ears, head	Firm well circumscribed nodules in dermis or subcutis, thickened overlying skin, hyperpigmentation, ulceration, may be alopecic	In German Shepherd Dogs associated with renal tumours and cysts
Acrochordon (acrochordonous plaque, skin tag, fibroepithelial polyp, fibromatous polyp, fibromatous plaque)	Common in dogs	Trunk, pressure points	Solitary or multiple, polypoid or filiform with thickened, alopecic and/ or pigmented epidermis	
Dermatofibroma	Usually less than 5 years old (dog or cat)	Head	Solitary circumscribed dermal nodule with alopecia and thickened epidermis	May be reactive rather than benign tumour: either way, surgery is curative
Nodular fasciitis	Uncommon: young dogs (not cats)	Any	Poorly demarcated mass, may be attached to deep fascia	Surgical excision curative
Fibroma	Quite uncommon, middle aged and older dogs	Head and limbs	Solitary rubbery circumscribed mass. Alopecia and atrophy of overlying dermis	Surgical excision if required
Fibrosarcoma	Gordon Setter, Golden Retriever, Irish Wolfhound, Dobermann, Brittany Spaniel	Trunk and limbs, feline injection sites	Firm, poorly circumscribed, may be multilobular. Alopecia/ulceration can occur	See text and Chapter 14
Myxoma/myxofibroma		Trunk or limbs	Soft mass, often ill defined	Can be difficult to differentiate histologically from myxofibrosarcoma
Feline sarcoid (fibropapilloma)	Rural cats only, mainly young males. Papillomavirus induced	Philtrum, nares, lip, digit, tail	Solitary or multiple nodules	Locally invasive, commonly recur after excision
Angiomatosis	Progressive form in young to middle-aged dogs or cats, scrotal form in older dogs	Digits, feet, limbs (any). Also scrotal type	Dark red macules and patches, with irregular margins	Progressive form in young dogs difficult to manage, scrotal type less rapidly progressive
Haemangioma	Many (short-haired, light-coated dogs vulnerable to solar induced)	Solar-induced on glabrous skin areas in dogs. Infiltrative haemangiomas in subcutaneous fat on trunk/proximal limbs. Head, legs, abdomen in cats	Solitary well circumscribed meaty masses, may be red to black/ bluish. Arise in dermis or subcutis	Infiltrative lesions difficult to excise surgically
Lymphangiomatosis/ lymphangioma	Rare; young animals	? Inguinal region	Poorly demarcated fluctuant swelling with ulcers/draining tracts	Probably mainly congenital malformation
Haemangiosarcoma	Uncommon. Older dogs and cats. Dogs with thin hair coat (Whippets). In dogs may arise from transformation of haemangiomas which are UV induced	Ventral abdomen, groin, axilla, any. Limbs and head in cats	Ill-defined red to dark blue plaques or nodules, invasive, friable, rapidly growing. May be soft/spongy, resembling haematoma	Surgical excision. Generally less metastatic than visceral counterparts, but still cause death due to local or distant disease. In cats, recurrence more common than metastases. Value of chemotherapy unclear (see text). (Lymphangiosarcomas behave similarly, but may be more metastatic)

12.11 Mesenchymal tumours of the skin and subcutaneous tissue in dogs and cats. (continues) ▶

Lesions (and pseudonyms)	Signalment/ predispositions	Predilection site	Clinical features	Possible treatment/ comments
Haemangiopericytoma [a]	Dogs only, usually older. Possible female predisposition	Trunk or limbs	Solitary deep dermal or s.c. multilobular masses. Often adherent to deep structures. Overlying skin may be alopecic, ulcerated, hyperpigmented	Surgical excision (see text)
Lipoma	Common in dogs. All breeds, older age	Trunk and limbs	Well circumscribed, freely mobile soft masses.	Surgical excision if required
Infiltrative lipoma	Uncommon in dogs, rare in cats. Labrador Retriever, Standard Schnauzer, Dobermann	Neck, trunk, legs	Large poorly defined deep subcutaneous and intramuscular lesions	May be difficult to excise. Possible role for adjunctive radiotherapy
Liposarcoma	Older dogs. Possible predisposition in Sheltie, Beagle. Rare in cats	Axial region, proximal limb	Variably circumscribed, soft to firm	Surgical excision (see text)
Leiomyoma	Rare	Vulva, perineum, groin, head, dorsum	Solitary well circumscribed firm masses	Surgical excision
Leiomyosarcoma	Rare	Perineum, trunk, legs, face, extremities	Small non-ulcerated dermal masses	Surgical excision (generally low metastatic potential)
Rhabdomyosarcoma	Rare	Feline injection site	Firm poorly demarcated multilobular s.c. mass, adhered to underlying tissue, skin	Surgical excision (generally low metastatic potential)
Benign peripheral nerve sheath tumour (schwannoma, neurofibroma) [a]	Uncommon, older cats and dogs	Trunk, distal limb in dogs, head and neck in cats	Circumscribed lobulated cutaneous or subcutaneous mass	Recurrence common after incomplete excision
Malignant peripheral nerve sheath tumour (malignant schwannoma) [a]	Uncommon, older cats and dogs	Trunk, distal limb in dogs, head and neck in cats	Circumscribed lobulated cutaneous or subcutaneous mass. Poorly circumscribed, adhered to underlying tissue, skin	Surgical excision (generally low metastatic potential, but some are metastatic especially in younger patients)

12.11 (continued) Mesenchymal tumours of the skin and subcutaneous tissue in dogs and cats. [a] See text re classification and nomenclature of these tumours.

metastases occur in 20% of cases. The syndrome is inherited in German Shepherd Dogs but can occur in other breeds.

The most commonly diagnosed soft tissue sarcomas of the skin and subcutis are fibrosarcoma (Figure 12.12) and haemangiopericytoma (peripheral nerve sheath tumour) (Figure 12.13). Fibrosarcomas account for 15–17% of feline skin tumours in cats and about 1.5% in dogs. Historically, haemangiopericytomas account for about 7% of canine skin tumours and about 13% of mesenchymal tumours. Recently it has been suggested that many tumours previously diagnosed as haemangiopericytomas are in fact peripheral nerve sheath tumours (there is currently no immunological marker for pericytes). Because of the conflicting terminology, some pathologists prefer to call these low-grade spindle cell tumours. For the soft tissue sarcomas, histological grade is prognostic for metastatic potential.

For all soft tissue sarcomas, treatment is by wide or compartmental excision and the first surgery is the most likely to achieve a cure: excisional biopsy is not recommended. Reported recurrence rate for

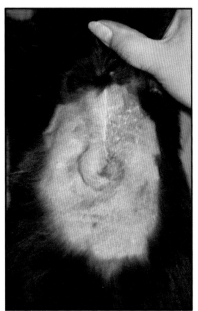

12.12 Recurrent fibrosarcoma (suspected injection-site sarcoma) after attempted excisional biopsy in a 10-year-old DSH cat.

139

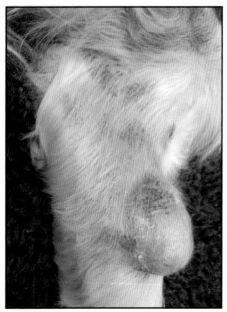

12.13 Haemangiopericytoma of the craniolateral elbow of a 9-year-old neutered crossbred bitch. The proximal limb is a common site for these tumours.

canine skin and subcutaneous sarcomas is 34% and for feline sarcomas in excess of 70%, illustrating both the difficultly in treating these tumours and consequences of inappropriate management. Radiation therapy can be used as an adjunctive therapy, and chemotherapy may delay the development of metastatic disease in high-grade tumours. The management of soft tissue sarcomas (including feline injection site sarcomas) is discussed in Chapter 14.

Round cell tumours

Cutaneous round cell tumours include mast cell, lymphoid and histiocytic tumours, and plasmacytoma. Mast cell tumours are discussed on pages 142–150.

Histiocytic tumours

Histiocytes are either macrophages (antigen-processing) or dendritic (antigen-presenting) cells. The phenotypes of these cells, and the tumours that arise from them, are summarized in Figure 12.14. Conditions that usually present as multiple lesions (cutaneous and systemic histiocytosis, malignant histiocytosis) are discussed in the section on multifocal skin tumours, below.

Canine cutaneous histiocytoma (CCH)

CCH is a common, benign tumour, accounting for up to 14% of canine skin tumours.

Aetiology, pathogenesis and predispositions: These tumours are thought to arise from the epidermal Langerhans' cells. CCH mainly affects dogs less than 3 years of age, but any age may be affected. Boxers, Dachshunds, Cocker Spaniels and Bull Terriers are predisposed.

Cell type	Phenotype (dog)	Phenotype (cat)	Disease state
Macrophage (from blood monocytes)	CD45 CD18 CD11d MCHC II CD68		Haemophagocytic histiocytic sarcoma
Dendritic cell (from CD34-positive haemopoietic stem cells)	CD45 CD18 CD1 CD11c CD11b MCHC II ICAM1 CD14	CD18 CD1 MHC II	Canine cutaneous histiocytoma (CD14 –ve) Cutaneous or systemic histiocyosis (CD14 +ve) Histiocytic sarcoma (CD14 +ve)
Langerhans' cell (epithelial dendritic cell)	E-cadherin		Canine cutaneous histiocytoma

12.14 Cells giving rise to histiocytic tumours and reactive histiocytoses in cats and dogs.

Presentation and clinical signs: Common sites are head, ears, neck and extremities. Clinically, CCHs are rapidly growing dome-shaped or plaque-like (or button-like) masses, which are often alopecic or ulcerated (Figure 12.15).

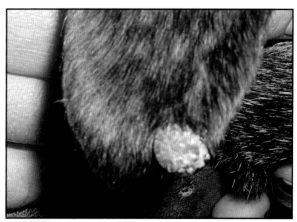

12.15 Histiocytoma on the ear of a 4-year-old male Boxer. (Courtesy of T. Nuttall)

Approach, management and prognosis: Diagnosis is usually easily achieved by FNA. Tumours may often resolve spontaneously (even if multiple). Langerhans' cells may migrate to the draining lymph node, resulting in lymphadenopathy, which will also regress. Surgical excision may be required for problematic lesions, or where cytology does not yield a definitive diagnosis.

Benign fibrous histiocytoma

Benign fibrous histiocytomas (reactive fibrohistiocytic nodule, juvenile xanthogranuloma, fibroxanthoma) are uncommon tumours in dogs, clinically similar to CCH.

Aetiology, pathogenesis and predispositions: These may represent reactive histiocytic proliferations rather than true tumours. They affect young dogs (2–4 years) of any breed, but Collies and Golden Retrievers may develop multiple lesions.

Presentation and clinical signs: Animals may present with solitary or multiple lesions on the face, legs and scrotum. Lesions are firm well circumscribed dermal nodules with normal or alopecic overlying skin.

Clinical approach, management and prognosis: Biopsy is required for diagnosis and these lesions are characterized by a swirling stroma embedded in the histiocytic and inflammatory cell population. Surgical excision is recommended. In multiple fibrous histiocytoma, lesions may also respond to immunosuppression (oral or intralesional glucocorticoids). The prognosis is good.

Histiocytic sarcoma

Localized histiocytic sarcoma is a focal soft tissue tumour. Pathologists are now diagnosing histiocytic sarcomas with increasing frequency, but immunohistochemistry is often required for absolute confirmation. Most tumours will be positive for CD18, as well as CD45 and CD11c. Fascin is also used but is not fully validated in the dog. Flat-coated Retrievers and Rottweilers are predisposed.

Presentation and clinical signs: Dogs most often present with a rapidly growing firm soft tissue mass, which may be ill-defined and usually infiltrates adjacent tissues. Any site can be affected, but subcutaneous lesions are common.

Clinical approach and management: These are managed in a similar way to other soft tissue sarcomas (see Chapter 14). Primary tumours are possibly more radiosensitive than other mesenchymal tumours. However, these tumours tend to be highly metastatic and many oncologists recommend adjunctive chemotherapy. Lomustine (CCNU) is currently the drug of choice. There may be a role for PEG-encapsulated doxorubicin.

Prognosis: MSTs after surgery alone are in the region of 5 months, but multimodality therapy may improve survival.

Feline histiocytic sarcoma

There are few data on histiocytic sarcoma in cats, though it may be that localized histiocytic sarcomas have been diagnosed as mesenchymal tumours in the past. Most cases in the literature have disseminated disease rather than cutaneous or subcutaneous lesions, and the prognosis is poor.

Plasma cell tumours

Cutaneous plasmacytoma/plasma cell tumours account for about 1.5% of all canine skin tumours and most often arise as a solitary mass, though multiple masses may occur.

Aetiology, pathogenesis and predispositions: The aetiology is unknown. Cocker Spaniels, Airedale Terriers, Kerry Blue Terriers, Scottish Terriers and Standard Poodles may be predisposed. Older animals are usually affected.

Presentation and clinical signs: Plasma cell tumours are usually sessile, firm, raised dermal masses, which may be alopecic. Common locations in dogs are the pinnae, lips, digits, chin, legs, trunk and oral cavity; mucosal lesions usually have an intact surface epithelium and are either pedunculated or have a broad base. In cats, similar sites are affected but also the tail, and lesions may be more likely to reflect systemic disease (plasma cell myeloma, see Chapter 19).

Clinical approach, management and prognosis: In dogs, most lesions are benign and can be cured by surgical excision. Where this is impossible, radiation therapy may be used. A minority are metastatic (initially to regional nodes) and infrequently patients present with multiple cutaneous lesions. There is no defined role for chemotherapy.

Melanocytic tumours

Lentiges

Lentiges are benign proliferations of melanocytes, common in dogs and cats.

Presentation and clinical signs: Lentiges are small (<5 mm), well demarcated, black, macular or slightly raised, smooth, well circumscribed lesions. In dogs, they occur almost exclusively on the nipples of older animals, while in cats they affect the lips, eyelid margins, nasal planum and pinnae and often arise in young animals.

Management and prognosis: No treatment is required. These lesions do not transform to malignancy.

Cutaneous melanoma

In dogs, two-thirds of cutaneous melanomas are benign (melanocytoma) and one-third malignant. Malignant transformation of benign lesions is thought to occur occasionally. In cats, cutaneous melanomas are rare, but at least half are malignant.

Aetiology, pathogenesis and predispositions: Canine and feline cutaneous melanomas are not thought to be UV-linked. Dogs with heavily pigmented skin and cats with black or grey hair coats are most at risk. Any age of animal may be affected, but most animals are older (8–12 years).

Presentation and clinical signs: Melanocytic tumours can occur anywhere on the body. Tumours of the nail bed and mucocutaneous junctions (and oral mucosa) are often malignant, while lesions on haired skin are more likely benign. Benign lesions are most often found on the head in cats, and on the head or trunk in dogs. Predilection sites for malignant tumours are lips, eyelids and legs (including nail beds) in dogs, and head, trunk and tail in cats. Benign melanomas are usually well circumscribed, pigmented, alopecic nodules (smooth to papillated, sessile, plaque-like or pedunculated). Most melanomas are at least partially pigmented. Ulceration and infiltration are common in malignant tumours.

Clinical approach, management and prognosis: Malignant melanoma patients should have staging to detect local and regional lymph node metastases, and distant metastases.

Treatment is surgical excision, but overall cure rate in dogs is only 35%, which is at odds with the reported rate of malignancy. Where complete excision of malignancy is impossible, radiotherapy may be of benefit. There is no proven role for chemotherapy and the melanoma vaccine has not been evaluated in these patients.

There is a relatively complex system of histological classification for melanomas but type is not of prognostic relevance. Higher mitotic index predicts more malignant behaviour, as do other proliferation markers (Ki67 and PCNA expression).

Mast cell tumours

MCTs in dogs

MCTs account for 7–21% of skin tumours in dogs, with an estimated annual incidence of 90–129 per 100,000 dogs. MCTs show variable biological behaviour. Metastatic rates of 10% to >95% are reported, and outcome correlates broadly with histopathological grade (Figure 12.16). These tumours can be challenging to manage and may require multimodality therapy. Treatment may be compromised by a lack of a diagnosis prior to therapy.

Aetiology, pathogenesis and predilections: The aetiology is unknown. A role for chronic inflammation has been suggested, but there is little evidence to support this.

The average age of dogs with MCTs is 8 years. Any age may be affected, but patients under 4 years are less common. Many breeds are predisposed; breed and site predispositions are summarized in Figure 12.17. The relative risk is 16.7 for Boxers and 8 for Boston Terriers.

Grade	Frequency of diagnosis	Metastatic potential	Recurrence potential	Recommended treatment	Prognosis
Well differentiated/ Grade I		<10%	Low	Surgical excision	Unlikely to cause death (up to 7–12%)
Intermediate grade/ Grade II	50% or more	5–22%	Variable	Surgical excision. Consider radiotherapy if complete excision impossible or nodal metastases; consider chemotherapy if MI >5	May cause death (17–56%) due to local treatment failure or metastatic disease
Poorly differentiated/ Grade III		> 80%	High	Chemotherapy; multimodality therapy	Likely to be cause of death

12.16 Summary of canine mast cell tumours by histopathological grade.

Breed	Predisposed sites	Other features
American Bull Terrier	Hindlimb	
Australian Cattle Dog		
Beagle		
Boston Terrier	Hindlimb	
Boxer	Hindlimb	High proportion of grade I or II tumours, predisposed to multiple tumours
Bulldog (American and English)		
Bullmastiff		
Dachshund		
Fox Terrier		
Golden Retriever		Predisposed to multiple tumours
Labrador Retriever		? High proportion of grade II tumours, predisposed to multiple tumours
Pug	Hindlimb	
Rhodesian Ridgeback	Tail	
Schnauzer		
Sharpei		High proportion of high-grade tumours (especially US population)
Staffordshire Bull Terrier		
Weimaraner		Predisposed to multiple tumours

12.17 Dog breed and site predispositions for mast cell tumours.

Presentation and clinical signs: Most dogs present with a cutaneous or subcutaneous mass. Although tumours are much more commonly solitary rather than multicentric, sequential or synchronous development of MCTs is common.

MCTs may develop anywhere on the body and may be cutaneous (dermal) or subcutaneous. Of cutaneous MCTs, 50–60% arise on the trunk, 25–40% on the extremities and 10% on the head and neck. The scrotum, perineum, back and tail are less commonly affected.

Occasionally, tumours occur in extracutaneous sites: the conjunctiva, or mucosa of the nasopharynx, larynx or oral cavity, GI tract or urinary tract. Spinal MCT is also reported. Visceral or systemic mastocytosis is described, but most often occurs where there is dissemination from an aggressive primary cutaneous tumour. Isolated visceral MCTs and primary mast cell leukaemias are very rare in dogs.

MCTs are often erythematous or oedematous (Figure 12.18) and may be alopecic, but their reputation as great imitators is well deserved and they have a wide variety of clinical appearances (Figure 12.19). Soft cutaneous or subcutaneous masses may mimic lipomas. Lack of investigation can result in late presentation of patients with more advanced disease that is clinically difficult to manage.

The gross appearance of MCTs does correlate to some extent with histological grade and a tumour that appears aggressive is almost certainly aggressive. However, a tumour that appears quiescent should not be assumed to be benign. The clinical features of aggressive MCTs are:

- Rapid growth
- Local irritation and inflammation
- Local infiltration/poor demarcation from adjacent tissues
- Ulceration
- Satellite nodules (Figure 12.20).

Patients may also present with urticarial swelling or diffuse oedema/inflammation (Figure 12.21) which may mimic cellulitis or acral lick dermatitis.

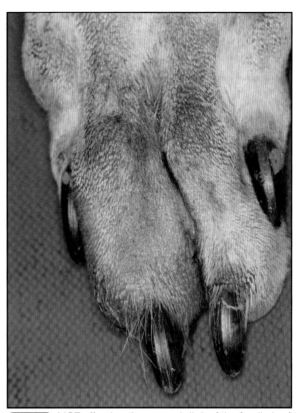

12.19 MCT affecting the second digit of the forelimb of a middle-aged crossbred dog. Differential diagnoses for this swollen digit would include infectious causes (nail-bed infection) and SCC.

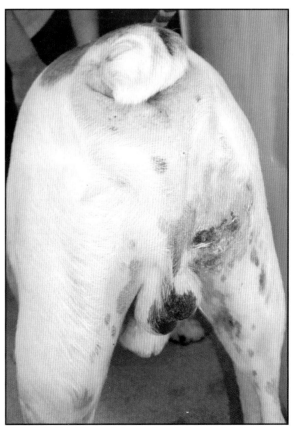

12.20 Satellite nodules and partial wound dehiscence after incomplete excision of a grade III MCT in a 2-year-old male Bulldog. The satellite nodules can be seen distal to the wound.

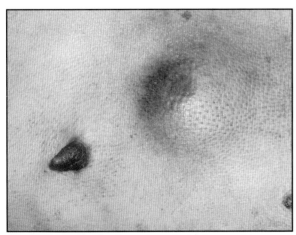

12.18 MCT on the thoracic wall of a 6-year-old neutered crossbred bitch, showing local erythema and oedema.

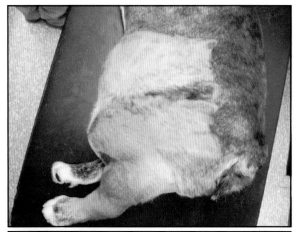

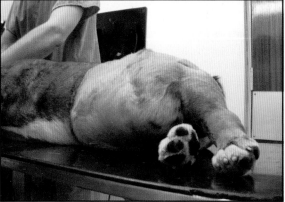

12.21 Extensive oedema and swelling around the surgical scar 3 months after excision of a grade II MCT from the flank of a 6-year-old male Bulldog. There is diffuse swelling over the left lateral abdomen extending from the last rib to the flank fold and, distally, down the left hindlimb to the stifle.

Complications resulting from the release of bioactive substances from MCTs occur in up to half of dogs with MCTs. Local effects of degranulation include erythema, inflammation and host irritation, local haemorrhage and poor wound healing (Figure 12.22).

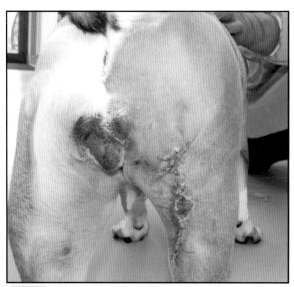

12.22 Wound breakdown following surgical removal of a grade III MCT from the thigh of a 5-year-old neutered Bulldog bitch.

Systemically, histamine release can result in gastrointestinal ulceration (due to H2 receptor stimulation by histamine, hyperacidity, vascular damage and hypermotility). Ulceration is found in 35–83% of dogs with MCTs at necropsy and is associated more commonly with higher-grade tumours or large-volume disease. Systemic release of other factors can result in so-called 'flashing syndromes', collapse or anaphylactic shock.

Clinical approach: FNA correctly diagnoses 92–96% of MCTs. Mast cell granules occasionally do not stain well with rapid modified Romanowsky-type stains, but this is uncommon and may be overcome by a longer fixation in alcohol. Although accurate cytological grading is not possible, particularly for grade I and II tumours, poorly differentiated tumours may be suspected based on cytological features. The approach to a mass confirmed cytologically to be a mast cell tumour is outlined in Figure 12.23. Histopathology is required for grading.

Imaging may assist assessment of the extent of the primary tumour; for example, an ultrasound examination may allow appreciation that the mass invades into the muscle layer deep to the tumour.

Metastasis is to the local lymph nodes, then spleen, liver or other visceral organs. The minimum recommended tumour staging is aspiration of local lymph nodes (even if palpably normal) and abdominal ultrasonography to assess the liver and spleen. Cytological evaluation of local nodes is the most important test. Diagnosis of metastases can be difficult, because normal mast cells may migrate to the node due to chemotaxis. It has been suggested that if >3% of cells are mast cells, metastasis should be diagnosed, but using this criteria up to 25% of normal lymph nodes would be positive. The presence of abnormal mast cells or aggregated cells is consistent with metastases.

Aspiration of ultrasonographically normal spleens is a low-yield procedure, but in the author's experience tumour metastases may be diagnosed in apparently normal spleens and this is highly significant for the individual patient. For high-grade tumours, aspiration of the spleen is recommended.

Pulmonary metastases are uncommon in MCTs, but thoracic radiographs may be indicated to evaluate for intrathoracic lymphadenopathy or pulmonary interstitial infiltrate. They may also be of value where there is a suspicion of concurrent disease or to rule out other significant pathology in older patients before expensive and involved treatment is undertaken (for example, surgery followed by radiation therapy).

Examining buffy coat smears from peripheral blood is not recommended, because mast cells are found more frequently in animals with inflammatory disease than in those with MCTs. The vast majority of dogs with MCTs do not have malignant mast cells in their circulation or bone marrow and this is very unlikely in patients without disseminated disease. Bone marrow aspiration should thus be reserved for animals with visceral and disseminated disease, although their poor prognosis might render the information of little clinical value.

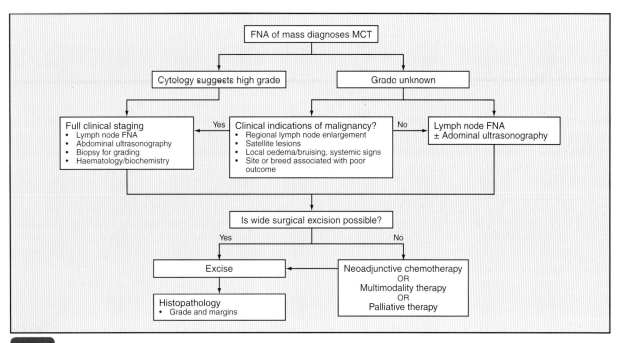

12.23 Approach to canine patients diagnosed with MCTs on the basis of cytology.

Decision making in MCT treatment is outlined in Figure 12.24.

Surgery: Surgery is the treatment of choice for primary grade I or II MCTs. The accepted ubiquitous dogma for MCT removal has been margins of 3 cm in two planes, and removal of one fascial plane deep to the tumour. However, recent studies have suggested that wide surgical margins may not be necessary for successful management of grade I and II MCTs up to 5 cm diameter, and suggest 2 cm lateral margins and a deep margin of one fascial plane as standard. A 2 cm/one facial plane option has not been evaluated for tumours >5 cm and will be inadequate in most grade III tumours.

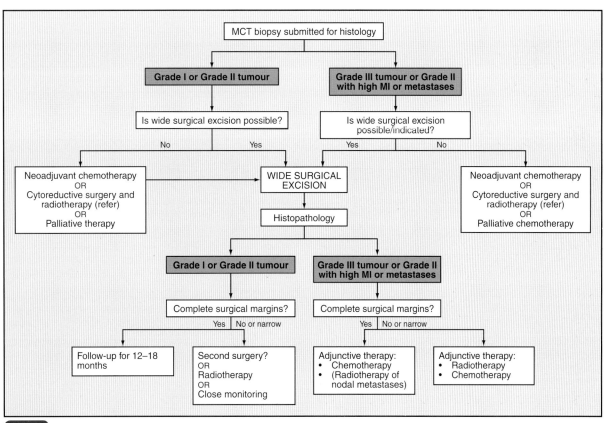

12.24 Approach to treatment of canine MCTs.

Radiation therapy: Radiation therapy is widely used in the treatment of MCTs, most often as a postoperative adjunctive therapy. This is best achieved where radiation is planned from the beginning, rather than as an afterthought following inadequate surgery. Radiation therapy is avoided as a sole therapy where there is bulky disease, due to the risk of radiation-induced mast cell degranulation and serious systemic effects: fatalities have been reported. Where there is gross disease, neoadjuvant chemotherapy or prednisolone will reduce the risk of significant degranulation events.

In order to maximize the chances of a good outcome, accurate recording of the presurgical tumour is required. Ideally, metal surgical clips should be placed at the surgical margins: these can be visualized by portal imaging and may also help to reduce the chance of a geographical miss, particularly on the trunk and body wall where there may be postsurgical tissue migration. The use of advancement flaps and grafting techniques may increase the field size for treatment and result in a delay in starting radiation therapy because of delayed wound healing or wound breakdown, and a simple surgery with primary closure may be preferable when postoperative radiation therapy is planned.

On the limbs, a strip of skin must be excluded from the radiation field to prevent late lymphoedema due to damage to the lymphatics. This means that the whole circumference of the limb cannot be irradiated, limiting margins, and where radiation is to be used postsurgically oblique and transverse incisions should be avoided.

Radiation therapy can also be used to treat local/regional nodal metastases.

The prognosis for MCTs treated with surgery and radiation is good, but the literature is difficult to interpret, given the low rate of recurrence reported with surgery alone, even when histological margins are incomplete; for example, one recent study reported 23% recurrence rate of incompletely excised grade II tumours (Séguin *et al.*, 2006). Adjuvant radiation therapy for intermediate grade MCTs results in a 1–2-year disease-free interval in 81–95% of cases, and disease-free intervals of 40 months have been reported for dogs with grade I/II tumours with regional lymph node metastases treated with surgery and radiation. Many different fractionation regimes are reported and the ideal protocol is unknown.

Traditional chemotherapy: Chemotherapy is used where systemic (rather than locoregional) therapy is required to treat disseminated, non-resectable and high-grade tumours. Chemotherapy is also sometimes used for residual microscopic disease where radiation therapy is not available.

For grade II tumours with a high mitotic index, grade III tumours or tumours where the pathologist suggests grade II/III features, chemotherapy is used to delay or prevent metastatic disease (in addition to surgical treatment of the primary site). Good outcomes have been reported in this setting, with all patients alive at 3 years in one study (Thamm *et al.*, 2006), though overall the prognosis is not as good for all high-grade cases.

Often first line therapy is vinblastine and prednisolone, and second line lomustine. Protocols alternating vinblastine and lomustine are also used. The commonest protocols are summarized in Figure 12.25. Good response rates are reported with combined vinblastine, cyclophosphamide and prednisolone, but the additional potential toxicity without proven survival advantage means that this protocol has not become established. There is only anecdotal evidence to support the use of other chemotherapeutic agents in the treatment of canine MCTs.

Drugs	Published response rate (measurable disease, complete and partial responses)	Protocol	Comment/toxicity	References
Vinblastine and prednisolone	47%	Vinblastine 2 mg/m^2 i.v. weekly for 4 weeks then fortnightly for 4 further treatments Prednisolone 2 mg/kg orally q24h for one week, then 1 mg/kg q24h for 2 weeks, then 1 mg/kg q48h	6–20% toxicity: myelosuppression and GI toxicity Can roll vinblastine out to 6 months Dose escalation of vinblastine may be possible in some cases	Thamm *et al.* (1999, 2006); Vickery *et al.* (2008)
Lomustine	44%	70 mg/m^2 orally q21d for 4 cycles	Lomustine is associated with myelosuppression, GI and hepatotoxicity Toxicity of longer-term monotherapy unknown if lomustine continued Lomustine often used as rescue therapy after vinblastine and prednisolone	Rassnick *et al.* (1999)
Vinblastine/lomustine and prednisolone (alternating vinblastine/lomustine, one treatment q14d)	Not published	Vinblastine 2 mg/m^2 i.v. week 1, then every 4th week Lomustine 70 mg/m^2 orally week 3, then every 4th week Prednisolone 0.5 mg/kg orally q24h	Protocol continues for 6 months	Welle *et al.* (2008)

12.25 Most commonly used chemotherapy protocols for canine MCTs. (continues) ▶

Drugs	Published response rate (measurable disease, complete and partial responses)	Protocol	Comment/toxicity	References
Vinblastine/lomustine (alternating vinblastine/lomustine, one treatment q14d)	57% overall response rate	Vinblastine 2 mg/m² i.v. week 1, then every 4th week Lomustine 60 mg/m² orally week 3, then every 4th week	Planned protocol 4–6 cycles Toxicity in 54% of cases, mainly myelosuppression	Cooper *et al.* (2009)
Vinblastine, cyclophosphamide, prednisolone	64% overall response	Vinblastine 2–2.2 mg/m² i.v. every 3 weeks Cyclophosphamide 200–250 mg/m² i.v. or orally day 8 of 21-day cycle Prednisolone 1 mg/kg orally q24h tapered and discontinued over 24–32 weeks	Protocol continues for 6 months 11–14% neutropenia	Camps-Palau *et al.* (2007)
Chlorambucil/prednisolone	38% overall response rate	Chlorambucil 5 mg/m² orally q48h Prednisolone 40 mg/m² orally q24h for 14 days then 20 mg/m² q48h	No toxicity	Taylor *et al.* (2009)

12.25 (continued) Most commonly used chemotherapy protocols for canine MCTs.

Neo-adjunctive chemotherapy, prior to surgery or radiotherapy, will often result in consolidation of the tumour mass and improve the likelihood of achieving complete excision, or make it easier and safer to irradiate the mass.

Information on the use of cytotoxic drugs is given in Chapter 7. Lomustine should be used with care: one recent study reported fatality in two of 12 dogs with mast cell tumours, due to hepatotoxicity (Hosoya *et al.*, 2009).

Tyrosine kinase inhibitors: Activation of the KIT receptor tyrosine kinase (TK) is associated with the development of canine MCTs. Activation is usually due to genetic mutations in the c-kit gene, which result in ligand-independent increased cell proliferation, and also alterations in migration, maturation and survival characteristics (see Chapter 9 for more details). Approximately 15–40% of canine MCTs harbour c-kit mutations. Mutations are more frequently found in higher grade tumours, and correlate with a poorer prognosis.

Recently, interest has focused on tyrosine kinase inhibitors (TKIs) for tumours bearing c-kit mutations, and the TKIs investigated so far (masitinib mesylate and toceranib phosphate (SU11654)) have most effect in MCTs with c-kit mutations. Both agents have been used without unacceptable toxicity in dogs, and controlled studies have demonstrated tumour response (toceranib) and delayed time to progression and increased survival (masitinib, toceranib) in selected grade II or III MCTs (Hahn *et al.*, 2008; London *et al.*, 2009). Interestingly, some tumours with wild type (normal) c-kit respond to these drugs, probably because these molecules also inhibit other TKs. These effects also explain the adverse effects seen with these agents. TKIs represent an exciting development in the treatment of canine MCTs but our understanding of their role is currently limited and much work remains to be done.

Supportive therapy: Patients with MCTs must be treated for systemic signs associated with the tumour. H2 antagonists such as cimetidine (licensed in the UK), ranitidine and famotidine are valuable treatments for patients with gastrointestinal signs associated with their tumour, or in asymptomatic patients at times of risk, e.g. when on high-dose prednisolone, or during and soon after radiation therapy. Sucralfate is also of benefit. H1 antagonists (e.g. chlorpheniramine) are seldom required on a continuing basis but are often recommend prior to manipulation of the tumour, for example during planned cytoreductive surgery, or radiotherapy.

Other treatments: Local intralesional therapy of primary MCTs has been described, using intralesional corticosteroids or deionized water, or brachytherapy (radioactive implants), with variable results. Experimental treatment with an immunomodulatory compound based on human chorionic gonadotrophin and bacillus Calmette–Guérin has resulted in responses in 28% of treated dogs (Henry *et al.*, 2007).

Prognostic indicators for MCTs: The most important prognostic factor is histological grade. The Patnaik system (based on extent, cellularity, cell morphology and nuclear features) is the most widely used. It has some limitations, particularly in dealing with well differentiated subcutaneous tumours or superficial dermal tumours (where cytological and architectural features result in conflicting grading), and suffers from subjectivity resulting in variation between pathologists in grading. Nevertheless, Patnaik grade I (well differentiated), grade II (intermediate grade) and grade III (poorly differentiated) tumours differ widely in their clinical behaviour and dictate different treatment and prognosis. Many studies have confirmed the behaviour of grade I (good) and grade III (bad) tumours, but for grade II tumours traditional histological grading is of limited value, because it does not identify those tumours that are likely to metastasize.

Clinical factors may be of prognostic relevance and are summarized in Figure 12.26.

Tumour features
• Rapid tumour growth • Large tumour size • Ulceration • Erythema • Irritation These features most often associated with higher-grade tumours
Systemic signs
• Gastrointestinal signs • Flashing syndromes • Anaphylaxis These features most often associated with higher-grade tumours
Tumour site
• Nail bed • Oral cavity • Muzzle • Inguinal • Preputial • Perineal • Mucocutaneous junctions Literature contradictory. Differences probably multifactorial and influenced by difficulty of achieving excision and/or propensity for high-grade tumours in some sites

12.26 Factors indicating poor prognosis in dogs with MCTs.

Tumour stage is prognostic, with more advanced disease generally having a poorer prognosis. Grade II tumours with metastases are controversial, as appropriate multimodality therapy may result in improved survival times for these patients compared with historical reports. The WHO staging system for MCTs is shown in Figure 12.27, but unfortunately stage and prognosis do not correlate directly in all clinical situations.

Proliferation indices such as mitotic index (MI), argyrophilic nucleolar organizer regions (AgNORs), Ki67 and proliferating cell nuclear antigen (PCNA) may offer prognostic information. These tests are summarized in Figure 12.28. MI has been shown to be a useful prognostic indicator: in one recent study, MST for dogs with a tumour with MI ≤5 per 10 high power fields was 70 months, compared with 2 months where MI was >5, irrespective of grade (Romansik *et al.*, 2007). This is supported by early work showing that patients with tumours with a mitotic index of 10 or more had a survival time of only 11 weeks (Bostock *et al.*, 1989). A cut-off MI of 7 rather than 5 has been proposed (Elston *et al.*, 2009), but further work exploring outcome for patients receiving adjunctive therapy on the basis of MI is required. The impact of MI on likelihood of recurrence is unclear. However, it is a useful marker that can be determined in most cases by standard histopathology.

Stage	Description

0	One tumour incompletely excised from the dermis, identified histologically, without regional lymph node involvement
	  a. Without systemic signs
	  b. With systemic signs

I	One tumour confined to the dermis, without regional lymph node involvement
	  a. Without systemic signs
	  b. With systemic signs

II	One tumour confined to the dermis, with regional lymph node involvement
	  a. Without systemic signs
	  b. With systemic signs

III	Multiple dermal tumours, or large infiltrating tumour with or without regional lymph node involvement
	  a. Without systemic signs
	  b. With systemic signs

IV	Any tumour with distant metastasis or recurrence with metastasis (including blood or bone marrow involvement)

12.27 World Health Organization staging system for canine MCTs.

Marker	Significance	Comment
Mitotic index (MI)	>5 prognostic for reduced survival independent of grade. Not proven to predict for recurrence	Useful test, can be carried out on routine histological sections. Some authors recommend 7 as cut-off rather than 5
Argyrophilic nucleolar organizer regions (AgNORs)	Higher AgNOR counts associated with increased likelihood of death, recurrence and metastasis	Not independent of histological grade
Ki67	High Ki67 expression (scores >1.8) associated with increased mortality, recurrence and metastasis. Prognostic factor independent of histological grade	Useful if available, as proven independent of grade
Proliferating cell nuclear antigen (PCNA)	Increased PCNA expression associated with increased mortality. Not consistently with increased risk of recurrence or metastasis	Not independent of histological grade

12.28 Markers of proliferation and MCT prognosis in dogs.

Margins of excision: Some studies have questioned whether there is any prognostic value in complete *versus* incomplete margins for MCTs. Certainly, in a significant proportion of tumours (probably 25% or more) with incomplete or narrow margins, *en bloc* resection of the scar reveals no mast cells, and one recent study reported only 23% recurrence rate of incompletely excised grade II tumours (Séguin *et al.*, 2006). This may reflect either that the mast cells seen at the margins were not neoplastic, or that the immune system had eradicated microscopic disease. The difficulties in assessing margins arise because MCTs release factors that are chemotactic for normal inflammatory mast cells, and while the tumour cells in high-grade tumours are readily differentiated from normal cells, those in grade I and II tumours are more difficult to differentiate from normal mast cells. Recurrence may occur even where margins have been reported as complete (local failure rates of 5–11% are reported in this situation) but is more likely where margins are incomplete or narrow.

Where margins are incomplete or narrow and there is macroscopic residual disease, recurrence or metastasis, clearly a 'wait and see' approach is not appropriate and where possible definitive surgery should be performed. In sites where surgical excision is difficult to achieve, neo-adjunctive chemotherapy (usually vinblastine and prednisolone, or prednisolone alone) may facilitate a complete excision, or postoperative radiotherapy may be used to deal with residual disease. Recurrent MCTs carry a poorer prognosis.

For grade I and most grade II tumours where incomplete margins are reported but there is no gross disease and the wound has healed uneventfully, the options are to perform an en bloc excision of the scar (preferred) or monitor the site and resect recurrent disease with adequate margins as soon as this is detected. If the second surgery achieves clean margins, no adjunctive therapy is given.

Dogs with multiple MCTs

Up to 44% of dogs cured of a previous MCT will develop further MCTs, and some dogs (probably >20%) develop multiple MCTs either within a relatively short time frame or sequentially throughout their lifetime, particularly Golden Retrievers and possibly Labrador Retrievers, Weimaraners and Boxers. These animals do not experience shorter survival than those with solitary tumours of the same grade, as the tumours represent *de novo* lesions rather than metastatic disease. There is no evidence that these dogs respond to systemic therapy, nor does systemic therapy prevent the development of further *de novo* lesions. Cutaneous metastases from MCTs tend to be seen only in association with aggressive high-grade tumours and are multiple, rapidly growing and often ulcerated (Figure 12.29).

MCTs in cats

MCTs are relatively common in cats (8–15% of skin tumours) but are poorly understood. Most are considered benign and well differentiated.

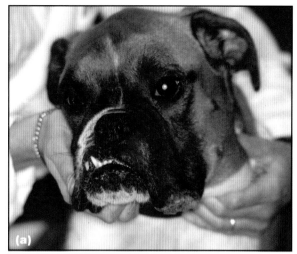
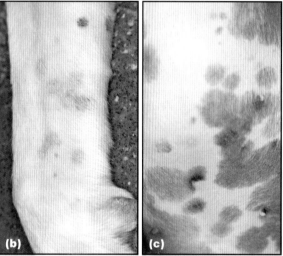
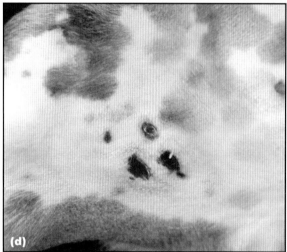

12.29 Metastases from a poorly differentiated MCT in a 6-year-old neutered female Boxer. The primary tumour affected the left upper lip **(a)** and there was marked enlargement of the left submandibular lymph node due to metastasis. Erythematous cutaneous metastatic lesions affected the skin of **(b)** the limbs and **(c)** the ventrum, and there were ulcerated lesions **(d)** on the medial thigh.

Aetiology, pathogenesis and predisposition: Cats with MCT are usually over 4 years of age, with an average of 9–11 years. A predisposition is reported in Siamese cats.

Clinical presentation and approach: Most often MCTs present as discrete firm alopecic nodules, which may be pale or tan in colour. Lesions may be solitary or multiple (approximately 25% are multiple at presentation). Distant metastasis is uncommon. Predilection sites are the head (Figure 12.30), limbs and tail. Cats can develop cutaneous metastases from visceral MCTs and animals presenting with multiple nodules (or palpable abdominal abnormalities) should always be clinically staged.

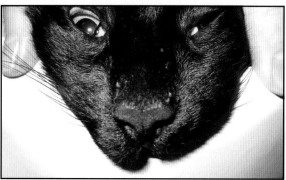

12.30 Diffuse MCT affecting the upper lip of an 11-year-old male DSH cat. (Courtesy of I Grant)

Treatment and prognosis: The treatment of choice for feline MCT is surgical excision. Tumours described histologically as diffuse require wider margins than those described as compact. There is no proven role for chemotherapy, but vinblastine, chlorambucil and lomustine are reported. Prednisolone is often included. There are limited data on radiation therapy.

Histopathological grading using Patnaik-type criteria does not predict prognosis. Histological classification as compact or diffuse tumours is useful: compact mastocytic tumours are commonest (70–85%), are minimally invasive and do not metastasize; but diffuse tumours are locally invasive and commonly have locoregional metastases (5–10%). Proliferation markers may offer some indication of prognosis.

'Histiocytic' MCTs
So-called histiocytic MCTs are not of histiocytic origin and are best described as atypical poorly granulated MCTs. These tumours most often present in young cats (6 weeks to 4 years). Again, Siamese cats are predisposed. These often present as multiple discrete relatively well circumscribed subcutaneous nodules. Lesions may be grouped together. The head is a predilection site. These lesions may regress spontaneously, suggesting a reactive rather than truly neoplastic process.

Spontaneous regression may occur, and steroid therapy does not enhance this. The prognosis is generally good.

Multifocal neoplastic skin disease

Multifocal neoplastic skin disease is an uncommon presentation in dogs and cats and must be differentiated from non-neoplastic disease (Figure 12.31). Diagnosis is often challenging and neoplasia is not suspected until more common differentials have been excluded. Neoplastic skin disease tends to affect older animals and, unlike allergic and endocrine skin disease, it is rarely symmetrical in distribution. Infrequently, animals may present with multifocal variants of tumours that are usually solitary: these are summarized in Figure 12.32.

Animals with multifocal neoplasia may present with multiple cutaneous masses, nodules or plaques. Lesions may also be erythematous, exfoliative, ulcerated and crusted and in some cases pruritic. Mucocutaneous lesions are relatively common in canine epitheliotrophic lymphoma.

Diagnosis depends on cytological or histological examination; and clinical staging and pre-treatment evaluation should be carried out as indicated by the tumour type.

Management is often difficult and the prognosis for multifocal skin neoplasia is generally guarded to poor.

Type	Neoplastic	Non-neoplastic
Multiple cutaneous masses, nodules or plaques	Lymphoma: • Non-epitheliotrophic lymphoma (D,C) • Epitheliotrophic lymphoma (D,C) Histiocytic disease: • Malignant histiocytosis (D,C) • (Multiple fibrous histiocytoma) (D) Others: • Multiple mast cell tumours (D,C) • Multiple squamous cell carcinoma/SCC *in situ* (C) Multiple fibrosarcoma (C) Cutaneous metastatic disease (D,C)	Infectious granulomas • Bacterial (D,C) • Mycobacterial (D,C) • Fungal (D,C) Hypersensitivity: • Eosinophilic granulomas/furunculosis (arthropod bites) (D,C) Immune-mediated: • Sterile nodular panniculitis (D,C) • Juvenile cellulitis and lymphadenitis (D) • Sterile nodular granuloma/pyogranuloma (D) • Plasma cell pododermatitis (C) Parasitic granulomas (D,C) Histiocytic disease: • Cutaneous histiocytosis (D) • Systemic histiocytosis (D) Multiple naevi/cysts (D)

12.31 Differential diagnosis of presentations of multifocal skin neoplasia in dogs (D) and cats (C). (continues) ▶

Type	Neoplastic	Non-neoplastic
Erythematous, exfoliative, alopecic and pruritic lesions	Lymphoma: • Epitheliotrophic (D,C) • (Non-epitheliotrophic) (D,C) Squamous cell carcinoma (C,D)	Hypersensitivity: • Flea allergic dermatitis (D,C) • Adverse food reaction (D,C) • Atopy (D,C) • Contact allergic/irritant dermatitis (D,C) Ectoparasites: • *Sarcoptes* (D,C) • *Cheyletiella* (D,C) • *Otodectes* (D,C) • Lice (D,C) • Harvest mites (D,C) • *Demodex* (D,C) • *Notoedres* (C) Immune-mediated: • Pemphigus complex (D,C) • Cutaneous lupus erythematosus (D,C) Infectious: • Pyoderma/bacterial folliculitis (D,C) • Dermatophytosis (D,C) • *Malassezia* (D,C) • Pox virus (C) Eosinophilic granuloma complex (C) Psychogenic alopecia (C)
Mucocutaneous lesions and multifocal facial ulcerations	Lymphoma: • Epitheliotrophic (D,C) • (Non-epitheliotrophic) (D,C) Squamous cell carcinoma (D,C)	Immune-mediated: • Pemphigus complex (D,C) • Cutaneous lupus erythematosus (D,C) • Drug eruptions (D,C) Hypersensitivity: • Eosinophilic granuloma complex (C) • Drug eruptions (D,C) Infectious: • Pyoderma/bacterial folliculitis (D,C) • Candidiasis (D,C) • (Subcutaneous and deep fungal infections) (D,C) (Toxic epidermal necrolysis) (D) (Erythema multiforme) (D)

12.31 (continued) Differential diagnosis of presentations of multifocal skin neoplasia in dogs (D) and cats (C).

Tumour (species)	Breed or sex predisposition	Predilection site	Clinical features	Possible treatment
Infundibular keratinizing acanthoma (intracutaneous cornifying epithelioma) (D)	Norwegian Elkhound, Kerry Blue Terrier, Lhasa Apso	Any	Multiple partially alopecic dermal nodules. May have central pore with protruding keratin	Isotretinoin 1–2 mg/kg/day
Squamous cell carcinoma (C,D)	Older	Digits, lips, external nares	Proliferative, erosive or ulcerated lesions	Surgical excision; radiation therapy (see text)
Lipoma (D,C)	(? Overweight female)	Any	Soft to firm slow-growing subcutaneous masses	Surgical excision
Haemangiosarcoma (D)	German Shepherd Dog	Any	Poorly circumscribed, invasive, friable, rapidly growing	Surgical excision Adjunctive chemotherapy
Fibrosarcoma (C)	Multiple fibrosarcomas only seen in young cats concurrently infected with FeLV and feline sarcoma virus: rare	Any	Firm, pale, rapidly growing, infiltrative or ulcerated cutaneous and subcutaneous masses	Biopsy to confirm diagnosis, clinical staging if appropriate. Disease progression rapid, no successful treatment
Perianal gland adenoma (D)	Male Samoyed, Cocker Spaniel, Bulldog, Beagle	Perianal region, perineum, tail, prepuce, thigh	Well circumscribed nodules, may ulcerate	Surgical excision Castration/hormonal therapy
Perianal gland adenocarcinoma (D)	Male	Perianal	Poorly circumscribed invasive masses, often ulcerated	Surgical excision ? Efficacy of radiation therapy/chemotherapy
Histiocytoma (D)	Often young (<3 years) Boxer, Bulldog, Dobermann, Dachshund	Head, limbs, feet	Well circumscribed nodule, may be hairless, may ulcerate	May spontaneously regress Surgical excision

12.32 Tumours that most commonly present as solitary lesions but may present in multifocal forms in dogs (D) and cats (C). Cases must be approached on an individual basis and treated as indicated by their clinical circumstances. (continues) ▶

Tumour (species)	Breed or sex predisposition	Predilection site	Clinical features	Possible treatment
Sebaceous adenoma/ epithelioma tumours (D)	Older dogs Cocker Spaniel, Kerry Blue Terrier, Boston Terrier, Beagle, Basset Hound, Dachshund, Siberian Husky, Miniature Poodle, Coonhound, Samoyed, Persian cats	Any, head, face	Dome-shaped or papillated nodule, fungiform mass, yellow opalescent or pigmented, may be alopecic or ulcerated	Surgical excision
Plasma cell tumour/ plasmacytoma (D)		Any, mucocutaneous junctions	Well circumscribed, usually non-ulcerated masses	Clinical staging to rule out cutaneous involvement in multiple myeloma. Surgical excision, radiotherapy (no proven chemotherapy)
Trichoepithelioma (D,C)	Basset Hound, Cocker Spaniel, German Shepherd Dog, Golden Retriever	Dorsal lumbar and lateral thoracic	Well circumscribed intradermal nodules	Surgical excision

12.32 (continued) Tumours that most commonly present as solitary lesions but may present in multifocal forms in dogs (D) and cats (C). Cases must be approached on an individual basis and treated as indicated by their clinical circumstances.

Primary cutaneous lymphoma

Cutaneous lymphomas account for only 3–8% of canine lymphomas (1% of canine skin tumours) and <3% of feline lymphomas (2.8% of feline skin tumours). Primary cutaneous lymphomas are classified histologically as either epitheliotrophic or non-epitheliotrophic, depending on whether the neoplastic infiltration is epidermal (epitheliotrophic) or dermal (non-epitheliotrophic). Epitheliotrophic lymphoma is more common than non-epitheliotrophic in dogs, and extremely rare in cats. Non-epitheliotrophic lymphoma is less common than epitheliotrophic lymphoma in dogs, but more common in cats, though rare.

Epitheliotrophic lymphoma (mycosis fungoides) is characterized by infiltration of neoplastic memory T cells into the epidermis, Pautrier's micro-abscesses (focal accumulations of tumour cells) and tropism of tumour cells for adnexal structures (Figure 12.33). In humans, epitheliotrophic lymphoma is further classified as in Figure 12.34, but in dogs these sub-classifications are more useful to pathologists than clinicians. The classical mycosis fungoides form is commonest in dogs.

Non-epitheliotrophic lymphoma is characterized by a diffuse infiltration of neoplastic lymphoid cells in the dermis, which may extend into the epidermis.

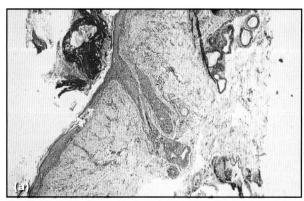 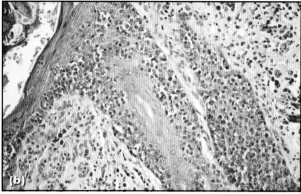

12.33 Epitheliotrophic lymphoma. The distribution of the tumour cell infiltrate in the epidermis and around the hair follicle is evident on low and high power. **(a)** H&E; ×20 original magnification; **(b)** H&E, ×100 original magnification. (Courtesy of A Jefferies)

Form of epitheliotrophic lymphoma	Subclassification	Characteristics (based on human data)	Dogs
Mycosis fungoides (MF)	Classic	Often characterized by orderly progression through eczematous to plaque to tumour stage	Commonest form, but no distinct progression through stages
	D'emblee	Sudden-onset nodular form with no pre-tumour stage	Clinically recognized in dogs
Pagetoid reticulosis (PR)	Woringer–Kolopp	Localized, often slowly progressive	One suspected case report
	Ketron–Goodman	Generalized form; differentiated from MF by histology	One case report
Sézary syndrome		Characterized by circulating neoplastic cells	Rare in dogs

12.34 Clinicopathological classification of epitheliotrophic lymphoma in humans, and relevance to dogs.

Aetiology, pathogenesis and predispositions: The aetiology of epitheliotrophic lymphoma is unknown. Chronic inflammation has been proposed as a possible risk factor in dogs. Chronic activation and stimulation of T lymphocytes by persistent environmental antigens or abnormalities in Langerhans' cell function may result in clonal expansion of activated lymphocytes giving rise to lymphoma. However, there is no clear evidence to support this in dogs.

The epitheliotrophic lymphomas are T-cell tumours. In both humans and dogs, these are tumours of the memory subpopulation of T cells, but in dogs the tumour cells have different cluster of differentiation (CD) antigen profiles and T-cell receptor gene rearrangements than in humans, suggesting a different molecular pathogenesis. Most (but not all) non-epitheliotrophic lymphomas in dogs and cats are also of T-cell origin. Although cats with this cutaneous lymphoma are usually FeLV-negative on p27 enzyme-linked immunosorbent assay (ELISA), tumour tissue may test positive for feline leukaemia virus antigen by immunohistochemistry or integrated retroviral elements on polymerase chain reaction (PCR), supporting the 'hit and run' theory of FeLV oncogenesis.

There is suggested breed predisposition for epitheliotrophic lymphoma in Cocker Spaniels and Boxers, but no sex predisposition. Older dogs tend to be affected (mean age 8–11 years). Non-epitheliotrophic lymphoma may be more common in Boxers, St Bernards, Basset Hounds, Irish Setters, Cocker Spaniels, German Shepherd Dogs, Golden Retrievers and Scottish Terriers.

Clinical signs: Cutaneous lymphoma can mimic many dermatides. In humans, there is a classical step-by-step progression of epitheliotrophic lymphoma from premycotic/eczematous to plaque to tumour stage. Dogs may present with lesions typical of any or all stages. Clinical features include:

- Exfoliative erythroderma, i.e. erythema, scaling, with or without loss of pigmentation and alopecia (Figure 12.35), which is often pruritic
- Mucocutaneous erythema, infiltration, depigmentation, alopecia or ulceration; multiple or solitary patches, plaques, or nodular masses, which may be scaly, crusty or erythematous (Figure 12.36)
- Infiltrative or ulcerative oral mucosal disease (Figure 12.37b,c).

Overall, erythema is present in about 80% of cases; plaques, scales and/or nodules each in 60% of cases; and erosions, ulceration, crusting, mucosal involvement and pruritus each in about 40% of cases. More than one form of lesion may be present in the same patient and involvement of the mucocutaneous junctions (especially lips) and oral cavity is common. Periocular tissues may also be affected. Disease progression to local and regional lymph nodes is common in dogs and systemic involvement of other lymphoid tissues may occur, resulting in lymphadenopathy and clinical signs associated with disseminated lymphoproliferative disease.

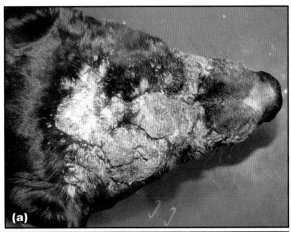

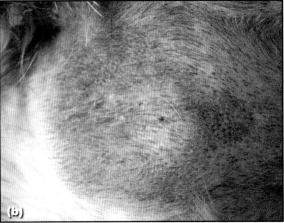

12.35 **(a)** A 14-year-old neutered male crossbred dog with cutaneous lymphoma with marked pruritus and scaling. **(b)** A proliferating erythematous scaling ulcerated lesion in an elderly pruritic crossbred dog with epitheliotrophic lymphoma. (b, Courtesy of L. Buckley)

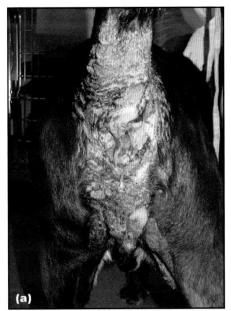

12.36 Mucocutaneous lesions in canine epitheliotrophic lymphoma. **(a)** The dog shown in Figure 12.35a, displaying perianal cutaneous and mucocutaneous erythema and ulceration, along with faecal staining due to pain (he would not allow the owners to clean the area). (continues) ▶

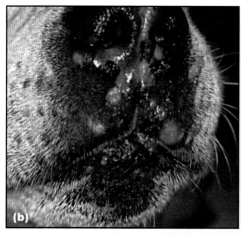
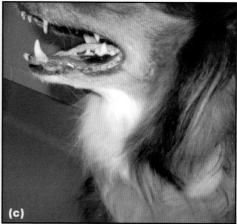

12.36

(continued) Mucocutaneous lesions in canine epitheliotrophic lymphoma. **(b)** Epitheliotrophic lymphoma on the muzzle of a middle-aged crossbred dog. **(c)** Lip lesion in a 9-year-old female Shetland Sheepdog.

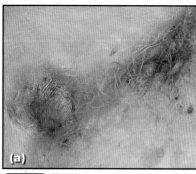
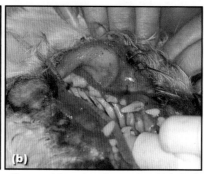
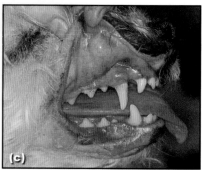

12.37 Epitheliotrophic lymphoma in an 8-year-old neutered crossbred bitch. **(a)** A raised reddened plaque-like lesion and erythematous nodular lesions in the groin. **(b)** Erythema, ulceration and a buccal mucosal plaque lesion. **(c)** The same patient on completion of radiation therapy: the plaque-like lesion has regressed and ulceration has resolved.

Clinical signs of non-epitheliotrophic lymphoma include:

- Generalized or multifocal nodular disease (Figure 12.38)
- Systemic involvement and signs of generalized lymphoproliferative disease (lesions progress rapidly and the clinical course is short).

Exfoliative erythroderma is present in only a minority of cases and pruritus is rare. Hypercalcaemia may be relatively common in non-epitheliotrophic lymphoma, so animals may have a history of polyuria/polydipsia, gastrointestinal signs and muscle weakness (see Chapters 4 and 19).

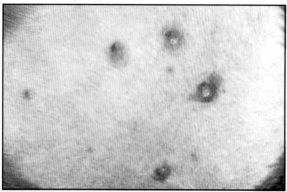

12.38 Non-epitheliotrophic lymphoma in a dog, showing multiple raised nodular lesions on the dorsum. (Courtesy of J Dobson)

Clinical approach: Diagnosis can only be confirmed by biopsy, where the microscopic distribution of the neoplastic cells can be appreciated, though the presence of a lymphoproliferative neoplasm may be apparent on cytology.

Clinical staging and pre-treatment evaluation should be carried out as with other lymphoma patients (see Chapter 19).

Management: Systemic combination chemotherapy (see Chapter 19) can be used to treat animals with cutaneous lymphoma, but response rates are generally low and median remissions of 1–11 months in dogs are reported, though there are occasional long-term survivors. There is no proven advantage of one combination protocol over any other for this form of lymphoma, but single agent lomustine has been reported to have high response rates (around 80%) as a primary or rescue drug. Long-term follow-up data are lacking and care must be taken when using lomustine. Cats respond less favourably than dogs to chemotherapy.

In human medicine, interferon alpha 2b (IFN) has been used in combination with local radiation therapy, photodynamic therapy or retinoid therapy. Interferon is thought to act as a biological response modifier and to up-regulate the host's immune response against the tumour. Currently, recombinant human IFN is available but not licensed for animal use: it has been used off-label in both cats and dogs and clinical response in epitheliotrophic lymphoma is reported. However, relatively rapid induction of antibodies to this foreign protein may limit its long-term value.

Retinoids (isotretinoin, etretinate) are vitamin A analogues that have been reported to produce clinical improvement in up to 50% of cutaneous lymphoma patients, though patients may show only an amelioration of clinical signs rather than a measurable tumour response. They are most commonly used in conjunction with corticosteroids or other treatments. Isotretinoin is used for dogs at 1–2 mg/kg/day, usually given as 1 mg/kg q12h, and for cats 2–3 mg/kg q24h. Care must be taken when handling these agents as they are powerful teratogens, and patients should be monitored for adverse effects.

Lymphoproliferative diseases are very radiosensitive and radiotherapy may be used to treat (for example) problematic oral lesions, to facilitate longer survival with a better quality of life, but the generalized nature of the disease means that radiation is not a suitable definitive therapy for most patients.

Prognosis: The prognosis for cutaneous lymphoma is guarded, with MSTs measured in terms of months, though there may be individual longer-term survivors. Localized forms of epitheliotrophic lymphoma, involving the lips or oral cavity, may carry a more favourable prognosis. These lesions may respond very well to surgical management or radiation therapy, which have the potential to be curative in truly localized disease. Sadly, solitary or localized tumours are uncommon.

Secondary cutaneous lymphoma

Lymphoma arising in another site (multicentric, cranial mediastinal, alimentary or extranodal) may disseminate to the skin during disease progression, giving rise to so-called secondary cutaneous lymphoma. Lesions may take any of the forms described above.

Cutaneous involvement should be confirmed cytologically or histologically. The immunophenotype reflects that of the original tumour, so that more B-cell tumours may be found. The animal should be appropriately evaluated for any rescue therapy considered.

Treatment is very difficult, as these animals have usually been extensively pretreated with combination chemotherapy and often exhibit multidrug resistance. Local radiotherapy may be considered for problematic lesions, where appropriate, but many animals have generalized relapse and rapidly progressive disseminated disease.

The prognosis for secondary cutaneous lymphoma is very guarded.

Multifocal histiocytic disease

There are three forms of multicentric histiocytic disease in dogs: cutaneous, systemic and malignant (also known as disseminated histiocytic sarcoma). Malignant histiocytosis has recently been described in cats, but the forms described here relate to dogs. Cutaneous and systemic histiocytoses are reactive histiocytoses, which result from reactive proliferation of dermal dendritic antigen-presenting cells as a consequence of immunodysregulation (see Figure 12.14) rather than neoplastic conditions.

Diagnosis of histiocytic disease requires cytological or histological (and occasionally immmunohistological) examination of cells. The differentiation between systemic and malignant histiocytosis depends on evaluation of cellular morphology: in malignant histiocytosis, the cells have features of malignancy, while the infiltrates in systemic histiocytosis are of apparently non-malignant cells. In both systemic and malignant histiocytosis, erythrophagocytosis may be a prominent feature.

It is important to stage these animals clinically, especially to differentiate cutaneous from systemic histiocytosis. Thorough clinical examination, imaging, haematology, biochemistry and bone marrow aspiration are recommended.

Cutaneous histiocytosis

Aetiology and predispositions: This reactive condition arises due to dysregulation of Langerhans' cells (see Figure 12.14). Cutaneous histiocytosis may affect any age or breed, but collies and spaniels seem predisposed.

Presentation and clinical signs: Dogs present with multiple cutaneous nodules, which are often depigmented. Predilection sites are the face (bridge of the nose, nose and muzzle), ears, neck, trunk, perineum and scrotum. Lesions are restricted to the skin. There is no lymph node or systemic involvement. Occasionally, involvement of the nasal mucosae may produce inspiratory stridor or sneezing, but involvement of other mucosal surfaces is uncommon.

Management and prognosis: The prognosis is variable and treatment should be regarded as palliative rather than curative. The clinical course may wax and wane, but around 50% of dogs will have a partial or complete response to immunosuppressive corticosteroids. Responders can often be weaned off therapy. Azathioprine or ciclosporin may be of value in refractory cases (Figure 12.39).

Drug	Dose	Side effects	Notes
Prednisolone	2–4 mg/kg q24h tapering to lowest effective dose q48h	Iatrogenic hyperadrenocorticism; GI effects; (pancreatitis)	Steroid side effects often underestimated
Azathioprine	2 mg/kg q24h for 7 days, then q48h	Myelosuppression; mild GI signs; (pancreatitis)	Monitor haematology for myelosuppression. *Cytotoxic drug: appropriate handling required*
Ciclosporin	Atopica 5 mg/kg q24h, then tapered to lowest effective dose q48h	Vomiting, diarrhoea (usually transient); anorexia; gingival hyperplasia; changes in hair coat; muscle cramps, weakness	Atopica not authorized for use for immunosuppression or treatment of histiocytic disorders but has licence for atopy in dogs

12.39 Immunomodulatory therapies used in multifocal skin disease in dogs.

Systemic histiocytosis

Aetiology, pathogenesis and predisposition: This reactive histiocytosis arises due to dysregulation of interstitial dendritic cells.

In Bernese Mountain Dogs, there is a polygenic inheritable trait and males are over-represented. Systemic histiocytosis had been reported in other breeds, including the Rottweiler and Golden Retriever.

Presentation and clinical signs: Cutaneous lesions are common but many non-cutaneous sites may be affected, including mucocutaneous junctions, the ocular and nasal mucosa, lymph nodes, liver, spleen, lung and bone marrow (Figure 12.40). Presentation depends on the organs involved and clinical signs include anorexia, weight loss, cutaneous nodules, stertorous respiration and scrotal dermatitis. Cutaneous nodules are again often found on the face, muzzle and around the nares. Ocular and periocular infiltrates may result in presentation with ocular or periocular signs such as intractable chemosis or episcleritis (Figure 12.41).

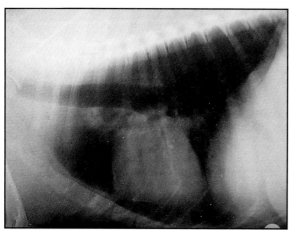

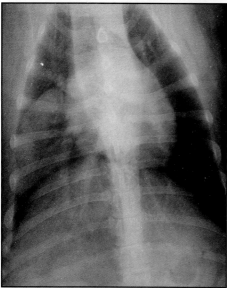

12.40 Systemic histiocytosis in a 5-year-old male Bernese Mountain Dog. Lateral and dorsoventral thoracic radiographs show consolidation of the right middle lung lobe, resulting in air bronchograms. FNA of the lesion revealed an infiltrate of histiocytic cells.

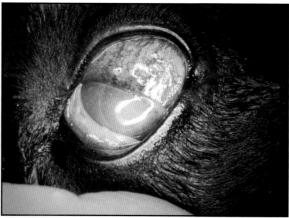

12.41 Ocular involvement in systemic histiocytosis, with conjunctival involvement and diffuse infiltrate resulting in uveitis-like signs.

Management: Systemic histiocytosis is generally slowly progressive with a waxing and waning clinical course, which makes it difficult to assess the impact of treatment on disease progression. Corticosteroid therapy alone is seldom sufficient and the addition of other immunosuppressive therapy is often required (see Figure 12.39). Dogs may be weaned off therapy, but relapse is common and the condition often becomes refractory. Many chemotherapeutic drugs have been used, including virtually all of the agents used against lymphoma, but the protracted and fluctuating nature of the disease course makes assessment of response difficult. Ocular disease may benefit from topical corticosteroids, but may be refractory.

Prognosis: The prognosis for systemic histiocytosis is guarded, with most animals succumbing to disease progression eventually, or in some cases the development of malignant histiocytosis.

Disseminated histiocytic sarcoma, malignant histiocytosis, haemophagocytic histiocytic sarcoma

These are truly neoplastic conditions. In malignant histiocytosis (MH) and disseminated histiocytic sarcoma, tumours arise from dendritic cells (CD18, 45 and 11c-positive), while in haemophagocytic histiocytic sarcoma there is a strong haemophagocytic component and the cell of origin is thought to be the CD11d-positive macrophage. Clinical features, breed predisposition and clinical course are similar and the prognosis is equally dismal.

Aetiology and predisposition: This disease affects predominantly Bernese Mountain Dogs, in which there is a poorly defined polygenic mode of inheritance, and MH accounts for up to 25% of tumours in this breed. There is a male predisposition. Flat-coated Retrievers, Golden Retrievers and Rottweilers are also predisposed, though it occurs in other breeds.

Presentation and clinical signs: Multiple organs are affected (spleen, liver, lymph nodes, lungs, bone marrow, kidneys) and there may be cutaneous or subcutaneous lesions, though these are often less clinically significant. Dogs present with vague clinical signs referable to the organs involved, including anorexia, weight loss, anaemia, dyspnoea and coughing. There is often pallor, lymphadenopathy and hepatic or splenic enlargement. Anaemia may be due to destruction of red cells in haemophagocytic histiocytic sarcoma, and bone marrow infiltration may result in neutropenia or thrombocytopenia. Animals may present with lameness or neurological signs due to the infiltration in joints or the central nervous system.

Management and prognosis: Malignant histiocytosis carries a grave prognosis: treatment rarely results in a sustained response, as the disease does not respond favourably to chemotherapy (though anthracylines and lomustine have been used). Successful treatment of dogs with a human cytotoxic T-cell line has been reported (Visonneau *et al.*, 1997), but has not proved repeatable and has not become an established therapy. Short-term maintenance with matched blood transfusions and corticosteroids may be possible in some cases.

Feline progressive dendritic cell histiocytosis

This is a progressive proliferation of non-Langerhans' dendritic cells. A small number of reports describe the development of multiple intradermal nodules over a protracted time course in cats. Distribution is usually generalized but often starts on the head and neck, or may be regional (e.g. one limb). There is no documented treatment and cats may progress to aggressive feline disseminated histiocytic sarcoma/malignant histiocytosis. Cats with truly malignant histiocytosis may present with anaemia, and splenomegaly may be prominent.

Metastatic digit tumours in cats: 'lung–digit syndrome'

This is a syndrome typically associated with primary lung tumours (SCC, bronchogenic carcinoma, pulmonary carcinoma) that metastasize to the digits.

Presentation and clinical signs: There is digital pain, swelling and ulceration and the nail may be lost. Cats are usually lame, or reluctant or unable to walk. Any digit or number of digits may be affected and the lesions may be asymmetric. Further metastatic lesions may be found in lymph nodes and other sites.

Clinical approach: Thoracic radiography should be carried out to identify the primary lesion (Figure 12.42). Radiography of the pedal lesions shows soft tissue swelling, lysis of the distal phalanges and sometimes irregular new bone formation. FNA of the pulmonary mass and digital lesions will often confirm the diagnosis, though biopsy of the digital lesions may be required in some cases.

Management and prognosis: There is no successful treatment and the prognosis for these cats is hopeless.

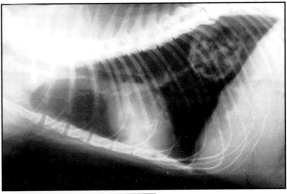

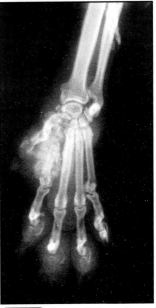

12.42 Lung–digit syndrome in an elderly neutered female DSH cat. On the lateral thoracic radiograph, a partially mineralized soft tissue mass is seen in the caudodorsal lung field, which was confirmed on FNA to be a carcinoma. The dorsopalmar view of the forepaw shows extensive soft tissue swelling on the medial aspect, with irregular new bone formation on the phalanges and metacarpi, accompanied by osteolysis. These lesions represent metastatic carcinoma. (Courtesy of S Corr)

Cutaneous metastases

The development of cutaneous metastatic disease may be seen with any malignancy and has been reported in a wide variety of tumours, including mammary adenocarcinoma in the cat, poorly differentiated soft tissue sarcomas, osteosarcoma, malignant melanoma, aggressive mammary carcinomas and seminoma in dogs and MCTs in both species. Cutaneous involvement may also be seen in lymphoproliferative disease.

Presentation and clinical signs: There is usually a known history of a malignancy, though occasionally animals present with the metastatic disease. Lesions are very variable in appearance, but may be nodular, erythematous, or ulcerated (Figure 12.43).

Clinical approach, management and prognosis: Biopsy or FNA is required for diagnosis. There is generally no effective therapy and the prognosis is grave.

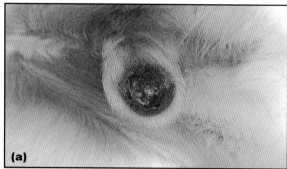

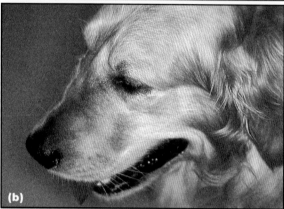

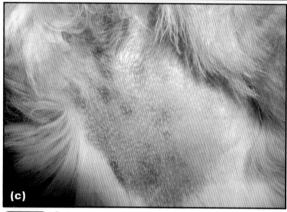

12.43 Cutaneous metastases. **(a)** An inflamed and ulcerated preputial metastatic lesion from **(b)** a primary anaplastic sarcoma on the bridge of the nose in a 4-year-old male Golden Retriever. **(c)** Metastases from a visceral haemangiosarcoma (the purplish lesions visible in the clipped area) in an elderly crossbred dog.

References and further reading

Bostock DE, Crocker J, Harris K and Smith P (1989) Nucleolar organiser regions as indicators of post-surgical prognosis in canine spontaneous mast cell tumours. *British Journal of Cancer* **59**, 915–918

Camps-Palau MA, Leibman NF, Elmslie R *et al.* (2007) Treatment of canine mast cell tumours with vinblastine, cyclophosphamide and prednisone: 35 cases (1997–2004). *Veterinary and Comparative Oncology* **5**, 156–167

Cooper M, Tsai X and Bennett P (2009) Combination CCNU and vinblastine chemotherapy for canine mast cell tumours: 57 cases. *Veterinary and Comparative Oncology* **7**, 196–206

Dobson JM and Scase TJ (2007) Advances in the diagnosis and management of cutaneous mast cell tumours in dogs. *Journal of Small Animal Practice* **48**, 424–431

Elston LB, Sueiro FAR, Cavalcanti JN and Metze K (2009) Letter to the editor. The importance of the mitotic index as a prognostic factor for survival of canine mast cell tumours: a validation study. *Veterinary Pathology* **46**, 362–365

Fontaine J, Bovens C, Bettenay S and Mueller RS (2009) Canine cutaneous epitheliotrophic T-cell lymphoma: a review. *Veterinary and Comparative Oncology* **7**, 1–14

Gross TL, Ihrke PJ, Walder EJ and Affolter VK (2005) Section two: neoplasms and other tumors. In: *Skin Diseases of the Dog and Cat: Clinical and Histopathologic Diagnosis, 2nd edn*, pp. 561–893. Blackwell Science, Oxford.

Hahn KA, Oglivie G, Rusk T *et al.* (2008) Masitinib is safe and effective for the treatment of canine mast cell tumors. *Journal of Veterinary Internal Medicine* **22**, 1301–1309

Henry CJ, Downing S, Rosenthal RC *et al.* (2007) Evaluation of a novel immunomodulator composed of human chorionic gonadotropin and bacillus Calmette-Guerin for treatment of canine mast cell tumours in clinically affected dogs. *American Journal of Veterinary Research* **68**, 1246–1251

Hosoya K, Kisseberth WC, Alvarez FJ *et al.* (2009) Adjuvant CCNU (lomustine) and prednisone chemotherapy for dogs with incompletely excised grade 2 mast cell tumors. *Journal of the American Animal Hospital Association* **45**, 14–18

London CA, Malpas PB, Wood-Follis SL *et al.* (2009) Multi-center, placebo-controlled, double-blind, randomized study of oral toceranib phosphate (SU11654), a receptor tyrosine kinase inhibitor, for the treatment of dogs with recurrent (either local or distant) mast cell tumor following surgical excision. *Clinical Cancer Research* **15**, 3856–3865

Murphy S (2006a) Skin neoplasia in small animals. 2. Common feline tumours. *In Practice* **28**, 320–325

Murphy S (2006b) Skin neoplasia in small animals. 3. Common canine tumours. *In Practice* **28**, 398–402

Murphy S, Sparkes AH, Smith KC, Blunden AS and Brearley MJ (2004) Relationships between the histological grade of cutaneous mast cell tumours in dogs, their survival and the efficacy of surgical resection. *Veterinary Record* **154**, 743–746

Padgett GA, Madewell BR, Keller ET, Jodar L and Packard M (1995) Inheritance of histiocytosis in Bernese mountain dogs. *Journal of Small Animal Practice* **36**, 93–98

Rassnick KM, Moore AS, Williams LE *et al.* (1999) Treatment of canine mast cell tumours with CCNU (lomustine). *Journal of Veterinary Internal Medicine* **13**, 601–605

Romansik EM, Reilly CM, Kass PH, Moore PF and London CA (2007) Mitotic index is predictive for survival for canine cutaneous mast cell tumours. *Veterinary Pathology* **44**, 335–341

Séguin B, Besançon MF, McCallan JL *et al.* (2006) Recurrence rate, clinical outcome, and cellular proliferation indices as prognostic indicators after incomplete surgical excision of cutaneous grade II mast cell tumours: 28 dogs (1994–2002). *Journal of Veterinary Internal Medicine* **20**, 933–940

Taylor F, Gear R, Hoather T and Dobson J (2009) Chlorambucil and prednisolone chemotherapy for dogs with inoperable mast cell tumours: 21 cases. *Journal of Small Animal Practice* **50**, 284–289

Thamm DH, Mauldin EA and Vail DM (1999) Prednisolone and vinblastine chemotherapy for canine mast cell tumor – 41 cases (1992–97) *Journal of Veterinary Internal Medicine* **13**, 491–497

Thamm DH, Turek MM and Vail DM (2006) Outcome and prognostic factors following adjuvant prednisone/vinblastine chemotherapy for high-risk canine mast cell tumour: 61 Cases. *Journal of Veterinary Medical Science* **68**, 581–587

Vickery KR, Wilson H, Vail DM and Thamm DH (2008) Dose-escalating vinblastine for the treatment of canine mast cell tumour. *Veterinary and Comparative Oncology* **6**, 111–119

Visonneau S, Cesano A, Tran T, Jeglum KA and Santoli D (1997) Successful treatment of canine malignant histiocytosis with the human major histocompatability complex nonrestricted cytotoxic T-cell line TALL-104. *Clinical Cancer Research* **3**, 1789–1707

Welle MM, Bley CR, Howard J and Rufenachts S (2008) Canine mast cell tumours: a review of the pathogenesis, clinical features, pathology and treatment. *Veterinary Dermatology* **19**, 321–339

13

Tumours of the skeletal system

William S. Dernell

Introduction

Osteosarcoma (OSA) is by far the most common primary bone tumour in dogs, accounting for up to 85% of malignancies originating in the skeleton. Primary OSA accounts for approximately 5% of all canine tumours and thus the practitioner can expect to see this tumour with some regularity. Although the diagnosis and treatment are straightforward, due to somewhat limited options, its biological aggressiveness makes successful treatment and follow-up challenging.

This chapter will focus on the diagnosis, treatment and follow-up of appendicular OSA, because of its prominence among bone malignances. Axial OSA and less common bone tumours will be discussed briefly, primarily in light of their differences to appendicular OSA.

Figures 13.1 and 13.2 list the differential diagnoses, clinical and radiographic features, biological

Tumour type	Clinical features	Radiographic features	Biological behaviour	Treatment options
Osteosarcoma: endosteal	Appendicular skeleton, metaphyseal locations	Lysis, unorganized periosteal response, osteoid production	90% micrometastatic at presentation	Surgery with adjuvant chemotherapy
Osteosarcoma: periosteal	Appendicular or axial skeleton	Bone surface lesion with cortical destruction	Locally invasive and presumed highly metastatic	Surgery with adjuvant chemotherapy
Osteosarcoma: parosteal or juxtacortical	Appendicular or axial skeleton	Osseous lesion adjacent to bone. No cortical destruction	Minimally invasive, variable (low) metastasis	Surgical resection
Chondrosarcoma	Primarily flat bones (skull)	Blastic, with features of slower growth	Locally invasive, moderate metastasis	Surgical resection
Haemangiosarcoma	Appendicular skeleton, variable locations	Lysis	90% micrometastatic at presentation	Surgery with adjuvant chemotherapy
Fibrosarcoma	Appendicular	Lysis without osteoid production	Locally invasive, low to moderate metastasis	Surgical resection
Multilobular osteochondrosarcoma	Flat bones, primarily skull	Lobular osteoid/fibrous tissue 'popcorn ball' appearance	Low to moderate invasion, low metastasis	Surgical resection
Bone cysts: aneurysmal, true cyst, pseudocyst	Metaphyseal locations, long bones	Thinned cortices, cystic appearance, may be expansile	Non-invasive, benign, can recur	Surgical curettage with filling or stabilization
Multiple cartilaginous exostoses	Any skeletal site, especially vertebrae	Circumscribed bony mass on surface	Benign, rare transformation	None, or surgical debulking
Osteoma	Flat bones, primarily skull	Dense, blastic response, smooth borders	Non-invasive	None, or surgical debulking

13.1 Features of the most common tumours of the skeletal system of the dog.

Tumour type	Clinical features	Radiographic features	Biological behaviour	Treatment options
Osteosarcoma	Appendicular or axial skeleton, variable sites	Often juxtacortical or parosteal	Moderate local invasion, low metastasis	Surgical resection, adjuvant chemotherapy for axial lesions
Multiple cartilaginous exostoses	Any skeletal site, especially vertebrae FeLV-positive	Circumscribed bony mass on surface, local destruction	Local invasion, malignant transformation	None or surgical removal for palliation
Chondrosarcoma, haemangiosarcoma, fibrosarcoma	As for dogs (see Figure 13.1)	As for dogs (see Figure 13.1)	Rare, assumed as for dogs (see Figure 13.1)	As for dogs (see Figure 13.1)

13.2 Features of the most common tumours of the skeletal system of the cat.

behaviour and treatment options for the most common tumours of the skeletal system for the dog and cat, respectively. Figure 13.1 also includes benign lesions that may present a similar radiographic appearance.

Osteosarcoma in dogs

Incidence and risk factors

OSA is estimated to occur in over 8000 dogs each year in the United States. It is largely a disease of middle-aged to older dogs, with a median age of 7 years. There is a wide range in age of onset, with a small peak in incidence at 18–24 months.

OSA is classically a cancer of large and giant breeds. Increasing weight and, more specifically, height appear to be the most predictive factors in the dog. The breeds most at risk are St Bernard, Great Dane, Irish Setter, Dobermann, German Shepherd Dog and Golden Retriever. The overall male/female ratio of OSA appears to be fairly equal, with a reported slightly increased incidence in males. In the Rottweiler, male and female dogs that underwent gonadectomy before 1 year of age had an approximately 1 in 4 lifetime risk for bone sarcoma and were significantly more likely to develop bone sarcoma than dogs that were sexually intact (Cooley *et al.*, 2002). There was a highly significant inverse dose–response relationship between duration of lifetime gonadal exposure and incidence rate of bone sarcoma, independent of adult height or body weight.

Overall, approximately 75% of OSA occurs in the appendicular skeleton, with the remainder occurring in the axial skeleton. The metaphyseal region of long bones is the most common primary site, with front limbs affected twice as often as rear limbs and the distal radius and proximal humerus being the two most common locations. It is rare for OSA to be located in bones adjacent to the elbow, but there is one report of 12 cases located at the proximal radius or distal humerus (Liptak *et al.*, 2004). No prognostic difference in these cases as compared with more common appendicular sites was found. In the rear limbs, tumours are fairly evenly distributed between the distal femur, distal tibia and proximal tibia, with the proximal femur a slightly less common site. Primary OSA distal to the antebrachiocarpal and tarsocrural joints is relatively rare in dogs.

In a study of 116 cases of canine primary OSA in the axial skeleton it was reported that 27% were located in the mandible, 22% in the maxilla, 15% in the spine, 14% in the cranium, 10% in ribs, 9% in the nasal cavity or paranasal sinuses and 6% in the pelvis (Heyman *et al.*, 1992). Documentable multicentric OSA at the time of initial diagnosis occurs in <10% of all cases.

Osteosarcoma of extraskeletal sites is rare, but primary OSA has been reported in mammary tissue, subcutaneous tissue, spleen, bowel, liver, kidney, testicle, vagina, eye, gastric ligament and adrenal gland.

Aetiology, pathology and natural behaviour

The aetiology of canine OSA is generally unknown. A simplistic theory proposes that multiple minor trauma and subsequent injury to sensitive cells in the physeal region may occur in large, fast-growing dogs. This may initiate the disease by inducing mitogenic signals increasing the probability for the development of a mutant lineage and subsequent tumour formation. There are reports of OSA associated with metallic implants used for fracture repair, chronic osteomyelitis and with fractures in which no internal repair was used (Figure 13.3). Exposure to ionizing radiation can induce OSA. Any chronic inflammatory process may cause sarcoma formation, and OSA is one of the histological tumour types reported with vaccine-associated sarcomas in cats. OSAs have been concurrently seen in dogs with bone infarcts, but it is not clear whether there is any causal relationship.

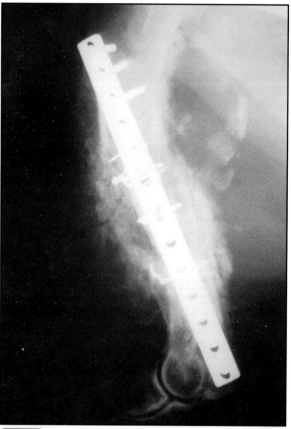

13.3 Lateral radiograph of a humeral osteosarcoma arising in association with longstanding internal fixation for fracture repair.

There has recently been a flurry of experimental work and clinical data to support molecular genetic models by which OSA may develop. Figure 13.4 lists some of the molecular and genetic factors that have been implicated in the formation or progression of OSA. As further research outlines the details, these features may prove useful in augmenting the present clinical techniques in diagnosis, prognosis and treatment options. Many similar approaches are being investigated and, in limited incidences, being applied for other cancer diseases in people and animals.

Factor	Comments	Prognostic relevance
p53	Mutated and/or over-expressed in several investigations	Expression predictive of outcome (related through MDR1)
IGF-1/IGF-1R	May contribute to the malignant phenotype	
HGF/c-Met	May contribute to the malignant phenotype	
erbB-2/HER-2	Over-expressed in several canine OSA cell lines	
PTEN	Mutated or down-regulated in high percentage of canine OSA cell lines	
sis/PDGF	Over-expressed in some canine cell lines	
Matrix metalloproteinases	Over-expressed in canine OSA cell lines	
Ezrin	A membrane–cytoskeleton linker associated with the metastatic phenotype in canine OSA	Expression predictive of metastasis and survival
COX-2	Expression up-regulated in some canine OSA; prognostic in some investigations, not in others	High expression predictive of poor outcome
Angiogenic factors	VEGF measurable in plasma of dogs with OSA; angiostatin present in urine of dogs with OSA	
Telomerase reverse transcriptase gene	Up-regulated in some canine OSA	

13.4 Molecular and genetic factors associated with OSA in dogs. (Adapted with permission from Dernell *et al.*, 2006)

OSA usually originates from elements within the medullary canal of bones (intraosseous OSA). There are rare forms that originate from the outside surface of bones: periosteal and parosteal (juxtacortical), the behaviour of which is described in Figure 13.1.

OSA is a malignant mesenchymal tumour of primitive bone cells. These cells produce an extracellular matrix of osteoid and the presence of tumour osteoid is the basis for the histological diagnosis differentiating OSA from other sarcomas of bone. The histological pattern may vary between tumours, or even within the same tumour. Small biopsy samples may lead to misdiagnoses such as chondrosarcoma, fibrosarcoma, haemangiosarcoma or simply reactive bone, depending on the section sampled. It is important to obtain histological analysis of the entire tumour following definitive excision to confirm the diagnosis. In addition, alkaline phosphatase staining has been shown to aid in differentiating OSA pathologically from other connective tissue tumours.

There are many histological subclassifications of OSA based on the type and amount of matrix and characteristics of the cells, including osteoblastic, chondroblastic, fibroblastic, poorly differentiated and telangiectatic OSA (a vascular subtype). In dogs, it has not been well established that there is a difference in the biological behaviour of the different histological subclassifications; however, histological grade, based on microscopic features, may be predictive for systemic behaviour (metastasis). Newer techniques designed to recognize molecular or genetic alterations are being evaluated to determine their potential use in predicting behaviour of OSA.

OSA has very aggressive local effects and causes lysis and/or production of bone (see Figure 13.5). The local disease is usually attended by soft tissue swelling. Pathological fracture of the affected bone can occur. Rarely, OSA will cross a joint surface. Although <15% of dogs have radiographically detectable pulmonary or osseous metastasis at presentation, approximately 90% will die with metastatic disease, usually to the lungs, within 1 year when amputation is the only treatment. Metastasis via the haematogenous route is most common, but on rare occasions extension to regional lymph nodes may occur. Although the lung is the most commonly reported site for metastasis, tumour spread to bones or other soft tissue sites occurs with some frequency. An increase in the incidence of bone metastasis following systemic chemotherapy has been documented in humans and is suspected in dogs. Some differences in metastatic behaviour have been observed based on the anatomical location of the primary OSA site. For example, mandibular OSA, and to a degree other calvarium locations, may have a less aggressive metastatic behaviour, but contradictory evidence exists (Straw *et al.*, 1992; Dickerson *et al.*, 2001).

History and clinical signs

Dogs with OSA of appendicular sites generally present with lameness or swelling (or both) at the primary site. Sometimes there is a history of mild trauma just prior to the onset of lameness and this can often lead to misdiagnosis as another orthopaedic injury. The pain is likely due to microfractures or disruption of the periosteum induced by osteolysis of cortical bone with tumour extension from the medullary canal. There may be a noticeable response to rest and analgesics, but recurrence of signs should prompt further evaluation. As the lameness worsens, a moderately firm to soft and variably painful swelling may arise at the primary site. Dogs may present with acute severe lameness associated with pathological fractures, though pathological fractures account for <3% of all fractures seen (Boulay *et al.*, 1987).

The signs associated with axial skeletal OSA are site-dependent, in general presenting with swelling and pain associated with function of the affected site. Dogs rarely have respiratory signs as the first clinical evidence of pulmonary metastasis; rather, their first signs are usually vague. With radiographically detectable pulmonary metastasis dogs may remain asymptomatic for many months, but most dogs develop decreased appetites and non-specific signs such as malaise within 1 month. Hypertrophic osteopathy may develop in dogs with pulmonary metastasis.

Clinical approach

In general, the basic approach to dogs with suspected OSA is a physical examination, radiography, biopsy and discussion of treatment options. In addition, due consideration should be given to obtaining blood work, thoracic radiography, abdominal ultrasonography and urinalysis, depending on the suspected health status of the patient and the possible or intended treatment.

Radiology: Initial evaluation of the primary site involves interpretation of lateral and craniocaudal radiographs. Special views may be necessary for lesions occurring in sites other than in the appendicular skeleton.

The overall radiographic abnormality of bone varies from mostly bone lysis to almost entirely osteoblastic or osteogenic changes (Figure 13.5). There is often soft tissue extension with an obvious soft tissue swelling, and new bone (tumour bone) may form in these areas in a palisading pattern perpendicular to or radiating from the axis of the cortex ('sun-burst' effect). As tumour invades the cortex, the periosteum is elevated and new bone is laid down by the cambium layer, providing a triangular deposition of dense new bone on the cortex at the periphery of the lesion. This periosteal new bone has been called 'Codman's triangle' but this is not pathognomonic for OSA. Osteosarcoma does not directly cross articular cartilage, but the tumours may extend into periarticular soft tissues, and adjacent bones are at risk by extension. Other radiographic changes that can attend OSA are loss of the fine trabecular pattern in the metaphysis, a vague transition zone at the periphery of the medullary extent of the lesion (rather than a sharp sclerotic margin) or areas of fine punctate lysis. Any one or combinations of these changes may be seen, depending on the size, histological subtype, location and duration of the lesion.

A presumptive diagnosis of OSA can be made based on signalment, history, physical examination and radiographic findings. Differential diagnoses of lytic, proliferative or mixed-pattern aggressive bone lesions identified on radiographs include: other primary bone tumours; metastatic bone cancer; multiple myeloma or lymphoma of bone; systemic mycosis with bony localization; and bacterial osteomyelitis. In cases where the travel or clinical history might support the possibility of osteomyelitis, a biopsy with submission for histology and culture may be warranted.

Cytology: Although cytology has not historically been thought to be definitive for diagnosis, recent evidence would support the use of fine-needle aspirate cytology in the preoperative diagnosis of OSA. Even if it is not diagnostic, it may support the tentative diagnosis and, combined with clinical features and radiographic appearance, there may be enough confidence in the diagnosis to move forward with discussion of treatment options.

Slight differences exist in the technique of obtaining samples as well as the interpretation of results. Since the presence of tumour osteoid is the hallmark feature of a definitive diagnosis, samples obtained using larger-gauge needles and true (negative suction) aspiration are often more successful than those obtained with smaller-bore needles, with or without aspiration. Because bone lesions are often more painful than soft tissue masses and as larger-bore needles are more often used, the use of systemic analgesics is indicated for patient comfort and to assure adequate sampling.

Specific cytological criteria in support of a definitive diagnosis have been described (Reinhardt *et al.*, 2005). In the majority of cases, the cytological diagnosis, if made, will be sarcoma, suggestive of OSA. This

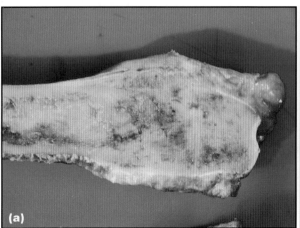
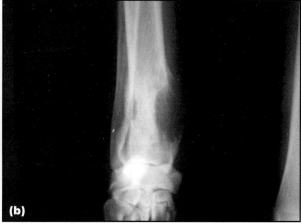

13.5 **(a)** Longitudinally split specimen of distal radial OSA in a dog, showing cortical destruction, soft tissue and osteoid neoplastic components. **(b)** Dorsopalmar radiograph of a similar lesion. Radiographic features include: Codman's triangle; cortical lysis; loss of trabecular pattern in the metaphases; and tumour bone extension into the soft tissues in a 'sunburst' pattern

diagnosis with supporting clinical and radiographic evidence may be considered definitive, depending on the individual case. If further confirmation is required, additional staining, such as with bone alkaline phosphatase, may increase the specificity of the results. Negative cytological results do not necessarily indicate that OSA is not present.

Tissue biopsy: If the clinical and radiographic features are typical for OSA, especially when there is little possibility of fungal or bacterial infection, and if the client is willing for treatment to be based on the presumptive diagnosis, confirmation of histological diagnosis following surgical treatment of local disease (amputation or limb sparing) can be considered. If histological confirmation is needed prior to treatment intervention, a tissue biopsy is indicated.

Bone biopsy may be performed as an open incisional, closed needle or trephine biopsy. The advantage of the open techniques is that a large sample of tissue is procured, which presumably improves the likelihood of establishing an accurate histological diagnosis. This advantage may be outweighed by the disadvantages of an operative procedure and risk of postsurgical complications, including pathological fracture. This underscores some of the advantages of a closed biopsy using a Jamshidi or similar type of bone marrow biopsy needle. Needle biopsy has an accuracy rate of 91.9% for detecting tumour versus other disorders and an 82.3% accuracy rate for diagnosis of specific tumour subtype (Powers *et al.*, 1988).

For bone biopsy (Figure 13.6), the centre of the radiographic lesion is chosen for sampling. Biopsy at the lesion periphery will often result in sampling the reactive bone surrounding the tumour growth. If there is a possibility of limb sparing, additional considerations exist (see later).

Material for culture and cytology may be taken from the samples prior to fixation. Generally, half of each sample is put in for culture and half for histology. It is crucial to the success of a limb-sparing surgery that the biopsy procedure is planned and performed carefully with close attention to asepsis, haemostasis and wound closure. The skin incision for the biopsy must be small and placed so that it can be completely excised with the tumour at limb sparing without compromising the procedure. Fluoroscopy or advanced imaging (computed tomography) can assist in obtaining needle-core biopsy samples of suspected bone lesions, especially for axial sites.

Staging and patient assessment: Examination for evidence of apparent spread of OSA is essential, since the presence of detectable metastases is the single most important prognostic indicator. Regional lymph nodes should be palpated and fine-needle cytology performed on any enlarged node.

Although some controversy exists, it is still considered important by most oncologists to have three radiographic views of the thorax, including both right and left lateral views. Pulmonary metastases from OSA are generally of a soft tissue density and cannot

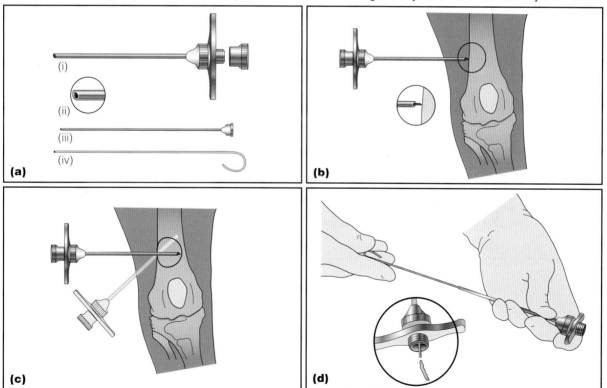

13.6 **(a)** The Jamshidi bone biopsy needle: (i) cannula and screw-on cap; (ii) tapered point; (iii) pointed stylet to advance cannula through soft tissues; and (iv) probe to expel specimen from cannula. **(b)** With the stylet locked in place, the cannula is advanced through the soft tissue until bone is reached. The inset is a close-up view showing stylet against bone cortex. **(c)** The stylet is removed and the bone cortex penetrated with the cannula. The cannula is withdrawn and the procedure repeated with redirection of the instrument to obtain multiple core samples. **(d)** The probe is then inserted retrograde into the tip of the cannula to expel the specimen through the base (inset). (Reproduced from *BSAVA Guide to Procedures in Small Animal Practice*)

be detected radiographically until the nodules are 6–8 mm in diameter (Figure 13.7). It is relatively rare (<10% of dogs) to detect pulmonary metastatic disease at the time of diagnosis but, to date, treatment recommendations and prognoses are based on the results of plain radiographs. Computed tomography (CT) may increase the number of dogs detected with lung lesions at presentation but is not widely used in veterinary patients, due to availability and cost constraints. In addition, the sensitivity of CT may result in a number of false-positive results.

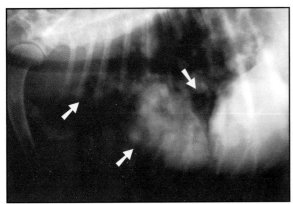

13.7 Lateral thoracic radiograph showing multiple soft-tissue dense metastatic osteosarcoma lesions.

Sites of bone metastasis may be detected by a careful orthopaedic examination, bone survey radiographs or nuclear scintigraphy (Figure 13.8). Due to the low incidence of scintigraphic lesions in most cases of OSA, the usefulness of nuclear scintigraphy (bone scan) for clinical staging of dogs with OSA is somewhat controversial. In one study of 70 patients, scintigraphy was not successful in detecting metastatic or synchronous lesions (Lamb *et al.*, 1990). Another study found secondary sites considered highly suspect of bony metastasis in 7.8% of (399) cases; however, most suspected lesions were not subjected to histological confirmation (Jankowski *et al.*, 2001). Scintigraphy can also be used to evaluate the degree of bone involvement from a primary bone tumour, with scintigraphy overestimating the length of OSA disease in limb-spare patients by 30%, allowing for adequate required margin definition (Leibman *et al.*, 2001).

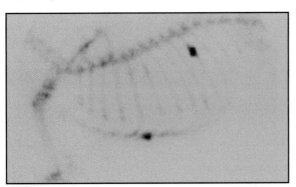

13.8 Scintigraphic view of an osteosarcoma patient following technetium[99M] hydroxymethylene diphosphonate injection. Increased uptake is noted in the sternum and 10th rib, suggestive of bone metastases.

CT or magnetic resonance imaging (MRI) can also be used to stage local disease, especially for axial tumour sites or for planning limb-sparing resection margins. In one study, MRI was more accurate than plain radiographs or CT in predicting length of tumour involvement for appendicular canine OSA (Wallack *et al.*, 2002).

The patient's overall health status requires careful assessment. Advancing years do not preclude treatment, but prolonged anaesthesia and chemotherapy may not be tolerated in dogs with organ compromise. Particular attention to the cardiovascular system is important. Coexisting cardiomyopathy or any degree of heart failure may lead to serious complications, particularly during fluid diuresis, anaesthesia or administration of certain chemotherapy agents.

Management
Treatment options for appendicular OSA and the predicted outcome are listed in Figure 13.9. Occult metastatic disease is present in approximately 90% of dogs at presentation and median survival is only 3–4 months if amputation is the only treatment; therefore, some form of systemic therapy is necessary if survival is to be improved. With no treatment at all, the condition becomes very painful because of extensive destruction of bone and surrounding tissue by primary tumours, and most owners elect for euthanasia for their pets soon after diagnosis if no treatment is given.

Surgery
Surgical options for primary bone tumours at different anatomical sites are set out in Figure 13.10.

Amputation of the affected limb is the standard treatment for canine appendicular OSA. Even large- and giant-breed dogs can function well after limb amputation and most owners are pleased with their pets' mobility and quality of life after surgery. Pre-existing degenerative joint disease at the level found in most older large-breed dogs is rarely a contraindication for amputation. Most dogs will readily compensate; although the osteoarthritis may progress more rapidly in the three-legged dog, this rarely results in a clinical problem. Severe pre-existing orthopaedic or neurological conditions may cause poor results in some cases, and careful preoperative examination is important.

It is generally recommended to perform a complete forequarter amputation for forelimb lesions and a coxofemoral disarticulation amputation for hindleg lesions. This level of amputation assures complete local disease removal and also results in a more cosmetic and functional outcome; and the more aggressive amputations reduce the weight to be carried by the animal. For proximal femoral lesions, a complete amputation and *en bloc* acetabulectomy is recommended to obtain proximal soft tissue margins.

Surgery alone must be considered palliative for OSA, but a study demonstrated significant improvement in survival times for dogs undergoing amputation in comparison with dogs undergoing no treatment (Zachos *et al.*, 1999), possibly due to the pain-alleviating nature of surgery.

Treatment option	Methods	Median survival	Mode of failure	Approximate cost (based on survival times)	Comments
Pain management	NSAIDs Narcotics 'Local' analgesics	2–4 months	Leg pain, lameness, pathological fracture	$100–$200	Often used in conjunction with other treatments
Palliative radiation	Megavoltage photons Strontium or samarium	2–6 months	Leg pain, lameness, pathological fracture Metastasis (lung) late	$600–$800	Addition of (platinum) chemotherapy improves response
Surgery alone	Amputation Limb sparing	3–6 months	Lung metastases	$1500 $3500–$5000	Potential complications of limb sparing make this option questionable without adjuvant therapy
Radiation and chemotherapy	Fractionated megavoltage with platinum chemotherapy	6–12 months (estimate)	Lung metastases	$4000–$8000 (cost dependent on chemotherapy regimen)	Data (immature) from one institution
Amputation and chemotherapy	Cisplatin, carboplatin, doxorubicin or combinations	10–14 months	Lung or bone metastases	$2500–$5000 (cost dependent on chemotherapy regimen)	Limb sparing may be an option in selected cases
Limb sparing and chemotherapy	Cisplatin, carboplatin, doxorubicin or combinations	12–16 months	Lung or bone metastases	$5000–$10,000 (cost dependent on chemotherapy regimen)	Survival improved in dogs with postoperative infection of allografts (Lascelles *et al.*, 2005)

13.9 Treatment options and predicted outcome for canine appendicular osteosarcoma. Approximate cost based on The Colorado State University Veterinary Teaching Hospital in 2002.

Site	Treatment options	Comments
Humerus, femur, tibia	Amputation Limb sparing in limited cases	Generally high complication rate for limb sparing. Diaphyseal locations amenable to intercalary allografts. Total hip sparing possible for proximal femoral lesions. Intraoperative extracorporal radiation technique may apply
Radius	Amputation Limb sparing (allograft; endosteal prosthesis; intercalary bone graft; ulnar transposition; bone transport osteogenesis; pasteurized autograft; intraoperative extracorporal radiation therapy)	Can combine radius/ulna resection (graft radius only)
Ulna	Amputation Ulnectomy	Often does not require allograft reconstruction
Scapula	Amputation Scapulectomy	Proximal lesions best. Complete scapulectomy described
Pelvis	Pelvectomy with or without amputation	Lateral portion of sacrum can be excised. May include body wall
Metacarpus/ metatarsus	Amputation Local resection	Limb-sparing function dependent on bone(s) involved
Mandible	Mandibulectomy	Often requires total hemimandibulectomy. Bilaterally limited to 4th premolar
Maxilla/orbit	Maxillectomy Orbitectomy	Limited by midline palate or cranial vault invasion. Combined approach may assist exposure
Calvarium	Resection ± radiation	Resection dependent on venous sinus involvement
Vertebrae	Decompression (palliative) ± radiation/chemotherapy	Vertebrectomy techniques not well developed. Limited local disease control
Rib	Rib resection	Requires removal of additional cranial and caudal rib

13.10 Surgical treatment options for OSA by site. (Adapted with permission from Dernell *et al.*, 2006)

Limb sparing

In some instances, limb sparing (limb salvage) may be considered and may be preferred to amputation for functional or cosmetic reasons. Examples would include extremely large or obese dogs or those with concurrent (severe) orthopaedic or neurological disease. To date, the majority of limb-sparing procedures have been performed because of owner reluctance to amputate.

Limb-sparing surgery aims to provide a functional pain-free limb for the patient after removal of the local disease. The bone or joint removed is most often replaced by an allograft, but newer techniques are being investigated. Function following limb sparing has been good in most patients. There is no significant difference in survival rates for dogs treated with amputation and cisplatin compared with dogs treated with limb sparing and cisplatin (Figure 13.11).

Case selection: Although limb sparing does not compromise patient survival when compared with amputation, the complication rate is high. Tumour recurrence, deep infections and other problems that are rare after amputation are not uncommon after limb-sparing operations. The cost and owner commitment for limb sparing is large when compared with amputation and these factors can multiply exponentially if complications occur. For these reasons, limb sparing cannot be considered as the treatment of choice for local disease control in most cases of appendicular bone tumours. Owners must be thoroughly informed of all factors involved with limb sparing before that commitment is made.

If biopsy is performed, planning the biopsy technique with specific attention to the site is essential to avoid compromise of limb sparing (see also section on biopsy, above). Both the skin incision and biopsy tract must be removed at the definitive limb sparing to avoid compromise of the resection with potential seeding of the tissues involved in the biopsy. Care must be taken to avoid contacting the ulna when sampling the radius (or to avoid the radius when sampling the ulna), to prevent iatrogenic tumour seeding. Discussion of biopsy technique with the surgeon or centre performing the limb-sparing surgery may be warranted.

Experience has assisted in case selection of limb-sparing candidates with a higher likelihood of short- and long-term success. Dogs with tumour confined to one site, with <50% of the length of the bone radiographically affected, are potential candidates. Length involvement of >50% makes implant fixation to the remaining host bone more difficult, potentially increasing the chance of orthopaedic failure.

A small to moderate soft tissue component is preferred when considering limb sparing. Tumour resection is less successful in cases presenting with large soft tissue components, due to the increased chance of tumour seeding of the operative site. Preoperative down-staging, using combinations of chemotherapy and radiation, can be considered in select patients.

Optimal outcome after traditional limb sparing of metaphyseal lesions has been limited to distal radial and ulnar sites (Figure 13.12). Limb sparing of proximal humeral and distal tibial sites has resulted in poor function and increased complications, primarily due to the need for arthrodesis of high-motion joints. Since functional outcome for amputees is generally good, with a low complication rate, this is presently recommended (with exceptions) for tumour sites other than distal radius or ulna. Limb sparing at other sites may become applicable as the technology for total joint replacement improves. Proximal femoral sites have been treated with resection followed by proximal femoral allograft placement and total hip arthroplasty (Figure 13.13).

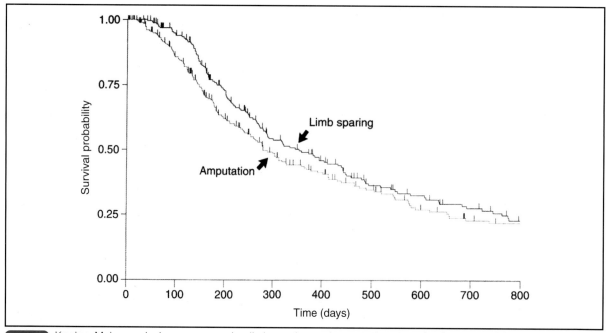

13.11 Kaplan–Meier survival curve comparing limb-sparing and amputation surgeries for canine OSA, followed by chemotherapy. No significant difference is evident in survival between the two surgeries. (Reprinted with permission from Straw and Withrow, 1992)

Site of tumour	No. of cases
Distal radius	297
Proximal humerus	27
Ulna	46
Femur	6
Tibia	15
Metacarpus	7
Scapula	22
Carpus	1

13.12 Limb-sparing treatments at Colorado State University from 1975 to 2002. (Adapted with permission from Dernell, 2002)

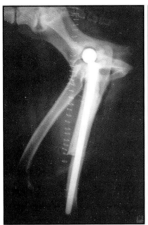
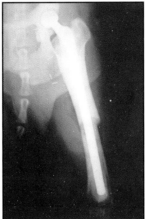

13.13 Lateral and craniocaudal radiographic views following limb sparing for a proximal femoral OSA resected with allograft fixation and total hip replacement.

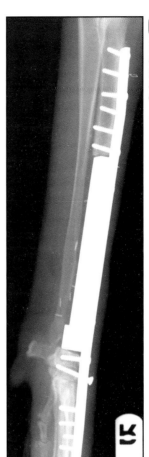

13.14 Lateral radiographic view after metal implant placement and carpal arthrodesis for a distal radial osteosarcoma in a dog.

Limb-sparing techniques for distal radial OSA: The following are the current options for limb-sparing techniques (following tumour resection) for the distal radial site.

- **Bone allograft replacement** is the traditional method of limb sparing in dogs. Following a marginal resection of the tumour bone, a bone allograft (either banked from previous harvest or purchased from a bank) is fitted to the defect and secured using a bone plate and including arthrodesis of the adjacent joint. This technique has been applied to numerous tumour locations, with the distal radius being the most common and the site resulting in the best outcome (LaRue *et al.*, 1986).
- **Metal implant** utilizes a commercially available metal implant to replace the bone defect with composite stabilization similar to that of the allograft technique. The primary advantage is that this technique avoids the need for allograft procurement (and/or storage). The primary disadvantage is the lack of autogenous repair and replacement and the permanent reliance on the (metal) implants for weight bearing (Figure 13.14) (Liptak *et al.*, 2004).

- **Autogenous replacement** involves replacement of the resected bone specimen after either heat (autoclave) sterilization or high-dose radiation sterilization of the tumour tissue. Only a few reports exist of this approach, the primary complication being orthopaedic failure secondary to collapse of the tumour bone implant (Morello *et al.*, 2003).
- **Vascularized ulnar transposition** involves the rotation of a vascularized portion of the ipsilateral ulna into the (radial) defect. The primary advantage of this technique is the rapid repair and remodelling of the vascularized bone. The primary disadvantage is the smaller implant size with increased risk of postoperative failure (Séguin *et al.*, 2003).
- **Bone transport osteogenesis** involves the application of distraction osteogenesis to fill the defect created by the resection. The primary advantage of the technique is the autogenous nature of the replacement bone. The primary disadvantage is the long-term application of external skeletal fixation devices (Ehrhart *et al.*, 2002).
- **Intraoperative extracorporal radiation** involves high-dose radiation of the bone *in situ*, which sterilizes the tumour while sparing joint tissues and subsequent function (the primary advantage). This technique is most applicable for high-motion joints and the primary complication is orthopaedic failure following implant collapse (Figure 13.15) (Liptak *et al.*, 2004).

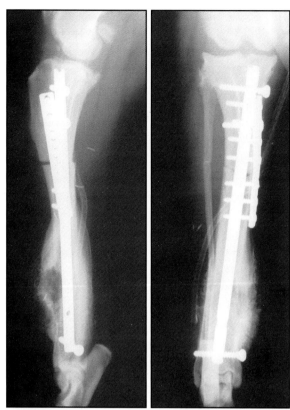

13.15 Postoperative lateral and craniocaudal radiographs after limb-sparing and joint-sparing surgery with intraoperative radiation for a distal tibial osteosarcoma in a dog. (Reprinted from Dernell, 2002, with permission of WB Saunders, Philadelphia)

Other limb-sparing sites: For distal **ulnar** sites, an ulnectomy is generally performed without allograft replacement. Salvage of the styloid process is recommended, if possible, with fixation of the remaining styloid to the distal radius. If the styloid process is removed, reconstruction of the lateral joint should be attempted. More proximal tumours are more difficult, due to the close association of the two bones at the level of the interosseous ligament, and amputation is generally recommended. Return to normal function after ulnectomy is generally rapid and complete within 2–4 weeks.

Techniques for limb sparing in dogs with **humeral** and **tibial** lesions have been described, but a high failure rate precludes recommendation to consider salvage of these sites, unless they occur in the diaphysis. Newer techniques for limb sparing, involving intraoperative radiation of the tumour bone, are being evaluated with an emphasis on maintaining joint function. Although these techniques show promise, evaluation is preliminary. Owners who desire limb-sparing options for sites other than distal radius or ulna can be considered on a case-by-case basis. Discussion with, or referral to, a centre performing limb-sparing procedures is recommended in these circumstances. The author has experience with two cases of limb salvage involving proximal femoral resection, allograft replacement and total hip replacement (see Figure 13.13).

Scapular lesions (Figure 13.16) can be treated with amputation or with partial or complete scapul-

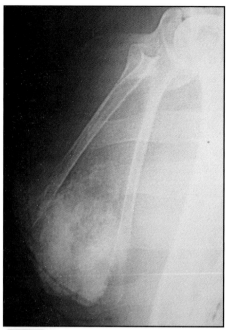

13.16 Preoperative radiograph of OSA of the proximal scapula.

ectomy. Contraindications to scapulectomy include disease that extends beyond the intrinsic musculature of the scapula or distal to the scapulohumeral joint. Reconstruction involves reattachment of dorsal muscles to ventral muscles or muscle reattachment to the remaining scapular bone or proximal humerus. Function is generally good after postoperative rehabilitation, though a mechanical limp often persists due to increased dorsal motion of the limb in reference to the body wall. Physiotherapy is important after scapulectomy to maintain muscle mass and to facilitate fibrous tissue formation, limb support and a rapid return to function.

Pelvic lesions usually require pelvectomy with hindlimb amputation, but in certain locations, and with small low-grade lesions, internal pelvectomy and limb sparing can be considered. Obtaining wide margins for aggressive malignancies often necessitates amputation with pelvectomy.

Metatarsal and **metacarpal** locations can be treated with local resections or amputation. Proximally located lesions are more difficult to resect completely, due to the proximity of adjacent bones. Experience at Colorado State University would support removal of a single bone or the central two bones in most dogs with good functional outcome. In small dogs, removal of the medial or lateral two bones can result in normal function. Resection to this extent has not been attempted in larger dogs.

Postsurgical patient follow-up therapy: The short-term survival with surgery alone supports the need for follow-up systemic therapy (see below). Overall, limb function has been satisfactory, with approximately 80% of dogs experiencing good to excellent limb function.

Immediate postoperative recommendations include frequent bandage changes and continuation of prophylactic antibiotics until systemic adjuvant chemotherapy is completed. Recommended follow-up includes leg and chest radiographs at 3-month intervals to evaluate for healing, local tumour recurrence and infection as well as distant metastasis.

The major complications related to surgery are recurrent local disease and infection. The incidence of local recurrence ranges from 20% to 30%. Local tumour recurrence can be difficult to differentiate from infection radiographically or clinically and so cytological or histological confirmation is recommended. Local disease control can be improved by pretreatment down-staging (discussed above). When a prolonged-release form of cisplatin is implanted at the time of tumour removal the incidence of local recurrence drops to 10%. Some dogs can have their locally recurrent disease resected en bloc and remain disease-free for an extended period, but recurrence generally warrants amputation for disease control.

In one study, 40% of dogs developed infections involving the allograft bone placement for limb sparing. Systemic antibiotics control the majority of infections with or without local antibiotic (antibiotic-impregnated PMMA beads) implantation. However, amputation may be required in a small number of dogs with uncontrolled infections.

An unexpected finding has been that dogs with allograft infections experience a statistically significant prolongation of overall survival times compared with dogs with limb sparing without infected allografts (Lascelles et al., 2009). The reason for this is unclear but could be related to activation of immune effector cells and a response to cytokines, such as interleukins or tumour necrosis factor, elaborated in the face of chronic bacterial infection.

Additional complications following limb sparing include implant failure, such as plate fracture or screw pullout. These rare occurrences are dealt with on a case-by-case basis.

Surgical approach at other sites: Mandibulectomy and maxillectomy are appropriate surgeries for bone tumour primaries of oral sites. Tumours of periorbital sites can be removed by orbitectomy. Rib tumours can be removed by thoracic wall resection and reconstruction.

Vertebral OSA sites are the most difficult with respect to adequate treatment of local disease. Techniques of complete vertebrectomy are not well established in veterinary medicine, and surgery is often an attempt to decompress dogs with neurological deficits and to obtain a diagnosis. Present recommendations are to perform surgery in cases that require decompression (with or without stabilization) and institute radiation therapy and chemotherapy.

Adjuvant treatment

Immunotherapy: Liposome/MTP-PE (LMTP-PE), a synthetic analogue of a fragment of *Mycobacterium* cell wall, has been shown to activate macrophages to destroy malignant cells. It has been studied in dogs and positive effects on prolonging survival were found.

Molecular targeted therapy: A combination of a growth hormone (GH) inhibitor (to lower insulin-like growth factor-1) in combination with carboplatin in OSA dogs following amputation has shown that lower IGF-1 has minimal enhancement of survival time (Khanna et al., 2002).

A number of reports have evaluated the potential therapeutic effects of bisphosphonates for canine OSA *in vitro* and *in vivo*. Both cytotoxic and cytostatic effects were seen in canine OSA cell lines exposed to pamidronate, alendronate and zoledronate *in vitro* in a dose-dependent manner (Poirier et al., 2003; Farese et al., 2004; Ashton et al., 2005). Additionally, surrogate biological activity was shown *in vivo* following pamidronate administration in dogs with gross primary OSA as assessed by reduction in urinary N-telopeptide excretion and enhanced bone mineral density (dual-energy X-ray absorptiometry) (Fan et al., 2005). Whether the *in vitro* and surrogate *in vivo* effects translate into survival advantages in dogs with OSA awaits investigation with controlled clinical trials.

In a prospective randomized clinical trial using dogs with naturally occurring appendicular OSA, the therapeutic potential of dexniguldipine, an inhibitor of protein-kinase-C (a potent stimulator of tumour cell proliferation), was evaluated. Dogs treated with dexniguldipine or cisplatin had longer median remission duration and survival time than untreated dogs, but dexniguldipine-treated dogs had a shorter survival time than cisplatin-treated dogs (Hahn et al., 1997). The combination of dexniguldipine and chemotherapy has not been investigated in dogs.

Chemotherapy: Figure 13.17 lists commonly reported adjuvant chemotherapy protocols and outcome for dogs following amputation for OSA (see Chapter 9 for more detailed discussions).

Cisplatin has been demonstrated to improve survival in dogs with OSA after amputation. There does not appear to be a significant influence of the timing of cisplatin chemotherapy (or with other chemotherapeutics) in reference to beginning preoperatively, immediately postoperatively or after a delay of up to 14 days postoperatively. It seems reasonable, however, to recommend the earliest possible administration of chemotherapy, which is usually at the time of amputation.

The recommended dose for cisplatin is 70 mg/m^2 body surface area. Saline diuresis helps to prevent nephrotoxicity, which is dose-limiting. Most studies involve the targeted administration of four doses of cisplatin; the administration of more than four doses appears to increase the incidence of (renal) toxicity.

Carboplatin is a second-generation platinum compound that is less nephrotoxic than cisplatin and can be given without diuresis with apparently similar anti-tumour effects as cisplatin. One multi-institutional study has supported its efficacy against canine OSA. More evaluations are ongoing. The drug can be given at amputation and in subsequent 21-day cycles provided that peripheral blood counts and renal function remain adequate. The dose recommended for use in dogs is 300 mg/m^2 administered every 3 weeks, with a target of four treatments, but the maximum tolerated cumulative dose has not been described.

Drug and no. of dogs in study	Dosage/regimen	Disease-free range	Survival range	Comments	References
Cisplatin (n = 26)	70 mg/m² i.v. on two occasions, every 21 days	Median 177–226 days	At 1 year: 38–43% At 2 years: 16–18% Median 262–282 days	No significant difference between survival data for dogs given cisplatin before amputation compared with those treated after amputation	Straw et al., 1991
Cisplatin (n = 22; some dogs treated with limb sparing)	60 mg/m² i.v. on 1 to 6 occasions, every 21 days	Not reported	At 1 year: 45.5% At 2 years: 20.9% Median 325 days	Apparent increase in treatment failures due to bone metastases	Berg et al., 1992
Cisplatin (n = 11)	40–50 mg/m² i.v. on 2 to 6 occasions, every 28 days	Median 165 days	Median 300 days		Shapiro et al., 1988
Cisplatin (n = 15)	50 mg/m² i.v. on 2 occasions, 2 and 7 weeks after amputation	Not reported	At 1 year: 30% Median 290 days		Thompson and Fugent, 1992
Cisplatin (n = 16)	50 mg/m² i.v. on up to 9 occasions, every 28 days	Not reported	At 1 year: 62% Median 413 days	Trend for dogs receiving higher cumulative doses of cisplatin to have longer survival times	Kraegel et al., 1991
Carboplatin (n = 48)	300 mg/m² on 4 occasions, every 21 days	Median 257 days	At 1 year: 35.4% Median 321 days	Maximum tolerated cumulative dose has not been described for dogs	Bergman et al., 1996
Doxorubicin (n = 35)	30 mg/m² on 5 occasions, every 2 weeks	Not reported	At 1 year: 50.5% At 2 years: 9.7% Median 366 days	Percentage necrosis of tumour predicted survival	Berg et al., 1995
Doxorubicin and cisplatin alternating sequentially (n = 19)	Doxorubicin at 30 mg/m² i.v. on day 1 and cisplatin at 60 mg/m² i.v. on day 21, cycle repeated once in 21 days	Median 210 days	At 1 year: 37% Median 300 days	No significant difference found between survival data from this study and from a single-agent cisplatin study	Mauldin et al., 1988
Doxorubicin and cisplatin concurrent (n = 102)	Doxorubicin at 15–20 mg/m² followed in 2 hours by cisplatin at 60 mg/m²	Not reported	At 1 year: 48% At 2 years: 28% Median 345 days	Twenty-two cases of dose reduction. No difference in postoperative versus preoperative chemotherapy	Berg et al., 1997
Doxorubicin and cisplatin concurrent (n = 14)	Cisplatin at 50 mg/m² on day 1 and doxorubicin at 15 mg/m² on day 2	Median 470 days	Median 540 days	Small sample size. Another trial looking at similar protocol with higher cisplatin dosing (60 mg/m²) and doxorubicin (25 mg/m²) was associated with unacceptable toxicity	Chun et al., 2000; DeRegis et al., 2003
Doxorubicin and carboplatin alternating sequentially (n = 32)	Carboplatin at 300 mg/m² on day 1 and doxorubicin at 30 mg/m² on day 21, alternating at 3-week intervals for 3 cycles (6 total treatments)	Median 227 days	At 1 year: 48% At 2 years: 18% Median 320 days	Includes both amputation and limb-salvage therapies for the primary tumour	Kent et al., 2004
Doxorubicin and carboplatin concurrent (n = 24)	Carboplatin at 175 mg/m² on day 1 and doxorubicin at 15 mg/m² on day 2, every 3 weeks for 4 treatments	Median 195 days	Median 235 days	The combination at these dosages was well tolerated in most cases	Bailey et al., 2003
Lobaplatin	35 mg/m² every 3 weeks for 4 treatments	At 1 year: 21.8%	At 1 year: 31.8%	No need for diureses with this platinum analogue	Kirpensteijn et al., 1999
OPLA-Pt (n = 37)	80 mg/m² implanted at time of amputation	Median 256 days	At 1 year: 41.2% Median 278 days	New trials ongoing with injectable polymer containing cisplatin	Withrow et al., 1995

13.17 Commonly used adjuvant chemotherapy agents and survival outcome for dogs with OSA where amputation has been performed. These data reflect single or multiple studies (combined) for the drug(s) listed. Note that few of these protocols include large numbers of dogs and fewer compare treatment protocols in a randomized prospective fashion; therefore evaluations of efficacy between the various protocols are subject to bias and should be compared with caution. (Adapted with permission from Dernell et al., 2006)

Lobaplatin is a new third-generation platinum compound. In an adjuvant study of 28 dogs treated with 35 mg/m² every 3 weeks for four treatments, the drug was well tolerated. However, those patients had a 32% 1-year survival rate – less than that seen in historical sets of dogs treated with carboplatin or cisplatin (Kirpensteijn *et al.*, 1999).

Doxorubicin had a poor response as a single agent in an older report of 16 dogs with OSA. In that study doxorubicin was given intravenously at a dosage of 30 mg/m² every 3 weeks, beginning 3 weeks after surgery. In a more recent study, doxorubicin was given at the same dosage but every 2 weeks for five treatments to 35 dogs with appendicular OSA (Berg *et al.*, 1995). The 1- and 2-year survival rates were 50.5% and 9.7%, respectively. No difference was found between dogs treated prior to or immediately following amputation. Subsequent trials have supported the efficacy data of these later studies.

It would seem reasonable that combinations of cisplatin or carboplatin and doxorubicin – drugs shown to be efficacious alone which work by different cytotoxic mechanisms – could further improve survival times. To date, however, results do not support increased response outcome for combination therapy when compared with single-agent platinum compounds. Reports of recent evaluations of combination protocols alternating cisplatin or carboplatin with doxorubicin are summarized in Figure 13.17.

Radiation

The combination of external beam radiation therapy and limb sparing has been described (Thrall *et al.*, 1990; Withrow *et al.*, 1993). It appears that radiation therapy can cause considerable necrosis of primary OSA in dogs. In this manner, radiation can be used in an effort to downstage the primary tumour to improve the success of local disease control following removal.

At present, the role of radiation therapy used to replace surgery, with or without systemic chemotherapy, is unclear. Currently, radiation therapy in dogs with appendicular OSA is primarily reserved for palliation of bone pain (see later). As a primary therapy, a median survival time of 209 days has been reported in 14 dogs with appendicular OSA treated with fractionated high-dose radiation (median dose of 57 Gy) to their primary tumour and systemic chemotherapy for micrometastasis (Walter *et al.*, 2005). Similar results are seen in people with extremity OSA treated with high-dose radiation with and without surgical stabilization.

Radiation therapy likely plays a role in the treatment of OSA of vertebrae. In a series of 14 dogs with vertebral OSA treated between 1986 and 1995, 12 had surgery to decompress the spinal cord, 7 were treated with OPLA-Pt implanted in a distant intramuscular site and 11 were given intravenous cisplatin. Nine dogs were treated with fractionated external beam radiation therapy. All dogs had surgery, radiation therapy or both, while no dog was treated with chemotherapy alone. Four dogs improved neurologically, four dogs worsened and six dogs remained the same. The median survival of 135 days after treatment was relatively short and local disease recurrence rather than metastasis was the usual cause of death (Dernell *et al.*, 2000).

Stereotactic radiosurgery or intensity modulated radiation therapy: Stereotactic radiosurgery (gamma knife therapy) has been performed as a means of limb-salvage surgery in 11 dogs (Farese *et al.*, 2004). In some cases, carboplatin was used immediately prior to treatment for its radiosensitizing potential in addition to its conventional cytotoxic qualities. Impressively, overall median survival was 363 days in this series, albeit numbers are still small.

Advantages of this technique include the normal tissue-sparing effects that stereotactic radiation potentially provides and the ability to avoid surgery. Disadvantages are that the technique involves equipment that is not typically available to veterinary surgeons.

Intensity modulated radiation therapy (IMRT) is a means of precisely delivering radiation therapy to tumours while conformally avoiding normal tissues. A form of IMRT, Tomotherapy®, utilizes a marriage of a CT scan and a linear accelerator and has been investigated in dogs with OSA and dogs with nasal tumours (Forrest *et al.*, 2004). While such techniques are investigational in dogs at present, they would allow delivery of significant doses of radiation therapy that theoretically could be locally curative while sparing normal structures.

Radioisotopes: The bone-seeking radioisotope samarium-153-ethylenediamine tetramethylene phosphonate ([153]samarium-EDTMP) has been used to treat OSA in dogs and humans. In high doses, samarium has been shown to deliver locally 20 to 200 Gy of radiation to normal bone and OSA tumours, respectively. The efficacy of samarium in canine OSA patients has been reported (Milner *et al.*, 1998; Aas *et al.*, 1999). Studies on the efficacy of samarium for OSA in dogs indicate that tumour doses equivalent to 20 Gy may be deposited in canine OSAs using low to moderate doses of samarium, and the ratio between tumour dose and dose to surrounding tissues is favourable. The treatment provides pain relief in canine patients and in some cases tumour growth delay but is not curative.

Isolated limb perfusion

Isolation of limb circulation and perfusion with chemotherapy has been used in people with sarcomas and melanomas as a sole treatment or to downstage local disease and allow limb sparing. Isolated limb perfusion (ILP) allows delivery of high concentrations of chemotherapy as well as delivery of compounds that are poorly tolerated systemically. Varying degrees of local toxicity are reported, depending on the drugs used. Successful use of ILP in canine OSA has been reported (Van Ginkel *et al.*, 1995). ILP may be a method to facilitate therapeutic drug concentrations in primary tumours for preoperative downstaging prior to limb salvage. Currently investigations are being conducted delivering the radioisotope samarium at high doses using ILP in dogs to assess whether a clinically meaningful percentage necrosis can be achieved prior to primary tumour removal.

Follow-up and prognosis after curative intent therapy

Once surgery and adjuvant therapy are completed, follow-up includes physical examination and thoracic radiographs to assess for metastases, recommended at 3-monthly intervals. Nuclear scintigraphy can be used for screening for suspicious bone lesions, with follow-up radiographs. Clients may consider follow-up academic, but early detection of metastasis (or other, non-tumour disease) can assist treatment effectiveness. In addition, the data gathered on response to treatment protocols are invaluable in improving the overall treatment success of the disease. With radiographically detectable pulmonary metastasis dogs may remain asymptomatic for many months, but most dogs develop decreased appetites and non-specific signs such as malaise within 1 month. Hypertrophic osteopathy may develop in dogs with pulmonary metastasis and may be the cause of the primary presenting complaint.

In a multi-institutional study of 162 dogs with appendicular OSA treated with amputation alone, dogs younger than 5 years of age had worse survival rates than older dogs (Spodnick et al., 1992). Additional studies have related large tumour size and humeral location to poor outcome. The only anatomical site that has an improved outcome is the mandible: dogs with OSA of the mandible treated with mandibulectomy alone had a 1-year survival rate of 71% in one study (Straw et al., 1996). In contrast, maxillary OSA has demonstrated a median survival of 5 months following maxillectomy (Hardy et al., 1967; Schwarz et al., 1991; Wallace et al., 1992). A study evaluating response to treatment for orbital OSA reported long-term survival following complete surgical excision (Hendrix and Gelatt, 2000).

OSA of the canine scapula has been reported to have a poor prognosis when treated with surgery and chemotherapy (Hammer et al., 1995; Trout et al., 1995). Survival of dogs with OSA distal to the antebrachiocarpal or tarsocrural joints was somewhat longer (median of 466 days) than survival of dogs with OSA of more common appendicular sites, but OSA in these sites is aggressive with a high potential for metastasis (Gamblin et al., 1995).

Although vertebral OSA is uncommon, reported cases indicate an aggressive local and systemic behaviour. In 15 dogs treated with a combination of surgery, radiation and chemotherapy, the median survival was 4 months (Dernell et al., 2000).

For OSA originating from flat bones, small dog size and capacity for the lesion to be excised completely were positive prognostic indicators. Extraskeletal (soft tissue) OSA sites also appear to have aggressive systemic behaviour that benefits from adjuvant therapy following surgical resection. Whilst there are differences in disease distribution and prevalence, documentation of improved survival for small dogs with OSA is lacking.

A negative prognosis can also be predicted by a higher tumour grade (Kirpensteijn et al., 2002). Dogs presented with stage III disease (measurable metastases) have a very poor prognosis and dogs with lymph node metastasis had short survivals with a median of only 59 days, compared with 318 days for dogs without nodal spread (Hillers et al., 2005).

In dogs, it has not been well established that there is a difference in the biological behaviour of the different histological subclassifications, but histological grade, based on microscopic features, has been shown to be potentially predictive for systemic behaviour (metastasis) (Kirpensteijn et al., 1999).

Elevated alkaline phosphatase has been associated with a poorer prognosis for dogs with appendicular OSA. A preoperative elevation of either the total (serum) or bone isoenzyme is associated with a shorter disease-free interval and survival. In one study, dogs that had elevated preoperative values that did not return to normal within 40 days following surgical removal of the primary lesion also failed earlier from disease (Ehrhart et al., 1998) (Figure 13.18). A rise in serum alkaline phosphatase after treatment has been shown to predict pulmonary metastatic failure, indicating that it could be used to screen patients for pending metastasis to assist pre-emptive treatment decisions (Dye et al., 2001).

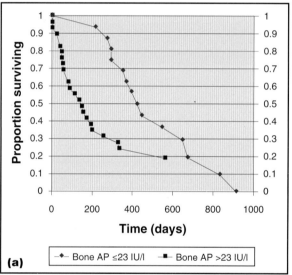

(a)

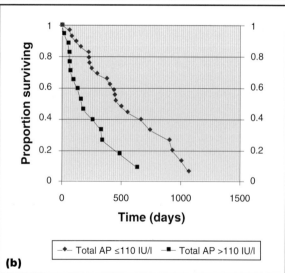

(b)

13.18 (a) Relation of disease-free interval in dogs treated for OSA and preoperative bone alkaline phosphatase levels. (b) Relation of survival outcome of dogs treated for OSA and preoperative serum alkaline phosphatase levels. (Reprinted with permission from Ehrhart et al., 1998)

Metastatic disease and its treatment

The usual cause of death in humans and dogs following amputation as the sole treatment for OSA is diffuse pulmonary metastasis. There is a report of 36 dogs treated with pulmonary metastasectomy for OSA (O'Brien *et al.*, 1993). Based on this study, the criteria established for case selection for pulmonary metastasectomy in order to maximize the probability of long survival periods are:

- Primary tumour in complete remission, preferably for a long relapse-free interval (>300 days)
- One or two nodules visible on plain thoracic radiographs
- Cancer only found in the lung
- Perhaps long doubling time (>30 days) with no new visible lesions within this time.

Metastasectomy may be indicated for dogs with solitary bone metastases and no evidence of cancer elsewhere, but the subsequent disease-free interval is generally short.

Cisplatin, doxorubicin and mitoxantrone chemotherapy appear to be ineffective for the treatment of measurable metastatic OSA in the dog, but may slow the progression of disease (Ogilvie *et al.*, 1993). A number of potential targeted therapies have been established for metastatic OSA, including inhalant Il-2, doxorubicin, paclitaxel and gemcitabine, and a liposome-DNA complex that codes for IL-2 (Khanna *et al.*, 1996, 1997; Micheau *et al.*, 1997; Hershey *et al.*, 1999; Poulaki *et al.*, 2001; Khanna and Vail, 2003; Koshkina and Kleinerman, 2005).

Palliative treatment

An alternative to curative-intent treatment is to treat metastatic bone lesions with palliative radiation. Various protocols have been reported, most using larger fraction sizes (6–10 Gy) with one, two or three treatments over time. Over 70% of dogs respond positively (improvement in clinical evidence of pain and lameness) for 2–4 months. Unfortunately, the lesions usually become symptomatic again within 2–4 months after radiation. Adding additional fractions beyond three (course) fractions has been successful for further temporary pain relief in a few dogs, but the potential for marked acute radiation toxicity is increased. Radiopharmaceuticals (such as strontium and samarium) have also been used to palliate pain from metastatic bone cancer in people. As mentioned above, [153]samarium-EDTMP is a radiopharmaceutical that has been used to treat metastatic and primary bone tumours in dogs (Lattimer *et al.*, 1990). Other therapies to palliate the pain associated with OSA are discussed in Chapter 11.

Other primary bone tumours of dogs

When only small amounts of biopsy tissue are evaluated it can be difficult to distinguish chondroblastic OSA from chondrosarcoma, or fibroblastic OSA from fibrosarcoma, or telangiectatic OSA from haemangiosarcoma. This makes interpretation of older reports difficult in terms of trying to establish the true incidence of the different types of primary bone tumours and it underscores the importance of evaluating the entire excised specimen to validate the preoperative biopsy. This is also true in cases where the initial biopsy might indicate low-grade disease.

Primary bone tumours other than OSA make up 5–10% of bone malignancies in dogs and include chondrosarcomas, haemangiosarcomas, fibrosarcomas, lymphomas and myelomas.

Chondrosarcoma

Chondrosarcoma (CSA) is the second most common primary tumour of bone in humans and dogs, and accounts for approximately 5–10% of all canine primary bone tumours. CSA occurs most commonly in flat bones, with the nasal cavity as the most common site.

CSAs are characterized histologically by anaplastic cartilage cells that elaborate a cartilaginous matrix. The aetiology is generally unknown, though CSA can arise in dogs with pre-existing multiple cartilaginous exostosis. CSA is generally considered to be slow to metastasize. Tumour location rather than histological grade may be prognostic, but histological grade has been found to be important for predicting survival for tumours of the same anatomical site of origin. The reported median survival of dogs with nasal CSA ranges from 210 days to 580 days with radiation therapy, or rhinotomy and radiation therapy, or rhinotomy alone. Metastatic disease is not a feature of nasal CSA in dogs.

The reported median survival for dogs with CSA of ribs varies widely, but appears to be prolonged (up to 1000 days) following curative-intent resection. The median survival for dogs with CSA of long bones was 201 days in one report of seven dogs treated with amputation with or without adjuvant chemotherapy and 540 days in another study of five dogs treated with amputation alone. Death was usually associated with metastatic disease. Response to chemotherapy is not known for canine CSA. Based on the treatment success of nasal CSA, adjuvant radiation therapy can be utilized for incompletely resected lesions, but response data are lacking.

Haemangiosarcoma

Primary haemangiosarcoma (HSA) of bone is rare and probably accounts for <5% of all bone tumours. This disease generally affects middle-aged to older dogs and can occur in dogs of any size. Similar to OSA, it is a highly metastatic tumour and virtually all dogs affected will develop measurable metastatic disease within 6 months of diagnosis without adjuvant therapy. Metastases can be widely spread throughout organs such as lungs, liver, spleen, heart, skeletal muscles, kidney and brain, and also other bones. Dogs can present with multiple lesions, making it difficult to determine the site of primary disease.

Histologically, HSA is composed of highly anaplastic mesenchymal cells which are precursors to vascular endothelium. The cells are arranged in chords separated by a collagenous background and may appear to be forming vascular channels or sinuses. Cellular pleomorphism and numerous mitotic figures are features of this highly malignant disease. There is profound bone lysis and the malignant cells aggressively invade adjacent normal structures. The lesion may be confused with telangiectatic OSA, especially if the diagnosis is based on small tissue samples. Often the dominant radiographic feature is lysis.

If HSA is diagnosed, the dog must be thoroughly staged with thoracic and abdominal films, bone survey radiography or bone scintigraphy and ultrasonographic evaluation, particularly of the heart and abdominal organs. Right atrial HSA may be present without clinical or radiographic signs of pericardial effusion. The prognosis is poor and even dogs with HSA clinically confined to one bony site have a <10% probability of surviving 1 year if the tumour can be completely excised. Cyclophosphamide, vincristine and doxorubicin have been used in combination as an adjuvant protocol and the reported median survival of dogs with non-skeletal HSA is 172 days (Hammer *et al.*, 1991; Ogilvie *et al.*, 1996).

Fibrosarcoma

Primary fibrosarcoma (FSA) of bone is a rare tumour in dogs and probably accounts for <5% of all canine primary bone tumours. The difficulty in distinguishing FSA from fibroblastic OSA histologically renders study of this tumour problematic. For example, in a study of 11 dogs thought to have FSA, the histological diagnosis was changed to OSA in six dogs upon review (Wesselhoeft *et al.*, 1991). Histological characteristics of FSA have been described as interwoven bundles of fibroblasts within a collagen matrix permeating cancellous and cortical bone but not associated with osteoid produced by the tumour cells.

Complete surgical resection of the primary lesion is recommended for dogs with FSA clinically confined to the primary site. This treatment may be curative, but metastatic potential may be variable. Data on the efficacy of adjuvant therapy are lacking due to the rare nature of the disease.

Multilobular osteochondrosarcoma

Multilobular osteochondrosarcoma (MLO) is an uncommon tumour in dogs that generally arises from the skull. These tumours have a characteristic radiographic appearance: generally the borders of the tumour are sharply demarcated, with limited lysis of adjacent bone, and there is a coarse granular mineral density throughout (Figure 13.19).

Histologically these tumours are composed of multiple lobules each centred on a core of cartilaginous or bony matrix that is surrounded by a thin layer of spindle cells. In one report of 39 dogs, slightly fewer than 50% of dogs had local tumour recurrence following resection at a median time of approximately 800 days (Dernell *et al.*, 1998a). A little over half the dogs developed slowly progressive metastases after treatment, with a median time to metastasis of 542 days. The median survival time was also 800 days.

Local tumour excision appears to offer a good opportunity for long-term tumour control, partially predicted by histological grade and the ability to

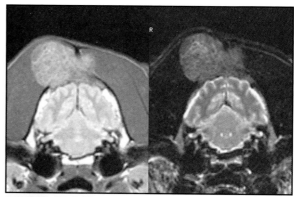

13.19 T2 (left) and T1 (right) MR images of a multilobular osteochondrosarcoma arising from the calvarium in a dog. These tumours have a granular appearance on radiography, often referred to as 'popcorn-ball'.

obtain histologically complete resection. Lesions of the cranium will often invade into the calvarium, displacing brain tissue causing central nervous system signs, but these tumours are rarely invasive into brain. Craniectomy will often result in rapid recovery and has the potential for long-term remission.

The role of chemotherapy and radiation therapy in the management of MLO is not well defined.

Metastatic tumours of bone

Almost any malignant tumour can metastasize to bone via the haematogenous route. The lumbar vertebrae, femur, humerus, rib and pelvis are common sites for primary bone tumour metastasis as well as from the common urogenital malignancies such as prostate, bladder, urethral and mammary cancer. Metastatic lesions in long bones frequently affect the diaphysis, probably because of the proximity to the nutrient foramen. Nuclear scintigraphy is a very sensitive technique to detect the usual multiple sites of bone metastasis.

Primary bone tumours of cats

Incidence and risk

Cancer involving feline bones is rare. An estimate of the incidence of all bone tumours in cats is 4.9 per 100,000 (Dorn *et al.*, 1968). Up to 90% of bone tumours in cats are histologically malignant. In one study, 50 of 90 skeletal OSA cases were appendicular and 40 of 90 were axial (Heldmann *et al.*, 2000).

OSA accounts for 70–80% of all primary malignant bone cancer in cats. The disease differs from that in dogs in that the primary lesions occur more often in hindlimbs in cats and the disease is far less metastatic. OSA generally affects both male and female older cats but the age range of reported cases is large (1–20 years).

Multiple cartilaginous exostosis (MCE) is a disease that occurs after skeletal maturity in cats. This is in contrast to dogs, where exostoses develop before closure of growth plates. Also in contrast to dogs, the lesions seldom affect long bones in cats, are rarely symmetrical and are probably of viral rather than familial origin. There does not appear to be any breed or sex predisposition. Affected cats range in age from 1.3 to 8 years (mean 3.2 years). Virtually all cats with multiple cartilaginous exostosis will test positive for the FeLV virus. This disease has an aggressive natural behaviour.

Pathology and natural behaviour

A histological feature of some feline OSA cases is the presence of multinucleate giant cells, which may be numerous. Reactive and remnant host bone are often present in specimens. Tumours are seen to be invasive, but some surrounding soft tissue may be compressed rather than infiltrated. There is often variation of the histological appearance within the tumour, with some portions having more fibrosarcomatous appearance and others more cartilaginous. Some authors have described subtypes that resemble those seen in dogs, but these features do not appear to confer any prognostic predictive value.

OSA in cats is more often of the juxtacortical (parosteal) type. In a recent large case study, 56 of 146 cases were extraskeletal in origin with the most common site being intrascapular (Heldmann *et al.*, 2000). In this subset, vaccination at the site was considered a predisposing factor. No mention was made of any differences in the pathology of these tumours in comparison with skeletal sites.

History and clinical signs

The most common signs of OSA are deformity and lameness, depending on the location of the lesion. The lesions may appear radiographically similar to OSA in dogs, or can arise from the periosteal surface (juxtacortical OSA). It is rare for cats to have metastatic OSA.

Cats with virally associated multiple cartilaginous exostosis have rapidly progressing conspicuous hard swellings over affected sites, causing pain and loss of function. Common sites for lesion development are the scapula, vertebrae and mandible, but any bone can become affected. Radiographically the lesions are either sessile or pedunculate protuberances from bone surfaces with indistinct borders. There may be a loss of smooth contour with evidence of lysis, particularly if there is malignant transformation.

Diagnostic work-up, therapy and prognosis

Both OSA and MCE may be suspected from the radiographic appearance of the lesions, and MCE from the FeLV status of the cat. Definitive diagnosis is confirmed by histopathological evaluation.

In cats with OSA of a limb where there are no clinically detectable metastatic lesions, amputation alone may be curative. In two studies of 15 cats, the median survival after amputation alone was 24 and 44 months (Turrel and Pool, 1982; Bitetto *et al.*, 1987). The metastatic potential is much less than for the same disease in dogs or humans. Axial sites carry a

poorer prognosis, presumably due to increased difficulty of local resection and control. Axial sites are best treated with combination therapy, and chemotherapy has shown a survival advantage in these cases (Heldmann *et al.*, 2000).

Cats with MCE have a guarded prognosis. Lesions may be removed surgically for palliation, but local recurrences are common or new painful debilitating lesions may occur. No reliably effective treatment is known for this condition in cats.

References

Aas M, Moe L and Gamlem H (1999) Internal radionuclide therapy of primary osteosarcoma in dogs, usi ng 153Sm-ethylene-diamino-tetramethylene-phosphonate (EDTMP). *Clinical Cancer Research* **5**, 3148s–3152s

Ashton JA, Farese JP, Milner RJ, Lee-Ambrose LM and van Gilder JM (2005) Investigation of the effect of pamidronate disodium on the in vitro viability of osteosarcoma cells from dogs. *American Journal of Veterinary Research* **66**, 885–891

Bailey D, Erb H, Williams L, Ruslander D and Hauck M (2003) Carboplatin and doxorubicin combination chemotherapy for the treatment of appendicular osteosarcoma in the dog. *Journal of Veterinary Internal Medicine* **17**, 199–205

Berg J, Gebhard MC and Rand WM (1997) Effect of timing on postoperative chemotherapy on survival of dogs with osteosarcoma. *Cancer* **79**, 1343–1350

Berg J, Weinstein MJ, Schelling SH and Rand WM (1992) Treatment of dogs with osteosarcoma by administration of cisplatin after amputation or limb-sparing surgery: 22 cases (1987–1990). *Journal of the American Veterinary Medical Association* **200**, 2005–2008

Berg J, Weinstein MJ, Springfield DS and Rand WM (1995) Response of osteosarcoma in the dog to surgery and chemotherapy with doxorubicin. *Journal of the American Veterinary Medical Association* **206**, 1555–1560

Bergman PJ, MacEwen EG, Kurzman ID *et al.* (1996) Amputation and carboplatin for treatment of dogs with osteosarcoma: 48 cases (1991–1993). *Journal of Veterinary Internal Medicine* **10**, 76–81

Bitetto WV, Patnaik AK, Schrader SC and Mooney SC (1987) Osteosarcoma in cats: 22 cases (1974–1984). *Journal of the American Veterinary Medical Association* **190**, 91–93

Boulay JP, Wallace LJ and Lipowitz AJ (1987) Pathologic fracture of long bones in the dog. *Journal of the American Animal Hospital Association* **23**, 297–303

Chun R, Kurzman ID, Couto G *et al.* (2000) Cisplatin and doxorubicin combination chemotherapy for the treatment of canine osteosarcoma: a pilot study. *Journal of Veterinary Internal Medicine* **14**, 495–498

Cooley DM, Beranek BC, Schlittler DL *et al.* (2002) Endogenous gonadal hormone exposure and bone sarcoma risk. *Cancer Epidemiology, Biomarkers and Prevention* **11**, 1434–1440

Davis GJ, Kapatkin AS, Craig LE, Heins GS and Wortman JA (2002) Comparison of radiography, computed tomography and magnetic resonance imaging for evaluation of appendicular osteosarcoma in dogs. *Journal of the American Veterinary Medical Association* **220**, 1171–1176

DeRegis CJ, Moore AS, Rand WM and Berg J (2003) Cisplatin and doxorubicin toxicosis in dogs with osteosarcoma. *Journal of Veterinary Internal Medicine* **17**, 668–673

Dernell WS (2002) Limb sparing surgery for dogs with bone neoplasia. In: *Textbook of Small Animal Surgery, 3rd edn*, ed. DM Slatter, pp. 2272–2285. WB Saunders, Philadelphia

Dernell WS, Ehrhart NP, Straw RC and Vail DM (2006) Tumours of the skeletal system. In: *Small Animal Clinical Oncology, 4th edn*, ed. SJ Withrow and DM Vail, pp.540–582. WB Saunders, Philadelphia

Dernell WS, Straw RC, Cooper MF *et al.* (1998a) Multilobular osteochondrosarcoma in 39 dogs: 1979–1993. *Journal of the American Animal Hospital Association* **34**, 11–18

Dernell WS, Van Vechten BJ, Straw RC *et al.* (2000) Outcome following treatment for vertebral tumors in 20 dogs (1986–1995). *Journal of the American Animal Hospital Association* **36**, 245–251

Dernell WS, Withrow SJ, Straw RC *et al.* (1998b) Clinical response to antibiotic impregnated polymethyl methacrylate bead implantation of dogs with severe infections after limb sparing with allograft replacement – 18 cases (1994–1996). *Veterinary Comparative Orthopedics and Traumatology* **11**, 94–99

Dickerson ME, Page RL, LaDue TA *et al.* (2001) Retrospective analysis of axial skeleton osteosarcoma in 22 large breed dogs. *Journal of Veterinary Internal Medicine* **15**, 120–124

Dorn CR, Taylor DON and Schneider R (1968) Survey of animal neoplasms in Alameda and Contra Costa Counties, California. II.

Cancer morbidity in dogs and cats from Alameda County. *Journal of the National Cancer Institute* **40**, 307–318

Dow S, Elmslie R, Kurzman I *et al.* (2005) Phase I study of liposome-DNA complexes encoding the interleukin-2 gene in dogs with osteosarcoma lung metastases. *Human Gene Therapy* **16**, 937–946

Dye TL, Kristal OM, Dernell WS *et al.* (2001) Alkaline phosphatase as a predictor of canine osteosarcoma metastasis. *Proceedings of the Veterinary Cancer Society, 21st Annual Meeting, Baton Rouge, LA*, 75 (abstract)

Ehrhart N, Dernell WS, Hoffmann WE *et al.* (1998) Prognostic importance of alkaline phosphatase activity in serum from dogs with appendicular osteosarcoma: 75 cases (1990–1996). *Journal of the American Veterinary Medical Association* **213**, 1002–1006

Ehrhart N, Eurell JC, Tommasini M *et al.* (2002) The effects of cisplatin on bone transport osteogenesis. *American Journal of Veterinary Research* **63**, 703–711

Fan TM, de Lorimier LP, Charney SC and Hintermeister JG (2005) Evaluation of intravenous pamidronate administration in 33 cancer-bearing dogs with primary or secondary bone involvement. *Journal of Veterinary Internal Medicine* **19**, 74–80

Farese JP, Ashton J, Milner R, Ambrose LL and Van Gilder J (2004) The effect of the bisphosphonate alendronate on viability of canine osteosarcoma cells in vitro. *In Vitro Cellular and Developmental Biology – Animal* **40**, 113–117

Farese JP, Milner R, Thompson MS *et al.* (2004) Stereotactic radiosurgery for treatment of osteosarcomas involving the distal portions of the limbs in dogs. *Journal of the American Veterinary Medical Association* **225**, 1548, 1567–1572

Forrest LJ, Mackie TR, Ruchala K *et al.* (2004) The utility of megavoltage computed tomography images from a helical tomotherapy system for setup verification purposes. *International Journal of Radiation Oncology Biology Physics* **60**, 1639–1644

Gamblin RM, Straw RC, Powers BE *et al.* (1995) Primary osteosarcoma distal to the antebrachiocarpal and tarsocrural joints in nine dogs (1980–1992). *Journal of the American Animal Hospital Association* **31**, 86–91

Hahn KA, Legendre AM and Schuller HM (1997) Amputation and dexniguldipine as treatment for canine appendicular osteosarcoma. *Journal of Cancer Research and Clinical Oncology* **123**, 34–38

Hammer AS, Couto CG, Filppi J, Getzy D and Shank K (1991) Efficacy and toxicity of VAC chemotherapy (vincristine, doxorubicin, and cyclophosphamide) in dogs with hemangiosarcoma. *Journal of Veterinary Internal Medicine* **5**, 160–166

Hammer AS, Weeren FR, Weisbrode SE and Padgett SL (1995) Prognostic factors in dogs with osteosarcomas of the flat or irregular bones. *Journal of the American Animal Hospital Association* **31**, 321–326

Hardy WD, Brodey RS and Riser WH (1967) Osteosarcoma of the canine skull. *Journal of the American Veterinary Radiology Society* **8**, 5–9

Heldmann E, Anderson MA, Sweet D and Wagner-Mann CC (2000) Feline osteosarcoma: 145 cases (1990–1995). *Journal of the American Animal Hospital Association* **36**, 518–521

Hendrix DV and Gelatt KN (2000) Diagnosis, treatment and outcome of orbital neoplasia in dogs: a retrospective study of 44 cases. *Journal of Small Animal Practice* **41**, 105–108

Hershey AE, Kurzman ID, Forrest LJ *et al.* (1999) Inhalation chemotherapy for macroscopic primary or metastatic lung tumors: proof of principle using dogs with spontaneously occurring tumors as a model. *Clinical Cancer Research* **5**, 2653–2659

Heyman SJ, Diefenderfer DL, Goldschmidt MH and Newton CD (1992) Canine axial skeletal osteosarcoma a retrospective study of 116 cases (1986 to 1989). *Veterinary Surgery* **21**, 304–310

Hillers KR, Dernell WS, Lafferty MHI, Withrow SJ and Lana SE (2005) Incidence and prognostic importance of lymph node metastases in dogs with appendicular osteosarcoma: 228 cases (1986–2003). *Journal of American Veterinary Medical Association* **226**, 1364–1367

Jankowski MK, Steyn PF, Lana SE *et al.* (2001) Clinical sensitivity and specificity of nuclear scanning with 99mTc-HDP for osseous metastasis in dogs with osteosarcoma. *Proceedings of the Veterinary Cancer Society, 21st Annual Meeting, Baton Rouge, LA*, 35 (abstract)

Kent MS, Strom A, London CA and Séguin B (2004) Alternating carboplatin and doxorubicin as adjunctive chemotherapy to amputation or limb-sparing surgery in the treatment of appendicular osteosarcoma in dogs. *Journal of Veterinary Internal Medicine* **18**, 540–544

Khanna C, Anderson PM, Hasz DE *et al.* (1997) Interleukin-2 liposome inhalation therapy is safe and effective for dogs with spontaneous osteosarcoma metastases. *Cancer* **79**, 1409–1421

Khanna C, Hasz DE, Klausner JS and Anderson PM (1996) Aerosol delivery of interleukin 2 liposomes is nontoxic and biologically effective: canine studies. *Clinical Cancer Research* **2**, 721–734

Khanna C, Prehn J, Jacob S *et al.* (2002) A randomized controlled trial of octreotide pamoate long-acting release and carboplatin versus carboplatin alone in dogs with naturally occurring osteosarcoma: evaluation of insulin-like growth factor suppression and chemotherapy. *Clinical Cancer Research* **8**, 2406–2412

Khanna C and Vail DM (2003) Targeting the lung: preclinical and comparative evaluation of anticancer aerosols in dogs with naturally occurring cancers. *Current Cancer Drug Targets* **3**, 265–273

Khanna C, Wan X, Bose S *et al.* (2004) The membrane–cytoskeleton linker ezrin is necessary for osteosarcoma metastasis. *Nature Medicine* **10**, 182–186

Kirpensteijn J, Kik M, Rutterman GR and Teske E (2002) Prognostic significance of a new histologic grading system for canine osteosarcoma. *Veterinary Pathology* **39**, 240–246

Kirpensteijn J, Steinheimer D, Park RD *et al.* (1998) Comparison of cemented and non-cemented allografts for limb sparing procedures in dogs with osteosarcoma of the distal radius. *Veterinary Comparative Orthopedics and Traumatology* **11**, 178–184

Kirpensteijn J, Teske E, Klenner TH, Kik M and Rutterman GR (1999) Surgery and loboplatin chemotherapy for treatment of canine appendicular osteosarcoma. *Veterinary Surgery* **28**, 396 (abstract)

Koshkina NV and Kleinerman ES (2005) Aerosol gemcitabine inhibits the growth of primary osteosarcoma and osteosarcoma lung metastases. *International Journal of Cancer* **116**, 458–463

Kraegel SA, Madewell BR and Simonson E (1991) Osteogenic sarcoma and cisplatin chemotherapy in dogs: 16 cases (1986–1989). *Journal of the American Veterinary Medical Association* **199**, 1057–1059

Lamb CR (1987) Bone scintigraphy in small animals. *Journal of the American Veterinary Medical Association* **191**, 1616–1622

Lamb CR, Berg J and Bengston AE (1990) Preoperative measurement of canine primary bone tumors, using radiography and bone scintigraphy. *Journal of the American Veterinary Medical Association* **196**, 1474–1478

LaRue SM, Withrow SJ and Wrigley RH (1986) Radiographic bone surveys in the evaluation of primary bone tumors in dogs. *Journal of the American Veterinary Medical Association* **188**, 514–516

Lascelles BDX, Dernell WS, Correa MT *et al.* (2005) Improved survival associated with postoperative wound infection in dogs treated with limb-salvage surgery for osteosarcoma. *Annals of Surgical Oncology* **12**, 1073-1083

Lattimer JC, Corwin LA, Stapleton J *et al.* (1990) Clinical and clinicopathologic response of canine bone tumor patients to treatment with samarium-153-EDTMP. *Journal of Nuclear Medicine* **31**, 1316–1324

Leibman N, Kuntz CA, Steyn P *et al.* (2001) The measurement of the proximal extent of canine osteosarcoma of the distal radius using radiography, nuclear scintigraphy and histopathology. *Veterinary Surgery* **30**, 240–245

Liptak JM, Dernell WS, Straw RC *et al.* (2004) Proximal radial and distal humeral osteosarcoma in 12 dogs. *Journal of the American Animal Hospital Association* **40**, 461–467

Mauldin GN, Matus RE and Withrow SJ (1988) Canine osteosarcoma treatment by amputation versus amputation and adjuvant chemotherapy using doxorubicin and cisplatin. *Journal of Veterinary Internal Medicine* **2**, 177–180

Micheau O, Solary E, Hammann A, Martin F and Dimanche-Boitrel MT (1997) Sensitization of cancer cells treated with cytotoxic drugs to fas-mediated cytotoxicity. *Journal of the National Cancer Institute* **89**, 783–789

Milner RJ, Dormehl I, Louw WK and Croft S (1998) Targeted radiotherapy with Sm-153-EDTMP in nine cases of canine primary bone tumours. *Journal of the South African Veterinary Association* **69**, 12–17

Morello E, Vasconi E, Martano M, Peirone B and Buracco P (2003) Pasteurized tumoral autograft and adjuvant chemotherapy for the treatment of canine distal radial osteosarcoma: 13 cases. *Veterinary Surgery* **32**, 539–544

Mullins MN, Lana SE, Dernell WS *et al.* (2004) Cyclooxygenase-2 expression in canine appendicular osteosarcomas. *Journal of Veterinary Internal Medicine* **18**, 859–865

O'Brien MG, Straw RC, Withrow SJ *et al.* (1993) Resection of pulmonary metastases in canine osteosarcoma: 36 cases (1983–1992). *Veterinary Surgery* **22**, 105–109

O'Brien MG, Withrow SJ, Straw RC, Powers BE and Kirpensteijn J (1996) Total and partial orbitectomy for the treatment of periorbital tumors in 23 dogs and 6 cats. *Veterinary Surgery* **25**, 471–479

Ogilvie GK, Krawiec DR and Gelberg HB (1988) Evaluation of a short-term saline diuresis protocol for the administration of cisplatin. *American Journal of Veterinary Research* **49**, 1076–1078

Ogilvie GK, Powers BE, Mallinckrodt CH and Withrow SJ (1996) Surgery and doxorubicin in dogs with hemangiosarcoma. *Journal of Veterinary Internal Medicine* **10**, 379–384

Ogilvie GK, Straw RC, Jameson VJ *et al.* (1993) Evaluation of single agent chemotherapy for the treatment of clinically evident osteosarcoma metastasis in dogs (1987–1991). *Journal of the American Veterinary Medical Association* **202**, 304–306

Poirier VJ, Huelsmeyer MK, Kurzman ID, Thamm DH and Vail DM (2003) The bisphosphonates alendronate and zoledronate are inhibitors of canine and human osteosarcoma cell growth *in vitro*. *Veterinary Comparative Oncology* **1**, 207–215

Poulaki V, Mitsiades CS and Mitsiades N (2001) The role of Fas and FasL as mediators of anticancer chemotherapy. *Drug Resistance Update* **4**, 233–242

Powers BE, LaRue SM, Withrow SJ, Straw RC and Richter SL (1988) Jamshidi needle biopsy for diagnosis of bone lesions in small animals. *Journal of the American Veterinary Medical Association* **193**, 205–210

Reinhardt S, Stockhaus C, Teske E, Rudolph R and Brunnberg L (2005) Assessment of cytological criteria for diagnosing osteosarcoma in dogs. *Journal of Small Animal Practice* **46**, 65–70

Schwarz PD, Withrow SJ, Curtis CR, Powers BE and Straw RC (1991) Partial maxillary resection as a treatment for oral cancer in 61 dogs. *Journal of the American Animal Hospital Association* **27**, 617–624

Séguin B, Walsh PJ, Mason DR *et al.* (2003) Use of an ipsilateral vascularized ulnar transposition autograft for limb-sparing surgery of the distal radius in dogs: an anatomic and clinical study. *Veterinary Surgery* **32**, 69–79

Shapiro W, Fossum TW and Kitchell BE (1988) Use of cisplatin for the treatment of appendicular osteosarcoma in dogs. *Journal of the American Veterinary Medical Association* **4**, 507–511

Spodnick GJ, Berg RJ, Rand WM *et al.* (1992) Prognosis for dogs with appendicular osteosarcoma treated by amputation alone: 162 cases (1978–1988). *Journal of the American Veterinary Medical Association* **200**, 995–999

Straw RC, Powers BE, Klausner J *et al.* (1996) Canine mandibular osteosarcoma: 51 cases, (1980–1992). *Journal of the American Animal Hospital Association* **32**, 257–262

Straw RC and Withrow SJ (1992) Limb-sparing surgery versus amputation for dogs with bone tumors. *Veterinary Clinics of North America* **26**, 135–143

Straw RC, Withrow SJ and Powers BE (1992) Partial or total hemipelvectomy in the management of sarcomas in nine dogs and two cats. *Veterinary Surgery* **21**, 183–188

Straw RC, Withrow SJ, Richter SL *et al.* (1991) Amputation and cisplatin for treatment of canine osteosarcoma. *Journal of Veterinary Internal Medicine* **5**, 205–210

Thompson JP and Fugent MJ (1992) *Journal of the American Veterinary Medical Association* **200**, 531–533

Thrall DE, Withrow SJ, Powers BE *et al.* (1990) Radiotherapy prior to cortical allograft limb sparing in dogs with osteosarcoma: a dose response assay. *International Journal of Radiation Oncology Biology Physics* **18**, 1354–1357

Trout NJ, Pavletic MM and Kraus KH (1995) Partial scapulectomy for management of sarcomas in three dogs and two cats. *Journal of the American Veterinary Medical Association* **207**, 585–587

Turrel JM and Pool RR (1982) Primary bone tumors in the cat: a retrospective study of 15 cats and a literature review. *Veterinary Radiology* **23**, 152–166

Van Ginkel RJ, Hoekstra HJ, Meutstege FJ *et al.* (1995) Hyperthermic isolated regional perfusion with cisplatin in the local treatment of spontaneous canine osteosarcoma: assessment of short-term effects. *Journal of Surgical Oncology* **59**, 169–176

Vasseur P (1987) Limb preservation in dogs with primary bone tumors. *Veterinary Clinics of North America* **17**, 889–993

Vignoli M, Ohlerth S, Rossi F *et al.* (2004) Computed tomography-guided fine-needle aspiration and tissue core biopsy of bone lesions in small animals. *Veterinary Radiology and Ultrasound* **45**, 125–130

Wallace J, Matthiesen DT and Patnaik AK (1992) Hemimaxillectomy for the treatment of oral tumors in 69 dogs. *Veterinary Surgery* **21**, 337–341

Wallack ST, Wisner ER, Werner JA *et al.* (2002) Accuracy of magnetic resonance imaging for estimating intramedullary osteosarcoma extent in pre-operative planning of canine limb-salvage procedures. *Veterinary Radiology and Ultrasound* **43**, 432–441

Walter WS, Dernell SM, LaRue SE *et al.* (2005) Curative-intent radiation therapy as a treatment modality for appendicular and axial osteosarcoma: a preliminary retrospective evaluation of 14 dogs with the disease. *Veterinary and Comparative Oncology* **3**, 1–7

Wesselhoeft Ablin L, Berg J and Schelling SH (1991) Fibrosarcoma in the canine appendicular skeleton. *Journal of the American Animal Hospital Association* **27**, 303–309

Withrow SJ, Straw RC, Brekke JH *et al.* (1995) Slow release adjuvant cisplatin for treatment of metastatic canine osteosarcoma. *European Journal of Experimental Musculoskeletal Research* **4**, 105–110

Withrow SJ, Thrall DE, Straw RC *et al.* (1993) Intra-arterial cisplatin with or without radiation in limb-sparing for canine osteosarcoma. *Cancer* **71**, 2484–2490

Yazawa M, Okuda M, Kanaya N *et al.* (2003) Molecular cloning of the canine telomerase reverse transcriptase gene and its expression in neoplastic and non-neoplastic cells. *American Journal of Veterinary Research* **64**, 1395–1400

Zachos TA, Chiaramonte D, DiResta GR *et al.* (1999) Canine osteosarcoma: treatment with surgery, chemotherapy and/or radiation therapy, the Animal Medical Center experience. *Proceedings of the Veterinary Cancer Society, 19th Annual Meeting, Woods Hole, MA*, 12 (abstract)

14

Soft tissue sarcomas

Nicholas Bacon

Introduction

Soft tissue sarcoma (STS) is a catch-all classification referring to tumours that arise from the embryonic mesoderm and, as such, can occur anywhere in the body. The term is most commonly used in reference to subcutaneous tissues, with other sites such as the alimentary and urogenital tracts being less frequently affected. This variable distribution leads to a huge range of histopathological subtypes. Generally, they are classified by histopathology or immunohistochemistry according to the presumed cell of origin, such as fibrosarcoma (FSA), peripheral nerve sheath tumour (PNST), myxosarcoma, liposarcoma, or leiomyosarcoma (Figure 14.1). Sometimes these distinctions are not clear and the generic terms soft tissue sarcoma and spindle cell sarcoma are employed. As tumours within this group tend to have similar biological behaviour, they are often treated as one. Some tumours of mesoderm behave in a much more aggressive and less predictable fashion and have a much higher rate of metastasis. These tend not to be included in STS; examples include visceral haemangiosarcoma (Chapter 19b), chondrosarcoma, and osteosarcoma (Chapter 13).

Aetiology and pathogenesis

Many subcutaneous soft tissue lesions are benign or inflammatory, but STSs comprise 15% of all skin and subcutaneous tumours in dogs and 7–9% in cats (Theilen and Madewell, 1979; Miller et al., 1991). No consistent sex or breed predisposition in dogs has been found, although spayed females were overrepresented in one study (Baker-Gabb et al., 2003). Middle-aged to old dogs of medium to large breeds seem to be most commonly affected. While STSs are less common in cats, there has been an increase in the number of feline sarcomas since 1991, particularly at anatomical sites used for vaccination. This was coincident with the shift from modified live to killed rabies vaccine products. Links with feline leukaemia virus vaccines, vaccination for other feline infectious diseases and non-vaccine injections in general have also been described.

Presentation and clinical signs

History

Many STSs are detected when still small, but are often not investigated as the owner or clinician assumes them to be benign. They are typically non-painful masses and, although they may be firm and attached to deeper tissues, many are soft and mobile, mimicking lipomas or other benign masses. Haemangiopericytomas in particular are slow growing, and may contain fluid pockets creating 'soft spots' on palpation.

A study of insured dogs in the UK identified lipomas in 318 per 100,000 dogs, with STS at 142 per 100,000 (Dobson et al., 2002). It is this greater incidence of benign lipomas that leads to incorrect assumptions that soft subcutaneous masses are not malignant and thus many malignant tumours go undiagnosed until they change their behaviour, cause clinical signs or cause concern for the owner.

Malignant	Benign
Liposarcoma	Lipoma
Fibrosarcoma	Fibroma
Haemangiosarcoma	Haemangioma
Myxosarcoma	Myxoma
Peripheral nerve sheath tumours (PNSTs) including: • Haemangiopericytoma • Neurofibrosarcoma • Malignant schwannoma	Neurofibroma
Lymphangiosarcoma	Lymphangioma
	Epidermal inclusion cyst
	Collagenous naevi
Malignant fibrous histiocytoma (MFH)	
Histiocytic sarcoma	Histiocytoma
Injection-associated sarcomas in cats: • Fibrosarcoma • Osteosarcoma	
Leiomyosarcoma	Leiomyoma
Gastrointestinal stromal tumour (GIST)	
Rhabdomyosarcoma	Rhabdomyoma
Synovial cell sarcoma	

14.1 Benign and malignant soft tissue tumours.

A history of a mass on the body wall or extremities (Figure 14.2) slowly growing over several years is not uncommon.

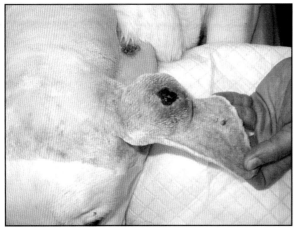

14.2 Soft tissue sarcomas eventually invade the overlying skin and become ulcerated. This often prompts veterinary attention, as with this long-standing STS of the pinna.

Feline injection-site sarcomas (ISSs) are seen 2–10 months after vaccination and are on average 23 cm³ in volume on palpation at diagnosis (McEntee and Samii, 2000), often with a history of rapid growth (Figure 14.3). Most resolve in 30–90 days. Only those that persist longer than 3 months should be investigated and possibly removed.

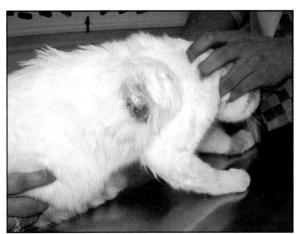

14.3 Feline injection site sarcomas (ISSs) typically occur over the interscapular area or body wall. To achieve a cure, 3 cm margins and a resection of at least one uninvolved fascial plane below/around the tumour is recommended at the first surgery.

Clinical signs
STSs are typically in the subcutaneous space and the skin overlying the mass is often freely mobile. Many STSs feel encapsulated and distinct from surrounding tissues. This is because they are surrounded by a pseudocapsule, which creates an easy plane of cleavage between tumour and surrounding tissues, allowing the masses to be 'shelled out'. The pseudocapsule arises because expanding tumours are histologically surrounded by a poorly defined reactive zone (Figure 14.4), consisting of some or all of:

- A vascular response (new blood vessels)
- Mesenchymal response (to physical presence of the tumour and abnormal local tissue forces)
- An inflammatory response (to necrosis or haemorrhage).

This reactive zone may be fractions of a millimetre wide in small low-grade tumours, but significantly wider in rapidly expanding high-grade tumours. The zone creates a visible and palpable 'edge' to the tumour, mimicking a fascial plane, but microscopically or immunohistochemically it is a three-dimensional 'halo' of malignancy. Dissections within the reactive zone (i.e. 'shelling out') are therefore marginal excisions; these commonly result in tumour cells extending to the edges of the resected tissue, or satellite deposits of tumour cells in the reactive zone being left in the wound.

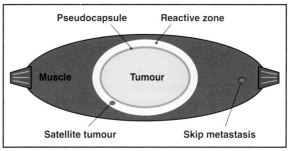

14.4 The reactive zone contains satellite deposits of cancer cells. These microscopic tumours are easily left behind in the wound if a marginal excision is performed by peeling the mass out.

STSs present as non-painful masses on the trunk or extremities. As they grow, they invade the skin and deeper tissue, causing them to become more fixed and often superficially ulcerated or infected (Figure 14.5). When sarcomas are confined within anatomical spaces, patients present with signs of pain due to increased compartmental pressure. Examples include STSs contained within muscle bellies, or expansile intermuscular tumours compressing neurovascular structures (e.g. thigh masses compressing the sciatic nerve).

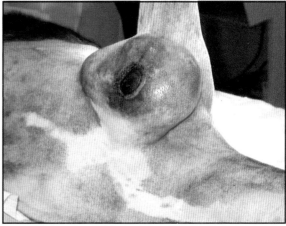

14.5 This slow-growing axillary grade I STS in an elderly Rottweiler had been present for 6 years, but was beginning to interfere with walking.

Feline ISSs historically arise in popular injection sites such as the dorsal interscapular area. Recent work has shown that, following publication of vaccine guidelines in the mid 1990s recommending vaccination in the extremities (to allow for amputation should a tumour arise), tumours are now arising with increasing frequency in the hindlimbs and caudal flank (the latter likely due to misplaced injections designed for the pelvic limbs in sitting cats) (Shaw *et al.*, 2009). Feline ISSs are locally invasive with an infiltrative growth pattern and will regrow following inadequate surgery. There are often centrally located micro- or macro-abscesses giving rise to a cystic centre, yielding fluid on fine-needle aspiration (FNA).

Clinical approach

Diagnostic investigation of a possible STS has three aims:

- To diagnose the tumour accurately before treatment
- To define the anatomical relations of the primary tumour to surrounding structures for surgery and/or radiation planning
- To identify the presence or absence of metastatic disease.

Biopsy

Fine-needle aspiration
FNA is of limited value in diagnosing STS, because cells do not exfoliate easily and clinical pathologists find it difficult to determine whether there is cancer present or not based on only a few cells. However, fine-needle aspirates have an important role in ruling out other subcutaneous differentials, such as lipomas, mast cell tumours or inflammatory lesions, all of which exfoliate cells easily. In a university setting, fine-needle aspirates of STSs yielded a correct diagnosis in 62.5% cases, were non-diagnostic in 22.5% cases, and an incorrect diagnosis was made in 15% (Baker-Gabb *et al.*, 2003). If an aspirate of a subcutaneous mass fails to yield many cells on the slide, the index of suspicion for an STS should be raised and should prompt a core biopsy.

Core biopsy
Percutaneous core biopsies (e.g. Tru-cut) are possibly the best technique for safely achieving an accurate diagnosis and can easily be performed with local anaesthesia and sedation. Tru-cut biopsies will reliably differentiate benign from malignant disease and in most cases will also give a good indication of grade. The simplicity and accuracy of core biopsy for STS means that incisional biopsies are infrequently indicated, therefore avoiding the added concerns of location and direction of scar, and tumour dissemination from post-incisional biopsy haematoma.

Evaluation of primary tumour and possible metastasis
Radiographs of the mass may yield some information regarding local behaviour (especially whether invasion of underlying bone is evident), but often only confirm that the mass is of soft tissue density (Figure 14.6).

Ultrasonography (especially Doppler) can be useful to ascertain degree of local vascularity, but cross-sectional imaging – computed tomography (CT) or magnetic resonance imaging (MRI) – is the imaging method of choice, if available, and is typically supportive of the diagnosis, in addition to identifying accurately the relationship of the mass to local vital structures. Whereas MRI is traditionally regarded as superior for soft tissue detail, CT (especially contrast CT) offers a fast, simple and accurate alternative for all but the most complex STSs (Figure 14.7). It is

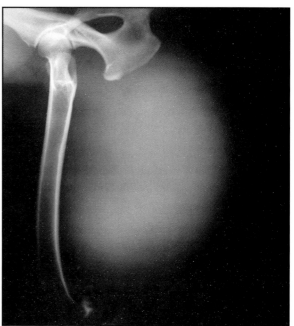

14.6 Plain radiographs of the extremities will show the mass to be of soft tissue rather than fat density, as in this STS of the caudal thigh.

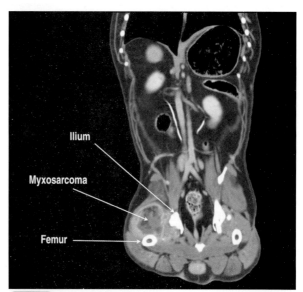

14.7 Contrast CT showing a grade II myxosarcoma of the proximal right thigh in a dog. The close anatomical relationship with both the femur and pelvis shows that amputation alone would not cure this dog: hemipelvectomy to remove the ilium would also be necessary.

often cheaper than MRI, is more intuitive to interpret if inexperienced (as the images are very similar to conventional radiographs) and it has the added advantage that imaging the thorax for metastatic disease can easily be performed at the same time.

STSs metastasize haematogenously and lymphatic involvement is unusual. Any firm, irregular or enlarged regional lymph nodes should be evaluated by FNA, Tru-cut biopsy or excisional biopsy.

Histological grading

STSs are graded into low (I), intermediate (II) and high (III), taking into account histological features such as mitotic rate, extent of necrosis, cellular differentiation and cellular pleomorphism. Grading of STS in dogs is considered more important for prognosis than the cell of origin, because grade significantly affects likelihood of metastasis (Powers *et al.*, 1995; Kuntz *et al.*, 1997). Reported metastatic rates for the dog are: grade I, 13%; grade II, 7%; and grade III, 41% (Kuntz *et al.*, 1997).

Silver staining techniques have demonstrated that increased AgNOR count in tissue specimens is a significant prognostic indicator for decreased survival time (Ettinger *et al.*, 2006). On the strength of this, AgNORs may become part of routine evaluation of malignancy of STS along with histological grading.

Grade plays an important role in tumours of the upper limb, chest wall and flank where wide excisions with tumour-free margins can be taken, but may have a lesser role when tumours involve the head and neck, retroperitoneum or distal limbs, where specific anatomical restraints at these sites prevent wide curative-intent excision. In these locations the amount of tumour excised or excisable may prove to be more important than grade.

Histological subtypes

Peripheral nerve sheath tumour (PNST) and haemangiopericytoma

This large group of tumours contains neurofibrosarcomas and malignant schwannomas in addition to PNSTs. Somewhat contentiously, haemangiopericytomas are also included under PNSTs. Most haemangiopericytomas do not stain with S100 (marker for peripheral nerve), and so many pathologists prefer to place haemangiopericytomas in a separate group of 'low-grade spindle cell tumours'. However, recent information has suggested that haemangiopericytomas are less frequent and more malignant than previously believed (Avallone *et al.*, 2007). Together, these tumours tend to be locally invasive but metastasize rarely, especially haemangiopericytomas.

PNSTs arise predominantly in the distal extremities and they can become large and adherent to the overlying skin (Figure 14.8). Infiltration between the flexor and extensor tendons is common, making many of these excisions marginal at best, leaving residual tumour disease behind. These tumours can also be derived from peripheral nerves close to the spinal column, most commonly in the brachial plexus.

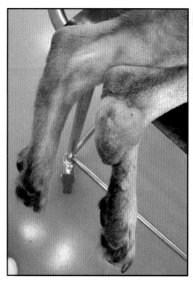

14.8 Grade I PNST over the hock in an elderly German Shepherd Dog.

Patients will present with muscle wasting, single forelimb lameness and often a firm painful mass deep in the axilla, or just an adverse reaction to axilla palpation. Because of the common occurrence of elbow and shoulder joint disease leading to lameness, many of these tumours go undiagnosed for several months. Electromyography to demonstrate muscle denervation and CT or MRI to plan surgery are recommended. Many cases have spinal cord invasion, and amputation combined with a laminectomy may be necessary.

Invasion into the spinal cord is also possible in cats, but much less common than in dogs, representing < 5% of cases (Marioni-Henry *et al.*, 2008).

Fibrosarcoma (FSA)

Originating from neoplastic fibroblasts, fibrosarcomas have a low–moderate metastatic rate. They occur most commonly on the flanks (dermal, subcutaneous and deep fascia) and oral cavity (see Chapter 15a). Non-oral FSAs behave like STSs.

A specific type of FSA, the 'hi-lo', is encountered in the mouth of young dogs, commonly Golden Retrievers. This is a biologically high-grade but histologically low-grade tumour, i.e. the biopsy can be misleading in terms of clinical behaviour and prognosis. Aggressive surgical excision and fractionated radiation therapy of a 'hi-lo' may still result in local recurrence and/or distant metastasis.

FSA in the cat is covered as a separate condition (see 'Feline sarcomas', below).

Myxosarcoma

A mesenchymal malignancy characterized by the production of mucinous matrix, myxosarcoma can grossly appear wet when biopsy sampled or sectioned and the tumours are generally softer to the touch than other STSs. Otherwise they behave biologically in a similar fashion to other STSs.

Rhabdomyosarcoma

An STS originating from striated skeletal muscle, rhabdomyosarcoma commonly arises in the head and neck, including the tongue, pharynx, larynx and trachea. Tumours have also been reported in the urethra, bladder and cardiac muscle. Occasionally feline injection site sarcomas will differentiate into rhabdomyosarcoma. Many rhabdomyosarcomas are low grade, especially in the larynx, and differentiation from rhabdomyoma may be difficult. Treatment options are similar to those for other STSs, though marginal excision of low-grade tumours in the neck may result in long disease-free intervals.

Synovial cell sarcoma

Arising within joints, synovial cell sarcoma is a locally aggressive tumour and therefore typically painful. Bone destruction is seen radiographically in many cases but is not always present. Metastatic rate is high, with up to 22% of dogs having metastases at presentation (Vail *et al.*, 1994). The stifle is the most commonly affected joint but any can be involved.

Synovial cell sarcomas are unlike other STSs in that lymph node involvement is frequently encountered and staging should include FNA of the draining lymph node along with chest radiographs. It is thought that this is found because many 'synovial cell sarcomas' are actually a histiocytic variety of sarcoma. Immunohistochemical staining for cytokeratin, CD18, and smooth muscle actin is recommended to make the diagnosis of either synovial cell sarcoma or histiocytic sarcoma, and thereby predict the behaviour of synovial tumours in dogs.

Any effort to preserve the joint by incomplete surgical excision typically results in rapid local regrowth and progression of disease and pain. Attempts to predict outcome in terms of grade, cytokeratin staining and epitheloid versus histiocytic tumours have been largely inconclusive. The most important prognostic factors are clean wide excision (typically amputation), lack of metastasis at time of surgery and histological type. In one study, the average survival time was 31.8 months for dogs with synovial cell sarcoma, 5.3 months for dogs with histiocytic sarcoma, 30.7 months for dogs with synovial myxoma and 3.5 months for dogs with other sarcomas (Craig *et al.*, 2002).

One poorly understood phenomenon seen with synovial cell sarcoma in particular is that of possible (but unlikely) local recurrence at the amputation site and owners should be warned of this. Again, this may well be due to the presence, in those cases, of the histiocytic sarcoma.

Leiomyosarcoma and gastrointestinal stromal tumours (GISTs)

Leiomyosarcoma is a tumour arising from smooth muscle cells and is predominantly found in the walls of the alimentary and urogenital tract, where it results in clinical signs due to its physical presence (luminal obstruction/organ deviation), or through ulceration (vaginal bleeding, melaena). Rarely it may involve overlying subcutaneous spaces or skin.

- Small-intestinal leiomyosarcoma treated by resection anastomosis with 3–5 cm margins usually results in tumour-free margins, but the draining mesenteric lymph nodes should be carefully inspected, and biopsy samples taken, or removed if firm or enlarged.
- Leiomyosarcoma of the oesophagus presents late in the course of the disease but appears to be low grade and has been treated with marginal excision with long-term resolution of clinical signs (Farese *et al.*, 2007).
- Leiomyosarcoma in the vagina may be managed by episiotomy and resection, and occasionally total vaginectomy if extensive disease is present.
- Paraneoplastic hypoglycaemia has been associated with leiomyosarcoma.

GISTs arise from the interstitial cells of Cajal (ICC), which are pacemaker cells believed to coordinate peristalsis in the intestinal tract. They are STSs that arise solely within the intestinal tract, most frequently the caecum (see also Chapter 15). Appearing similar to leiomyosarcoma on H&E histopathology, they have subtle immunohistochemical differences (GISTs express CD117), but this has not been shown to translate into a different prognosis.

Studies have shown no significant difference in survival between tumour subtypes or whether the tumour is small intestinal or caecal. An important difference, however, is that dogs with GISTs are significantly more likely to be older, and to present with caecal perforation and septic peritonitis, than dogs with intestinal leiomyosarcomas, and this might result in GISTs having a higher perioperative mortality (Maas *et al.*, 2007; Russell *et al.*, 2007).

Adipose tumours

Lipoma

Lipoma is a well circumscribed soft mass within a thin capsule and can occasionally grow to considerable size. Although the subcutaneous site is the most common, lipomas have been diagnosed in the thoracic and abdominal cavities and pelvic canal. Indications for removal include sudden rapid growth, recent change in texture, causing clinical signs due to its space occupying nature, bothering the animal, bothering the owner, or interfering with normal function. Lipomas in cats are rare.

Infiltrative lipoma

Most commonly reported in the limbs and flank, and occasionally associated with joints, infiltrative lipomas are poorly demarcated tumours, with the macroscopic appearance of mature fat, but microscopically the fat infiltrates muscle fibres. There is no obvious tumour capsule and CT or MRI is necessary to adequately plan surgery and identify potential risks (McEntee and Thrall, 2001). Infiltration between muscle bellies and around neurovascular structures makes surgery an intra-lesional dissection (Figure 14.9). Cobalt radiation therapy has been used with some success to control local disease following debulking surgery, with a median survival of 40 months reported (McEntee *et al.*, 2000). These tumours do not metastasize.

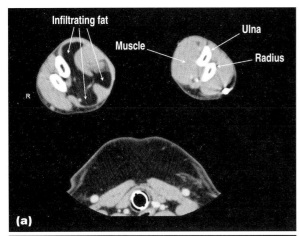

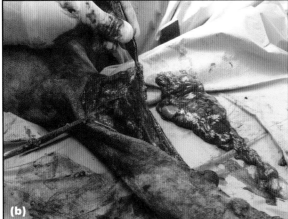

14.9 Infiltrative lipoma. **(a)** CT images show an area of fat density pushing between the muscles of the right limb. **(b)** Intra-lesional excision. Umbilical tape can be seen retracting and protecting a nerve. Gross tumour will be left behind and postoperative radiation should be considered.

Liposarcoma

A malignant mesenchymal tumour derived from adipocytes, liposarcoma can occur equally on the flanks and the limbs and occasionally in body cavities. The tumours are locally invasive and median size at presentation is 4 cm. Recent work has indicated that their metastatic potential may be lower than previously believed. A wide excision is associated with a median survival of 1188 days, compared with 649 days for a marginal excision (Baez *et al.*, 2004).

Haemangiosarcoma

Visceral HSA

HSA is most often considered a visceral disease, with internal organs such as the spleen, liver and heart being commonly affected. It is a highly malignant tumour, with death typically occurring within 6 months through widespread systemic metastases, despite the use of chemotherapy (see Chapter 19).

Dermal and subcutaneous HSA

Dermal HSA is biologically much more benign than the aggressive visceral form. It is reported more frequently in breeds such as Irish Wolfhound, Whippet, Saluki, Bloodhound and pointers. Lightly pigmented,

sparsely haired dogs (Beagle, white Bulldog, English Pointer and Dalmatian) have also been reported as predisposed to the development of cutaneous and subcutaneous HSA. It is possible that unpigmented skin in cats may also be predisposed to developing dermal HSA. It has been suggested that cutaneous haemangiomas may undergo malignant transformation to HSA, but this appears less likely with the subcutaneous form.

In dogs, most cutaneous HSAs are well defined superficial masses that are amenable to local excision and that metastasize slowly, if at all. Subcutaneous HSA tends to be a more locally invasive, problematic tumour. Infiltrative tumours, plus those with hypodermal or muscular involvement, seem to have a high recurrence rate and incidence of metastasis.

In cats, dermal and subcutaneous HSAs are more common than the visceral form and are treated primarily by surgery. Attaining a tumour-free margin following surgery is more likely with a well defined dermal mass and this translates into a longer recurrence-free interval, whereas margins of normal tissue can be difficult to identify with subcutaneous HSA because of localized bleeding and bruising. In one study 50% cats with subcutaneous HSA suffered local recurrence following surgery, while none of the cats with dermal HSA had recurrence (Johannes *et al.*, 2007). Subcutaneous HSA is particularly difficult to manage when it arises in the ventral (Figure 14.10) or inguinal areas as these tumours are often too large to treat by the time of diagnosis (McAbee *et al.*, 2005). A high mitotic count (>3/10 hpfs) is associated with a poorer survival in cats (Johannes *et al.*, 2007). It is likely that the metastatic rate of feline subcutaneous HSA is higher than previously thought (Kraje *et al.*, 1999).

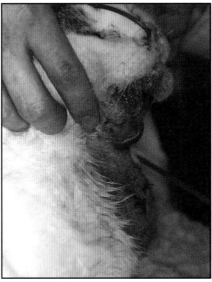

14.10 Subcutaneous HSA of the ventral neck in a cat. Chest radiographs revealed disseminated metastatic disease.

Radiation therapy for unresectable or incompletely excised dermal or subcutaneous HSA has been poorly reported in dogs and cats. A recent report described the use of palliative radiation to treat non-splenic HSA in dogs: 20 patients were given doses of either 6 or 8 Gy to a maximum of 24 Gy; a subjective reduction in tumour size was seen in 70% and a complete response seen in 20%, but the median survival time (MST) was only 95 days (Hillers *et al.*, 2007). Chemotherapy for subcutaneous tumours has been described, with commonly used agents being doxorubicin, vincristine and cyclophosphamide, but there is little evidence to show any benefit.

Although the prognosis for dermal HSA in both dogs and cats is good, no difference in overall survival in dogs has been found between visceral and subcutaneous HSA, whereas in cats the subcutaneous form is less aggressive than the visceral form (Sorenmo *et al.*, 1993; Johannes *et al.*, 2007). Stage 1 HSA (tumour <5 cm, does not invade beyond dermis) has a long MST with surgery alone of 780 days in dogs and 36 months in cats. Stage 2 (invades subcutaneous tissue) and stage 3 (invades adjacent muscle) carry a poorer prognosis.

Lymphangiosarcoma

In addition to behaving like any STS where older patients are more at risk, lymphangiosarcomas can also affect younger dogs and cats, often with soft fluctuant swellings arising along the ventral body wall, the inguinal area or around the proximal thigh. The masses are soft and easily compressible, sometimes adopting the feel of 'bubble-wrap'. Clear transudate can be easily expressed from any skin puncture (e.g. through a needle tract for Tru-cut biopsy). Due to anatomical location, often wide excision means amputation and reconstruction with myocutaneous flaps. The prognosis is guarded due to risk for local recurrence at the amputation site, and reportedly increased risk of metastasis. There is no known benefit to giving chemotherapy.

Histiocytic sarcoma

Arising from myeloid dendritic cells, these rare malignant tumours behave like other STSs, but tend to have a higher metastatic potential (see later). They should not be confused with histiocytomas (benign cutaneous round cell tumours often seen in juvenile dogs that can undergo spontaneous regression within 3 months). Histiocytic sarcomas are localized masses arising in the subcutaneous tissues, but primary tumours affecting joints have also been described (Craig *et al.*, 2002). They are locally invasive tumours, are graded according to STS guidelines and are primarily treated surgically.

They may represent an early form of the disseminated disease, malignant histiocytosis, which is a rapidly progressive systemic form most commonly seen in the Bernese Mountain Dog; Rottweiler and retrievers are also affected. Dogs with disseminated disease present with anorexia, weight loss and often pulmonary signs and are poorly responsive to therapy. It carries a grave prognosis (Fulmer and Mauldin, 2007).

Malignant fibrous histiocytoma (MFH)

These are often confused with histiocytic sarcomas, but are a separate member of the STS family,

reportedly arising in the subcutaneous tissues and spleen. Rottweiler and Golden Retriever are the breeds more commonly affected (Goldschmidt and Hendrick, 2002). Long-term local control is possible with surgery alone, or combined with radiation (McKnight *et al.*, 2000).

Feline sarcomas

Three types of sarcoma are seen in cats: viral-induced; non-viral non-vaccine; and injection site sarcoma.

Viral-induced (feline sarcoma virus, FeSV)

These are seen in cats also positive for feline leukaemia virus (FeLV). FeSV oncogenes transform fibroblasts and produce FSA. These are rare, accounting for 2% of FSA; they are seen in young cats and are typically multicentric. A rapid doubling time (12–72 hours) is possible. Surgery will not benefit these patients.

Non-viral, non-vaccine

Usually seen in older cats, these sarcomas affect the head, neck and extremities (Figure 14.11).

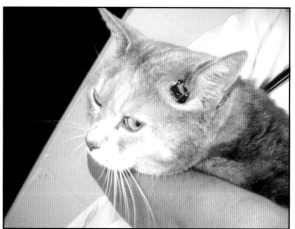

14.11 Fibrosarcoma on the rostral edge of the pinna in an elderly cat. This was treated by 3 cm excision, pinnectomy and total ear canal ablation, and closed with a single-pedicle advancement flap from the dorsal neck.

Feline injection site sarcoma (ISS)

Feline ISS (see Figure 14.3) is also referred to as vaccine-associated sarcoma in some parts of the world. This is due to the proven statistical link to vaccination injections, particularly FeLV and rabies virus vaccines, enhancing the risk of ISS by 2–5-fold. Cats are younger than those in the non-vaccine sarcoma group. There is an increased risk with increasing number of vaccinations, and with repeated vaccination at the same site (Kass *et al.*, 1993, 2003). Tumours usually arise 2–10 months after vaccination, and a risk of 0.32 sarcomas/10,000 doses given has been reported (Gobar and Kass, 2002). However, ISSs have also been seen following other injections in cats.

ISSs are mostly fibrosarcomas, but rhabdomyosarcoma, osteosarcoma, chondrosarcoma etc. are also seen. MSTs for cats with FSA or PNST are significantly longer than median time for cats with MFH (Dillon *et al.*, 2005). An inflammatory reactive granuloma is seen 11.8 times/10,000 doses of vaccine in cats, but it is not necessary to remove these masses unless malignant behaviour is apparent or they persist over 3 months (Gobar and Kass, 2002). ISSs are not linked to FeLV or FIV infection, but the aluminium adjuvant may play a role in carcinogenesis, as might the inflammation induced by any component of the injectate.

ISSs are graded from I (least aggressive) to III (most malignant) depending on mitotic index, differentiation and necrosis. Multinucleated giant cells are seen in the more malignant tumours, and most have peritumoral lymphocyte inflammation and increased vascular density. Recent evidence has suggested that a higher grade (i.e. grade III) is associated with an increased risk of metastasis (Romanelli *et al.*, 2008).

Management and prognosis

Surgical resection is the most effective treatment for primary localized STSs, as they are relatively chemo-insensitive, and radiotherapy is more effective at treating microscopic disease than unresectable gross disease. The aim of curative-intent surgery is to widely excise the primary tumour (3 cm wide and 3 cm or a fascial plane deep) and achieve histopathological margins clear of tumour cells (Figure 14.12).

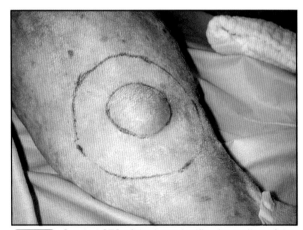

14.12 Grade I STS of the lateral stifle. An outline of the subcutaneous mass is drawn, followed by a 3 cm skin margin. This type of preoperative planning helps in choosing reconstructive options before excising the tumour *en bloc*.

The great variation in possible location, factored with variable size and grade, can present significant problems when designing a treatment plan and it is complicated by anatomical constraints, the need to maintain local function, biological characteristics of the tumour, and length and cost of surgery and reconstruction. Whenever concerns exist about the feasibility of a single curative excision due to the site or size of the mass, it is best to consult with a radiation oncologist prior to definitive surgery, as preoperative radiation to sterilize the tumour edges may allow for a smaller surgery to be performed.

Margins for surgical resection

Our understanding of margins for excising STSs is based on Enneking's pioneering work in musculoskeletal tumours in humans, whereby he classified resection margins as intralesional/intracapsular, marginal, wide or radical (Enneking *et al.*, 1980).

- An **intracapsular** margin is achieved by piecemeal removal ('debulking') of a lesion from within the capsule. This is also used if the capsule is accidentally entered during dissection as the surgical field is now contaminated. *Gross and/or microscopic disease remains.* Examples include incisional biopsy and infiltrative lipomas (see Figure 14.9b).
- A **marginal** margin is achieved by an extracapsular dissection through the reactive zone around the STS. Classically these are termed 'shell-outs' and involve peeling the mass out from its tissue bed and off local attachments. Both benign and malignant lesions may have extracapsular microextensions of disease, microsatellites (in the reactive zone), and 'skip' metastases of high-grade lesions (in normal tissue of the same compartment; see Figure 14.4). These have implications for marginal excisions in terms of potential for local recurrence (Figure 14.13).
- A **wide** margin is achieved by *en bloc* removal of the lesion, its capsule and the surrounding reactive zone but always working in normal uncontaminated tissue within the compartment of the lesion. Non-neoplastic, non-reactive intracompartmental normal tissue is left at the margins and there is the possibility of 'skip' metastases arising in the remaining portion of the compartment (e.g. high-grade STS).
- A **radical** margin removes the lesion, reactive zone and all the tissue of the associated compartment. There is no potential for residual neoplasm locally. The typical example is amputation, along with variants such as hemipelvectomy.

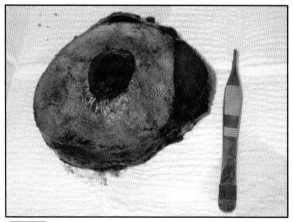

14.13 A marginal excision of the mass shown in Figure 14.5. The deep margin of the mass was peeled off the pectoral muscles. Residual disease was assumed. Given the age of the dog and the slow-growing history of the mass, the owner opted for a conservative palliative surgery to improve quality of life.

Upper limb

The abundance of skin on the neck and flanks of most patients means that wide resections of the upper limb or flank are possible and complex reconstructive techniques are often only indicated in awkward anatomical locations, for example around the perineum. Radiation has a very valuable role if incomplete margins are found and if further revision surgery is declined. Because extensive reconstructions result in often very large radiation fields being required postoperatively if the resection was incomplete, complicated and extensive reconstructive techniques are in general avoided where possible until the completeness of resection is known. It must be remembered that radiation in the area of the axial skeleton can have late side effects.

Distal limb

In the distal limbs (at/below the stifle and at/below the elbow), where a wide surgical margin of skin is usually only achievable using free skin grafts or various skin flaps, options such as amputation or marginal resection and radiation are the primary methods of tumour control. Both options have drawbacks in terms of altered function, morbidity and cost. Whereas amputation could be expected to cure a patient, the limb might be spared with marginal excision of the STS and radiation, but this is costly and results in a local recurrence rate of 19–35%.

Tissue slip

Following some resections it can be seen that the various components of the resected tissue move over each other (slip). For example, the tissues deep to a tumour that were resected may slip away, exposing the base of the tumour. In order to get accurate information from an examination of margins, many surgeons suggest reconstructing the resected tissue into the position and form present in the animal. This is done using sutures through the various layers at the margins. Edges of the resected tissue (skin margin and deep margin) should then be identified by painting with a thin layer of India ink (Figure 14.14), left to dry, and then placed into 10% formalin to fix, at a

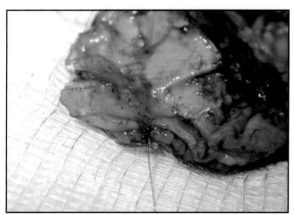

14.14 To prevent 'tissue slip', the deep fascia is sutured to the skin edge to ensure that ink does not 'under-run' the fascial layer, giving misleading results on tumour margins. A thin layer of India ink (*colours other than red recommended*) is applied to the cut surfaces with a cotton bud.

ratio of at least 1 part mass to 10 parts formalin. On processing and interpretation, inked margins assist in orientation of the resected tissue. Additionally, identifying tumour cells in inked tissue represents tumour at the wound edge, and so an incomplete excision. Larger tissue masses may need to be 'bread-loafed' prior to fixing, as the formalin cannot diffuse to a tissue depth of >1 cm. Alternatively, some surgeons prefer to tie small suture knots at locations where concern exists over the width of the normal tissue margin, to encourage the pathologist to examine these areas more critically.

Treatment of extremity STS

Treatment options for a histologically diagnosed extremity STS include:

- **Amputation**
- **Curative-intent excision plus radiation** if tumour cells extend to the edge of resected tissue microscopically (see notes above on extensive reconstruction)
- **Preoperative radiation** to sterilize tissue around the tumour, with **marginal excision** of mass 4 weeks later
- **Planned marginal excision** of mass, then **postoperative radiation** to sterilize residual tumour in the wound bed 2 weeks later
- **Skin-sparing surgery** – planned marginal excision to microscopic disease, including fascia where possible, but ensuring wound can be closed without advanced reconstruction.

The first four options are curative-intent plans and local recurrence is unlikely. Skin-sparing surgery is a palliative plan, and the owner accepts that local recurrence is a possibility. For many geriatric patients with low-grade STS, this is a viable option with the expectation that the patient will die of something else before the tumour has a chance to recur or metastasize.

Planned marginal excision

Without presurgical biopsies, inadvertent shell-out procedures on masses assumed to be benign that subsequently turn out to be malignant represent an unfortunately common but easily avoidable clinical scenario. The difference between planned and unplanned marginal excisions is as follows.

- In **planned marginal excisions**, typically in the distal extremities, the surgeon has performed a biopsy of the mass and is aware that the surgery is an incomplete excision of an STS. Local recurrence is anticipated and so the surgeon attempts wherever possible to work outside the pseudocapsule to excise the infiltration of the tumour into the surrounding tissues. Wide margins are not possible without reconstructive techniques (which have been discussed and declined by the owner) and so the aim is to remove as much tumour as possible, but still close the skin over the wound. This skin-sparing surgery may still involve excising fascia beneath the mass. At some point during the surgery the pseudocapsule is entered (normally when peeling tumour off skin) and so the surgery is classified as marginal. A recurrence rate in dogs of 11% for this technique has been reported when performed by experienced surgeons and all STSs were grade I (Stefanello *et al.*, 2008).

- An **unplanned marginal excision** is a true 'shell-out', working in the pseudocapsule of an unknown mass. Fascia is not taken, and small macroscopic disease may remain. As no attempt is made to reduce the chance of recurrence by wider dissection, local recurrence is considered likely.

Incomplete excision

If faced with an incompletely excised STS (so-called 'dirty margins'), treatment options include: amputation (if on a limb); postoperative radiation; re-excision; or 'wait and see'.

Amputation (if on a limb): This should be locally curative, assuming the scar and previous tumour-contaminated surgical wound are not entered during amputation. The risk of metastasis remains.

Postoperative radiation to sterilize tumour bed: Several studies have reported the results of adjunctive radiotherapy in the management of STS with surgically incomplete margins and its success has generally been measured by its long overall survival times. The effect on local tumour control, however, has been variable, with recurrence rates ranging between 17% and 31% (Figure 14.15) (Forrest *et al.*, 2000; McKnight *et al.*, 2000).

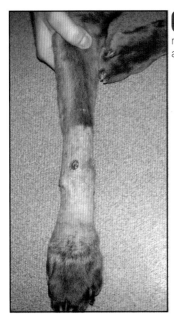

14.15 Recurrence of an STS in the radiation field on the antebrachium of a dog.

Re-excision of scar with local closure techniques: Even in the distal limbs, where there is little available soft tissue, re-excision of the scar with as wide a margin as possible (still to close the wound primarily) can result in clean margins of excision in over 90% of cases and a local recurrence rate of

15% (Figure 14.16). Tumour may be found in only 22% of resected scars on histopathology but its presence cannot be used to predict which dogs will have local recurrence (Bacon *et al.*, 2007).

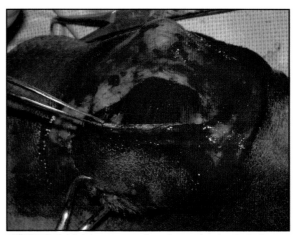

14.16 A 'dirty' scar over the elbow of a dog is being excised with 3 cm margins. The antebrachial fascia (in forceps) is forming the deep margin. The residual tumour was completely excised.

Wait and see: For many owners this is an understandable choice. The failure rate for marginal excisions in dogs is historically quoted as 60–70%, based on work performed 20–30 years ago on grade III sarcomas with unknown margin status, but much has changed since in terms of understanding tumour biology and especially earlier intervention by owners. Marginal excision of grade I sarcomas may have a local recurrence rate as low as 11%, and so the rate for grade II tumours is likely to be somewhere between 11% and 70%.

Chemotherapy

STSs are not considered chemosensitive. It is known that > 40% of dogs with grade III STS will develop distant metastatic disease (Kuntz *et al.*, 1997) and so the addition of conventional chemotherapy drugs to try to control this systemic spread is sensible. Little evidence exists, however, to show a beneficial effect of chemotherapy on overall survival. Doxorubicin as a single agent failed to improve disease-free interval or overall survival in dogs with grade III STS (Selting *et al.*, 2005). Recent work following dogs with incompletely excised STS receiving daily oral low-dose cyclophosphamide (10 mg/m^2) and full-dose piroxicam (0.3 mg/kg) showed it to be very effective at delaying local recurrence compared with a control population and could be considered in dogs with 'dirty' wounds (Elmslie *et al.*, 2008).

Radiotherapy

Use of radiotherapy as a sole treatment for unresectable STS has received recent attention. A study of dogs with macroscopic STS receiving four fractions of radiation (total dose 32 Gy) in a palliative setting showed that the treatment was well tolerated, with an overall response rate of 50%, but this was a short-lived improvement as median time to progression was 155 days (Lawrence *et al.*, 2008). Cobalt radiation was administered in three fractions (total dose 24 Gy) to dogs with non-resectable STS, and median time to progression was 263 days (Plavec *et al.*, 2006)

Management of feline ISS

The presence of metastasis has been shown to significantly decrease survival time in cats with ISS (Cohen *et al.*, 2001; Sorensen *et al.*, 2004), underlying the importance of preoperative staging prior to radical surgery. Three-view chest radiographs are a minimum and cross-sectional imaging such as contrast CT or MRI is recommended to delineate the tumour. From a practical point of view, the veterinary surgeon who is likely to perform the surgery should ensure that the cat is placed in an appropriate normal anatomical position during cross-sectional imaging, so that the relationship between the tumour and anatomical landmarks can be assessed accurately. This aids in surgical planning (Figure 14.17). Palpation may suggest a discrete mass, but post-contrast CT often shows the true extent of infiltrative disease, which cannot be appreciated by feel alone. Radical first excision of ISS yielded significantly longer median time to first recurrence (325 days) than did marginal first excision (79 days) (Hershey *et al.*, 2000). MST is significantly longer in cats with tumours <2 cm in diameter compared with those with tumours 2 cm in diameter (Dillon *et al.*, 2005).

Surgery for feline ISS

The general approach of surgical margins 2–3 cm wide and one fascial plane deep to the tumour bed has been adopted for ISS in cats, but even this may not be adequate considering historical rates of local recurrence. Some surgeons are suggesting more radical methods, including surgical margins of ≥3 cm and 1–2 fascial planes deep to the tumour, along with partial scapulectomy, osteotomy of spinous processes (Figure 14.18) or hemipelvectomy when indicated (Cohen *et al.*, 2001; Séguin, 2002; Kobayashi *et al.*, 2002; Davis *et al.*, 2007; Romanelli *et al.*, 2008).

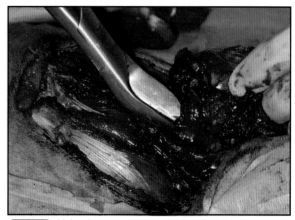

14.18 Using bone cutters to cut the dorsal spinous processes in a cat during ISS resection. The surgeon is moving from cranial to caudal. The dorsal border of the scapula in the foreground has also been resected.

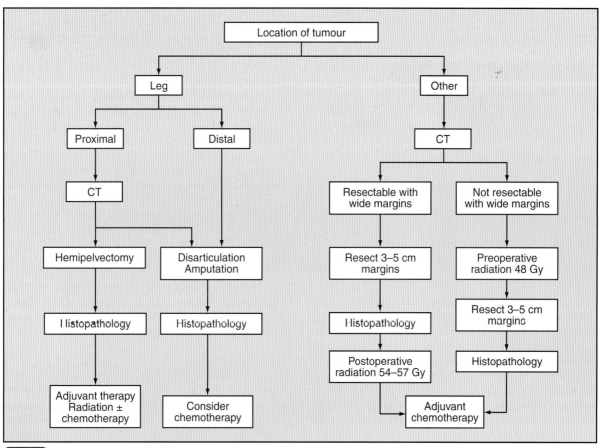

14.17 Treatment planning in feline ISS.

Currently, the Vaccine-Associated Sarcoma Task Force recommends multimodal treatment, including surgical resection with at least 2 cm margins in all planes, with mention of use of 3–5 cm surgical margins for exclsion (VASTF, 2005). When such large surgeries are performed, epidural analgesia, local tissue infiltration with bupivacaine prior to closure, and a constant rate infusion (CRI) of fentanyl, or fentanyl patches, should be used.

Chemotherapy for feline ISS
Although there are isolated reports of ISS responding to drugs such as doxorubicin, cyclophosphamide, mitoxantrone and carboplatin, there is little evidence in larger numbers of cats with ISS that adjuvant chemotherapy improves overall survival (Bregazzi et al., 2001; Martano et al., 2005). However, it may delay local recurrence in cats also receiving curative intent radiation therapy (Hahn et al., 2007).

Radiation therapy for feline ISS
Although ISS response to external beam radiation can be unpredictable, it plays an important role in large fixed tumours where CT shows that achieving tumour-free margins by surgery alone will be difficult.

- Preoperative radiation will sterilize the reactive zone and surrounding 'clean' tissues and so allow for a potentially smaller resection to be performed.
- Postoperative radiation can be used when a curative-intent surgery has been unsuccessful and residual tumour disease remains (see Figure 14.17).

The orientation of the scar is an important factor in limiting radiation side effects: a scar in the midline parallel to the spine will result in minimal dose to the spinal cord, as the beams can be targeted from laterally to 'skyline' the scar. If the scar runs perpendicular to the spine and extends down over the thoracic wall on both sides, then there is a much greater risk of including the spinal cord within the planned treatment volume.

The postoperative treatment is started 10–14 days after surgery when the surgical site has already healed. If radiation is given preoperatively, the dose is often lower to avoid overly damaging the skin and so reduce the risk of creating a non-healing wound following surgery.

Prognosis: Using preoperative cobalt 60 in combination with surgery, median time to recurrence was 2.7 years following complete excision and 0.8 years if incompletely excised (Kobayashi et al., 2002). Surgery followed by megavoltage radiation gave median survivals of 23–24 months, but time to recurrence and survival were decreased when time to surgery and starting radiation was increased (Bregazzi et al., 2001; Cohen et al., 2001).

Reported rates of local recurrence range from 25% to 60% (Kobayashi et al., 2002; Martano et al., 2005; Banerji and Kanjilal, 2006; Hahn et al., 2007; Romanelli et al., 2008) after various combinations of surgery, radiation (pre- or postoperative) and chemotherapy. Rates of metastasis range from 5.6% to 22.5% (Cohen et al., 2001; Kobayashi et al., 2002; Poirier et al., 2002; Romanelli et al., 2008). Pulmonary metastasis is most commonly reported, with other sites including regional lymph nodes, skin, intestine, spleen, epidural and ocular infiltration, or multi-organ involvement (Hershey et al., 2000; Kobayashi et al., 2002; Cohen et al., 2003; Chang et al., 2006).

Prevention of feline ISS
Preventive measures include:

- Not over-vaccinating
- Keeping detailed vaccination records
- Vaccinating in locations that can be easily resected in the future (e.g. mid-distal thigh, treatable by amputation)
- Excising or biopsying vaccine-site reactions that:
  o Persist over 4 months
  o Are >2 cm in diameter
  o Increase in size 1 month after vaccination (Hershey et al., 2000).

References and further reading

Al-Sarraf R (1998) Update on feline vaccine-associated fibrosarcomas. *Veterinary Medicine* **93**, 729–735
Avallone G, Helmbold P, Caniatti M et al. (2007) The spectrum of canine cutaneous perivascular wall tumours: morphologic, phenotypic and clinical characterization. *Veterinary Pathology* **44**, 607–620
Bacon NJ, Dernell WS and Ehrhart N (2007) Evaluation of primary re-excision after recent inadequate resection of soft tissue sarcomas in dogs: 41 cases (1999–2004). *Journal of the American Veterinary Medical Association* **230**, 548–554
Baez J, Hendrick M, Shofer F et al. (2004) Liposarcomas in dogs: 56 cases (1989–2000) *Journal of the American Veterinary Medical Association* **224**, 887–891
Baker-Gabb M, Hunt GB and France MP (2003) Soft tissue sarcomas and mast cell tumours in dogs; clinical behaviour and response to surgery. *Australian Veterinary Journal* **81**, 732–738
Banerji N and Kanjilal S. (2006) Somatic alterations of the p53 tumor suppressor gene in vaccine-associated feline sarcoma. *American Journal of Veterinary Research* **67**, 1766–1772
Bregazzi VS, LaRue SM, McNiel E et al. (2001) Treatment with a combination of doxorubicin, surgery, and radiation versus surgery and radiation alone for cats with vaccine-associated sarcomas: 25 cases (1995–2000). *Journal of the American Veterinary Medical Association* **218**, 547–550
Chang HW, Ho SY, Lo HF et al. (2006) Vaccine-associated rhabdomyosarcoma with spinal epidural invasion and pulmonary metastasis in a cat. *Veterinary Pathology* **43**, 55–58
Cohen M, Sartin EA, Whitley EM et al. (2003) Ocular metastasis of a vaccine-associated fibrosarcoma in a cat. *Veterinary and Comparative Oncology* **1**, 232–240
Cohen M, Wright JC, Brawner WR et al. (2001) Use of surgery and electron beam irradiation, with or without chemotherapy, for treatment of vaccine-associated sarcomas in cats: 78 cases (1996–2000). *Journal of the American Veterinary Medical Association* **219**, 1582–1589
Craig LE, Julian ME and Ferracone JD (2002) The diagnosis and prognosis of synovial tumors in dogs: 35 cases. *Veterinary Pathology* **39**, 66–73
Cronin K, Page RL, Spodnick G et al. (1998) Radiation therapy and surgery for fibrosarcoma in 33 cats. *Veterinary Radiology and Ultrasound* **39**, 51–56
Davidson EB, Gregory CR and Kass PH (1997) Surgical excision of soft tissue fibrosarcomas in cats. *Veterinary Surgery* **26**, 265–269
Davis KM, Hardie EM, Lascelles BD et al. (2007) Feline fibrosarcoma: perioperative management. *Compendium: Continuing Education for Veterinarians* **29**, 712–729
Dernell WS, Withrow SJ, Kuntz CA et al. (1998) Principles of treatment for soft tissue sarcoma. *Clinical Techniques in Small Animal Practice* **13**, 59–64

Dillon CJ, Mauldin GN and Baer KE (2005) Outcome following surgical removal of nonvisceral soft tissue sarcomas in cats: 42 cases (1992–2000). *Journal of the American Veterinary Medical Association* **227**, 1955–1957

Dobson JM, Samuel S, Milstein H *et al.* (2002) Canine neoplasia in the UK; estimates of incidence rates from a population of insured dogs. *Journal of Small Animal Practice* **43**, 240–246

Doddy FD, Glickman LT, Glickman NW *et al.* (1996) Feline fibrosarcomas at vaccination sites and non-vaccination sites. *Journal of Comparative Pathology* **114**, 165–174

Elmslie RE, Glawe P and Dow SW (2008) Metronomic therapy with cyclophosphamide and piroxicam effectively delays tumor recurrence in dogs with incompletely resected soft tissue sarcomas. *Journal of Veterinary Internal Medicine* **22**, 1373–1379

Enneking WF, Spanier SS and Goodman MA (1980) A system for the surgical staging of musculoskeletal sarcoma. *Clinical Orthopaedics and Related Research* **153**, 106–120

Ettinger S, Scase T and Oberthaler K (2006) Association of argyrophilic nucleolar organizing regions, Ki-67, and proliferating cell nuclear antigen scores with histologic grade and survival in dogs with soft tissue sarcomas: 60 cases (1996–2002). *Journal of the American Veterinary Medical Association* **228**,1053–1062

Farese JP, Bacon NJ, Ehrhart NP *et al.* (2007) Oesophageal leiomyosarcoma in dogs: surgical management and clinical outcome of four cases. *Veterinary and Comparative Oncology* **6**, 31–38

Forrest LJ, Chun R, Adams WM *et al.* (2000) Postoperative radiotherapy for canine soft tissue sarcoma. *Journal of Veterinary Internal Medicine* **14**, 578–582

Fulmer AK and Mauldin GE (2007) Canine histiocytic neoplasia: an overview. *Canadian Veterinary Journal* **48**, 1041–1050

Gobar GM and Kass PH (2002) World wide web-based survey of vaccination practices, postvaccinal reactions, and vaccine site-associated sarcomas in cats. *Journal of the American Veterinary Medical Association* **220**, 1477–1482

Goldschmidt MH and Hendrick MJ (2002) Tumors of the skin and soft tissues. In: *Tumors in Domestic Animals, 4th edn*, ed. DJ Meuten, pp. 89–91. Iowa State Univ Press, Ames, Iowa

Hahn K, Endicott M, King G *et al.* (2007) Evaluation of radiotherapy alone or in combination with doxorubicin chemotherapy for the treatment of cats with incompletely excised soft tissue sarcomas: 71 cases (1989–1999). *Journal of the American Veterinary Medical Association* **231**, 742–745

Hargis AM, Ihrke PJ, Spangler WL *et al.* (1992) A retrospective clinicopathological study of 212 dogs with cutaneous hemangiomas and hemangiosarcomas. *Veterinary Pathology* **29**, 316–328

Hendrick MJ, Shofer FS, Goldschmidt MH *et al.* (1994) Comparison of fibrosarcomas that developed at vaccination sites and at non-vaccination sites in cats: 239 cases (1991–1992). *Journal of the American Veterinary Medical Association* **205**, 1425–1429

Hershey AE, Sorenmo KU, Hendrick MJ *et al.* (2000) Prognosis for presumed feline vaccine-associated sarcoma after excision: 61 cases (1986–1996). *Journal of the American Veterinary Medical Association* **216**, 58–61

Hillers KR, Lana SE, Fuller CR *et al.* (2007) Effects of palliative radiation therapy on nonsplenic hemangiosarcoma in dogs. *Journal of the American Veterinary Animal Hospital Association* **43**, 187–192

Johannes CM, Henry CJ and Turnquist SE (2007) Hemangiosarcoma in cats: 53 cases (1992–2002). *Journal of the American Veterinary Medical Association* **231**, 1851–1856

Kass PH, Barnes WG, Spangler WL *et al.* (1993) Epidemiologic evidence for a causal relation between vaccination and fibrosarcoma tumorigenesis in cats. *Journal of the American Veterinary Medical Association* **203**, 396–405

Kass PH, Spangler WL, Hendrick MJ *et al.* (2003) Multicenter case-control study of risk factors associated with development of vaccine-associated sarcomas in cats. *Journal of the American Veterinary Medical Association* **223**, 1283–1292

Kobayashi T, Hauck ML, Dodge R *et al.* (2002) Preoperative radiotherapy for vaccine associated sarcoma in 92 cats. *Veterinary Radiology and Ultrasound* **43**, 473–479

Kraje AC, Mears EA, Hahn KA *et al.* (1999) Unusual metastatic behavior and clinicopathologic findings in eight cats with cutaneous or visceral hemangiosarcoma. *Journal of the American Veterinary Medical Association* **214**, 670–672

Kuntz CA, Dernell WS, Powers BE *et al.* (1997) Prognostic factors for surgical treatment of soft-tissue sarcomas in dogs: 75 cases (1986–1996). *Journal of the American Veterinary Medical Association* **211**, 1147–1151

Lawrence J, Forrest L, Adams W *et al.* (2008) Four-fraction radiation therapy for macroscopic soft tissue sarcomas in 16 dogs. *Journal of the American Veterinary Medical Association* **44**, 100–108

Maas CPHJ, Ter Haar G, Van der Gaag I *et al.* (2007) Reclassification of small intestinal and cecal smooth muscle tumors in 72 dogs: clinical, histologic, and immunohistochemical evaluation. *Veterinary Surgery* **36**, 302–313

Macy DW and Hendrick MJ (1996) The potential role of inflammation in the development of postvaccinal sarcomas in cats. *Veterinary Clinics of North America: Small Animal Practise* **26**, 103–109

Marioni-Henry K, Van Winkle TJ and Smith SH (2008) Tumors affecting the spinal cord of cats: 85 cases (1980–2005) *Journal of the American Veterinary Medical Association* **232**, 237–243

Martano M, Morello M, Ughetto M *et al.* (2005) Surgery alone versus surgery and doxorubicin for the treatment of feline injection-site sarcomas: a report on 69 cases. *The Vet Journal* **170**, 84–90

McAbee KP, Ludwig LL, Bergman PJ *et al.* (2005) Feline cutaneous hemangiosarcoma: a retrospective study of 18 cases (1998–2003). *Journal of the American Animal Hospitals Association* **41**, 110–116

McEntee MC and Thrall DE (2001) Computed tomographic imaging of infiltrative lipoma in 22 dogs. *Veterinary Radiology and Ultrasound* **42**, 221–225

McEntee MC, Page RL, Mauldin GN *et al.* (2000) Results of irradiation of infiltrative lipoma in 13 dogs. *Veterinary Radiology and Ultrasound* **41**, 554–556

McEntee MC and Samii VF (2000) The utility of contrast enhanced computed tomography in feline vaccine associated sarcomas: 35 cases [abstract]. *Veterinary Radiology and Ultrasound* **41**, 575

McKnight JA, Mauldin GN, McEntee MC *et al.* (2000) Radiation treatment for incompletely resected soft-tissue sarcomas in dogs. *Journal of the American Veterinary Medical Association* **217**, 205–210

Miller MA, Nelson SL, Turk JR *et al.* (1991) Cutaneous neoplasia in 340 cats. *Veterinary Pathology* **28**, 389–395

Plavec T, Kessler M, Kandel B *et al.* (2006) Palliative radiotherapy as treatment for non-resectable soft tissue sarcomas in the dog – a report of 15 cases. *Veterinary Comparative Oncology* **4**, 98–103

Poirier VJ, Thamm DH, Kurzman ID *et al.* (2002) Liposome-encapsulated doxorubicin (Doxil) and doxorubicin in the treatment of vaccine-associated sarcoma in cats. *Journal of Veterinary Internal Medicine* **16**, 726–731

Powers BE, Hoopes PJ and Ehrhart EJ (1995) Tumor diagnosis, grading and staging. *Seminars in Veterinary Medicine and Surgery* **10**, 158–167

Romanelli G, Marconato L, Olivero D *et al.* (2008) Analysis of prognostic factors associated with injection-site sarcomas in cats: 57 cases (2001–2007). *Journal of the American Veterinary Medical Association* **232**, 1193–1199

Russell KN, Mehler SJ, Skorupski KA *et al.* (2007) Clinical and immunohistochemical differentiation of gastrointestinal stromal tumors from leiomyosarcomas in dogs: 42 cases (1990–2003). *Journal of the Veterinary Medical Association* **230**, 1329–1333

Séguin B (2002) Injection site sarcomas in cats. *Clinical Techniques in Small Animal Practice* **17**, 168–173

Selting KA, Powers BE and Thompson LJ (2005) Outcome of dogs with high-grade soft tissue sarcomas treated with and without adjuvant doxorubicin chemotherapy: 39 cases (1996–2004). *Journal of the American Veterinary Medical Association* **227**, 1442–1448

Shaw SC, Kent MS, Gordon IK *et al.* (2009) Temporal changes in characteristics of injection-site sarcomas in cats; 392 cases (1990–2006). *Journal of the American Veterinary Medical Association* **234**, 376–380

Sorenmo KU, Jeglum KA and Helfand SC (1993) Chemotherapy of canine hemangiosarcoma with doxorubicin and cyclophosphamide. *Journal of Veterinary Internal Medicine* **1993**, 370–376

Sorensen KC, Kitchell BE, Schaeffer DJ *et al.* (2004) Expression of matrix metalloproteinases in feline vaccine site-associated sarcomas. *American Journal of Veterinary Research* **65**, 373–379

Stefanello D, Morello E, Roccabianca P *et al.* (2008) Marginal excision of low-grade spindle cell sarcoma of canine extremities: 35 dogs (1996–2006). *Veterinary Surgery* **37**, 461–465

Theilen GH and Madewell BR (1979) Tumours of the skin and subcutaneous tissues. In: *Veterinary Cancer Medicine*, ed. GH Theilen and BR Madewell, pp. 123–191. Lea and Febiger, Philadelphia

Vaccine-Associated Feline Sarcoma Task Force (2005) The current understanding and management of vaccine-associated sarcomas in cats. *Journal of the American Veterinary Medical Association* **226**, 1821–1842

Vail DM, Powers BE, Getzy DM *et al.* (1994) Evaluation of prognostic factors for dogs with synovial sarcoma: 36 cases (1986–1991). *Journal of the American Veterinary Medical Association* **205**, 1300–1307

Ward H, Fox LE, Calderwood-Mays MB *et al.* (1994) Cutaneous hemangiosarcoma in 25 dogs: a retrospective study. *Journal of Veterinary Internal Medicine* **8**, 345–348

Oral tumours

B. Duncan X. Lascelles

Introduction

Oral tumours are common in both cats and dogs, with cancers of the oral cavity accounting for 3–12% and 6% of all tumours in these species, respectively.

The most common malignant tumours of the mandible and maxilla in dogs are, in descending order, malignant melanoma, squamous cell carcinoma (SCC) and fibrosarcoma (FSA). Other malignant oral tumours include osteosarcoma (OSA), chondrosarcoma, anaplastic sarcoma, multilobular osteochondrosarcoma, intraosseous carcinoma, myxosarcoma, haemangiosarcoma, lymphoma, mast cell tumour (MCT), and transmissible venereal tumour. SCC is the

most common oropharyngeal cancer in cats and the most frequently diagnosed tumour in the tongue of dogs. A summary of the common oral tumours is given in Figure 15.1. Oral tumours cannot be distinguished by appearance alone (Figure 15.2), emphasizing the importance of biopsy early in the evaluation of oral masses.

It is important to remember that benign tumours are probably at least as common as malignant tumours in the dog, and so biopsy is always indicated prior to any definitive treatment. Benign tumours include the 'epulis' group, as well as viral papillomatosis, ameloblastoma and non-neoplastic gingival hyperplasia.

	Dogs				Cats	
	Malignant melanoma	Squamous cell carcinoma	Fibrosarcoma	Epulides	Squamous cell carcinoma	Fibrosarcoma
Frequency (of all oral tumours)	15–20%	8–15%	5–12%	40–50%	70–80%	15–20%
Average age (years) at presentation	12	8–10	7–9	Variable	10–12	10
Sex predisposition	Male (slight)	None	Male	None	None	None
Animal size	Smaller	Larger	Larger	None	no data	no data
Sites of predilection	Gingiva Buccal and labial mucosa	Rostral mandible	Maxillary gingiva Hard palate	Rostral mandible	Tongue Pharynx Tonsils	Gingiva
Lymph node metastasis	Common (40–75%)	Rare (<40%) Tonsillar SCC up to 73%	Occasional (10–30%)	None	Rare	Rare
Distant metastasis	Common (15–90%)	Rare (<35%)	Occasional (0–70%)	None	Rare	Rare (<20%)
Gross appearance	Pigmented (67%) or amelanotic (33%); ulcerated	Red; cauliflower, ulcerated	Flat, firm, ulcerated	Variable	Proliferative; ulcerated	Firm
Bone involvement	Common (60%)	Common (80%)	Common (60–70%)	Common (80–100%) with acanthomatous; does not occur with fibrous and ossifying types	Common	Common

15.1 Summary of presentation of common oral tumours in the dog and cat.

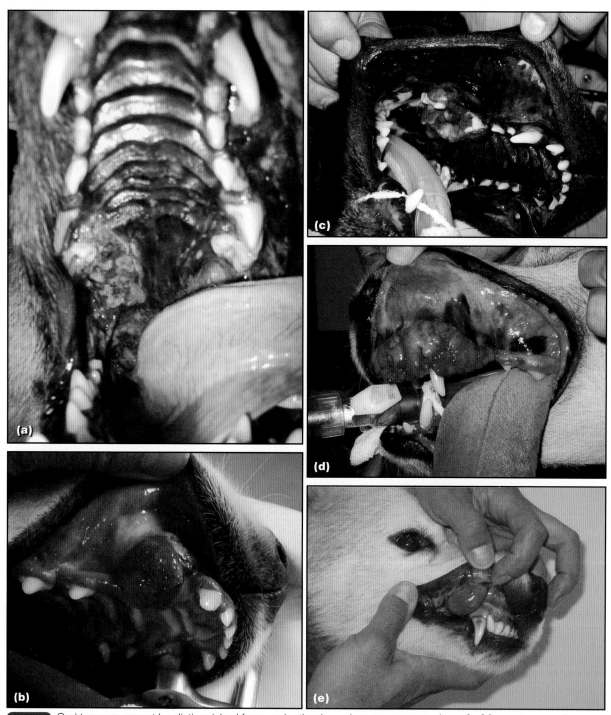

15.2 Oral tumours cannot be distinguished from each other based on appearance alone: **(a,b)** squamous cell carcinoma; **(c)** melanoma; **(d)** fibrosarcoma; **(e)** mast cell tumour.

Tumour types and behaviour

Oral tumours in dogs

Malignant melanoma

In contrast to other malignant oral tumours, malignant melanoma tends to occur in smaller breeds as well as some large breeds, with an average age of 11 years. Cocker Spaniel, Miniature Poodle, Anatolian Sheepdog, Gordon Setter, Chow Chow and Golden Retriever are over-represented. Malignant melanoma can be difficult to diagnose if the tumour or biopsy section does not contain melanin; amelanotic melanomas represent up to one-third of all oral melanomas in dogs. Underlying melanoma can be present with a returned histopathological diagnosis of undifferentiated or anaplastic sarcoma, or even of epithelial cancer. If the clinician is suspicious of this, melan A is an immunohistochemical stain with a high sensitivity and specificity for the diagnosis of melanoma in dogs and can be used along with S100 and HMB45 to differentiate melanoma from other poorly differentiated oral tumours (see also Chapter 2).

Melanoma of the oral cavity is a highly malignant tumour that frequently metastasizes (reported in up to 80% of dogs). The metastatic rate depends on site, size and stage. Malignant melanoma is a highly immunogenic tumour, and molecular approaches to treatment, particularly genetic immunotherapy, is an active area of research and treatment.

Squamous cell carcinoma

SCC is the second most common oral tumour in dogs and frequently invades bone. The metastatic rate for non-tonsillar SCC in dogs is approximately 20%, but the metastatic risk is site-dependent, with rostral tumours having a low metastatic rate and the caudal tongue and tonsil having a high metastatic potential. The tonsillar and lingual sites are the most important non-gingival sites in the dog. Tonsillar lesions metastasize to the regional (retropharyngeal) nodes in almost all cases. Distant metastasis may develop in patients that survive for longer.

Fibrosarcoma

Oral FSA is the third most common oral tumour in dogs. It tends to occur in large breeds, particularly the Golden and Labrador Retriever, with a median age of about 8 years, and there may be a male predisposition. Oral FSA may appear surprisingly benign histologically and, even with large biopsy samples, the pathologist will often diagnose fibroma or 'low-grade FSA'. This syndrome, which is common on the hard palate and maxillary arcade between the canine and carnassial teeth of large-breed dogs, has been termed 'histologically low-grade but biologically high-grade' FSA (Ciekot *et al.*, 1994). Treatment should be aggressive, especially if the cancer is rapidly growing, recurrent or invading bone. FSA is very locally invasive, but metastasizes to the lungs and, occasionally, regional lymph nodes in <30% of dogs.

Osteosarcoma

OSA of axial sites is less common than appendicular OSA (axial represents approximately 25% of all OSA), and about 25% of axial OSAs occur in the mandible and maxilla. The prognosis for dogs with oral OSA is better than that for dogs with appendicular OSA because of a lower metastatic potential, but this finding is controversial.

Epulides

Epulides are relatively common in dogs. Epulides are benign gingival proliferations arising from the periodontal ligament and appear similar to gingival hyperplasia. In general, four types of epulides have been described in the dog: fibromatous; ossifying; acanthomatous; and giant cell. However, the nomenclature is confusing, and varied, and the clinician is encouraged to speak directly to the pathologist if there are any questions over terminology. The term 'epulis' strictly refers to any tumour that arises from the gingiva but for a long time has been used to designate tumours that arise from the periodontal ligament. These were further described as being one of three main forms – fibromatous, ossifying or acanthomatous. However, more recently it has been shown that some of these tumours do not involve the periodontal ligament, with many of the fibromatous and ossifying types being derived from the gingiva. Acanthomatous epulis has been referred to as basal cell carcinoma and, more recently, as acanthomatous ameloblastoma, although the term acanthomatous epulis is still used. Adamantinoma is another term that has also been used for either ameloblastoma or acanthomatous ameloblastoma.

Acanthomatous epulis is a benign tumour but with an aggressive local behaviour and frequent invasion into bone of the underlying mandible or maxilla. The rostral mandible is the most common site. They do not metastasize. Acanthomatous epulis is the preferred term, but some pathologists will refer to these tumours by other terms (see above).

Fibromatous and ossifying epulides are benign oral tumours that, unlike acanthomatous epulides, do not tend to invade into underlying bone. They are slow-growing, firm masses and are usually covered by intact epithelium. Ossifying epulides usually have a broad base of attachment and are less pedunculated than fibromatous epulides. These two epulides are histologically differentiated by the presence or absence of bone within the tumour.

Oral tumours in cats

Squamous cell carcinoma

SCC is the most common oral tumour in cats. Reported risk factors for the development of oral SCC include flea collars, high intake of either canned food in general or canned tuna fish specifically, and exposure to household smoke (Bertone *et al.*, 2003). Bone invasion is frequent and is usually severe and extensive. Paraneoplastic hypercalcaemia has been reported in two cats with oral SCC. The metastatic rate in the cat is unknown, since so few cats have their local disease controlled to allow observation of the long-term metastatic potential.

Odontogenic tumours

These originate from epithelial cells of the dental lamina, and account for up to 2.4% of all feline oral tumours. They are broadly classified into two groups depending on whether the tumours are able to induce a stromal reaction – inductive and non-inductive. Inductive odontogenic tumours include ameloblastic fibroma, dentinoma, and ameloblastic, complex and compound odontomas. Ameloblastomas and calcifying epithelial odontogenic tumours are examples of non-inductive odontogenic tumours.

Inductive fibroameloblastoma is the most common odontogenic tumour in cats, occurring in cats less than 18 months of age and often in the region of the upper canine teeth and maxilla. Radiographically, there are varying degrees of bone destruction, production, and expansion of the mandibular or maxillary bones. Smaller lesions are treated with surgical debulking and cryosurgery or premaxillectomy. Larger lesions will respond to radiation. With aggressive local treatment, control rates are good and metastasis has not been reported.

Eosinophilic granuloma

Eosinophilic granuloma (rodent ulcer or indolent ulcer) occurs more commonly in female than in male cats, with a mean age of 5 years. The aetiology is unknown. Any oral site is at risk but the tumour is most common on the upper lip near the midline. The history is usually that of a slowly progressive (months to years) erosion of the lip. Biopsy is often necessary to differentiate the condition from true cancers. Care should be taken to rule out any underlying hypersensitivity as a cause. Various treatments have been proposed, including: oral prednisone (1–2 mg/kg q12h for 30 days) or subcutaneous methylprednisolone (20 mg/cat every 2 weeks); megestrol; hypoallergenic diets; radiation therapy; surgery; immunomodulation; or cryosurgery. The prognosis for complete and permanent recovery is fair, and rare cases may undergo spontaneous regression.

Other tumour types

Oral FSA is the second most common oral tumour in cats but very little is reported on its biological behaviour. Epulides have also been reported in cats. The most common are the fibromatous and giant cell epulides; acanthomatous and ossifying epulides are rare in cats.

Presentation and clinical signs

Most cats and dogs with oral cancer present with a mass in the mouth noticed by the owner. Cancer in the caudal pharynx, however, is rarely seen by the owner, and the animal is often presented at a later stage of disease, which results in fewer options for treatment. The animal may present with signs of hypersalivation, exophthalmos or facial swelling, epistaxis, weight loss, halitosis, bloody oral discharge, dysphagia or pain on opening the mouth, or occasionally cervical lymphadenopathy (especially in SCC of the tonsil). Loose teeth, especially in an animal with generally good dentition, may be indicative of underlying neoplastic bone lysis, especially in cats. *A complete examination of the oral cavity during annual health checks is recommended* to screen for oropharyngeal masses, as this may permit earlier diagnosis, better treatment and improved prognosis.

Clinical approach

Diagnosis and clinical staging

Biopsy

Biopsy is required for definitive diagnosis and will assist the clinician in determining biological behaviour and prognosis. Indeed, the author recommends biopsy before any other staging, as the tumour type will influence the staging required. Touch or aspiration cytology preparations are usually not rewarding, and can result in an incorrect diagnosis since many oral tumours are associated with a high degree of

necrosis and inflammation. A large incisional biopsy is recommended. Cautery should only be used for haemostasis after blade incision or punch biopsy, so as not to damage the specimen. Care must be taken not to contaminate normal tissue that cannot be removed with surgery or included in the radiation field. If the lesion is small and an excisional biopsy is performed, detailed notes should be recorded about exactly where the sample was taken from (possibly with supporting photographs) so that any follow-up therapy that is required can be targeted to the correct area.

Clinical staging

Local tumour imaging: Regional radiographs of the skull, or dental films, can be useful in delineating the extent of disease, but bone lysis is not radiographically evident until 40% or more of the cortex is destroyed and hence apparently normal radiographs do not exclude bone invasion. Advanced imaging modalities are now widely available and these are recommended for imaging of oral tumours, particularly tumours arising from the maxilla, palate and caudal mandible. Computed tomography (CT) scans are generally preferred to magnetic resonance imaging (MRI) because of superior bone detail, but both CT and MRI provide more information on the local extent of the tumour than regional radiographs. This information is important for planning the definitive surgical procedure (or radiation therapy if indicated).

Regional lymph nodes: Regional lymph nodes should be carefully palpated for enlargement or asymmetry. However, caution should be exercised when making clinical judgements based on palpation alone, as lymph node size is not an accurate predictor of metastasis. In one study of 100 dogs with oral melanoma, 40% of dogs with normal sized lymph nodes had metastasis and 49% of dogs with enlarged lymph nodes did not (Williams and Packer, 2003). Furthermore, the regional lymph nodes include the mandibular, parotid and medial retropharyngeal lymph nodes. *En bloc* resection of the regional lymph nodes has been described and, although the therapeutic benefit of this approach is unknown, it may provide valuable staging information (Herring *et al.*, 2002; Smith, 1995).

Distant metastasis: Three-view thoracic radiographs (right and left lateral plus dorsoventral or ventrodorsal views) are generally recommended to evaluate animals for thoracic metastasis; right and left lateral views are the minimum requirement. Helical CT scans should be considered for animals with highly metastatic tumour types, such as oral malignant melanoma, since CT scans are significantly more sensitive than radiographs for detecting pulmonary metastatic lesions.

Based on these steps, oral tumours are then clinically staged according to the World Health Organization (WHO) staging scheme (Figure 15.3).

T – Primary tumour	
Tis	Tumour *in situ*
T1	Tumour <2 cm in diameter at greatest dimension
T1a	Without evidence of bone invasion
T1b	With evidence of bone invasion
T2	Tumour 2–4 cm in diameter at greatest dimension
T2a	Without evidence of bone invasion
T2b	With evidence of bone invasion
T3	Tumour >4 cm in diameter at greatest dimension
T3a	Without evidence of bone invasion
T3b	With evidence of bone invasion
N – Regional lymph node status	
N0	No metastasis to regional lymph nodes
N1	Movable ipsilateral lymph nodes
N1a	No evidence of lymph node metastasis
N1b	Evidence of lymph node metastasis
N2	Movable contralateral lymph nodes
N2a	No evidence of lymph node metastasis
N2b	Evidence of lymph node metastasis
M – Distant metastasis	
M0	No distant metastasis
M1	Distant metastasis [specify sites]

(a) TNM classification.

I	T1	N0, N1a, N2a	M0
II	T2	N0, N1a, N2a	M0
III	T3	N0, N1a, N2a	M0
	Any T	N1b	M0
IV	Any T	N2b, N3	M0
	Any T	Any N	M1

(b) Stage grouping.

15.3 Clinical staging (TNM) of oral tumours in dogs and cats.

Management

Clinical series have been reported of over 500 dogs with various oral malignancies, treated with either mandibulectomy or maxillectomy. The majority of these were treated with surgery alone, indicating the important role surgery plays in the management of oral tumours. Other surgical procedures include hard palate resection and partial/total glossectomy. In general, maxillofacial surgery should be referred to a specialist veterinary surgeon. Detailed surgical approaches are described and illustrated in other books, including the *BSAVA Manual of Canine and Feline Head, Neck and Thoracic Surgery.*

Surgery

Surgical excision is the most commonly used modality for treatment of the local oral tumour, and surgical approach depends on tumour type and location. Except for fibromatous and ossifying epulides, the majority of tumours involving the mandible, maxilla and hard palate have some underlying bone involvement, and surgical resection of these should include bony margins to increase the likelihood of complete excision. Radical surgeries such as mandibulectomy and maxillectomy are well tolerated by cats and dogs (see Chapter 13). These procedures are indicated for oral tumours involving the mandible and maxilla, particularly lesions with extensive bone invasion and tumour types that have poor sensitivity to radiation therapy.

A detailed knowledge of the regional anatomy is important for a successful outcome and to minimize the risk of complications. The anatomy should be reviewed prior to surgery, in combination with either CT or MRI images of the patient, to plan the surgical approach, resection and reconstruction. Cat and dog skulls should be available for intraoperative orientation and planning.

Effective pain management is of paramount importance in any surgery (see Chapters 6 and 11).

Margins

Minimum margins of at least 2 cm, and preferably 3 cm, have been recommended for malignant cancers such as SCC, malignant melanoma and fibrosarcoma in the dog, but this is unrealistic in most cases. It is the author's opinion that most of the published work has involved margins of 0.5–1.0 cm (see below). Likewise, it has been suggested that SCC in the cat should be treated with surgical margins >2 cm because of high local recurrence rates. This is not usually realistic; such margins may not be possible without significant morbidity because of the extent of the tumour. While such recommended margins would be likely to improve tumour control, the reality is that the reported outcomes of oral surgery for neoplasia are based on narrower margins – approximately a full centimetre of normal tissue beyond the gross margin. Therefore, although wider margins may result in longer disease-free intervals, a working goal of 1 cm is what the clinician should strive for: a 1 cm margin of normal tissue beyond *either* the grossly visible tumour *or* the extent of the tumour as determined by imaging, whichever is greater, is recommended for malignant oral tumours. For benign tumours, a margin of 0.5–1.0 cm is recommended.

Instruments and suture materials

An oscillating saw is preferred for mandibular osteotomies, although pneumatic burrs, Gigli wire and bone cutters can also be used. Osteotomes should be avoided for all non-symphyseal mandibular osteotomies because of the risk of bone shattering.

Monofilament absorbable suture material (e.g. polydioxanone) is recommended for closure of oral defects because it maintains adequate tensile strength for prolonged periods and is relatively inert, which minimizes mucosal irritation and inflammation. Two-layer closure is preferred to one-layer closure because of a reduced risk of incisional dehiscence. Suture material should be passed through bone tunnels if possible, particularly in the hard palate and maxilla, because of increased holding power compared to soft tissue (Figure 15.4).

Outcome

Over 85% of owners are satisfied with the postoperative cosmetic and functional results in terms of eating, drinking and ability to hold objects in the mouth (Lascelles *et al.*, 2003; Northrup *et al.*, 2006). Results should be discussed with owners, preferably using representative postoperative images (e.g. Figures 15.5 to 15.8) prior to obtaining consent for surgical

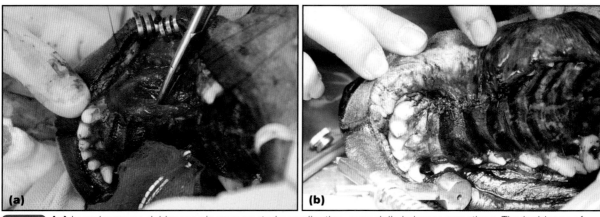

15.4 **(a)** In oral surgery, dehiscence is an expected complication, especially in larger resections. The incidence of dehiscence can be decreased by using holes drilled in bony edges through which to secure sutures.
(b) Closure of the defect has been completed using a two-layer closure. Polydioxanone has been used to close the oral layers; although this is stiffer than polyglactin 910, and potentially more irritating, its more gradual loss of tensile strength results in a longer-lasting suture and decreased dehiscence.

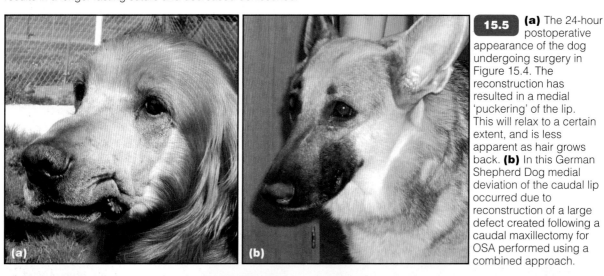

15.5 **(a)** The 24-hour postoperative appearance of the dog undergoing surgery in Figure 15.4. The reconstruction has resulted in a medial 'puckering' of the lip. This will relax to a certain extent, and is less apparent as hair grows back. **(b)** In this German Shepherd Dog medial deviation of the caudal lip occurred due to reconstruction of a large defect created following a caudal maxillectomy for OSA performed using a combined approach.

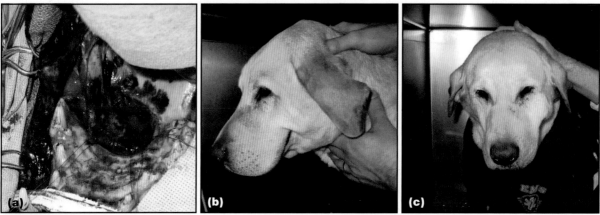

15.6 **(a)** Complete excision of a relatively small, low-grade FSA using full thickness resection of the caudal hard palate. **(b)** Reconstruction was performed using a labial mucosal flap, and the closure of this defect resulted in 'dimpling' of the lateral face. **(c)** Head and neck surgery readily results in swelling.

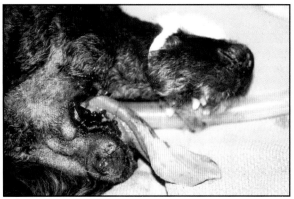

15.7 Postoperative appearance can be dramatically altered following radical oral surgery, such as in this dog with a bilateral rostral mandibulectomy to the level of the 3rd premolar. However, function in this dog was excellent. During surgery, care was taken to avoid the hypoglossal nerve to avoid any functional compromise of the tongue.

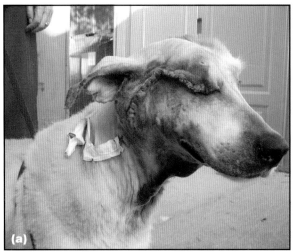

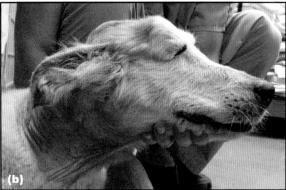

15.8 This dog underwent resection of the zygomatic arch, vertical ramus and caudal maxilla and a partial orbitectomy (including orbital contents) for a low-grade multilobular osteochondrosarcoma. Due to the extent of surgery and some postoperative bleeding, the immediate postoperative appearance of the dog **(a)** is startling. Note the analgesic catheter on the lateral aspect of the neck of the dog – a technique that ensures the dog is kept maximally comfortable postoperatively. Owners should be over-warned about the postoperative alteration of their pet's features. **(b)** After several weeks, however, the appearance of the dog is very reasonable. Part of the pigmented tissue around the eyelid had been left in place as this was considered cosmetically more acceptable to the owner, and did not compromise the resection.

treatment. The cosmetic appearance is usually very good following most mandibulectomy and maxillectomy procedures, but can be challenging with aggressive bilateral rostral mandibulectomies and radical maxillectomies (Lascelles *et al.*, 2003).

Complications

Blood loss and hypotension are the most common intraoperative complications, particularly during caudal maxillectomy (Lascelles *et al.*, 2003). Postoperative complications are uncommon but include incisional dehiscence (Figure 15.9), epistaxis, increased salivation, mandibular drift and malocclusion, and difficulty prehending food. Enteral feeding tubes are not usually required following oral surgery in dogs, but are recommended for cats treated with any type of mandibulectomy as eating can be difficult for 2–4 months following surgery (Figure 15.10).

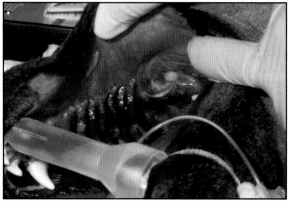

15.9 Dehiscence can occur following oral surgery. It is minimized by adhering to appropriate surgical principles and by minimizing tension. Pre- or postoperative radiation therapy increases the chance of dehiscence occurring, as in the patient shown here. In this case, multiple surgical attempts to close the small oronasal fistula were unsuccessful, and so a 'nasal septal button' was placed to 'plug' the fistula. This was a permanent placement, and the dog died several years later of disease unrelated to the oral tumour.

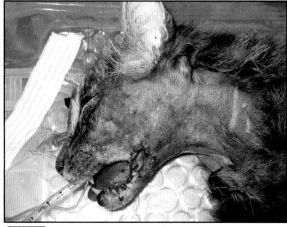

15.10 Although dogs generally function extremely well after radical resections, cats tend not to function as well, and feeding tubes should always be placed after radical oral surgery. Owners should be warned that cats may not learn to eat on their own, and may require their owners to groom them.

Multimodal management

Radiation therapy

This can be effective for locoregional control of oral tumours. It can be used as a primary treatment, with palliative or curative intent, or as an adjunct for incompletely resected tumours or those with an aggressive local behaviour, e.g. oral FSA. Malignant melanoma, canine oral SCC, and some benign tumours, such as the acanthomatous epulides, are known to be responsive to radiation, and radiation therapy can be considered in the primary treatment of these tumours (although surgery is still the treatment of choice due to the risk of osteonecrosis developing following radiation treatment).

For canine oral SCC, dental tumours and FSA, daily and alternate-day protocols have been described, consisting of 2.7–4.2 Gy per fraction with a total dose ranging from 48 to 57 Gy. Tumour control is better for smaller lesions (T1 and T2 tumours) treated with radiation alone. Local tumour control and survival time can be improved by combining radiation therapy with surgery, especially for tumours considered to be radiation-resistant, such as canine oral FSA and feline oral SCC. Radiation sensitizers, such as etanidazole and gemcitabine, have been suggested to result in improved response rates in cats with oral SCC, and platinum drugs have been used as radiation sensitizers in dogs with oral melanoma (Jones *et al.*, 2003, Proulx *et al.*, 2003), but their true benefit is controversial.

Oral melanoma is responsive to coarse fractionation protocols. In human patients doses >4 Gy per fraction are recommended, as response rates are significantly better with fractions >8 Gy compared to <4 Gy. However, in one study of dogs with oral melanoma that compared two hypofractionated protocols of 9–10 Gy per fraction with a fully fractionated protocol of 2–4 Gy per fraction, there were no significant differences in either local recurrence rates or survival time (Proulx *et al.*, 2003). Coarse fractionation of oral melanoma has been described in a few cats with limited success, including one complete response and two partial responses.

Acute radiation side effects are common but self-limiting. They include alopecia and moist desquamation, oral mucositis, dysphagia and ocular changes such as blepharitis, conjunctivitis, keratitis and uveitis. Acute side effects of coarse fractionation are less severe than with full-course protocols. Late complications are rare (<5% of cases) but can include permanent alopecia (Figure 15.11), skin fibrosis, bone necrosis and oronasal fistula formation, development of a second malignancy within the radiation field, keratoconjunctivitis sicca, cataract formation and ocular atrophy (see Chapter 8).

Chemotherapy

The major problem with most oral tumours is control of local disease. Chemotherapy would be indicated for some tumours in principle because of their high metastatic potential (e.g. oral melanoma in dogs, tonsillar SCC in cats and dogs) but chemosensitivity is low.

Expression of COX-2 has been noted in feline oral tumours (mainly SCC) (Hayes *et al.*, 2006; DiBernardi *et al.*, 2007) but non-steroidal anti-inflammatory drugs (NSAIDs) such as piroxicam have not been effective in the management of SCC in cats in preliminary unpublished studies. Piroxicam does have some effect against oral SCC in dogs and this response rate is improved when piroxicam is combined with cisplatin (Boria *et al.*, 2004).

Immunotherapy

Malignant melanoma is a highly immunogenic tumour. The use of immunotherapy agents and biological response modifiers is an emerging and exciting approach for the adjunctive management of dogs with oral melanoma. Biological response modifiers, such as *Corynebacterium parvum* and liposome muramyl tripeptide phosphatidylethanolamine (L-MTP-PE), have shown encouraging results compared to control groups in controlled clinical studies. Others, such as bacillus Calmette-Guérin (BCG) and levamisole, however, have failed to improve survival times in dogs with malignant melanoma.

Genetic immunotherapy is an active area of research and current approaches have resulted in significant improvements in local control rates and survival times. These approaches include: systemic administration of interleukin-2 (IL-2) and tumour necrosis factor (TNF); autologous vaccines from

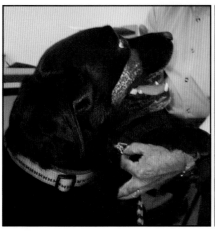
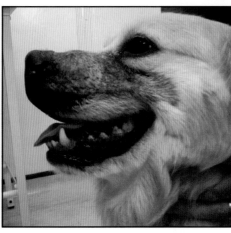

15.11 Radiation of oral tumours can result in side effects. These two dogs show permanent alopecia in the radiation field.

irradiated tumour cells transfected with human recombinant (hr) granulocyte-macrophage colony-stimulating factor (GM-CSF) – a potent haemopoietic and proinflammatory cytokine; direct injection of DNA into tumours to induce expression of staphylococcal enterotoxin B (a superantigen) in combination with either GM-CSF or IL-2; and DNA vaccination with murine or human tyrosinase, which can result in cytotoxic and T-cell responses, with or without hrGM-CSF.

Preliminary results suggest immunotherapeutic approaches, in combination with either surgery and/ or radiation therapy, are promising in the management of oral melanoma. A DNA vaccine with human tyrosine is now commercially available (under restricted licence) for the adjunctive treatment of dogs with completely excised oral malignant melanoma (see Chapter 9).

Prognosis

Figure 15.12 summarizes prognostic data for the common malignant oral tumours in dogs and cats.

With surgical treatment
Overall, the lowest rates of local tumour recurrence and best survival times are reported in dogs with acanthomatous epulis and SCC, while FSA and malignant melanoma are associated with the poorest results (Kosovsky *et al.,* 1991; Schwarz *et al.,* 1991a,b; Wallace *et al.,* 1992a,b). Most of these reports suggest that histologically complete resection

and rostral location are favourable prognostic factors. In two studies of 142 dogs treated with either mandibulectomy or maxillectomy, tumour-related deaths were 10–21 times more likely with malignant tumors, up to 5 times more likely with tumours located caudal to the canine teeth, and 2–4 times more likely following incomplete resection (Schwarz *et al.,*1991a,b). Fibrosarcoma has a high local recurrence rate, whereas melanoma is controlled locally in 75% of cases but metastatic disease caused the death of most dogs. Improved exposure of the tumour to be resected appears to result in improved outcome (Lascelles *et al.,* 2003).

With radiation therapy
For dogs treated with megavoltage radiation, tumour size is the most important factor in local tumour control for both benign and malignant oral tumours. Local recurrence is reported in up to 30% of cases and, compared to T1 tumours (<2 cm diameter), recurrence is three times more likely in T2 tumours (2–4 cm diameter) and up to eight times more likely in T3 tumours (>4 cm diameter). Tumour size is also associated with survival in dogs with malignant oral tumours, with 3-year progression-free survival rates of 55%, 32% and 20% for T1, T2 and T3 tumours, respectively.

Tumours of the tongue
The prognosis for tongue tumours appears to depend on the site, type and grade of cancer. In a recent retrospective study 42 cases of lingual tumours in

	Dogs				Cats	
	Malignant melanoma	Squamous cell carcinoma	Fibrosarcoma	Epulides	Squamous cell carcinoma	Fibrosarcoma
Response to surgery:	Fair to good	Good	Fair to good	Excellent	Poor	Fair
Local recurrence	0–60%	0–50%	30–60%	0–10%	no data	no data
MST	5–17 months	9–26 months	10–12 months	>28–64 months	45 days	no data
1-year survival rate	20–35%	60–90%	20–50%	70–100%	<10%	no data
Response to radation therapy:	Good	Good	Poor to fair	Excellent	Poor	Poor
MST	4–12 months	16–36 months	7–26 months	37+ months	90 days	no data
1-year survival rate	35–70%	70%	77%	85%	40 days	no data
Optimal therapy	Surgery and/or radiation ± immunotherapy	Surgery and/or radiation	Surgery and/or radiation	Surgery	Surgery and/or radiation ± sensitizer	Surgery and/or radiation
Overall prognosis	Poor to fair	Moderate to good	Moderate to good	Excellent	Poor	Fair
Cause of death	Distant metastasis	Local disease or distant metastasis	Local disease	Rarely tumour-related	Local disease	Local disease

15.12 Summary of prognosis for common malignant oral tumours in dogs and cats.

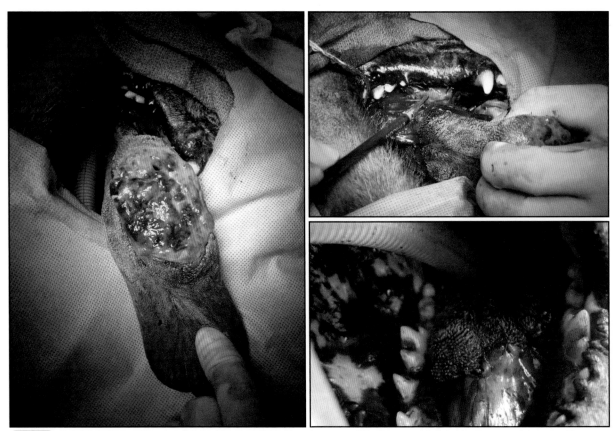

15.13 Subtotal glossectomy performed for a malignant melanoma of the tongue. Histologically, complete resection was achieved and the dog learned to 'suck' up food of a slurry consistency. A surgically placed gastrostomy tube was placed at the time of surgery and used over a 1-month period while the dog learned to suck up food.

dogs were evaluated (Syrcle *et al.,* 2008): 27 (64%) were malignant and 15 (36%) were benign. The overall median survival time (MST) for dogs with benign tumours was >1607 days, compared to 286 days for malignant tumours. Complete resection (Figure 15.13), small tumour size and and benign tumours were associated with increased survival. Short-term morbidity associated with glossectomy included ptyalism and dehiscence. Long-term morbidity included minor changes in eating and drinking habits.

Multilobular osteochondrosarcoma
Multilobular osteochondrosarcoma is an infrequently diagnosed bony and cartilaginous tumour, which usually arises from the canine skull, including the mandible, maxilla and hard palate. Surgery is recommended for management of the local tumour, although there are anecdotal reports that multilobular osteochondrosarcoma may also be responsive to radiation therapy. The overall rate of local recurrence following surgical resection is about 50% and is dependent on completeness of surgical resection and histological grade. The median disease-free interval for completely resected multilobular osteochondrosarcoma is almost 4 years, and significantly better than the 11 months reported for incompletely excised tumours. The local recurrence rate is significantly worse with higher grade. The tumour has a moderate metastatic potential, particularly to the lungs, which is grade-dependent but usually occurs late in the course of disease. Metastasis is significantly more likely following incom-

plete surgical resection, with a 25% metastatic rate in completely excised tumours and 75% following incomplete resection; metastasis is also more likely with higher histological grade. There is no known effective chemotherapy treatment for metastatic disease. Tumour location appears to have prognostic significance, as the outcome for dogs with mandibular multilobular osteochondrosarcoma is significantly better than for tumours at other sites.

References and further reading

Bertone ER, Snyder LA and Moore AS (2003) Environmental and lifestyle risk factors for oral squamous cell carcinoma in domestic cats. *Journal of Veterinary Internal Medicine* **17**, 557–562

Boria, PA, Murry DJ, Bennett PF *et al.* (2004) Evaluation of cisplatin combined with piroxicam for the treatment of oral malignant melanoma and oral squamous cell carcinoma in dogs. *Journal of the American Veterinary Medical Association* **224**, 388–394

Ciekot PA, Powers BA, Withrow SJ et al. (1994) Histologically low-grade, yet biologically high-grade, fibrosarcomas of the mandible and maxilla in dogs: 25 cases (1982–1991). *Journal of the American Veterinary Medical Association* **15**, 610–615

DiBernardi L, Dore M, Davis JA *et al.* (2007) Study of feline oral squamous cell carcinoma: potential target for cyclooxygenase inhibitor treatment. *Prostaglandins Leukotrienes and Essential Fatty Acids* **76**, 245–250

Hayes A, Scase T, Miller J *et al.* (2006) COX-1 and COX-2 expression in feline oral squamous cell carcinoma. *Journal of Comparative Pathology* **135**, 93–99

Herring ES, Smith MM and Robertson JL (2002) Lymph node staging of oral and maxillofacial neoplasms in 31 dogs and cats. *Journal of Veterinary Dentistry* **19**, 122–126

Jones PD, de Lorimier LP, Kitchell BE and Losonsky JM (2003) Gemcitabine as a radiosensitizer for nonresectable feline oral squamous cell carcinoma. *Journal of the American Animal Hospital Association* **39**, 463–467

Kosovsky JK, Matthiesen DT, Marretta SM and Patnaik AK (1991) Results of partial mandibulectomy for the treatment of oral tumors in 142 dogs. *Veterinary Surgery* **20**, 397–401

Lascelles BD, Thomson MJ, Dernell WS *et al.* (2003) Combined dorsolateral and intraoral approach for the resection of tumors of the maxilla in the dog. *Journal of the American Animal Hospital Association* **39**, 294–305

Northrup NC, Selting KA, Rassnick KM *et al.* (2006) Outcomes of cats with oral tumors treated with mandibulectomy: 42 cases. *Journal of the American Animal Hospital Association* **42**, 350–360

Proulx DR, Ruslander DM, Dodge RK *et al.* (2003) A retrospective analysis of 140 dogs with oral melanoma treated with external beam radiation. *Veterinary Radiology and Ultrasound* **44**, 352–359

Schwarz P, Withrow S, Curtis C, Powers B and Straw R (1991a) Mandibular resection as a treatment for oral cancer in 81 dogs. *Journal of the American Animal Hospital Association* **27**, 601–610

Schwarz PD, Withrow SJ, Curtis CR, Powers BE and Straw RC (1991b) Partial maxillary resection as a treatment for oral cancer in 61 dogs. *Journal of the American Animal Hospital Association* **27**, 617–624

Smith MM (1995) Surgical approach for lymph node staging of oral and maxillofacial neoplasms in dogs. *Journal of the American Animal Hospital Association* **31**, 514–518

Syrcle JA, Bonczynski JJ, Monette S and Bergman PJ (2008) Retrospective evaluation of lingual tumors in 42 dogs: 1999–2005. *Journal of the American Animal Hospital Association* **44**, 308–319

Wallace J, Matthiesen DT and Patnaik AK (1992) Hemimaxillectomy for the treatment of oral tumor in 69 dogs. *Veterinary Surgery* **21**, 337–341

Williams LE and Packer RA (2003) Association between lymph node size and metastasis in dogs with oral malignant melanoma: 100 cases (1987–2001). *Journal of the American Veterinary Medical Association* **222**, 1234–1236

15b

Tumours of the salivary glands

Brian J. Trumpatori and Richard A.S. White

Introduction

Tumours of the salivary glands are unusual in the dog, with an overall incidence reported as 0.2% (Koestner and Buerger, 1965; Carberry *et al.*, 1987; Spangler and Culbertson, 1991; Head *et al.*, 2003). In a report of histological evaluation of salivary tissue from both dogs and cats, 30% of the 245 submissions were neoplastic (Spangler and Culbertson, 1991). The mean age of affected dogs and cats is above 10 years. Spaniels were reported to be at greater risk than other breeds (Karbe and Schiefer, 1967) but subsequent studies have not substantiated this. Tumours at this site are equally uncommon in the cat, although one report indicates that Siamese may be over-represented, suggesting a possible breed predisposition (Hammer *et al.*, 2001).

All major glands may be affected, but the mandibular and parotid glands appear to be most frequently involved. Tumours may also be derived from the minor salivary glands scattered throughout the mucosa of the tongue and orpharyngeal surfaces.

Salivary gland tumours can be either benign or malignant, with most of epithelial origin and malignant in nature. Benign salivary tumours are very unusual; they include adenoma and lipoma (Stubbs *et al.*, 1996; Brown *et al.*, 1997; Shimoyama *et al.*, 2006).

Most malignant salivary tumours in the dog and cat are simple adenocarcinomas (Hammer *et al.*, 2001). Other less important histological types include squamous cell carcinoma, basal cell adenocarcinoma, mast cell tumours, osteosarcoma, malignant fibrous histiocytoma, malignant myoepithelioma, oncocytoma, carcinoma ex pleomorphic adenoma, carcinosarcoma (malignant mixed tumour) and complex, anaplastic, mucoepidermoid or clear cell carcinomas. Some obscure tumours of complex origin may require immunohistochemical techniques to identify keratin or vimentin expression for more accurate typing (Perez-Martinez *et al.*, 2000).

Salivary gland tumours may be locally invasive and locoregional lymph node metastasis is common in both dogs and cats. Distant metastasis is less common and may be slower to develop. Reported sites of distant metastasis include, eyes, lung, kidneys and bone. In one study, 17% and 8% of dogs had lymph node and distant metastasis, respectively, at the time of initial diagnosis (Hammer *et al.*, 2001).

Presentation and clinical signs

The most common presenting sign for salivary gland tumours is a palpable mass noticed by the owner (Figures 15.14 and 15.15). The mass is normally non-painful and the patient is otherwise asymptomatic. The location of the swelling may vary depending on the gland involved and may be located at the cranioventral cervical region (mandibular, sublingual glands), base of the ear (parotid gland), upper lip or maxilla (zygomatic gland), or within the mucosa of the upper lip or tongue (accessory salivary tissue). Alternatively, there may be a history of rapidly developing salivary mucoceles caused by erosion or obstruction of the salivary duct (Stubbs *et al.*, 1996). Halitosis and dysphagia may be seen in patients with large masses that have intra-oral involvement. Tumours of the zygomatic gland usually present with exophthalmos. Differential diagnoses for salivary gland masses or enlargement include mucoceles, abscesses, sialadenitis, sialadenosis, necrotizing sialometaplasia, obstructive sialolithiasis and regional lymphadenopathy. Cats are reported to present with more advanced lesions than dogs (Hammer *et al.*, 2001).

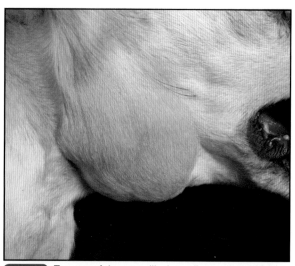

15.14 Tumour of the mandibular salivary gland with associated mucocele.

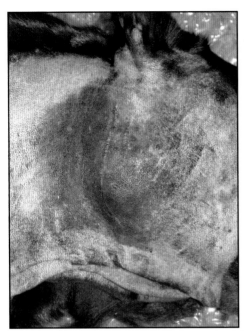

15.15 Tumour of the parotid salivary gland. Surgical biopsy revealed the mass to be an adenocarcinoma.

Clinical approach

Primary lesions should be carefully palpated to assess their infiltration into local tissues. The mandibular and sublingual glands are easy to palpate, but the margins of the parotid gland are more diffuse and, therefore, difficult to assess. Assessment of zygomatic lesions by palpation is not normally possible, due to their location within the orbit. Plain film radiography may reveal periosteal reaction on adjacent osseous structures or distortion of regional anatomy, but alone it is generally insufficient for evaluation of extent or invasiveness.

Diagnostic imaging (Figure 15.16), particularly ultrasonographic examination, may be helpful in further assessment of the mass. When surgical management is contemplated, it may be appropriate to consider contrast-enhanced CT or MRI of the region to assess involvement of the infiltration of surrounding soft tissue structures.

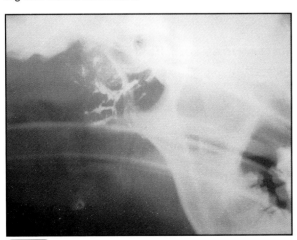

15.16 Sialogram of a parotid adenocarcinoma.

Early diagnosis and treatment are reported to improve survival times significantly in dogs (Hammer *et al.*, 2001). Fine-needle aspiration (FNA) of the primary mass is recommended to differentiate neoplastic from non-neoplastic disease and has been reported for the diagnosis of adenocarcinoma in the dog (Militerno *et al.*, 2005). If this does not provide the necessary answer, incisional wedge biopsy can be performed to obtain a definitive diagnosis. However, the surgeon should ensure that the surgical incision is positioned within the field of subsequent resection. In some cases, tumour-like (but non-neoplastic) lesions such as necrotizing sialometaplasia may be difficult to differentiate from neoplasia even with the aid of histopathology (Militerno *et al.*, 2005).

The regional lymph nodes should be examined initially using palpation and FNA, but subsequent imaging procedures (CT, MRI) may reveal enlargement of regional lymph nodes not readily accessible by palpation. A search for distant metastatic disease that includes thoracic radiographs and abdominal ultrasonography should be made, but in view of the wide distribution of potential target tissues it may be difficult to rule out secondary tumours entirely.

Management

Surgery

Aggressive surgical resection is the treatment of choice for benign and non-metastasized salivary tumours. Due to the invasive nature of most malignant salivary neoplasms, and the close association with vital structures of the head and neck, wide excision may not be possible in many cases. Tumours of the mandibular and sublingual chain are normally amenable to conventional sialoadenectomy, although there is little tissue available for the resection of additional margins of surrounding tissue. Several different surgical techniques may be used.

Mandibular/sublingual sialoadenectomy

Lateral approach: The lateral approach gives more immediate access to the mandibular and intracapsular sublingual glands than the ventral approach, but it is restricted in its exposure of the more rostral portion of the sublingual chain.

1. Position the dog in lateral recumbency with a pack placed under the cervical spine.
2. Make a curved skin incision caudal to, but following the angle of, the mandible.
3. Split the platysma (panniculus) muscle in the direction of its fibres, allowing the linguofacial and maxillary veins to be identified.
4. Isolate the capsule of the mandibular gland from the surrounding connective tissue; it should remain intact throughout the dissection.
5. Ligate vessels on the medial aspect of the gland.
6. Apply traction to the mandibular gland and duct; this will elevate the sublingual chain from below the digastricus muscle. Small artery forceps can

be placed one after another to help to elevate the duct, which may be sectioned without ligation once the oral mucosa is reached.

Ventral approach: The major advantage of this approach is the excellent access it provides to the rostral portion of the sublingual chain (Ritter *et al.*, 2006).

1. Position the dog in dorsal recumbency.
2. Make an incision medial to the mandible and lateral to the larynx to permit the mandibular gland to be identified.
3. The capsule of the mandibular gland should remain intact (as far as possible) while the sublingual gland is dissected rostrally. The salivary chain runs ventral to the digastricus muscle and must be passed beneath this muscle during the dissection.
4. Identify the rostral component of the chain by traction on the distal section and resect by blunt dissection.

Parotid sialoadenectomy

Resection of the normal parotid gland is a difficult and prolonged procedure that is complicated by its indistinct margins and the proximity of the facial nerve. Fragments of the gland are frequently left *in situ*, due to the difficulty of recognizing the limits of the salivary tissue. Furthermore, good margins of normal tissue are very rarely available (Figure 15.17). Removal of parotid gland tumours is, therefore, something of a surgical challenge. Resection of the facial nerve is a possible complication.

The difficulty of achieving sufficient surgical margins has led to the exploration of radiation therapy as a postoperative adjuvant for parotid lesions (Evans and Thrall, 1983).

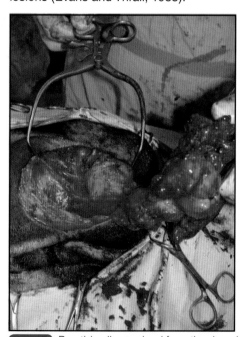

15.17 Parotid salivary gland from the dog shown in Figure 15.15, after resection of the adenocarcinoma. The dissection is complex and there are minimal surgical margins available.

Zygomatic sialoadenectomy

1. Approach zygomatic lesions via a skin incision made along the dorsal brim of the zygoma.
2. Reflect the orbital fascia dorsally and the masseter muscle ventrally.
3. It may be necessary to resect the zygoma and replace it later, or to cut a dorsal 'window' in the bone to expose the gland in the orbit.
4. Tumours of the gland can normally be easily dissected, although it is sometimes difficult to distinguish the tumour from surrounding orbital fat.
5. Replace or discard the sectioned zygoma.
6. Repair the periosteum and close the skin.

Other modalities

Although radiation therapy (Evans and Thrall, 1983; Carberry *et al.*, 1987) and chemotherapy (Hammer *et al.*, 2001) have both been used in the treatment of salivary tumours, too few cases have been reported to allow any significant conclusions regarding efficacy to be drawn.

Prognosis

The prognosis for salivary gland tumours is variable and is likely to be worse in patients with advanced disease or in those for which complete surgical excision cannot be performed. There are few reports of survival data for large numbers of salivary tumours. Clinical experience based on small numbers of cases would seem to indicate that incomplete resection alone is likely to result in local recurrence; however, incomplete resection followed by radiation therapy may result in acceptable local control and long-term survival. Histopathological features were not found to be of prognostic importance in one study (Hammer *et al.*, 2001), although clinical stage was predictive. The MSTs for dogs and cats with salivary malignancies have been reported as 550 days and 516 days, respectively (Hammer *et al.*, 2001). In another study of six dogs with salivary carcinomas in particular, the MST was 74 days, with all dogs eventually developing pulmonary metastatic disease (Hahn and Nolan, 1997).

References and further reading

Brown PJ, Lucke VM, Sozmen M and Wyatt JM (1997) Lipomatous infiltration of the canine salivary gland. *Journal of Small Animal Practice* **38**, 234–236

Carberry CA, Flanders JA, Anderson WI and Harvey HJ (1987) Mast cell tumour in the mandibular salivary gland in a dog. *Cornell Veterinarian* **77**, 362–366

Evans SM and Thrall DE (1983) Postoperative orthovoltage radiation therapy of parotid gland adenocarcinoma in three dogs. *Journal of the American Veterinary Medical Association* **182**, 993–994

Hahn KA and Nolan ML (1997) Surgical prognosis for canine salivary gland neoplasms. *Proceedings, American College of Veterinary Radiology and Veterinary Cancer Society*

Hammer A, Getzy D, Ogilivie G *et al.* (2001) Salivary gland neoplasia in the dog and cat: survival times and prognostic factors. *Journal of the American Animal Hospital Association* **37**, 478–482

Head KW, Cullen JM, Dubielzig RR *et al.* (2003) Histological classification of salivary gland tumors of domestic animals. In: *Histological Classification of Tumors of the Alimentary System of*

Domestic Animals, 2nd Series, Vol. 10, pp 58–72. Armed Forces Institute of Pathology, American Registry of Pathology, and The World Health Organization Collaborating Center for Worldwide Reference on Comparative Oncology, Washington, DC

Karbe E and Schiefer B (1967) Primary salivary gland tumours in carnivores. *Veterinary Journal* **8**, 212–215

Koestner A and Buerger L (1965) Primary neoplasms of the salivary glands in animals compared to similiar tumors in man. *Veterinary Pathology* **2**, 201–226

Militerno G, Bazzo R and Marcato PS (2005) Cytological diagnosis of mandibular salivary gland adenocarcinoma in a dog. *Journal of Veterinary Medicine, Series A* **52,** 514–516

Perez-Martinez C, Garcia Fernandez RA, Reyes Avila LE *et al.* (2000) Malignant fibrous histiocytoma (giant cell type) associated with a malignant mixed cell tumor in the salivary gland of a dog.

Veterinary Pathology **37**, 350–353

Ritter MJ, von Pfeil DJF, Hauptman JG and Walshaw R (2006) Mandibular and sublingual sialoceles in the dog: a retrospective evaluation of 41 cases, using the ventral approach for treatment. *New Zealand Veterinary Journal* **54**, 333–337

Shimoyama Y, Yamashita K, Ohmachi T *et al.* (2006) Pleomorphic adenoma of the salivary gland in two dogs. *Journal of Comparative Pathology* **134**, 254–259

Spangler WL and Culberston MR (1991) Salivary gland disease in dogs and cats: 245 cases (1985–1988) *Journal of the American Veterinary Medical Association* **198**, 465–469

Stubbs WP, Voges AK, Shiroma JT and Wolf J (1996) What is your diagnosis? Infiltrative lipoma with chronic salivary duct obstruction. *Journal of the American Veterinary Medical Association* **209**, 55–56

15c

Tumours of the oesophagus

Brian J. Trumpatori and Richard A.S. White

Introduction

Primary tumours of the oesophagus are extremely rare in both dogs and cats. In Europe, primary oesophageal neoplasia is so rare that it is difficult to assess its true rate of occurrence. In regions of the world where oesophageal sarcoma occurs secondary to infestation with the parasite *Spirocerca lupi,* the incidence is still reported to be only 0.5% of all tumours, making *S. lupi*-associated sarcomas the major cause of oesophageal neoplasia.

In general, most oesophageal tumours are locally invasive and metastasize by haematogenous, lymphatic or direct extension.

Primary tumours of the canine oesophagus are most commonly malignant. They include squamous cell carcinoma (SCC), osteosarcoma (OSA), fibrosarcoma (FSA) and leiomyosarcoma (Campbell and Pirie, 1965; Carb and Goodman, 1973; Ridgeway and Suter, 1979; McCaw *et al.*, 1980; Farese *et al.*, 2008). Sarcomas associated with *Spirocerca* infection are most commonly OSA, followed by FSA and undifferentiated sarcoma. These particular tumours have been reported to occur more commonly in the bitch (Ranen *et al.*, 2008). In the cat, SCC has been reported to occur in the mid-thoracic oesophagus, most commonly in queens. Metastatic disease from malignant lesions may be found in the regional nodes or lungs, as well as in various abdominal organs.

Benign tumours, including leiomyomas and plasmacytomas, are encountered infrequently and are most commonly located at the terminal oesophagus and gastric cardia at the level of the lower oesophageal sphincter.

Secondary invasion of the oesophagus is sometimes encountered in association with cervical peri-oesophageal tumours (e.g. thyroid) or with tumours of the mediastinum and thorax (e.g. thymoma, heart base, lung).

Aetiology and pathogenesis

Oesophageal tumours associated with *Spirocerca lupi* infection are encountered in areas of the world where the parasite is endemic; this includes parts of the south-eastern USA, Africa, Israel, Turkey, India, Pakistan and areas of Asia. Dogs infested with the parasite pass embryonated eggs in their faeces, which are then ingested by dung-eating beetles. The eggs develop to an infective third stage and encyst in the beetle; this may then be ingested by the dog directly or there may be a paratenic host such as a snake or rat. Once in the primary host, the larvae migrate within 3 weeks through the stomach wall to the arterial supply and thence to the thoracic aorta, where they remain for 2–3 months. The larvae then move to the oesophageal wall, where they become surrounded by a cystic granulomatous nodule and also become sexually mature. These granulomas communicate with the oesophageal lumen via fistulae, through which eggs pass periodically into the alimentary tract.

S. lupi may damage a variety of tissues along its migratory tract. Injury to the aortic wall may promote the development of aneurysms, potentially leading to rupture of the vessel. Gastrointestinal granulomas may also rupture, with fatal consequences. Oesophageal or pulmonary lesions can give rise to neoplastic lesions, which are usually sarcomas. Occasionally, patients may develop hypertrophic pulmonary osteopathy secondary to thoracic oesophageal or pulmonary lesions, and signs of this may precede those associated with the primary site.

The aetiology of other oesophageal tumours is unclear due to their rarity, although ingestion of carcinogens has been shown experimentally to induce cancer in dogs (Sasaki *et al.*, 1984).

Presentation and clinical signs

Important signs associated with oesophageal neoplasia reflect luminal obstruction and include dysphagia, discomfort on swallowing, regurgitation and aspiration. Weight loss and cough are seen in more advanced cases. Patients may be presented for the investigation of orthopaedic signs or lameness when affected by hypertrophic pulmonary osteopathy associated with *S. lupi*-induced lesions. Clinicopathological changes associated with *S. lupi* infection include non-regenerative anaemia, neutrophilic leucocytosis, hyperproteinaemia and elevated alkaline phosphatase (Mylonakis *et al.*, 2006). A recent retrospective study comparing benign and malignant lesions associated with *S. lupi* infection found that anaemia and leucocytosis were more severe with malignant than with benign tumours. Additionally, older dogs, spayed females, and those with hypertrophic osteopathy were more likely to have malignant tumours (Dvir *et al.*, 2008).

Clinical approach

Radiography

Radiographic investigation is indicated in patients with regurgitation or dysphagia and in all patients presenting with hypertrophic osteopathy. Thoracic views may demonstrate a soft tissue mass within the thorax, the presence of an abnormal gas shadow within the oesophageal lumen, dilatation of the oesophagus proximal to the mass, or compression of the oesophageal lumen.

Masses associated with *S. lupi* usually affect the terminal portion of the oesophagus but cranially located masses have also been described (Dvir *et al.*, 2001). Spondylitis of the thoracic vertebrae is considered a pathognomonic finding for *S. lupi* infection, the underlying pathogenesis of which is unknown. Aortic mineralization secondary to small aneurysms can also be identified in cases of *S. lupi* infection. Secondary conditions including tracheal or bronchial displacement, pleural effusion, aspiration pneumonia, mediastinitis and pneumothorax may also be identified.

Positive contrast radiographic (Figure 15.18) and/or fluoroscopic evaluation studies of the upper gastrointestinal tract will help to identify the level, location and nature of the lesion and highlight the mass. The lungs, mediastinal and bronchial lymph nodes should also be evaluated radiographically for evidence of secondary disease.

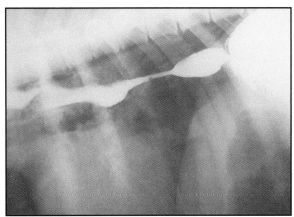

15.18 Lateral thoracic radiograph demonstrating compression of the distal oesophagus associated with primary oesophageal leiomyoma.

Endoscopy

Direct observation and biopsy of the mass can be achieved using oesophagoscopy. Most malignant lesions appear ulcerated. Rare benign lesions may be asymptomatic, and comparatively large lesions may be detected incidentally.

A biopsy sample may be taken using endoscopy: malignant lesions may be amenable to having a sample taken from their ulcerated surface. To ensure a representative sample, several specimens should be obtained, as ulcerated masses often contain areas of inflammation and necrosis on histopathology. When the luminal surface is intact (as may be the case with smooth muscle lesions), obtaining a representative biopsy sample via endoscopy can be difficult.

Advanced imaging

Advanced imaging modalities including CT and MRI should be considered in patients suspected of having malignant disease, to determine the extent of local invasion and to evaluate for regional and distant metastases. In the event that attempts to obtain a biopsy sample via endoscopy are unsuccessful, cervical, thoracic or abdominal exploration may be required for confirmation of the diagnosis.

Other

If infection with *Spirocerca lupi* is suspected, a faecal analysis should be performed.

Management

Medical management

Oesophageal granulomas associated with *S. lupi* may progress to malignant disease; they are reported to respond well to treatment with oral doramectin (Berry, 2000; van der Merwe *et al.*, 2008). The use of chemotherapy for treatment of oesophageal sarcoma has not been clinically evaluated but in one recent report the histological scores of lung metastases in several dogs receiving doxorubicin for oesophageal sarcomas were noted to be significantly lower than those of the primary tumours at the time of necropsy, suggesting that the role of chemotherapy deserves further evaluation (Ranen *et al.*, 2008).

Similarly, the role of radiation therapy is currently unknown, but it is felt that it would be of limited value due to the potential for undesirable effects to the surrounding structures. Palliative treatment typically includes nutritional support via oesophagostomy or gastrostomy tube feeding.

Surgery

Access to the oesophagus is obtained via cervical midline incision or intercostal thoracotomy. In some cases benign smooth muscle tumours may be removed at thoracotomy, if there is minimal disturbance of the mucosal surface (Figure 15.19).

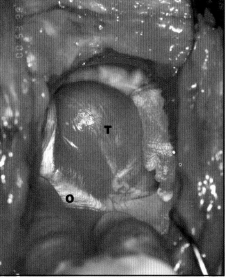

15.19 Resection of oesophageal leiomyoma via thoracotomy. O, oesophagus; T, tumour mass.

Exposure of caudal lesions via lateral thoracotomy is normally excellent, while mid-thoracic sections are more difficult to access. In some cases of benign smooth muscle tumours, complete excision may be performed via thoracotomy or coeliotomy.

In contrast, however, because of the advanced nature of disease at presentation, patients with malignant lesions rarely represent realistic surgical candidates. Intrathoracic resections are often made more difficult by poor surgical exposure, the need to resect a large segment of oesophagus and the resultant defect in oesophageal length. The major complication of such resections is tension across the anastomosis site, leading to dehiscence and infection. A variety of solutions have been described in order to recruit or substitute tissue for reconstruction, including patching of deficits with pericardium, vascularized intercostal muscle, or packing with omentum, and the use of Gortex stents (Straw *et al.*, 1987). Replacement by microvascular anastomosis using jejunum or colon has been described for oesophageal tumours in human patients, but has only rarely been reported in small animals (Gregory *et al.*, 1988; Kuzma *et al.*, 1989). Expandable chrome/cobalt stents have also been used as a temporary palliative measure in humans to maintain oesophageal patency. Advancement of the stomach through the diaphragm or the creation of an iso- or antiperistaltic gastric tube may be used for resection of lesions affecting the distal oesophagus or cardia.

Prognosis

The prognosis for benign smooth muscle tumours of the oesophagus is excellent (Hamilton, 1994; Rolfe, 1994). However, the outlook for primary malignancies has historically been considered universally poor, since adequate surgical resection and reconstruction is rarely feasible.

In a report of six dogs treated by partial oesophagectomy for *Spirocerca*-associated sarcomas, the MST was 267 days; five of the six dogs also received concurrent chemotherapy with doxorubicin (Ranen *et al.*, 2004a,b).

More recently, the outcome of marginal resection of low-grade oesophageal leiomyosarcomas was reported in four dogs. In three of these dogs, tumour margins were considered 'dirty'; in the fourth, the margins were clean but close. Two of the dogs died from causes unrelated to their neoplasm and the remaining two were alive at 388 and 405 days, respectively, demonstrating the potential for prolonged survival with marginal resection of malignant smooth muscle tumours (Farese *et al.*, 2008).

A histological grading scheme has recently been proposed for oesophageal sarcomas but in a report of 32 dogs (Ranen *et al.*, 2008) there was no apparent correlation noted between survival and grade or tumour type. A total of 19 dogs underwent surgery. The MST for the 10 dogs that survived the immediate postoperative period was 278 days; 6 of those cases received adjuvant chemotherapy with doxorubicin (plus carboplatin in 1 case).

The long-term development of metastatic disease from oesophageal malignancies is not well recorded, but in the report by Ranen *et al.* (2008) 53% of dogs undergoing necropsy demonstrated various abdominal organ metastases (renal, stomach, spleen, pancreas, adrenal, heart, tongue and lymph node) and pulmonary metastasis. Local recurrence was noted in two of three dogs that had undergone resection of the primary tumour.

Tumours arising from peri-oesophageal structures may be amenable to management, in which case the outlook is normally dependent on the prognosis for the primary tumour.

References and further reading

Berry WL (2000) *Spirocerca lupi* esophageal granulomas in 7 dogs: resolution after treatment with doramectin. *Journal of Veterinary Internal Medicine* **14**, 609

Campbell J and Pirie H (1965) Leiomyoma of the oesophagus in a dog. *Veterinary Record* **77**, 624

Carb A and Goodman D (1973) Oesophageal carcinoma in the dog. *Journal of Small Animal Practice* **14**, 91

Dvir E, Kirberger RM and Malleczek D (2001) Radiographic and computed tomographic changes and clinical presentation of spirocercosis in the dog. *Veterinary Radiology and Ultrasound* **42**, 119–129

Dvir E, Kirberger RM, Mukorera V *et al.* (2008) Clinical differentiation between dogs with benign and malignant spirocercosis. *Veterinary Parasitology* **155**, 80–88

Farese JP, Bacon NJ, Ehrhart NP *et al.* (2008) Oesophageal leiomyosarcoma in dogs: surgical management and clinical outcome of four cases. *Veterinary and Comparative Oncology* **6**, 31–38

Gregory CR, Gourley IM, Bruyette DS and Schulz LJ (1988) Free jejunal segment for treatment of cervical esophageal stricture in a dog. *Journal of the American Veterinary Medical Association* **193**, 230–232

Hamilton TA and Carpenter JL (1994) Oesophageal plasmacytoma in a dog. *Journal of the American Veterinary Medical Association* **204**, 1210–1211

Kuzma AB, Holmberg DL, Miller CW, Barker I and Roth J (1989) Esophageal replacement in the dog by microvascular colon transfer. *Veterinary Surgery* **18**, 439–445

McCaw D, Pratt M and Walshaw R (1980) Squamous cell carcinoma of the oesophagus in the dog. *Journal of the American Animal Hospital Association* **16**, 561–563

Mylonakis M, Rallis T, Koutinas AF *et al.* (2006) Clinical signs and clinicopathologic abnormalities in dogs with clinical spirocercosis: 39 cases (1996–2004) *Journal of the American Veterinary Medical Association* **228**, 1063–1067

Ranen E, Dank G, Lavy E *et al.* (2008) Oesophageal sarcomas in dogs: histological and clinical evaluation. *The Veterinary Journal* **178**, 78–84

Ranen E, Lavy E, Aizenburg I *et al.* (2004a) Spirocercosis-associated esophageal sarcomas in dogs: a retrospective study of 17 cases (1997-2003). *Veterinary Parasitology* **119**, 209–221

Ranen E, Shamir MH, Shahar R et al. (2004b) Partial esophagectomy with single layer closure for treatment of esophageal sarcomas in 6 dogs. *Veterinary Surgery* **33,** 428–434

Ridgeway RL and Suter PF (1979) Clinical and radiographic signs in primary and metastatic esophageal neoplasms of the dog. *Journal of the American Veterinary Medical Association* **174**, 700–704

Rolfe DS, Twedt DC and Seim HB (1994) Chronic regurgitation or vomiting caused by oesophageal leiomyoma in three dogs. *Journal of the American Animal Hospital Association* 30, 425–430

Sasaki O, Saito T, Matsukuchi T *et al.* (1984) Endoscopic study of chronological changes leading to cancer in the esophagus of dogs induced by *N*-ethyl-*N'*-nitro-*N*-nitrosoguanidine. *Gastroenterology Japan* **19**, 456–463

Straw RC, Tomlinson JL, Constantinescu G, Turk MAM and Hogan PM (1987) Use of a vascular skeletal muscle graft for canine esophageal reconstruction. *Veterinary Surgery* **16**, 155–156

van der Merwe LL, Kirberger RM, Clift S *et al.* (2008) *Spirocerca lupi* infection in the dog: a review. *The Veterinary Journal* **176**, 294–309

Tumours of the stomach

Jonathan Bray and Reto Neiger

Introduction

Neoplasia of the stomach is uncommon in the dog, accounting for <1% of all tumours. Most stomach tumours are malignant, and adenocarcinoma represents the majority (42–72%) of cases. Other malignant tumour types that have been reported in dogs include fibrosarcoma, leiomyosarcoma and lymphosarcoma. Benign tumours (leiomyoma, most commonly) have also been recorded, and may occur at the cardia or caudal oesophageal region. A variety of other sporadic tumours have been reported, including plasmacytoma, polyps, squamous cell carcinoma and carcinoid tumours (from the enterochromaffin cells). Although tumours of the stomach may arise anywhere, sites of predilection include the incisure angularis and the pyloric antrum.

In the cat, B-lymphocytic lymphoma is the most common tumour of the stomach; affected cats are typically negative for feline leukaemia virus.

Aetiology and predispositions

Helicobacter pylori infection has been strongly associated with development of gastric adenocarcinoma and mucosal-associated lymphoid tissue (MALT) lymphoma in humans. In dogs, there is no indication that gastric *Helicobacter* spp. are an increased risk factor for gastric tumours. However, a study in cats suggested that *Helicobacter* spp. might be responsible for MALT lymphomas (Bridgeford *et al.*, 2008).

In humans, a variety of dietary substances have been implicated as risk factors in the development of gastric tumours, e.g. salt, starch, mycotoxins and polycyclic hydrocarbons found in smoked meat and fish. Experimental studies showed that long-term administration of nitrosamines can induce carcinomas in the dog. Duodenogastric reflux has been shown to be a risk factor for gastric cancer in a murine model.

Some breed predispositions are noted. Belgian Shepherd Dogs have a higher than average incidence of gastric carcinoma and the disease seems to have a heritable component (h2 = 0.09 ± 0.02). Collies and Staffordshire Bull Terriers are also reported to be at increased risk of gastric carcinoma.

Tumour behaviour

Carcinomas

Histologically, carcinomas can be subclassified into signet ring cell carcinoma, undifferentiated carcinoma, tubular adenocarcinoma and scirrhous adenocarcinoma, but the clinical behaviour of these is very similar. Carcinomas infiltrate the gastric mucosa and extend into submucosa, muscularis and serosa. This results in a very tough, scirrhous lesion that is sometimes called a 'linitis plastica' because of its non-distensible nature. Later, a central ulcer is commonly found. At the time of diagnosis, most gastric carcinomas have spread to the regional lymph nodes, lung, liver and spleen.

Adenomas

Adenomatous polyps can cause outflow obstruction due to the close proximity to the pylorus. In humans, they are considered to be premalignant lesions.

Lymphomas

Gastric lymphomas arise from the submucosa or from the mucosa-associated lymphoid tissue (MALT). They can be either diffusely infiltrative or localized, or may be seen as part of more generalized lymphoma.

Mesenchymal tumours

Mesenchymal tumours can be divided into gastrointestinal stromal tumours (GISTs) and leiomyomas on the basis of histological features and cell differentiation.

In humans GISTs arise from the interstitial cells of Cajal. They constitute the majority of mesenchymal tumours of the gastrointestinal tract and can occur anywhere, though are most common in the stomach and small intestine. GISTs have a spectrum from small benign tumours to frankly malignant sarcomas. They typically express KIT (CD117). In dogs, GISTs seem to occur more commonly in the colon and small intestine, whereas only 19% of them are located in the stomach.

Leiomyomas are composed of well differentiated smooth muscle cells that are typically positive for smooth muscle actin and desmin, markers for differentiation. These tumours are negative for CD117 and typically have an indolent clinical course. In dogs, leiomyoma occurs most commonly in the stomach of geriatric animals, with a predilection for males.

Presentation and clinical signs

Patients with gastric cancer typically present with a history of chronic vomiting, but may otherwise appear to be healthy. The vomiting may be intermittent and may be typified by the emission of partially digested food at a time when the stomach would normally considered to be empty (6–8 hours after feeding). The history is usually chronic, with signs developing insidiously over a period of weeks or months. In some patients, fresh or digested blood (haematemesis) may be seen in the vomitus on occasion.

There may be weight loss in chronic cases due to a combination of poor digestion, anorexia, protein and blood loss from the ulcer, and cancer cachexia. Metastatic disease may result in other systemic abnormalities.

Clinical approach

Diagnosis

Confirmation of the diagnosis of gastric neoplasia requires ruling out metabolic or concurrent disease using physical examination, haematology and biochemistry. Rarely is physical examination and abdominal palpation of benefit. Because the stomach is completely protected by the costal arch, most dogs may have no detectable abnormalities on physical examination, though some cranial abdominal pain may be evident in late stages.

Imaging

Plain radiographs are often insensitive to the subtle changes associated with gastric neoplasia but may be helpful to assess other abdominal organs. In some cases, however, plain films may demonstrate a markedly distended stomach, with caudal extension of the gastric fundus and body, and increased dimension of the pylorus if outflow obstruction is present. Positive contrast studies may demonstrate filling defects. Fluoroscopy is useful in evaluating gastric peristalsis and pyloric sphincter function.

Ultrasonography is more helpful than radiography and may show thickening and disruption of the normal layering of the gastric wall (Figure 15.20). It is also important to check for evidence of regional lymph node enlargement or more distant metastasis to other abdominal organs, especially the liver. When an obvious lesion is evident with ultrasound, it may be possible to obtain guided aspiration samples for cytological evaluation.

Flexible gastroscopy permits direct visualization of and biopsy from the gastric mucosal surface, and is perhaps the most effective method for identifying a lesion affecting the stomach lumen. Gross findings may include a proliferative mass on the mucosal wall of the stomach or a deep ulceration of the mucosal surface (Figure 15.21). More subtle changes may occur with lymphoma, with the mucosal surface developing a generalised smooth or lightly cobble-stoned appearance.

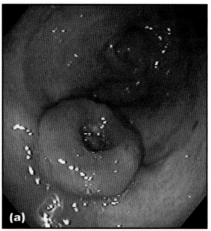

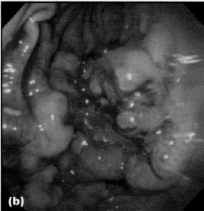

15.21 **(a)** Endoscopic view of a gastric mass shown by biopsy to be a plasmacytoma. (Reproduced from *BSAVA Manual of Canine and Feline Gastroenterology, 2nd edn*) **(b)** Endoscopic view of a gastric adenocarcinoma. (Courtesy of E Hall)

Histology

Due to the superficial necrosis and inflammation that is often associated with malignant lesions, it is important to perform multiple biopsies in order to obtain representative neoplastic tissue. Taking samples from ulcerated, necrotic or haemorrhagic areas should be avoided. False-negative histopathological results are not uncommon. The clinician should endeavour to take multiple samples from several locations about the lesion to improve diagnostic accuracy.

15.20 Ultrasound image showing markedly thickened gastric mucosa and loss of the typical mucosal layer due to lymphoma in a 10-year-old Labrador Retriever. (Courtesy of P Mantis)

Staging

Staging of gastric tumours is mainly done by diagnostic imaging (ultrasonography, thoracic radiography) and by endoscopy. The WHO staging for gastric adenocarcinomas (Figure 15.22) suggests that there might be a worse prognosis for local infiltration and metastatic disease. No histological grading system is used. Gastric lymphomas are staged as described in Chapter 19.

T – Primary tumour	
T0	No evidence of primary tumour
T1	Tumour not invading serosa
T2	Tumour invading serosa
T3	Tumour invading neighbouring structures
N – Regional lymph node status	
N0	No evidence of lymph node involvement
N1	Regional lymph nodes involved
N2	Distant lymph nodes involved
M – Distant metastasis	
M0	No evidence of distant metastasis
M1	Distant metastasis detected

15.22 WHO classification of gastric tumours.

Management

Surgery

For gastric neoplasia (except gastric lymphoma), wide surgical resection is indicated. Due to the insidious and non-specific nature of the clinical signs, malignant gastric tumours can be of considerable size and may have already metastasized prior to surgery. In these patients, tumour resection would require extensive reconstructive surgery. End-to-end gastroenteric re-anastomosis with a gastroduodenostomy (Bilroth I; see *BSAVA Manual of Canine and Feline Abdominal Surgery*) can be used if the tumour involves only parts of the antrum/pylorus. Unfortunately, in many patients, the tumour is so advanced that surgical excision is precluded. Extensive surgery, such as a gastrojejunostomy (Bilroth II), which is sometimes performed in humans, results in high morbidity in dogs and should be performed only in exceptional cases. Survival times are extremely poor (14 days, on average) and the post-surgical course is complicated with a high morbidity. Whilst total gastrectomy has been described, it is also associated with numerous complications and considerable morbidity.

Benign neoplasms and discrete tumours located in the fundus or body of the stomach can often be excised completely, but the surgeon must try to take adequate margins (at least 1–2 cm of normal tissue beyond obviously abnormal tissue) to ensure good long-term survival. Partial gastrectomy is indicated if a large section of the fundus is involved.

Radiation therapy

Radiation therapy for gastric tumours is not well tolerated in small animals, due to the sensitivity of the gastrointestinal tract and the associated organs to radiation toxicity.

Chemotherapy

Cytotoxic drug therapy for gastric carcinomas has not been seen to be effective in dogs and cats. In human medicine, intraperitoneal 5-fluorouracil or cisplatin plus intravenous 5-fluorouracil has been used, but with little success.

Treatment of gastric lymphomas

Gastric lymphomas are only treated surgically if perforation is likely without surgical intervention. They are usually treated with a standard chemotherapy protocol although they rarely respond well. Whether partial resection of localized lymphoma is prognostically advantageous is not known. Eradication of *H. pylori* often reverses MALT lymphoma in human patients, but it is unclear whether eradication of *Helicobacter* spp. in animals with lymphoma might have a similar effect.

Prognosis

In general the prognosis for gastric tumours is poor. The MST for gastric adenocarcinoma is 2 months, despite surgical excision of the tumour; very rare cases may survive longer (3 years). In contrast, leiomyosarcomas have a better prognosis if they can be resected completely and no complications arise during the postoperative period; for patients who survive the immediate surgical intervention (2 weeks), the MST is 12 months (Kapatkin *et al.*, 1992). Leiomyomas and other benign tumours have a good prognosis after complete resection, with the possibility of the disease being cured. The prognosis for gastric lymphomas in dogs is poor, significantly worse than that of multicentric lymphoma.

References and further reading

Bridgeford EC, Marini RP, Feng Y *et al.* (2008) Gastric *Helicobacter* species as a cause of feline gastric lymphoma: a viable hypothesis. *Veterinary Immunology and Immunopathology* **123**, 106–113
Kapatkin AS, Mullen HS, Matthiesen DT and Patnaik AK (1992) Leiomyosarcoma in dogs: 44 cases (1983–1988). *Journal of the American Veterinary Medical Association* 201, 1077–1079

15e

Tumours of the small intestines

B. Duncan X. Lascelles and Richard A.S. White

Introduction

Most intestinal tumours in small animals are malignant, with adenocarcinoma being most common in the dog, and lymphoma most common in the cat. Tumours of the large intestine are more common, with the rectum considered to be the most common site (see Chapter 15f).

The dog

The small intestines are an uncommon site of neoplasia in the dog and account for <1.0% of all malignant tumours. The jejunum, ileum and caecum are reported to be the most common sites, and the important histological types include adenocarcinoma, gastrointestinal stromal tumours (GISTs), leiomyosarcoma, leiomyoma and lymphoma (Birchard et al., 1986; Maas et al., 2007).

Half of all gastrointestinal tumours in the dog are adenocarcinomas; there is a mean age of 9 years at presentation. Collies, German Shepherd Dogs and Boxers may be at increased risk for this disease; males are also at increased risk. Adenocarcinomas cause luminal obstruction: usually through development in an annular pattern of growth, thereby causing constriction of the bowel; or, less commonly, through intraluminal intrusion. Histological classification into acinar, solid, mucinous and papillary groups has been linked with the pattern of growth. Both lymphatic and vascular metastases may develop from adenocarcinomas and can be found in the mesenteric lymph nodes, peritoneal cavity, omentum, liver, kidneys and lungs.

Recently, it has been recognized that tumours previously classified as leiomyosarcomas and leiomyomas may in fact be GISTs. This new information regarding classification may help define improved treatments in the future, though one recent study concluded that there were no significant differences in survival for these three tumour types, histological or immunohistochemical characteristics (Maas et al., 2007). In general, these tumour types affect slightly older dogs (10–11 years); there is no reported breed predisposition. When these tumours occur in the small intestine, they tend to develop secondary disease more slowly; although nodal disease may occur, the disease is often less aggressive than adenocarcinoma.

Lymphoma accounts for approximately 10% of all gastrointestinal canine malignancies and affects younger dogs, with a mean age of 7 years. There is predilection for the male; no breed predisposition has been recorded.

The cause of most small intestinal tumours in the dog remains unclear. Diet has been demonstrated to have an important causal relationship in several types of human intestinal cancer, but its role in animal tumours is uncertain.

The cat

Intestinal tumours are also unusual in the cat; the mean age of affected animals is 11 years. Lymphoma is by far the most common type of tumour in the small intestine, with the jejunum and ileum being involved most frequently. Lesions of small intestinal lymphoma in the cat may be solitary or diffuse. Mesenteric lymph node involvement is commonly found with diffuse lesions; some reports also suggest that renal involvement is common (Turk et al., 1981). Fewer than 25% of cats with small intestinal lymphoma are found to be positive for feline leukaemia virus.

Mast cell tumours (MCTs) are occasionally found in the small intestine of older cats (mean age 13 years). Intestinal MCTs in cats behave aggressively and commonly metastasize to the mesenteric lymph nodes, the liver, the spleen and other sites. Adenomatous polyps have been recorded in the duodenum of oriental cats (MacDonald et al., 1993).

Adenocarcinomas are reported to be found in the ileum and ileocaecal region, although one report indicates the jejunum to be the more important site (Kosovsky et al.,1988). The Siamese is reported to be at increased risk for adenocarcinomas. Metastatic spread at the time of diagnosis is seen in three-quarters of cats, and transabdominal spread giving rise to invasion of adjacent abdominal organs is commonly encountered (Figure 15.23).

Presentation and clinical signs

The clinical signs of small intestinal neoplasia are varied and non-specific. Discrete lesions (e.g. adenocarcinomas) are often annular and commonly give rise to signs of obstruction, including vomiting, anorexia, abdominal pain and weight loss. Melaena, diarrhoea and microcytic normochromic anaemia may be seen in patients with ulcerated lesions. A palpable abdominal mass is present in some cases.

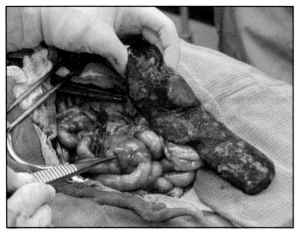

15.23 Laparotomy in a cat with what was found to be metastatic adenocarcinoma spreading to the spleen, liver and local lymph nodes. Following resection of the intestinal mass and splenectomy, the cat survived another 14 months with no other treatment.

The onset of clinical signs is often chronic and insidious over many weeks, although acute presentation of animals with complete obstruction, or perforation that has led to peritonitis, is possible. These signs may be seen with either benign or malignant lesions. One recent study of smooth muscle tumours in dogs found that dogs with caecal tumours were more likely to present with perforation and peritonitis than when the tumour was located more proximally in the small intestines (Maas *et al.,* 2007).

Diffuse or infiltrating tumours (e.g. lymphoma) tend to cause less acute signs and may cause more chronic signs of malabsorption, weight loss, hypoproteinaemia or intermittent diarrhoea (due to altered motility patterns).

Involvement of mesenteric lymph nodes may result in obstructed lymphatic drainage and lymphangiectasia.

Rarely, tumours may release biologically active agents such as histamine (e.g. MCTs), which may give rise to cutaneous changes or acute diarrhoea.

Clinical approach

In all cases of small intestinal neoplasia, a thorough evaluation of all signs associated with the disease (e.g. anaemia, hypoproteinaemia, occult faecal blood) should be combined with a search for regional and distant metastatic disease. Biochemical investigations may reveal electrolyte abnormalities resulting from intestinal obstruction or low serum protein levels resulting from infiltrating tumours.

Imaging

Diagnostic imaging is the most effective diagnostic tool for the identification of neoplastic lesions of the small intestines. Common radiological signs associated with small intestinal neoplasia include:

- Signs of ileus associated with luminal obstruction
- An abnormal transit time (increased or decreased)

- Thickening of the intestinal wall and reduction in luminal diameter
- Ulceration of the intestinal wall.

Ultrasonographic examination is often helpful, both for detecting mass lesions and for providing an appreciation of increased bowel wall thickness. It may also show a loss of layering of the intestinal wall in the case of infiltrative tumours such as lymphoma. However, a recent report of idiopathic eosinophilic masses of the gastrointestinal tract in dogs highlighted that diffuse thickening can be seen with non-neoplastic disease (Lyles *et al.,* 2009). Involvement of other abdominal sites, resulting in mesenteric lymphadenopathy, hepatomegaly or splenomegaly may also be readily identified. Ultrasound-guided fine needle aspirates can be retrieved from intestinal sites and from other abdominal organs, such as the liver and the spleen.

Coeliotomy and biopsy

Definitive diagnosis and clinical staging of small intestinal tumours may be achieved at coeliotomy. The mesenteric lymph nodes and, in particular, the liver should be carefully inspected for any evidence of metastatic disease before resection is attempted. Suspected metastatic disease should prompt biopsy. A positive biopsy result does not preclude reasonable survival following resection of the primary lesion, and suspected metastatic disease is rarely a compelling reason to cease treatment at this stage of evaluation, but biopsy results may be information owners would like in order to decide whether to proceed further.

Coeliotomy is also indicated in the case of infiltrating tumours of the small intestine to permit multiple biopsies to be taken for confirmation of the diagnosis. Biopsy sites should be carefully closed and omental patches applied.

Management

Surgery

The extent of the resection necessary for removal of the primary lesion should be assessed following biopsy; surgical technique is covered in the *BSAVA Manual of Canine and Feline Abdominal Surgery.* In most instances, wide local resection with margins extending 2–4 cm on either side of the tumour can be performed by enterectomy and anastomosis. Resections should be performed between bowel clamps (Figure 15.24) (or with an assistant's fingers acting to clamp the bowel) and extended through the supporting mesentery. Where appropriate, regional lymph nodes should be included in an *en bloc* resection. This is not possible and should not be attempted when affected lymph nodes are intimately involved with mesenteric vessels supplying unaffected parts of the bowel. *En bloc* resection of this kind is possible with more aggressive resections of the iliocaecocolic junction area. Mesenteric vessels supplying the affected segment of bowel should be ligated, as well as the vessels supplying the mesenteric borders of

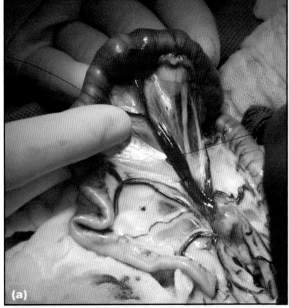

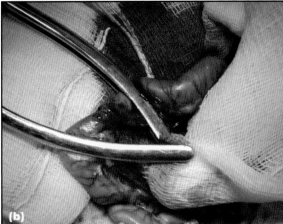

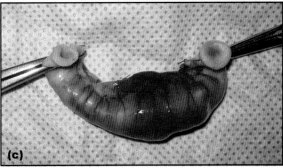

15.24 Resection and anastomosis of an adenocarcinoma in the mid intestine of a cat. **(a)** The mesenteric vessels are ligated. **(b)** The resection is complete. Anastomosis is initiated by placing the mesenteric and antimesenteric sutures. Note the Doyen forceps in place – often these are too large for smaller animals, and an assistant's clamped fingers work better. **(c)** Resected specimen. Note that the margin of grossly normal tissue on the left is considered barely sufficient (1.5 cm).

the two ends to be anastomosed. These vessels should be carefully looked for; if they are not ligated, significant bleeding can occur following surgery. Some surgeons prefer to resect any everting mucosa to ensure accurate apposition of the two cut ends although, with practice, this is rarely important.

The type of suture pattern used for bowel anastomoses in the dog and cat is probably best limited to a simple approximating type. The simple interrupted pattern is a non-crushing technique that causes minimal tissue ischaemia at the anastomotic site. This technique calls for accurate and atraumatic placement of the sutures and apposition of the two segments of bowel in a gentle manner. This is technically simple and is recommended for general use in all anastomoses in small animals. Crushing techniques result in more local ischaemia than simple interrupted sutures, but are reported to allow more rapid mucosal regeneration and less scar formation (Brown, 2003). The two techniques provide similar immediate resistance to bursting pressure, and their long-term healing results show little difference. The use of a continuous suture pattern has been described; this results in less mucosal eversion and more precise apposition of the submucosal layer than interrupted patterns (Weisman *et al.*, 1999).

The choice of suture material tends to be a matter for the individual surgeon. Synthetic absorbable materials will far outlast the healing period and there is no indication, even in cachexic hypoproteinaemic cancer patients, to use permanent materials. The use of monofilament suture materials rather than braided materials is considered to result in less trauma to the intestine as the suture is passed through it, and to provide less risk of bacterial 'wicking' from the lumen. Conversely, however, it is worth bearing in mind that braided materials allow for substantially greater knot stability. Since many more patients experience postoperative complications through dehiscence of the anastomosis than ever succumb to infection resulting from bacterial migration along suture material, this may be the more compelling argument.

Anastomosis using surgical stapling instruments is undoubtedly a much less time-consuming option, although it is more expensive. Good outcomes have been reported in clinical cases (White, 2008), although only 5 of those 15 cases underwent resection and anastomosis for intestinal tumours.

Irrespective of the suture material and pattern chosen for the anastomosis, meticulous care in technique is very important. Ischaemic damage is an important factor leading to failure of the surgery. Once the intestinal anastomosis is complete, the supporting mesentery should be carefully repaired to ensure that incarceration cannot occur.

Only rarely is the resection compromised by lack of adjacent normal tissue, but small intestinal surgery may be beset by a variety of other problems:

- Duodenal lesions may be complicated by the problems inherent in preserving the biliary and pancreatic ducts, and margins may need to be modified to accommodate this
- Adhesions associated with tumour growth are common and may require extensive resection of involved mesentery
- Perforations of neoplastic bowel may be encountered with resulting localized or,

occasionally, generalized, peritonitis and may require the use of peritoneal lavage and drainage procedures.

Resection and anastomosis is associated with a risk of dehiscence. One study evaluated 115 cases of intestinal anastomosis in dogs and cats and concluded that preoperative factors significantly associated with development of anastomotic leakage in dogs included preoperative peritonitis, low serum albumin concentration, neutrophilia, and the presence of an intestinal foreign body (Ralphs *et al.,* 2003). Subsequent work found hypoproteinaemia not to be a risk factor (Shales *et al.* 2005). Discriminant analysis showed that dogs with two or more of the following factors were predicted to develop anastomotic leakage: preoperative peritonitis; intestinal foreign body; low serum albumin concentration. Dogs with gastrointestinal tumours rarely present for foreign bodies, but the other factors are likely significant risk factors in cancer cases.

Chemotherapy

While some lymphoma lesions of the small intestine are sufficiently localized to allow surgical resection, many intestinal lymphomas are more suitable to chemotherapeutic management. However, in the treatment of large masses (especially in the large bowel), aggressive cytotoxic therapy can result in rapid perforation of the intestine. In these instances, surgical resection or cytoreductive surgery prior to medical therapy is preferred, to reduce the risk of this complication. Various protocols have been reported for the treatment of small intestinal lymphoma in cats (see Chapter 19a). The use of chemotherapy for other small intestinal neoplasia is unproven in small animals.

Radiation therapy

Radiotherapy has very limited application in the management of small intestinal malignancy because of the difficulty of irradiating the affected area accurately using external beam therapy and the high risk of radiation-associated complications such as perforation and adhesions.

Prognosis

In the dog, wide resection of well differentiated, non-metastasized small intestinal adenocarcinomas provides a favourable prognosis; local recurrence or secondary extension of the disease is unlikely. However, lesions that have metastasized do not have the same favourable prognosis. Small intestinal leiomyomas, leiomyosarcomas and GISTs have been found to be associated with a good prognosis

following surgical resection (Maas *et al.,* 2007). Following excision, 1- and 2-year recurrence-free periods were 80% and 67% for small intestinal tumours. No difference in survival was noted for tumour type, location, histological grade or immunohistochemical characteristics. This is similar to previous reports of gastrointestinal leiomyosarcomas (Cohen *et al.,* 2003).

In one report of small intestinal adenocarcinoma in the cat, two distinct survival groups were noted: about 50% died within 2 weeks of surgery, while the average survival time for those cats surviving longer was 15 months (Kosovsky *et al.,* 1988). Extended survival (MST 12 months) was seen in some cats with detectable nodal disease at surgery, suggesting that advanced disease is not necessarily consistent with a grave prognosis. High-grade small intestinal lymphoma that is not amenable to surgical resection may be treated medically with cytotoxic drugs, but with little expectation of long-term survival. Few cats experience remissions for >6 months. Cats with low-grade, diffuse alimentary lymphoma often respond favourably to chemotherapy and achieve long periods of remission.

References and further reading

Birchard SJ, Couto CG and Johnson S (1986) Non-lymphoid intestinal neoplasia in 32 dogs and 14 cats. *Journal of the American Animal Hospital Association* **22**, 533–537

Brown DC (2003) Small intestines. In: *Textbook of Small Animal Surgery, 3rd edition,* ed. D Slatter. WB Saunders, Philadelphia

Cohen M, Post GS and Wright JC (2003) Gastrointestinal leiomyosarcoma in 14 dogs. *Journal of Veterinary Internal Medicine* **17,** 107–110

Kosovsky JG, Matthiesen DI and Patnaik AK (1988) Small intestinal adenocarcinoma in cats: 32 cases. *Journal of the American Veterinary Medical Association* **192**, 233–235

Lyles SE, Panciera DL, Saunders GK and Leib MS (2009) Idiopathic eosinophilic masses of the gastrointestinal tract in dogs. *Journal of Veterinary Internal Medicine* **23**, 818–823

Maas CP, ter Haar G, van der Gaag I and Kirpensteijn J (2007) Reclassification of small intestinal and cecal smooth muscle tumors in 72 dogs: clinical, histologic, and immunohistochemical evaluation. *Veterinary Surgery* **36**, 302–313

MacDonald JM, Mullen HS and Moroff SD (1993) Adenomatous polyps of the duodenum in cats: 18 cases (1985–1990). *Journal of the American Veterinary Medical Association* **202**, 647–651

Ralphs SC, Jessen CR and Lipowitz AJ (2003) Risk factors for leakage following intestinal anastomosis in dogs and cats: 115 cases (1991–2000). *Journal of the American Veterinary Medical Association* **223**, 73–77

Shales CJ, Warren J, Anderson DM, Baines SJ and White RAS (2005) Complications following full-thickness small intestinal biopsy in 66 dogs: a retrospective study. *Journal of Small Animal Practice* **46**, 317–321

Turk MAM, Gallina AM and Russel TS (1981) Non-hemopoietic gastrointestinal neoplasia in cats. *Veterinary Pathology* **18**, 614–620

Weisman DL, Sweak DD, Birchard SJ and Zweigart SL (1999) Comparison of a continuous suture pattern with a simple interrupted pattern for enteric closure in dogs and cats: 83 cases (1991–1997). *Journal of the American Veterinary Medical Association* **214**, 1507

White RN (2008) Modified functional end-to-end stapled intestinal anastomosis: technique and clinical results in 15 dogs. *Journal of Small Animal Practice* **49**, 274–281

15f

Tumours of the colon and rectum

Jonathan Bray

Introduction

Although cancer of the gastrointestinal tract in dogs and cats is uncommon, the majority of tumours that do occur will develop within the rectum or colon of the dog. Tumours of the large intestine represent 36–60% of all gastrointestinal neoplasms in the dog, and 10–15% of all feline gastrointestinal neoplasms. Tumours are more likely to affect the older animal, with male animals more at risk of developing carcinoma. Polyps occur with equal frequency in males and females. Collies and German Shepherd Dogs have an increased prevalence of carcinoma, as does the Siamese cat. Histological tumour types include epithelial, mesenchymal, neuroendocrine and round cell.

Aetiology

In humans, nearly 800,000 new colorectal cancer cases are believed to occur globally every year. Colorectal cancer accounts for approximately 10% of all incident cancers. The annual worldwide mortality rate from colorectal cancer is estimated at nearly 450,000. In the USA, colorectal cancer accounts for nearly 10% of cancer mortality. The majority of colorectal cancer in humans is an age-related disease, and sporadic colorectal cancer increases dramatically above the age of 45–50 years for all groups. In humans, a genetic predisposition to colorectal cancer is well recognized, and some family lines inherit gene mutations that make their likelihood of developing colorectal cancer almost inevitable (e.g. *APC* gene). For the majority of the population, however, the aetiology of colorectal cancer is complex, and involves interplay of environmental and genetic factors. Obesity and total caloric intake are independent risk factors for colorectal cancer, as revealed by cohort and case-control studies. Ingestion of red meat but not white meat is associated with an increased colorectal cancer risk. It has been established that genetic and environmental factors will conspire to change the normal mucosa to a premalignant adenomatous polyp and then to a frank colorectal cancer over the course of many years (Figure 15.25).

A similar level of molecular detail has not been elucidated in small animal patients to indicate whether the progression of colorectal cancer shares

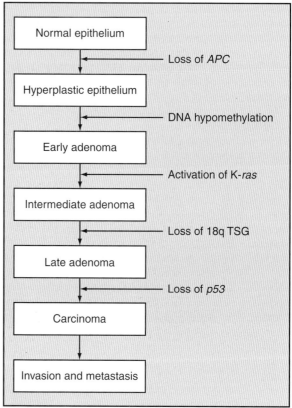

15.25 The stepwise progression of cancer development for proceeding from dysplasia to an outright invasive malignant neoplasm has been well described in humans. Genetic and environmental factors conspire to change the normal mucosa to a premalignant adenomatous polyp and on to a frank colorectal cancer over the course of many years.

characteristics with human disease. All colorectal adenomas and about 50% of all carcinomas in dogs demonstrate increased B-catenin activity. Based on the results of one study, however, malignant progression in canine intestinal tumours does not appear to be dependent on a loss of E-cadherin or B-catenin expression, nor is it strongly associated with overexpression of p53. Positive staining for increased p53 expression was observed in about 44% of tumour types, including hyperplastic polyps (50%), adenomas (48%), carcinoma *in situ* (41%), adenocarcinomas (75%), and invasive carcinomas (35%). However, there was no significant relation between MST and p53 immunoreactivity.

Tumour types

Epithelial tumours

Polyps

Adenomatous polyps are a non-neoplastic condition that may be detected occasionally, mainly In the dog. They are usually located at the anorectal junction, but may be found several centimetres within the rectum. Although benign in behaviour, many have evidence of early malignant transformation on histological assessment. The characteristic feature of polypoid disease is the absence of invasion beneath the lamina muscularis on biopsy, so gross evaluation alone is insufficient to achieve a diagnosis. Polyps may be single or multiple, and are usually pedunculated from the mucosal surface. Occasionally, a thick 'carpet' of sessile polypoid tissue may be found extending a variable length about the circumference of the rectal wall.

Carcinoma

Carcinoma is the most commonly encountered tumour affecting the colorectal region of the dog. It may occur anywhere along the length of the colon, though a mid-rectal location is most common. Histological descriptions include adeno- (gland-forming), mucinous, signet ring and undifferentiated or solid forms. Grossly, the tumour may be intraluminal (pedunculated, frequently multiple, usually ulcerated; Figure 15.26) or annular. With progressive invasion about the circumference of the rectum, annular lesions will ultimately cause circumferential narrowing of the colon. The mucosal surface of annular

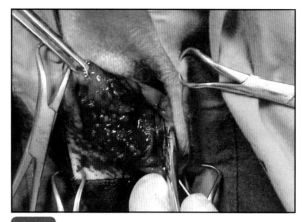

15.26 Sessile mucosal carcinoma in a dog.

tumours may be irregular and ulcerated, but there is frequently no intraluminal 'mass' evident and the misdiagnosis of stricture may therefore be made.

Colorectal carcinoma is a malignant tumour, with metastasis to regional nodes and lung (and other sites) occurring. Direct extension of disease through the serosa of the colon into the abdominal cavity can also occur (Figure 15.27).

Mesenchymal tumours

Leiomyomas are benign tumours of smooth muscle cells between the serosa and submucosa and form extraluminal masses. They can grow to a considerable size before they cause recognizable clinical signs. Signs are usually due to the physical size of the mass causing occlusion of the intestinal lumen.

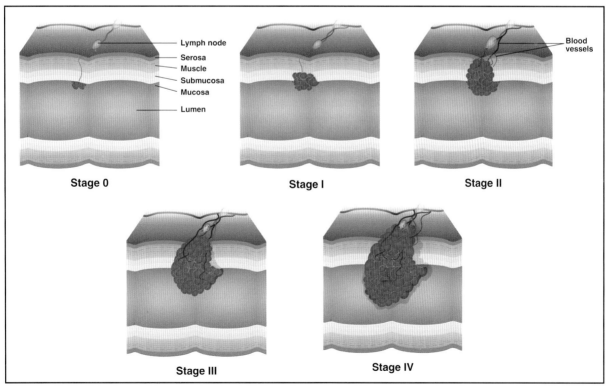

15.27 Epithelial colorectal tumours develop initially on the surface of the mucosa and are thus amenable to local resection with a margin of surrounding mucosa, provided there is sufficient local tissue available for closure. Colorectal carcinoma shows malignant potential to invade deeper into the underlying tissues. Once the tumour has invaded through the submucosa, full-thickness resection of the rectal wall will be necessary to achieve adequate local management.

In seven cases of colorectal leiomyoma, two were asymptomatic at the time of tumour detection and five showed clinical signs such as tenesmus or abnormal stool formation. The mucosa over the tumour usually remains intact and so ulceration and haemorrhage are uncommon.

In humans, most tumours previously diagnosed as leiomyosarcoma are now classified as gastrointestinal stromal tumours (GISTs), which are believed to arise from the cells of Cajal and are characterized by high vimentin immunoreactivity, low alpha smooth muscle actin reactivity and expression of the receptor tyrosine kinase KIT (CD117). GISTs have been recognized in the dog (see Chapter 15d).

Round cell tumours

Lymphoma tends to affect the small intestine (see Chapter 15e) of both cats and dogs more commonly than the colorectal region. Extramedullary plasmacytomas can occur rarely in the colorectal region. They are usually solitary with no systemic signs.

Presentation and clinical signs

Clinical signs relate to the physical presence of the mass, the effects of mucosal ulceration, and pain associated with tumour infiltration into the intestinal muscle wall. Because the surface of the mass is likely to be friable, frank blood may be seen on the surface of the stool, or the dog may bleed spontaneously from the rectum. Occasionally, the owner may report a visible mass protruding from the anus during defecation, and constipation. Additional signs that may occur include anorexia, weight loss, vomiting, and diarrhoea.

Clinical approach

Because some of the clinical signs described are similar to those reported for inflammatory or obstructive disease, a careful investigation is essential to differentiate the two. Due to the non-specific nature of the clinical signs, diagnosis of a colorectal cancer is often made very late in the course of disease. Early diagnosis and prompt management of most colorectal cancers, particularly epithelial cancer, is more likely to be associated with a good clinical outcome.

Physical examination

A complete physical examination is important. Rectal examination should always be performed, as the majority of colorectal tumours are within digital reach. It may be possible to prolapse the mass for visual inspection in the sedated animal (Figure 15.28). The presence of a painful, circumferential stricture should prompt consideration of annular carcinoma.

Imaging

Rigid proctoscopy or endoscopy (performed under general anaesthesia) will enable a more detailed inspection of the colorectal canal. Preoperative

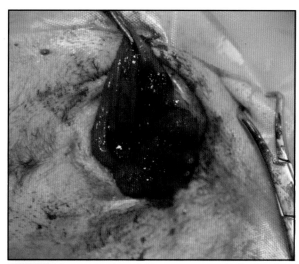

15.28 As most colorectal tumours occur in the last few centimetres of the colon, it is usually possible to assess the lesion with rigid proctoscopy or (as here) by gentle eversion of the rectal mucosa.

evacuation of stool using a warm water enema may be required, depending on the location of the mass. The size, location, distribution and appearance of the lesion should be noted.

Abdominal and thoracic radiographs should also be obtained. Although they are unlikely to reveal much morphological information on an intraluminal mass, the radiographs can be assessed for evidence of tumour extension (localized peritonitis) or metastasis (enlarged sublumbar nodes, presence of thoracic lesions).

Ultrasonography is probably the most effective and least invasive diagnostic modality available to detect and evaluate masses within the intestinal tract. The limitation with colorectal masses, however, is their caudal location, and the inability to scan beyond the pubic brim. Pararectal scanning may provide a reasonable acoustic window, but overall evaluation of the last few centimetres of the rectum is poor. Ultrasonographic features of certain tumours may assist in diagnosis:

- Transmural thickening, with the loss of normal gastrointestinal wall layering, is characteristic of intestinal adenocarcinoma (Figure 15.29)
- Leiomyosarcomas have been reported to have an eccentric growth pattern, with a lack of regional lymphadenopathy. When the lesion extends over 4 cm in length, the presence of poorly echogenic cavities is common
- Transmural circumferential thickening with complete loss of layering, associated with moderate or severe lymphadenopathy, has been reported for feline and canine lymphoma.

Ultrasonography may also assist in determining the extent of a lesion and thus in surgical planning.

The use of CT or MRI has not been specifically described in colorectal cancer in the dog or cat, although it may be of value to assess the extent and local invasiveness of large intrapelvic stromal tumours to assist surgical planning (Figure 15.30).

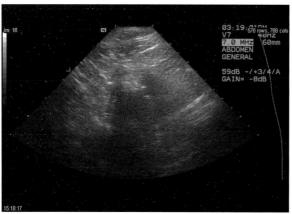

15.29 Transmural thickening with the loss of normal gastrointestinal wall layering is characteristic of intestinal adenocarcinoma. A large intraluminal mass is also evident.

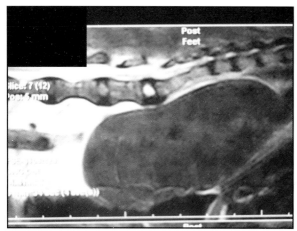

15.30 A T2-weighted sagittal image of a large rectal leiomyoma. The size of the mass made evaluation of resectability difficult on palpable characteristics alone. The information obtained by imaging in this case indicated that the mass was not invasive into surrounding structures, and surgery (via a combined dorsal rectal and abdominal approach) proceeded uneventfully.

Biopsy

Incisional biopsy should be performed on any lesions that are present. Biopsy samples should include the submucosal layer to allow the pathologist to assess the extent of tumour invasion; the small samples obtained using endoscopic forceps may thus fail to reveal the true invasive potential of many large colorectal masses. Ultrasound can be useful to guide biopsy of intestinal masses and enlarged lymph nodes, for tumour diagnosis and staging purposes.

Management

Surgery

Surgical excision is the treatment of choice for all colorectal lesions other than lymphoma. The extent of surgery required will be indicated by the tumour diagnosis. Recommended margins for resection vary from 1–2 cm for rectal polyps to a minimum of 2–8 cm for malignancies. As well as having a potential to spread to regional lymph nodes (and thence to other

parenchymal organs such as lung and liver), adenocarcinoma also has a tendency to invade through the layers of the intestine. Once it has invaded through the serosa, it may continue to progress by transcoelomic spread.

Risk factors

There are several factors associated with the anatomy and function of the colon that predispose it to significant operative and postoperative complications.

- Many of the tumours that occur within the rectum are located within the last 6 cm of the bowel. Surgical access to this location can be impeded by the pelvis. A variety of surgical routes have been described that facilitate access but, in almost all cases, the working room for the surgeon is greatly constrained.
- Preservation of continence is a significant challenge whenever surgery is contemplated on the terminal rectum. Sphincter continence can usually be retained provided a short cuff (1–1.5 cm) of rectal muscularis and the external anal sphincter is preserved. In addition, during dissection, it is vital to protect the pelvic plexus, pudendal nerves and rectal nerves, by staying as close to the rectal serosa as possible. Whenever a full-thickness resection of the rectum is contemplated, it is likely that some or all of these elements will be disrupted which can result in profound postoperative incontinence.
- Postoperative tenesmus and postoperative scarring can be a problem in some patients, particularly when the lumen is small. This can also complicate surgical recovery in some cases.
- The bacterial content of the colon is high and surgical stimulation of the colon results in a high level of collagenase activity. This effectively prolongs the 'lag phase' of healing to 5–7 days postoperatively before gains in tensile strength of the wound are seen. This can result in a weakened suture line and subsequent dehiscence if any surgical errors have been made. Excessive tissue trauma, vascular compromise or strangulation of tissues with suture, may potentiate the risk of dehiscence.

Surgical strategies

Surgical options for management of colorectal tumours will be dictated by the location and biological behaviour of the mass and by considerations regarding postoperative complications (see above). Typically, there is a trade-off between an aggressive 'curative intent' resection with a higher rate of potential complications, and a more conservative strategy that may result in inadequate oncological management. Underlying any decision regarding surgical dose is the fundamental issue that most colorectal tumours will be malignant and thus may already have escaped any hope of curative management, regardless of the extent of surgical intervention. Being certain of tumour stage is, therefore, critical if undertaking surgery that may be associated with a high risk of postoperative complications.

Surgical strategies described for the management of colorectal cancer may be divided into those where the resection is performed entirely within the lumen of the rectum (so-called 'intraluminal') and those where full-thickness resection and anastomosis of the colon is performed. Further information on many of these techniques is available in the *BSAVA Manual of Canine and Feline Abdominal Surgery*.

Intraluminal procedures: Intraluminal procedures only enable resection of the mucosa and submucosal lining of the rectum, and are thus most appropriate for lesions arising from the mucosal surface (i.e. epithelial tumours, <Stage 2). Once the tumour has invaded into the muscular wall of the rectum, intraluminal surgery is unlikely to provide curative tumour control.

- **Rectal pull-out, or mucosal eversion:** A simple and effective technique for management of most solitary benign lesions (e.g. pedunculated masses) only. The mucosal lining is progressively everted from the anus, using atraumatic forceps, until the mass and a section of surrounding mucosa can be readily viewed. The tissues are maintained in an exteriorized position using stay sutures. A resection of the mass is then performed, trying to maintain about 1–2 cm margins about the edge of the grossly visible mass. Resection occurs at the level of the muscularis, with no attempt to achieve a deeper margin. Primary reconstruction of the mucosal defect is performed using simple interrupted absorbable suture material. The use of stapling equipment has also been described to enable rapid but effective resection and closure of the defect.
- **Transanal endoscopic treatment:** Removal of polypoid masses with electrocautery has been described for tumours affecting 2–13 cm of the rectal mucosal length (Holt, 2007).

Full-thickness resection and anastomosis:

- **Rectal 'pull-through' resection:** The rectum is everted and several stay sutures are placed though the rectum cranial to the mucocutaneous junction. The rectal wall is then circumferentially transected, leaving the stay sutures attached to the most cranial section of the resected bowel to enable manipulation. A minimum of 1–1.5 cm of normal distal rectum should remain attached to the anal ring distally in order to preserve continence. The rectum is mobilized by continuing blunt dissection along its adventitial surface, extending as far cranially as the cranial rectal artery if required. After sufficient colon cranial to the lesion is identified, the abnormal tissue and 1–2 cm of normal tissue proximal and distal to the lesion is excised and the rectal ends anastomosed. The anastomosis can be performed in stages by incising a section of the rectum and suturing the corresponding normal tissue to the distal rectal cuff left at the mucocutaneous junction. The anastomosis

should be made with one or two layers of simple interrupted sutures.
- **Colonic resection and anastomoses:** For lesions located within the colon or at the colorectal junction, a ventral midline laparotomy combined with a pubic osteotomy/symphysiotomy can be performed. This access provides opportunity for extensive resection of colonic lesions and allows a more conventional end-to-end anastomosis (EEA) to be performed. Surgical access remains limited and the use of EEA stapling equipment can therefore be helpful to perform the anastomosis safely.

Colostomy: In humans, the use of colostomy systems is relatively commonplace to overcome the inevitable consequences of extensive resection of colorectal cancer affecting the distal sections of the large bowel. Colostomy provides the patient with an ability to manage their toilet functions in a hygienic and accessible manner following resection of the distal sections of the colon. In veterinary patients, the use of colostomy following colorectal resections has been isolated to a small number of patients. Stoma management in human patients can be a major consideration and has been associated with significant reduction in quality of life outcomes in affected patients. It is unclear whether this strategy has a realistic role in veterinary patients.

Pararectal lesions: The dorsal approach to the rectum and pelvic canal provides access to the dorsal pelvic canal, and lesions within the caudal and middle rectum. Access for manipulation is limited, and performance of anastomoses can be difficult. A high incidence of complications is reported (20%, mostly infection), due to the high potential for contamination and limited drainage from this region.

Chemotherapy

Apart from lymphoma, most colorectal tumours respond poorly to conventional chemotherapy. Doxorubicin has been shown to improve survival in cats with colonic adenocarcinoma (MST 280 days *versus* 56 days without chemotherapy; Slawienski *et al.*, 1997). Very few other studies exist to determine benefit from adjuvant chemotherapy following resection of intestinal tumours in dogs and cats.

The use of anti-inflammatory drugs for the management and prevention of colorectal cancer has been reported increasingly in both human and veterinary fields. It has been suggested that the drugs exert a direct antineoplastic activity via inhibition of COX-2 receptors. However, despite clear evidence for pro-apoptotic and antiproliferative effects in tumours, the mechanism by which NSAIDs cause protective and direct antitumour effects is still to be determined. *In vitro* studies with both piroxicam and meloxicam have suggested that the concentrations required to obtain significant cytotoxic effects appear higher than could be achieved *in vivo* through regular systemic delivery at recommended doses and intervals of both drugs. Topically applied medication may, however, enable high local drug concentrations to be achieved without systemic toxicity being a concern. The use of piroxicam suppositories (0.3 mg/kg) has been shown to provide significant palliative benefit for patients with colorectal adenocarcinoma (Knottenbelt *et al.,* 2000), with excellent control of clinical signs, whilst systemic piroxicam at similar doses was associated with a undesirable rate of renal and gastrointestinal complications. Topical treatment can also reduce the bulk and friability of the rectal mass supporting a direct antineoplastic property of the drug. Anecdotal benefit has been reported for systemic meloxicam but large clinical studies have not been reported.

Prognosis

Epithelial tumours

The prognosis for patients with colorectal cancer is influenced significantly by tumour type, size, location and clinical stage. However, irrespective of the cancer type being treated, long-term survival has been shown to be significantly influenced by the ability to achieve a clean surgical margin. Because there is a varied 'menu' of treatment options, the choice of technique for tumour management must weigh up the prospect of achieving a complete surgical resection, against the potential complications associated with the chosen approach.

Rectal eversion

Due to limited access and the conservativism of resection, mucosal eversion was traditionally reserved for localized benign lesions. However, in 2006, Danova *et al.* described the results for 23 dogs with a variety of primary rectal tumours, including adenocarcinoma, adenomatous polyps and plasmacytoma. Incomplete microscopic margins were obtained for a mucinous carcinoma in one dog, but no tumour recurrence was recorded in this dog 38 months after resection. Tumour recurrence occurred in two dogs 16 and 24 months after the original surgery, despite apparently clean histological margins. Resections were repeated in these two dogs, providing further disease-free intervals of 86 and 14 months, respectively. For the 18 dogs followed up in this paper (mean follow-up 33 months, range 5–84 months), a disease-free interval of 34.8 months (range 5–84 months) was reported. Half of the dogs died for reasons unrelated to their cancer. Complications were observed in 10 dogs but were limited to rectal bleeding and mild tenesmus, which resolved spontaneously within 7 days. Wound infections, rectal stricture or faecal incontinence were not observed. The results of this study suggest that the anal approach may be an effective solution for many non-infiltrative lesions affecting the caudal rectal lumen.

Transanal cautery

The use of transanal cautery was described in 13 dogs by Holt (2007). Five animals were cured of their disease, with follow-up ranging from 1.3 to 5.5 years, whilst three dogs had their clinical signs successfully palliated for 19 months to 4 years. Unfortunately, fatal complications occurred in three dogs due to rectal perforation and peritonitis.

Rectal pull-through

Results for this procedure were first described by White and Gorman (1987), who reported results for nine dogs with epithelial tumours affecting the colorectal region. Two dogs died in the immediate postoperative period, but seven dogs remained alive at the close of the study, with follow-up times ranging from 8 to 20 months. Two dogs developed local recurrences (at 3 and 11 months following surgery) and one dog developed a local lymph node metastasis. Resection of these recurrent lesions permitted further palliation of signs and prolonged survival. Several cases developed postoperative stenosis of the colorectal repair, which was managed by bougienage dilation. Faecal incontinence was not reported in any dog, though resection was limited to the last 6 cm of the terminal rectum.

More recently, Morello *et al.* (2008) reported results for 11 dogs with extensive pull-through resections for colorectal adenocarcinoma and *in situ* carcinoma. An abdominal approach was combined with a transanal resection in four patients to enable removal of tumours located in the mid-cranial region of the rectum to the level of the descending colon. Mean disease-free and overall survival times were 44.3 and 44.6 months, respectively, indicating that prolonged survival times are possible with complete *en bloc* resection. Incontinence occurred in two dogs for a period of 1–5 months after surgery. Two dogs developed fatal complications in the postoperative period.

Colonic resection (pubic symphysiotomy)

There are limited clinical reports on the outcome following resection of adenocarcinoma via this route. Yoon and Mann (2008) reported no postoperative ambulatory complications associated with the approach through the pubis. Neurological complications (faecal/urinary) were not reported in the small number of cases in their study, but follow-up times were too short in this study to comment on long-term outcome. Resection margins were not described.

Mesenchymal tumours

The prognosis for leiomyoma following resection is considered to be very good, with 'curative' management likely in the majority of cases. Because the tumour is typically non-invasive, it usually 'shells-out' from the wall of the intestine. Malignant leiomyosarcoma may occur, which may demonstrate a higher potential for metastasis (up to 30%); further clinical data on this tumour type are limited, however.

Round cell tumours

The prognosis for plasmacytomas is usually excellent following excision, provided tumour-free margins have been obtained. Repeat surgery should be considered if incomplete margins are obtained. Where further surgery is not possible, adjunctive chemotherapy (with melphalan) may be considered. The patient should be monitored for evidence of local recurrence, or development of multiple myeloma in the future.

Details for lymphoma are covered in Chapter 19a.

presentation – but are rarely adherent or fixed to surrounding structures. Malignant lesions may diffusely infiltrate the anal area and will be adherent to deeper tissues on palpation; their rate of growth tends to be faster and they are frequently associated with clinical signs of dyschezia and anal pain.

Anal sac apocrine adenocarcinoma

Tumours may be detected for a variety of reasons, although frequently (40%) they may be recognized incidentally during routine examination. The majority of dogs remain apparently healthy, with only a third showing evidence of ill health. Perianal swelling and/or faecal tenesmus are the most common signs, and some dogs may also lick frequently at the anal area. Other signs can include polyuria/polydipsia, hindlimb weakness, lethargy and weight loss. Typically, signs relate to the size of the tumour or whether paraneoplastic hypercalcaemia is present. Careful rectal palpation is necessary as up to 50% of tumours are not detectable on external examination alone. However, tumour size can be considerable (Figure 15.32), with some extending round more than 50% of the anal circumference. During rectal assessment it may be possible to detect lymphadenopathy of the iliac lymph nodes.

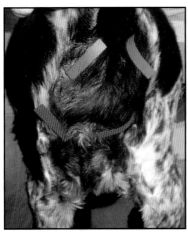

15.32 Anal sac adenocarcinomas can be very large. Paper strips have been used to outline the size of the mass on this dog.

Paraneoplastic hypercalcaemia, originally considered a common occurrence with this tumour, is now shown to be less common (20%) than originally suspected. Presenting signs are usually those of hypercalcaemia and include anorexia, polydipsia, polyuria, depression, weakness and weight loss.

Clinical approach

Perianal sebaceous adenoma and adenocarcinoma

Preoperative evaluation should include a thorough digital and rectal examination of the mass to determine its size, and degree of infiltration into the surrounding tissues; the sublumbar nodes should also be carefully evaluated. Caudal abdominal radiography and, if possible, ultrasound examination of the sublumbar nodes should be performed if adenocarcinoma is suspected. As most affected patients are elderly, a routine geriatric work-up is essential prior to anaesthesia.

Distinguishing between benign and malignant disease is important, as the tumour forms have a very different biological behaviour and patient outcome. Cytology has not been found to be reliable in differentiating perianal gland adenoma from perianal gland adenocarcinoma.

Anal sac apocrine adenocarcinoma

Blood tests, combined with a measure of ionized blood calcium, are important to determine the patient's general health status. Confirmation of clinical diagnosis can usually be achieved by cytology of a fine-needle aspirate from the enlarged perianal mass (Figure 15.33).

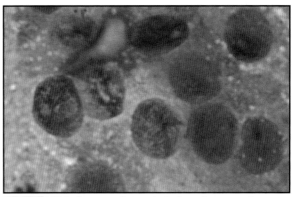

15.33 This fine-needle aspirate from the mass in Figure 15.32 shows that this is an epithelial tumour with obvious features of malignancy. (Diff-Quik, original magnification X40)

Staging

Diagnostic evaluation of anal sac adenocarcinoma requires accurate staging of the disease and assessment of the systemic effects of hypercalcaemia, if present. The size of the primary tumour should be measured with calipers, especially when it is large as this may have an influence on prognosis. The extent of local invasion, including its degree of local fixation and proximity to the rectal wall, will also assist evaluation of surgical risk. A tumour staging system proposed by Polton and Brearley (2007) (Figure 15.34) has been shown to demonstrate statistically significant relevance to clinical decision-making. The WHO staging scheme for anal sac adenocarcinoma is presented in Figure 15.35.

The tumour is likely to have metastasized to the regional iliac and sublumbar lymph nodes in >50% of cases. Rarely is the full extent of lymphadenopathy evident on physical examination alone. Caudal abdominal radiography is also insensitive, with >60% of lesions failing to be detected (Figure 15.36).

A full abdominal ultrasound examination is essential to quantify the extent of disease present. Lymphadenopathy may appear as multiple discrete masses, located adjacent to the iliac bifurcation, and can extend on either side of the aorta/vena cava to the level of the kidneys. Confluent masses, especially when there is evidence of invasion into the sublumbar muscles, present difficulties for surgical resection.

Advanced coaxial imaging may also be used to reveal the extent of lymph node involvement (Figure 15.37).

Clinical stage	T – tumour	N – node	M – metastasis	Median survival time (MST)
Stage 1	<2.5 cm max diameter	None	None	>1205 days
Stage 2	>2.5 cm max diameter	None	None	>722 days
Stage 3a	Any T	Present (<4.5 cm max diameter)	None	448–492 days
Stage 3b	Any T	Present (>4.5 cm max diameter)	None	294–335 days
Stage 4	Any T	Any N	Present	71–82 days

15.34 Clinical staging system for anal sac adenocarcinoma proposed by Polton and Brearley (2007).

T – Primary tumour	
Tis	Preinvasive carcinoma (carcinoma *in situ*)
T0	No evidence of tumour
T1	2 cm max diameter, superficial or exophytic
T2	2.5 cm maximum diameter, or with invasion of the subcutis, irrespective of size
T3	Tumour invading other structures such as fascia, muscle, bone, or cartilage
N – Regional lymph nodes	
N0	No evidence of regional lymph node involvement
N1	Movable ipsilateral nodes
	a – Nodes not considered to contain growth
	b – Nodes considered to contain growth
N2	Movable contralateral or bilateral nodes
	a – Nodes not considered to contain growth
	b – Nodes considered to contain growth
N3	Fixed nodes
M – Distant metastasis	
M0	No evidence of distant metastasis
M1	Distant metastasis detected

15.35 WHO TNM classification for canine tumours of epidermal or dermal origin (excluding lymphosarcoma and mastocytoma).

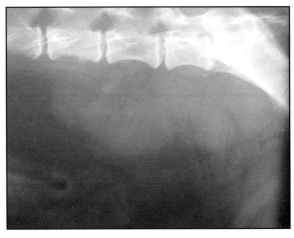

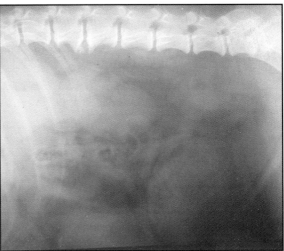

15.36 Although radiographs of the sublumbar spine are not always sensitive enough to reveal the full extent of lymph node involvement, these two radiographs both show obvious lymph node enlargement.

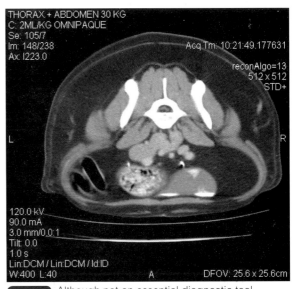

15.37 Although not an essential diagnostic tool, coaxial imaging can provide very detailed information on the extent and discreteness of the metastatic burden. This computed tomography 'slice' reveals a large cluster of lymph node enlargements about the iliac bifurcation.

Thoracic radiography may reveal evidence of pulmonary metastasis (Figure 15.38) in up to 20% of cases. Dogs with evidence of pulmonary metastasis have a significantly shorter survival following treatment, than those who do not.

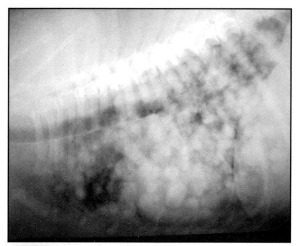

15.38 Thoracic metastasis detected radiographically in a dog with anal sac apocrine adenocarcinoma.

Management

Perianal sebaceous adenoma and adenocarcinoma

Adenomas

The majority (95%) of adenomas can be managed by castration alone. Attempts to resect the tumour itself are often complicated by its friable character, resulting in haemorrhage and unnecessary surgical trauma. The response to castration is usually brisk and the mass should be considerably smaller and less friable by the time of suture removal. Surgical resection may be necessary for tumours in females, for tumours that persist following castration, for large uncomfortable tumours, or when the owners do not consent to castration. Pre-treatment with anti-testosterone medications may reduce the size of mass to limit the surgical intervention necessary.

Adenocarcinomas

Surgical resection of adenocarcinomas is often difficult due to the diffusely infiltrative nature of the tumour. They do not respond to castration. Local recurrence is common, as most 'shell-out' resections are incomplete. For this reason, if malignancy is suspected preoperatively, a biopsy would be advisable to ensure the mass is removed with adequate margins. Adjunctive radiotherapy following cytoreductive surgery may prolong the disease-free interval, but is rarely curative. Regional lymph node excision should be considered if metastatic disease is suspected.

The development of regional or distant metastasis may take several years. Numerous palliative local surgeries can therefore be justified if local recurrence occurs.

Anal sac apocrine adenocarcinoma

A variety of therapeutic options exist, depending on the size and stage of the tumour, the physical status of the patient, and the availability of adjunctive therapeutic modalities. Surgical resection of the tumour, combined with metastatectomy where necessary, has been associated with good long-term survival. Most authors have not shown any statistically significant difference in survival time between dogs treated with surgery alone, radiation therapy alone, surgery and radiotherapy, surgery and chemotherapy, or a combination of surgery, chemotherapy and radiotherapy. However, strict interpretation of these findings is difficult due to the small numbers in each study, the heterogeneity of the populations studied, and differences in chemotherapy administered. Williams *et al.* (2003) demonstrated that there was a survival advantage for dogs who received any type of surgery as part of their treatment. Polton and Brearley (2007) considered that chemotherapy may be of greatest benefit for Stage 3b tumours.

Local surgery

Tumours arise from the apocrine component of the anal sac glands located adjacent to the anal sac, and extend variably into the surrounding connective tissues. The lumen of the anal sac is typically not infiltrated by the tumour but may be compressed by the surrounding growth. The tumours are often highly infiltrative. Marginal excision of the tumour (Figure 15.39) is advised, as attempts at wide surgical excision are more likely to induce complications such as faecal incontinence. Occasionally, invasion by the tumour into the rectal wall may necessitate partial resection of the mucosa at this site, with subsequent primary closure of the luminal defect. Where the tumour is very large, surgical management can be complicated and the case should be discussed with someone experienced with this type of surgery. For these larger masses, particular care must be taken to close the considerable dead space that develops in the pararectal fossa to prevent redundancy in the rectal wall.

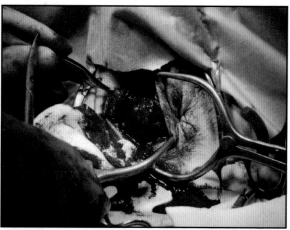

15.39 Surgical management of the anal sac mass requires gentle excision about the infiltrative border of the mass, taking care not to damage remaining anal sphincter muscle, neural elements and the rectal wall.

Metastatectomy

Abdominal exploration and sublumbar lymphadenectomy should be performed in all cases where lymph node metastases have been detected, to reduce tumour burden. If pelvic lymphadenopathy is present, these glands may be better approached via a dorsal rectal dissection.

Exposure of the sublumbar fossa is achieved by utilizing the duodenal or colic manoeuvre and packing intestinal content with moistened laparotomy sponges. The enlarged lymph nodes are normally palpable as they extend along the aorta and vena cava and their iliac bifurcations. Masses are typically discrete and can be removed from their fascial bed with gentle dissection (Figure 15.40). Care is required to ensure all enlarged lymph nodes are removed; in some cases there may be as many as 9–12 separate nodes. When they are confluent, with invasion into the sublumbar muscles, attempts to remove them are ill advised, due to the potential for neurological injury, haemorrhage and other complications.

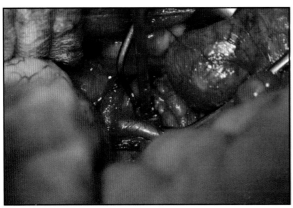

15.40 Removal of sublumbar lymph node deposits requires careful dissection of the lymph node swellings from the sublumbar fascia. The median iliac artery is visible towards the bottom of the surgical field. The suction tip is sitting on top of the enlarged lymph node.

The close proximity to major vessels and the expansile, confluent nature of the lymphadenopathy indicates that surgical management of metastatic disease should only be undertaken by surgeons experienced with this type of procedure. Most animals are in clinically good health despite their tumour burden, so exposing them to unnecessary surgical risk as a result of surgical inexperience is not justifiable.

Chemotherapy

A variety of chemotherapeutic agents have been described for the management of anal sac adenocarcinoma, with treatment employed either as the primary modality or, more commonly, as an adjunct to surgery. As a primary treatment, no significant differences have been identified between different drugs or combination protocols, though patient numbers are low.

Polton and Brearley (2007) intimated that neoadjuvant treatment with carboplatin might be useful at reducing tumour volume and should therefore be considered for higher-stage presentations in particular. In this context, even if complete remission does not occur, the patient may be sufficiently 'downstaged' to become a more suitable surgical candidate. Bennett et al. (2002) reported MSTs of about 7–8 months (Figure 15.41).

Drug	Number of dogs treated	Response to treatment	Number showing that response
Cisplatin	13	PR	4 (31%)
		SD	1 (8%)
		PD	8 (61%)
Carboplatin	3	PR	1 (33%)
		SD	2 (67%)
Doxorubicin	4	SD	2 (50%)
		PD	2 (50%)
Dactinomycin	4	PD	4 (100%)
5-Fluorouracil	2	PD	2 (100%)
Mithramycin	1	PD	1 (100%)
Vincristine and cyclophosphamide	1	PD	1 (100%)
Melphalan	1	PD	1 (100%)
Epirubicin	1	PD	1 (100%)
Mitoxantrone	1	PD	1 (100%)

15.41 Responses to chemotherapy in dogs with anal sac adenocarcinoma. PR = partial remission (≥50% reduction in tumour size); SD = stable disease (<50% change in size of tumour within a 1-month period); PD = progressive disease (≥50% increase in tumour size within one treatment period, or any new tumour lesions). (Data from Bennett et al., 2002)

Radiotherapy

The role of radiotherapy in the management of anal sac adenocarcinoma is unclear, with insufficient data available to validate its use. Adjuvant fractionated radiotherapy in association with either surgery or mitoxantrone chemotherapy has been shown to provide prolonged tumour control.

Palliative care

Where specific tumour treatment is declined by the owners, palliative medical management may be of value. Palliative management is directed at the management of faecal tenesmus, using laxatives and other dietary aids, or at limiting the effects of hypercalcaemia with a combination of short-term intravenous fluids, prednisolone and furosemide. Survival times between 2 days and 9 months (MST 8.7 months; 95% confidence intervals 3.6–9.6 months) were achieved in 10 dogs managed in this way alone.

Repeated metastatectomy

Following initial lymphadenectomy, some patients can develop further lymph node enlargements. Repeated exploratory laparotomy to extirpate grossly evident tumour can be effective in these patients to continue palliation of their disease. Because surgery is associated with comparatively low morbidity, some patients may undergo three to five exploratory procedures during their lifetime. A limiting factor with subsequent surgeries is the mature perivascular fibrosis that develops as a consequence of previous dissection events, combined with progressive invasion of the tumour into the underlying musculature and perivascular stroma. When the metastatic lesions are confluent and not amenable to debulking, or when extirpation may be associated with life-threatening haemorrhage from the aorta, vena cava or associated vasculature, the procedure should be abandoned.

Prognosis

Perianal sebaceous adenoma and adenocarcinoma

The prognosis for adenomas is excellent.

The prognosis for adenocarcinoma is unfavourable due to local recurrence and metastasis. Survival times of >2 years have been recorded in 70% of patients that were node-negative at the time of the initial surgery.

Anal sac apocrine adenocarcinoma

Previously, a grave prognosis was given for dogs with this disease, with survival times of <12 months. However, recent work suggests that good tumour control is possible in many animals, even when metastatic spread to regional lymph nodes is present.

- Williams *et al.* (2003) reported an MST of 544 days (range 0–1873 days) for all patients, regardless of treatment method, with a 37% probability of surviving 2 years or more.
- Polton and Brearley (2007) reported MSTs of 479–508 days, with close correlation of survival times with clinical stage determination. Removal of metastatic lymph nodes was statistically associated with improved survival.
- Emms (2005) reported an MST of 20 months (range 5–42 months) but did not identify any difference in survival between dogs with differing stage disease (i.e. those with sublumbar lymph node metastasis compared to those without).
- Hobson *et al.* (2006) described survival in one dog for 50 months after diagnosis by performing repeated metastatectomy on four further occasions after original management.
- The importance of metastatectomy in improving survival was also illustrated by Bennett *et al.* (2002), who reported a poorer MST of 8.7 months (range 2 days to 41 months). Lymphadenectomy was uncommonly performed in this study (36%), even though regional lymph node enlargements were present in 91% of patients undergoing surgery. A high local recurrence following resection was also common, which may have had an impact on overall survival figures in the study.

Apart from Bennett *et al.* (2002), who described a 45% local recurrence rate, tumour recurrence as a cause of death is rarely reported, even with conservative surgery.

Hypercalcaemia

Signs associated with hypercalcaemia should resolve quickly (1–2 days) if all tumour is removed. Persistence, or recurrence, of hypercalcaemia is indicative of metastatic disease. Williams *et al.* (2003) identified the presence of hypercalcaemia as being a significant ($p = 0.002$) independent predictor of survival, with MSTs of 256 days for hypercalcaemic dogs, compared with 584 days for normocalcaemic dogs. However, these findings are not supported by other studies. Polton (2008) considered that hypercalcaemia *per se* was not an independent risk factor, but was a confounding effect due to clinical stage.

Tumour size

The size of the primary tumour may be an independent predictor of survival. The MST for dogs with tumours ≥10 cm^2 was 292 days, compared with 584 days for smaller tumours ($p = 0.04$). It is possible that large tumour size may present an obstacle to management due to concerns regarding complications, but where surgery is performed by experienced specialist soft tissue surgeons such risks seem to be minimal. Neoadjuvant chemotherapy may be a consideration to attempt reduction in tumour volume when the initial tumour size presents a surgical concern.

Recurrences

Tumour recurrence should be considered inevitable in almost all cases of anal sac adenocarcinoma, with tumour being considered the cause of death in almost all clinical studies. Tumour recurrence should be suspected whenever hypercalcaemia-related polyuria/polydipsia recurs, or when faecal tenesmus recurs. Other signs of distant metastatic disease may also occur (e.g. exercise intolerance or dyspnoea with pulmonary metastasis).

References and further reading

Bennett PF, DeNicola DB, Bonney P, Glickman NW and Knapp DW (2002) Canine anal sac adenocarcinomas: clinical presentation and response to therapy. *Journal of Veterinary Internal Medicine* **16**, 100–104

Emms SG (2005) Anal sac tumours of the dog and their response to cytoreductive surgery and chemotherapy. *Australian Veterinary Journal* **83**, 340–343

Hobson P, Brown MR and Rogers KS (2006) Surgery of metastatic anal sac adenocarcinoma in five dogs. *Veterinary Surgery* **35**, 267–270

Polton G (2008) Anal sac gland carcinoma in cocker spaniels. *Veterinary Record* **163**, 608

Polton GA and Brearley MJ (2007) Clinical stage, therapy and prognosis in canine anal sac gland carcinoma. *Journal of Veterinary Internal Medicine* **21**, 274–280

Williams LE, Gliatto JM, Dodge RK *et al.* (2003) Carcinoma of the apocrine glands of the anal sac in dogs: 113 cases (1985–1995). *Journal of the American Veterinary Medical Association* **223**, 825–831

Tumours of the liver

Jonathan Bray

Introduction

The liver is the largest parenchymous organ in the body and receives blood from both portal and systemic sources. Possibly because of these factors, 46% of all tumours that occur in the liver of the dog are of metastatic origin (Figure 15.42). In one study, up to a third of all dogs with a malignant primary tumour had evidence of liver involvement on postmortem examination; this contrasts with the lungs, which may be involved in just 24% of cases. Haemopoietic tumour types account for up to two-thirds of all metastases, followed by an approximately equal amount of epithelial and mesenchymal tumours.

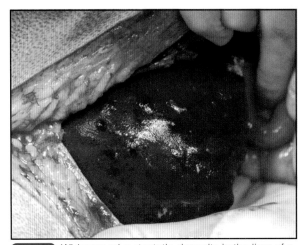

15.42 Widespread metastatic deposits in the liver of a 12-year-old Rhodesian Ridgeback with a splenic haemangiosarcoma.

Primary tumours of the liver are less common and account for 0.6–1.3% of canine tumours and 1.0–2.3% of all feline tumours. In the dog, approximately 25% of all liver tumours are of primary (hepatic or biliary tissue) origin, 25% are of haemopoietic origin and almost 50% are metastatic. In the cat, haemopoietic tumours (principally lymphoma) predominate, representing 75% of all liver tumours in this species.

Hepatic neoplasia is most common in the geriatric patient, with the mean age of occurrence being 10–11 years. In one study, cats with malignant hepatic masses were significantly younger than those with benign masses.

Tumour types and behaviour

There are four general tissue types from which primary hepatic tumours may be derived: hepatocellular; bile duct; neuroendocrine (carcinoid); and mesenchymal. Almost irrespective of origin, a primary hepatic tumour may develop according to three morphological subtypes: massive; nodular; or diffuse:

- Massive is defined as a large solitary mass confined to one liver lobe
- Nodular tumours are multifocal and may involve multiple lobes
- Diffuse disease includes multifocal or coalescing nodules affecting all lobes, often causing effacement of normal hepatic parenchyma.

An important differential for all liver masses is nodular hyperplasia (Figure 15.43), which may be found in 15–60% of geriatric dogs. Lesions can be solitary or multiple, and range from 0.1 to 5 cm in diameter. They are difficult to differentiate from other hepatic tumours; biopsy is therefore important.

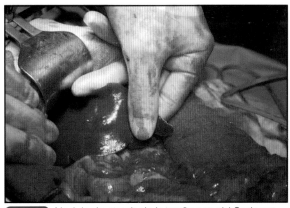

15.43 Nodular hyperplasia in an 8-year-old Springer Spaniel. This condition is an important differential for all liver masses.

Hepatocellular tumours

Hepatocellular tumours include hepatocellular carcinoma (HCC), hepatocellular adenoma and hepatoblastoma. HCC is the most common hepatic neoplasm in the dog and may account for up to 48% of all cases of primary hepatic tumours. Morphologically, over two-thirds of HCCs are massive (Figure 15.44), with the remainder either diffuse or

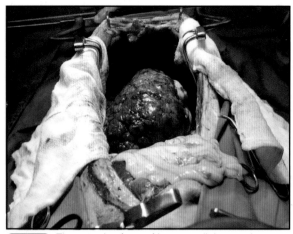

15.44 The massive form of hepatocellular carcinoma in a dog.

nodular. Metastasis is more common with nodular or diffuse HCC (93% and 100%, respectively), whilst solitary tumours are thought not to have such a high rate of metastatic spread (0–37%).

Hepatocellular adenomas (hepatomas) are typically an incidental finding at necropsy, and only rarely cause clinical signs. They can be seen in the living animal, however, as multiple nodules or pedunculated masses, and distinguishing them from a more generalized metastatic disease is therefore important. Some solitary adenomas can attain a considerable size, where their encroachment on other organs can result in non-specific clinical signs. Large adenomas may be friable, with intermittent bleeding from the surface causing anaemia and haemorrhagic ascites. In cats, hepatocellular adenoma occurs more frequently than HCC.

Bile duct tumours

Carcinoma of the bile duct (biliary carcinoma or cholangiocellular carcinoma; Figure 15.45) is the most common malignant non-haemopoietic hepatic tumour in cats and the second most common in dogs. These tumours principally arise from intrahepatic bile duct epithelium, although they can occur in the extrahepatic bile ducts or gallbladder. Intrahepatic tumours

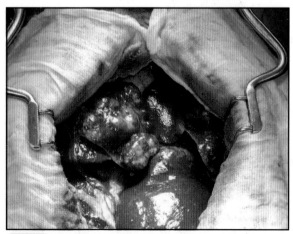

15.45 Carcinoma of the bile duct, a common malignant non-haemopoietic hepatic tumour in dogs. (Courtesy of Julius Liptak)

are more common in dogs, whereas there is an even distribution of intrahepatic and extrahepatic tumours in cats. The morphological distribution includes massive (37–46%), nodular (up to 54%), and diffuse (17–54%) forms. Metastasis is reported to be as high as 88% in dogs and 78% in cats, occurring most often in the regional lymph nodes, lungs or peritoneum.

Benign adenoma affecting the bile duct have also been called biliary or hepatobiliary cystadenomas, due to their cystic appearance (Figure 15.46). Bile duct adenomas may account for >50% of all feline primary hepatic tumours, affecting mainly domestic short-haired cats over 10 years of age. They typically do not cause clinical signs until they are large enough to compress adjacent tissues.

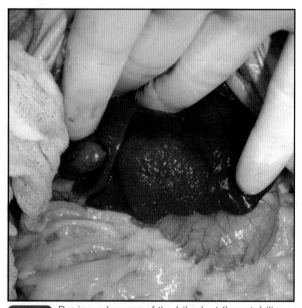

15.46 Benign adenoma of the bile duct (hepatobiliary cystadenoma) in a dog, showing the cystic appearance. (Courtesy of Julius Liptak)

Neuroendocrine tumours

Neuroendocrine tumours, also known as hepatic carcinoids, are infrequently reported in dogs and cats. Arising from neuroectodermal cells, they are embryologically similar to the cells responsible for insulinomas and gastrinomas. They tend to occur at a younger age than other hepatic tumours (7 years *versus* 10 years). Carcinoids have an aggressive biological behaviour and are not usually surgically resectable, as the majority are morphologically diffuse.

Mesenchymal tumours

Primary tumours of mesenchymal origin are rare in dogs and cats. The most common primary sarcomas are leiomyosarcoma, haemangiosarcoma and fibrosarcoma. Other sarcomas include rhabdomyosarcoma, liposarcoma, osteosarcoma and malignant mesenchymoma. Males appear predisposed, but there is no known breed association. Massive and nodular morphology have been reported in 33% and 67% of cases, respectively. Diffuse disease has not been reported. Sarcomas are aggressive biologically, with metastasis reported in 86–100% of cases.

Tumours of the exocrine pancreas

Brian J. Trumpatori and Reto Neiger

Introduction

Cancers of the exocrine pancreas are extremely rare in dogs and cats, accounting for <3% of all abdominal neoplasms in dogs; in cats, the incidence is even lower. In one study evaluating ultrasonography for pancreatic neoplasia in the dog, only 1 of 16 tumours was of exocrine origin, with the remainder either endocrine or metastatic in nature (Lamb *et al.*, 1995). Usually older animals are affected (mean age 10.5 years); and there is possibly an increased prevalence in bitches. There may be a breed predisposition in Cocker Spaniels, Airedale Terriers, Labrador Retrievers and Boxers.

Almost all tumours of the exocrine pancreas are epithelial, with adenocarcinomas (most common) arising from either acinar or duct cells. Other reported non-endocrine tumour types include squamous cell carcinoma, lymphoma, lymphangiosarcoma, spindle-cell sarcoma and various metastatic neoplasms (Hecht *et al.*, 2007). Early metastasis is very common and is presumed to have occurred at the time of diagnosis, mostly into regional lymph nodes, liver, omentum, peritoneum, diaphragm, lung and bones. Other reported sites include the heart, thyroid glands, central nervous system, adrenals and ovaries.

Benign conditions such as nodular hyperplasia, pancreatic pseudocysts, abcessation and adenomas have been reported as common, and sometimes incidental findings (Van Enkevort *et al.*, 1999).

Tumours of the endocrine pancreas are discussed in Chapter 20.

Presentation and clinical signs

Clinical signs are non-specific and include weight loss, anorexia, depression and vomiting. If biliary obstruction or hepatic metastasis is present, animals may become jaundiced. Rarely, signs might be due to diabetes mellitus and exocrine pancreatic insufficiency, caused by complete destruction of the pancreatic parenchyma. Ascites can be present if there is metastatic spread into the peritoneum.

Abdominal pain or an abdominal mass may be found on physical examination. In cases of destruction of the pancreas with necrotizing steatitis, the animal can present with signs of an 'acute abdomen'. Dermatological signs, such as paraneoplastic alopecia or subcutaneous swellings with discharging sinuses due to steatitis, have been reported in cats and dogs with malignant pancreatic neoplasms (Brown *et al.*,1994; Pascaltenorio *et al.*, 1997); following successful surgical resection, the alopecia may resolve but can then return upon regrowth of the carcinoma (Tasker *et al.*,1999).

Clinical approach

Diagnosis of exocrine pancreatic neoplasia is challenging, due to non-specific or absent clinical signs and clinicopathological changes. The final diagnosis is usually made by exploratory laparotomy. Histopathological confirmation of a neoplasm is important, as chronic pancreatitis can mimic a pancreatic tumour clinically.

Haematology and biochemistry
Haematology and serum biochemistry results are non-specific but may show a neutrophilia due to inflammation and a non-regenerative anaemia due to chronic disease. Increased serum amylase and lipase are inconsistently seen, while increased alkaline phosphatase and bilirubin can be found in cases of cholestasis. In severe cases, signs of exocrine pancreatic insufficiency may be identified (Bright, 1985).

Cytology
Aspiration of peritoneal effusion, if present, may reveal the presence of neoplastic cells on cytological evaluation.

Imaging
Plain abdominal radiographs may reveal a mass in the right cranial abdomen or decreased contrast serosal detail in cases with ascites (Hecht *et al.*, 2007). Abnormal gastric motility or, infrequently, invasion or compression of the duodenum may be seen on barium contrast series.

Abdominal ultrasonography is extremely helpful and is the most common modality used to evaluate the pancreas in dogs and cats. A tumour of the pancreas may be seen as an ill-defined hypoechoic mass between the duodenum and stomach (Figure 15.50). The area might also show mixed echogenicity if steatitis is present. However, differentiation between pancreatitis or nodular hyperplasia and pancreatic tumours is normally impossible ultrasonographically (Bennett *et al.*, 2001; Hecht *et al.*, 2007). Potential challenges to diagnostic imaging of pancreatic neoplasms include masses arising from adjacent structures, the presence of concurrent pancreatitis, abnormal lymph nodes in close proximity to the pancreas and the similar appearance of many pancreatic diseases, making definitive diagnosis difficult (Hecht and Henry, 2007). In a recent imaging study of pancreatic disease in cats, the only ultrasonographically unique feature of malignant disease was the presence of a single nodule or a mass exceeding 2 cm in at least one dimension; however, the authors noted a significant overlap between the appearance of nodular hyperplasia and neoplasia (Hecht *et al.*, 2007). While helpful, ultrasonography is highly operator-dependent. Lymphatic drainage of the pancreas is provided by the splenic, hepatic, pancreaticoduodenal and jejunal lymph nodes, each of which drains additional organs, making accurate assessment of metastatic disease difficult (Robben *et al.*, 2005; Hecht and Henry, 2007). The usefulness of ultrasound-guided FNA to diagnose pancreatic tumours has not been reported.

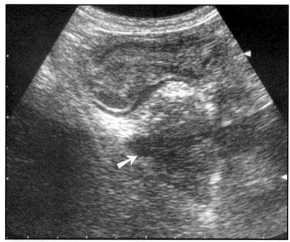

15.50 Ultrasonographic appearance of a hyperechogenic pancreas with a 1.3 cm hypoechogenic nodule (arrowed) in an 11-year-old American Cocker Spaniel. The dog was euthanased due to oesophageal rupture, and a pancreatic adenoma and chronic pancreatitis were found on histopathology. (Courtesy of J Lang)

The use of computed tomography for evaluation of the canine and feline pancreas has been reported for other conditions such as pancreatitis and endocrine neoplasia. While the use of advanced imaging modalities has not been specifically reported for diagnosis of exocrine neoplasia of the pancreas, CT is likely to be helpful in surgical planning, and may provide information about the status of regional lymph nodes and the presence of abdominal metastatic disease.

The use of magnetic resonance imaging for the diagnosis of benign and malignant pancreatic disease is common in humans, but has not yet been reported in veterinary medicine.

Management and prognosis

Since most tumours of the exocrine pancreas have either metastasized by the time of diagnosis or become locally invasive, extensive or 'heroic' surgery is often contraindicated. Complete pancreatectomy or pancreaticoduodenectomy is possible, but both carry a high risk of morbidity and mortality. To alleviate clinical signs, a palliative gastrointestinal bypass is an option. Most patients benefit from the placement of a jejunostomy or gastrostomy feeding tube. Radiation and chemotherapy have been shown to be ineffective for pancreatic tumours.

The prognosis for cancer of the exocrine pancreas in dogs and cats is grave, with a survival time of between 3 and 90 days.

References and further reading

Bennett PF, Hahn KA, Toal RL and Legendre AM (2001) Ultrasonographic and cytopathological diagnosis of exocrine pancreatic carcinoma in the dog and cat. *Journal of the American Animal Hospital Association* **37**, 466–473

Bright JM (1985) Pancreatic adenocarcinoma in a dog with maldigestion syndrome. *Journal of the American Veterinary Medical Association* **187**, 420–421

Brown PJ, Mason KV, Merrett DJ, Mirchandani S and Miller RI (1994) Multifocal necrotizing steatitis associated with pancreatic carcinoma in 3 dogs. *Journal of Small Animal Practice* **35**, 129–132

Hecht S and Henry G (2007) Sonographic evaluation of the normal and abnormal pancreas. *Clinical Techniques in Small Animal Practice* **22**, 115–121

Hecht S, Penninck DG and Keating JH (2007) Imaging findings in pancreatic neoplasia and nodular hyperplasia in 19 cats. *Veterinary Radiology and Ultrasound* **48**, 45–50

Lamb CR, Simpson KW, Boswood A and Matthewman LA (1995) Ultrasonography of pancreatic neoplasia in the dog: a retrospective review of 16 cases. *Veterinary Record* **137**, 65–68

Pascaltenorio A, Olivry T, Gross TL, Atlee BA and Ihrke PJ (1997) Paraneoplastic alopecia associated with internal malignancies in the cat. *Veterinary Dermatology* **8**, 47–52

Tasker S, Griffon DJ, Nuttal TJ and Hill PB (1999) Resolution of paraneoplastic alopecia following surgical removal of a carcinoma in a cat. *Journal of Small Animal Practice* **40**, 16–19

Robben JH, Pollak YW, Kirpensteijn J *et al.* (2005) Comparison of ultrasonography, computed tomography, and single-photon emission computed tomography for the detection and localization of canine insulinoma. *Journal of Veterinary Internal Medicine* **19**, 15–22

Van Enkevort BA, O'Brien RT and Young KM (1999) Pancreatic pseudocysts in 4 dogs and 2 cats: ultrasonographic and clinicopathologic findings. *Journal of Veterinary Internal Medicine* **13**, 309–313

16

Tumours of the mammary glands

Henrik von Euler

Canine mammary tumours

General considerations

Mammary tumours (MTs) are the most common type of neoplasia in entire female dogs, representing approximately 50% of all tumours reported, although recently quoted to be as high as 70% of all cancer types (Merlo *et al.*, 2008). Bitches are 62 times more likely to develop mammary gland tumours than male dogs, in which mammary tumours are predominantly benign.

The canine MT malignancy rate is about 50% and half of these will metastasize. Mean age of onset of MT is approximately 8 years. Dobson *et al.* (2002) reported a standardized incidence rate for MT of 205/100,000 dogs/year, based on a defined population of insured dogs in the UK.

In a Swedish study based on an insured dog population of 80,000 female dogs, the overall MT rate was 154 dogs a year at risk (DYAR) (Egenvall *et al.*, 2005). The incidence increased with age and varied by breed, from 319 DYAR in the English Springer Spaniel to only 5 DYAR in the Rough-Haired Collie, clearly showing both high-risk and potentially preventive (genetic) phenotypes. High-risk breeds vary, depending on study and geographical location. Toy and Miniature Poodles, English Springer Spaniel, Brittany Spaniel, Cocker Spaniel, Puli, English Setter, pointers, German Shepherd Dog, Maltese, Yorkshire Terrier and Dachshund have all been reported to be predisposed.

It is well established that sex hormone stimulation increases the risk of mammary tumours in dogs, as well as other species (including humans). Ovariohysterectomy prior to 2 years of age greatly reduces the risk of mammary tumours. There is no protective effect, however, for bitches that are spayed after the second heat. Ovariectomy before the first oestrus reduces the risk of mammary neoplasia to 0.5% of the risk in intact bitches; ovariectomy after the first oestrus reduces the risk to 8%. Although disputed, the importance of *timing* of spaying on survival of dogs with MTs has been claimed (Sorenmo *et al.*, 2000): bitches that were spayed less than 2 years before MT surgery had a significantly longer overall survival compared with intact bitches and those that were spayed more than 2 years before MT treatment. These data are contradicted by other studies showing no clinical benefit with ovariohysterectomy at (or in proximity to) mastectomy. Obesity at a young age and consumption of homemade meals have been associated with increased risk of developing MT.

Pathogenesis

The canine mammary tumour model supports the idea of the neoplastic progression as a continuum from preneoplastic lesions to fully invasive carcinomas, as also described in human breast cancer (Antuofermo *et al.*, 2007; Sorenmo *et al.*, 2009). This implies adenosis, sclerosing adenosis, intraductal papilloma, sclerosing papilloma, ductal hyperplasia, atypical ductal hyperplasia and ductal carcinoma *in situ*. Malignant foci are also found in otherwise benign tumours. Large tumours (longer growing time) are more often of a malignant phenotype and carry a worse prognosis; sex hormone receptor status changes with increased malignancy; and finally multiple tumours in the same individual often carry a different histopathological grade.

Histopathological classification

The highly detailed current World Health Organization (WHO) histological classification system aims to standardize terminology and nomenclature of canine MTs internationally (Misdorp *et al.*, 1999) (Figure 16.1). With the abundance of different malignant types it may be hard to get a clinically relevant overview, but it does show how an accurate histopathological diagnosis can aid in prognosis and define treatment options and approaches. In general there is a favourable prognosis for benign tumours as well as for 'unclassified' types.

The WHO classification follows the dedifferentiation process, starting with the malignant tumours most closely resembling the normal structure of the mammary gland and ending with the poorly differentiated tumours with no glandular structure. It has been shown that prognosis is closely correlated with the level of differentiation. This is very important to recognize in a clinical situation, so that prognosis and treatment planning may be communicated more easily (Figure 16.2).

- The malignant tumours with the best prognosis consist of highly differentiated glandular structure with secretory epithelium containing alveoli, tubuli and myoepithelium. These tumours are classified as **complex adenocarcinomas**. They seldom metastasize and with complete excision the prognosis is usually good.

Malignant tumours
• Non-infiltrating (*in situ*) carcinomas
• Complex carcinoma
• Simple carcinoma:
o Tubulopapillary carcinoma
o Solid carcinoma
o Anaplastic carcinoma
• Special types of carcinoma:
o Spindle cell carcinoma
o Squamous cell carcinoma
o Mucinous carcinoma
o Lipid-rich carcinoma
• Sarcoma:
o Fibrosarcoma
o Osteosarcoma
o Other sarcomas
• Carcinosarcoma
• Carcinoma or sarcoma in benign tumour

Benign tumours
• Adenoma:
o Simple adenoma
o Complex adenoma
o Basaloid adenoma
• Fibroadenoma
• Benign mixed tumour
• Duct papilloma

Unclassified
• Duct hyperplasia
• Lobular hyperplasia
• Cyst
• Ductectasia
• Local fibrosis
• Gynaecomastia

16.1 Histological classification of canine mammary tumours. (Adapted from Misdorp *et al.*, 1999)

Positive factors
• Small breeds (reported to have more benign tumours)
• Express oestrogen and progesterone receptors
• Male (reported to have more benign tumours)

Negative factors
• Tumour >3 cm diameter
• Ulceration or fixation
• Lymph nodes involved
• Distant metastasis present
• Do not express oestrogen and progesterone receptors
• Histological subtype (carcinoma – poorly differentiated, simple, solid, anaplastic, inflammatory carcinoma, sarcomas)
• Vascular or lymphatic invasion
• Index of proliferation: high AgNOR, Ki-67 or PCNA count; high p53 gene mutation or DNA aneuploidy

16.2 Prognostic factors involved in canine mammary gland tumours.

- If the myoepithelial cells are absent the tumours are called **simple adenocarcinomas**, often divided into alveolar, tubular, tubuloalveolar, papillary or papillary–cystic adenocarcinomas. These tumours are invasive and can lead to distant spread. If this has not occurred, surgical removal still gives a fair prognosis.
- If the tumour is lacking luminal structures, it is described as **solid carcinoma**. This type is more invasive and is prone to metastasize early. The prognosis is more guarded.
- The most poorly differentiated neoplasms, with a heterogenic disorganized tissue appearance, are the most malignant (Figure 16.3). These tumours are often called **anaplastic** and have a strong tendency to invade lymph and blood vessels. The invasion of cutaneous lymph vessels makes the skin appear inflamed, thus the clinical descriptive term 'inflammatory' adenocarcinoma. The prognosis for these patients is always poor, even with radical surgery. They are termed stage IV according to the clinical staging scheme (Figure 16.4) (Owen, 1980; see also Chapter 3).
- **Squamous cell carcinoma** in the mammary gland is sometimes seen and carries a grave prognosis, often metastasizing early to regional lymph nodes.
- The incidence of **sarcomas** varies between studies, but is commonly 5–10%. The majority are primary extraskeletal osteosarcomas (Figure 16.5). or fibrosarcomas These always carry a poor prognosis and 75% of the sarcomas give rise to metastases, most commonly through haematogenous spread. The mammary gland is the second most common place for primary osteosarcomas in intact females after the skeletal manifestation, and they behave just as malignantly. If there are malignant neoplastic cells of both epithelial and mesenchymal origin (very rare) the tumour is called **carcinosarcoma**. These MTs are always very aggressive and have a similar prognosis to the anaplastic carcinomas.

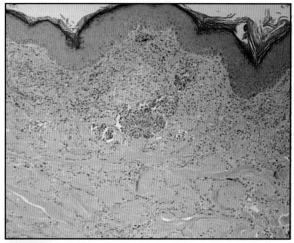

16.3 Histological specimen showing skin infiltration and neoplastic thrombi and skin ulceration in an anaplastic carcinoma. (Original magnification X100) (Courtesy of Dr Arman Shokrai, National Veterinary Institute, Uppsala, Sweden)

T – primary tumour size	
T1	<3 cm maximum diameter
T2	3–5 cm maximum diameter
T3	>5 cm maximum diameter
T4	Inflammatory carcinoma
N – regional lymph node status	
N0	No metastasis [a]
N1	Metastasis to ipsilateral node
N2	Metastasis to contralateral lymph node
M – distant metastasis	
M0	No distant metastasis
M1	Distant metastasis

(a) TNM classification. [a] Evidence of lymph node involvement based upon cytological or histological analysis.

I	T1	N0	M0
II	T0–1	N1	M0
	T2	N0–1	M0
III	T3	Nx	M0
	Tx	N2	M0
IV	Tx	Nx	M1
	T4	Nx	Mx

(b) Stage grouping.

16.4 Clinical staging of canine malignant mammary tumours. (Modified from Owen, 1980)

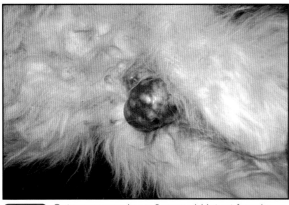

16.5 Osteosarcoma in an 8-year-old intact female Bichon Havanais.

Immunohistochemistry

In parallel with breast cancer in humans, there have been several reports showing the benefit of predicting prognosis with different immunohistochemistry markers. Prognostic markers include:

- Sex hormone receptor status
- Mitotic index (AgNOR, Ki-67 and PCNA)
- HER-2/neu expression
- BRCA1
- p53
- E-cadherin.

Sex hormone receptor status: The most obvious marker is the expression of sex hormone receptors: oestrogen receptor (ER) and progesterone receptor (PR). There is a clear tendency towards worse prognosis and higher malignancy grade with lower expression of ERs and PRs. This might explain the poor results of ovariohysterectomy in conjunction with mastectomy. Moreover, the metastases rarely express ERs or PRs. Sexual hormones, and in particular progestins, are believed to act via activation of growth hormone (GH) (van Garderen and Schalken 2002). Progestin-induced biosynthesis of GH occurs in the canine mammary gland tissue and is crucial for the normal cyclical development of the mammary gland, but may also promote mammary tumorigenesis by stimulating proliferation of susceptible, and sometimes transformed, epithelial cells. As the presence of PR often is reduced or even lost during malignant transformation, the GH stimulation may also act independently of sexual hormones.

Mitotic index: Higher mitotic indices recorded with either the proliferation marker Ki-67, argyrophilic nucleolar organizer region (AgNOR) or proliferating cell nuclear antigen (PCNA) all show that the higher the proliferation the poorer is the prognosis and the more likely a higher histological grade (Kumaraguruparan *et al.*, 2006).

HER-2/neu expression: Human epidermal growth factor receptor 2 (HER-2/neu)-positive canine mammary tumours are associated with indicators of poor prognosis such as histological grade III, invasive type of growth, simple histological type and absence of steroid hormone receptor. These findings are in agreement with those observed in human breast carcinoma, as over-expression of HER-2 also associates with features indicative of worse prognosis.

BRCA1: Loss of nuclear expression of the cell cycle-regulating phosphoprotein BRCA1 correlates with high Ki-67 proliferation and ER-negative tumours. The reduction and aberrant distribution of BRCA1 in canine mammary tumours are significantly associated with malignant characteristics.

p53: Probably the best known tumour suppressor gene is *p53*, which is a key player in cell cycle regulation. Alterations in *p53* have been reported in canine tumours, as both somatic and germ-line mutations. Many studies have also indicated that *p53* mutation is associated with progression and predicts increased malignant potential and worse prognosis in canine mammary tumours (Wakui *et al.*, 2001).

E-cadherin: Cadherins, and particularly E-cadherin (E-cad), a calcium-dependent epithelial cell adhesion molecule, are important during embryonic development and for the maintenance of adult tissue architecture. The reduction or loss of E-cad has been associated with tumour dedifferentiation, invasiveness and metastatic propensity and has been correlated with a significantly shorter overall survival and disease-free period (Gama *et al.*, 2008).

Cytology

Although aspiration cytology is easy to perform, aspirates of a mammary tumour unfortunately have little value in predicting malignancy in dogs (Figure 16.6). This is probably due to the highly variable morphology of the normal canine mammary cells in different stages of the oestrous cycle. The normal proliferation and involution of the gland give rise to cell morphology ranging from hyperplastic to apoptotic. However, occult tumours, such as mastocytomas, malignant lymphomas and melanomas, can be verified by this simple diagnostic tool. In these cases it will suggest other staging procedures as well as treatment regimens.

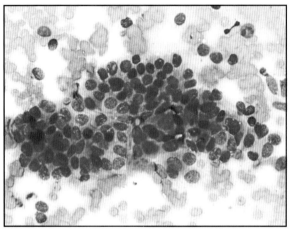

16.6 Cytological specimen from a dog with tubulopapillary adenocarcinoma. Cytology is rarely helpful in confirming degree of malignancy or type in canine mammary gland tumours, but inflammation, hyperplasia and non-mammary gland malignancies can often be differentiated. As with other carcinomas, features of malignancy include anisokaryosis, anisocytosis, increased basophilia, cellular piling, and large prominent and/or multiple nucleoli. Sometimes acinar structures can be seen. (Original magnification X100)

Clinical staging

Clinical staging (see Chapter 3) is important in determining prognosis. Bitches with high-stage disease according to the WHO TNM staging criteria (see Figure 16.4) carry a poor prognosis. Thus treatment planning should always rely on a proper staging procedure.

The general physical examination will ascertain whether the tumour is mobile in the mammary tissue or infiltrative involving the adjacent skin or the underlying fascia, or even the abdominal wall, which has been shown to imply a more guarded prognosis. If mammary hyperplasia is present this may be a sign of pseudopregnancy but may also indicate the presence of a hormone-producing ovarian tumour. In more malignant lesions there may be erythema of the skin, elevated temperature and sometimes ulceration and lymph oedema, all of which are features of the most aggressive canine mammary tumour, anaplastic (inflammatory) carcinoma, in which survival is only a few weeks despite aggressive surgery. Tumour size is a significant parameter predicting clinical outcome, according to TNM.

Most carcinomas metastasize through lymphatic spread. The two caudal glands (4–5) communicate with the superficial inguinal lymph node, whereas the two cranial glands (1–2) communicate with the axillary node. Mammary carcinomas that occur in the inguinal (5) gland may show retrograde metastasis via the lymphatic plexus in the subcutis of the inner thigh to the popliteal lymph nodes. The third gland usually drains via the inguinal route, but may also drain via the axillary. Palpation of the regional lymph nodes should always be performed, as detected lymph node metastasis carries a worse prognosis. If nodes are enlarged, an aspiration should be performed to detect metastasis on cytology prior to surgical planning.

The second most common organ for metastasis is the lungs. In 25% of the carcinomas and in the majority of the sarcomas, pulmonary metastasis usually occurs as the disease progresses (Figure 16.7). Three-view chest radiography is recommended, although a recent study on 375 MTs showed low specificity and sensitivity of detecting pulmonary metastases in dogs (Djupsjobacka and Eksell, 2003). It was found that the chance of detecting thoracic metastases was only 3% in dogs younger than 8 years with a tumour size of 1 cm. In these cases abdominal ultrasonography, screening for example the superficial inguinal and the medial iliac lymph nodes, might be more appropriate to detect possible metastasis earlier (Nyman *et al.*, 2005).

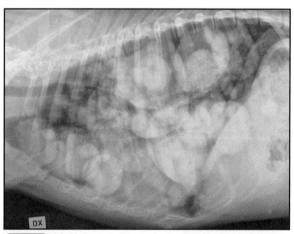

16.7 Multiple metastases in the lungs of a dog with adenocarcinoma simplex. (Courtesy of the Division of Diagnostic Imaging, University Small Animal Hospital, Uppsala, Sweden)

Other organs/systems reported to harbour MT metastasis are the liver, kidneys, spleen, skeleton (Figure 16.8), central nervous system and pleura. Occasional cases of retrograde metastatic spread by mammary carcinomas to the vagina have also been reported in bitches. Although rarely abnormal, it is prudent to perform haematology, biochemistry and urinalysis before surgery, as dogs with mammary tumours are often older and may carry undetected concomitant diseases important for planning the anaesthetic procedure. Finally, hypocalcaemia is reported as being a (rare) paraneoplastic finding in canine MTs.

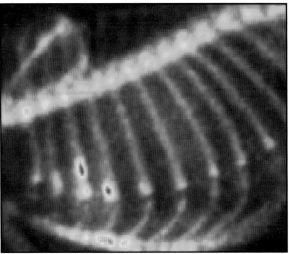

16.8 Skeletal metastasis is much more frequent in humans with breast cancer than in canine mammary tumours. This scintigraphy examination revealed a rib metastasis in a dog with a highly aggressive anaplastic carcinoma. (Courtesy of the Division of Diagnostic Imaging, University Small Animal Hospital, Uppsala, Sweden)

Management and prognosis

A management flow chart for both canine and feline MTs is given in Figure 16.9.

Surgery

The treatment of choice for canine MTs is surgery, the extent ideally being guided by clinical stage and histological grade. The different types of surgery proposed for defined tumour characteristics are shown in Figure 16.10.

Type of surgery	Tumour characteristics
Lumpectomy or partial mammectomy	<0.5 cm in diameter
Simple mastectomy	Tumour involves central areas or majority of the gland
Regional mastectomy	Multiple tumours in adjacent glands or tumour located between two glands
Radical mastectomy	Several tumours throughout the chain
Staged bilateral mastectomy	Multiple tumours in both chains

16.10 Recommended surgery for canine mammary tumours of different location and extent.

It is important to bear in mind that overall survival is (surprisingly) not influenced by the extent of the surgical procedure. If the surgery does not obtain clean margins, the outcome is always worse. The chosen surgical procedure should always aim to

16.9

An approach to management of canine and feline mammary tumours.

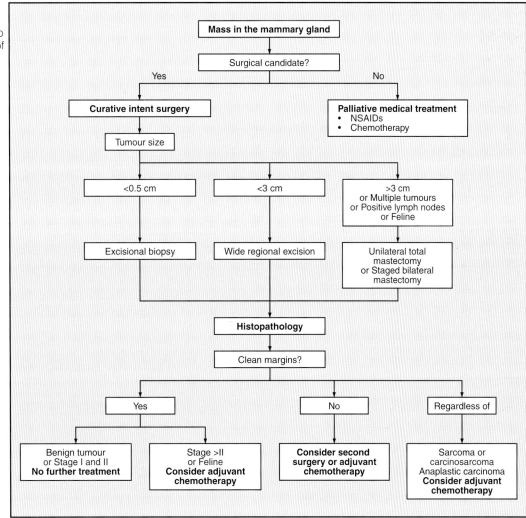

obtain free surgical margins with a suggested margin of 2 cm of grossly normal tissue.

Delaying surgery is not advisable, as tumour size is a significant prognostic marker. Tumours <1 cm in diameter have a favourable overall survival; tumours 2–3 cm in diameter still have a fair prognosis, with reported overall survival of 22 months. Conversely, the outcome is more guarded for tumours >3 cm, with reported survival times of approximately 1 year after surgery (Philibert *et al.*, 2003). All tumours >0.5 cm in diameter should be excised and submitted for histopathological review. If the tumour has a high grade or is reported to have incomplete margins, new and more aggressive surgery should be performed as soon as possible.

- **Mammectomy** may be performed if the tumour is small (>0.5 cm in diameter). Any signs of fixation to skin or underlying fascia should increase the amount of tissue excised, to obtain tumour-free margins. Mammectomy may often be more complicated to perform than a more extensive regional mastectomy.
- Based on the lymphatic drainage, **regional mastectomies** are generally recommended to include either glands 1–3 or glands 4–5. In the case of tumours in gland 3, an approach where at least resection of one normal gland flanking the affected part is recommended.
- The most radical approach with a **unilateral total mastectomy**, including all glands and the superficial lymph node (the axillary lymph node is only resected if palpably enlarged or proven cytologically positive), is recommended if several tumours are present. This will also decrease the risk of tumour recurrence in unaffected glands.
- If a **bilateral mastectomy** is needed, this should be performed as a staged procedure at least 3 weeks apart, to allow wound healing and skin relaxation. This is to decrease the risk of increased post-surgery intra-abdominal pressure, discomfort and wound dehiscence.

Adjuvant therapy

Although common in human breast cancer and proven to increase progression-free survival as well as overall survival in women, the use of chemotherapy, hormone therapy, immuno- and/or radiotherapy in dogs has shown little clinical benefit compared with surgery alone. However, it is obvious that in a certain subset of malignant tumours the current surgical treatment is clearly insufficient for long-term survival and hence calls for new treatment modalities.

Chemotherapy

Adjunct chemotherapy (see Chapter 7) in canine mammary tumours has yet to be proven as beneficial as it is in human breast cancer. It is possible that small sample size, retrospective studies and the large number of benign tumours have made it hard to show any significant benefits compared with surgery alone.

The most commonly used drugs in human breast cancer are cyclophosphamide, doxorubicin, gemcitabine and taxanes. These have all been used in canine mammary tumours. Bitches with malignant tumours treated with 5-fluorouracil and cyclophosphamide were reported to respond favourably when treated in an adjuvant postoperative setting compared with bitches treated by surgery alone. More recently, 12 bitches with invasive mammary gland tumours were treated with doxorubicin or docetaxel after mastectomy; however, the outcome was not significantly improved by chemotherapy (Simon *et al.*, 2006). In a prospective clinical trial (Marconato *et al.*, 2008) in which dogs with aggressive mammary carcinoma of clinical stages IV and V were treated with surgical excision (*n* = 9) or with surgery and adjuvant weekly gemcitabine (*n* = 10) for at least four cycles at a dose of 800 mg/m^2, there were no significant differences between the groups on either response or overall survival. However, in the dogs receiving adjuvant chemotherapy, the number of gemcitabine treatments was positively correlated with overall survival.

Radiotherapy

Although currently considered state-of-the-art treatment in certain subtypes of human breast cancer, adjuvant radiation therapy has not shown any benefits compared with surgery alone in dogs. Anecdotal case reports describe palliative protocols (8 Gy in 2–3 fractions) in non-resectable disease. Larger prospective trials are needed to determine the potential role of radiation therapy for canine mammary tumours. However, the anatomical location of the mammary glands leads to a high risk of inducing radiation therapy side effects, preferentially in the gastrointestinal tract.

Hormonal therapy

Early spaying prevents the development of mammary neoplasms. Most available literature states that spaying later or at the time of mastectomy has no impact on overall survival. In women with BRCA mutations, postpubertal oophorectomy significantly decreases the risk of developing breast cancer in the subsequent 15 years, particularly if performed before 40 years of age. Current studies within the dog genome project may find support for trials investigating the benefits of sex hormone ablation within a subset of dogs with mammary neoplasia.

Anti-oestrogens such as tamoxifen have been tested both *in vitro* and *in vivo* in dogs with mammary tumours. The adjuvant anti-tumour activity seen in women with breast cancer has not been reproduced in the canine trials. Most of the dogs had to stop medication prematurely due to oestrogenic side effects such as vulvular swelling, vaginal discharge, incontinence, urinary tract infection, stump pyometra, signs of oestrus and thus a higher interest from male dogs (Morris *et al.*, 1993). Simultaneously, the anti-tumour effects were marginal. Currently, the use of tamoxifen cannot be advised in dogs.

Comparative medicine and genetics

Gene arrays

The particularly high disease incidence reported in certain canine breeds suggests a significant genetic component. The identification of genetic risk factors is critical to improvements in prevention, diagnosis and treatment of these tumours.

In recent years there has been significant progress in developing the tools and reagents necessary to analyse the canine genome. This has culminated in a high-quality draft genome sequence, single nucleotide polymorphism (SNP) map and an SNP array for genome-wide association (GWA) analysis (Lindblad-Toh *et al.*, 2005; Karlsson *et al.*, 2007). These tools provide an unprecedented opportunity to characterize the genetic influences in canine diseases such as cancer, eventually allowing exploration of more effective therapies.

Expression analysis in canine MT

cDNA microarrays have been used to profile the gene expression patterns of nearly all major tumours in humans – including breast cancer – and have changed the way they are diagnosed, classified and treated. In contrast, very few expression studies have been published on canine MTs, most focusing on single, or in the best case a handful of, predetermined transcripts (Kumaraguruparan *et al.*, 2006). Although highly interesting, research on just a few genes at a time risks being biased, as cancer is a complex disease. A multimarker cDNA microarray study found 31 over-expressed genes out of 174 tested, based on a human breast cancer cDNA array (von Euler *et al.*, 2005). Among the genes over-expressed, many were associated with similar findings in human breast cancer. These findings were confirmed in a dog-specific cDNA array in 2008 where different canine mammary tumour cell lines were investigated (Rao *et al.*, 2008).

With the high homology of the dog genome to the human counterpart (higher than, for example, mouse *versus* human), molecular genetic and clinical comparisons are undertaken. In the post-genomic era, techniques that reflect gene expression are used as powerful tools, for example to detect molecular subclassification in tumours. It is hoped that this may also be useful in comparisons to enhance the understanding of tumorigenesis and metastatic pathways in both dogs and humans.

Feline mammary tumours

General considerations

Mammary tumours in cats are more often malignant than in the dog. The frequency of malignancy is reported to be at least 80%. Mammary tumours are the third most common cancer, outnumbered only by haemopoietic neoplasms and skin tumours. There are few reports on incidence compared with dogs and humans, but approximately 20% of tumours in the female cat consist of mammary tumours – half the incidence reported in humans and dogs.

Siamese and Domestic Short-hair cats are reported to have a higher incidence rate than other breeds. For the Siamese cat a two-fold increase in risk compared with other breeds is reported.

Mammary neoplasia has been reported in cats from 9 months to 23 years of age, with a mean age of occurrence of 10–12 years. Siamese cats are reported to have a slightly earlier onset. As in dogs, the majority of affected cats are intact females, although mammary neoplasia is also seen in late-spayed females and, rarely, in male cats. In contrast to male dogs, the majority of the mammary tumours found in male cats are malignant. The mean age at tumour diagnosis, around 13 years, is also slightly higher than that reported in queens (Skorupski *et al.*, 2005).

Hormonal importance

Hormonal influence is also reported to be part of the pathogenesis in feline mammary tumours. The risk of developing mammary tumours is seven times higher in intact than in oophorectomized cats. A recent report stated that cats spayed prior to 6 months of age and cats spayed between 6 months and 1 year of age had only 9% and 14%, respectively, of the risk of developing MT compared with intact cats (Overley *et al.*, 2005). No protective effect of spaying was seen if this was performed after 2 years of age.

There are many reports on the role of testosterone, oestrogen and progesterone receptors in the development of feline MTs. There is a strong association between the prior use of progesterone-like drugs and the development of benign and malignant MTs. Melengestrol acetate (MGA), a potent synthetic progestin, has been used as a contraceptive in zoo felids, and mammary gland carcinomas have been linked to this treatment. In one study, 90% of zoo felids with mammary tumours had been treated with MGA (McAloose *et al.*, 2007).

Only 10% of feline mammary tumours are reported to express oestrogen receptors, far lower than in dogs and humans. This reflects the higher percentage of malignant tumours seen in the cat, as the rate of tumour cells staining positive for steroid receptors decreases with increased malignancy (de las Mulas *et al.*, 2000).

Clinical presentation

Mammary tumours in cats can occur as single or multiple masses in one or many glands simultaneously. The tumours are generally considered to be equally located in the cranial (axillary) or the caudal (inguinal) glands. Most tumours present as a firm, well defined mass on palpation, but they may also be soft or ill-defined and infiltrative. More aggressive types often adhere to the skin and to the abdominal wall and may be ulcerated.

The aggressive nature also reflects the high frequency of lymphatic and lymph node invasion, visible at necropsy. The metastatic rate is high and occurs mostly in the regional lymph nodes and lungs. Metastases to the liver, skeleton, pleura, spleen and kidneys have all been reported.

Histopathology

The most common histological classification is adeno-carcinoma, accounting for >85% of tumours. The most common subtypes are tubular, tubulopapillary, solid or cribriform. Other malignant tumours less frequently reported are sarcomas, mucinous carcinomas, duct papillomas and adenosquamous carcinomas. Complex carcinomas showing a biphasic nature, with both neoplastic epithelial and myoepithelial cells, are reported to be less aggressive, with a better prognosis and also occurring at a younger age than other feline mammary carcinomas (Seixas *et al.*, 2008). Vascular invasion and, to an even higher degree, lymphatic invasion may be present upon histological examination and are of prognostic significance as they suggest metastatic propensity. The rare benign mammary gland dysplasias are important as differential diagnoses and because they may present as a severe clinical condition.

Hyperplasias

Non-inflammatory hyperplasia is generally either lobular hyperplasia or fibroepithelial hyperplasia.

Lobular hyperplasia: Lobular hyperplasia occurs infrequently as palpable masses in one or more glands. It has been reported in cats from 1 to 14 years of age (median 8 years). Most reports are from intact females. The most common type of lobular hyperplasia involves one or more enlarged lobules with a cystic or dilated ductal component. Mammary hyperplasia may also on rare occasions signify the presence of a hormone-producing ovarian tumour.

Fibroepithelial or fibroadenomatous hyperplasia: This will usually occur in young, cycling or pregnant queens. It is a benign, non-neoplastic lesion associated with progesterone stimuli. Apart from endogenous progesterone production, it is also seen in old intact females and in males given megestrol.

Clinically, most affected cats exhibit mammary gland hyperplasia 1–2 weeks after their first oestrus or 2–6 weeks after exogenously administered megestrol. The glands are generally significantly enlarged with a rapid clinical onset. The skin is sometimes erythematous and can become necrotic (Figure 16.11a). Also oedema of the skin and subcutis, and of both hindlegs, may be present. This condition can easily be confused with an acute mastitis or a fast-growing malignant tumour. The heat and pain present upon palpation generally seen at mastitis together with discomfort are rarely present to the same extent in fibroadenomatous hyperplasia. Moreover, a malignant tumour is seldom as fast growing and the anamnesis of recent progesterone administration, or a young animal and the involvement of many glands or the entire mammary chain, helps to distinguish this benign condition from a rapidly evolving malignancy. An incisional biopsy is generally diagnostic (Figure 16.11b,c).

As these conditions are thought to be associated with hormonal stimulation of the glandular tissue, ovariohysterectomy or non-renewal of progesterone treatment is generally curative, though the clinical

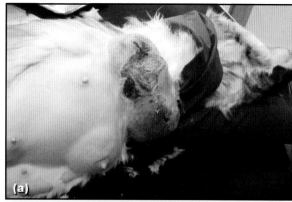
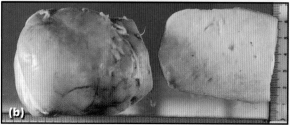
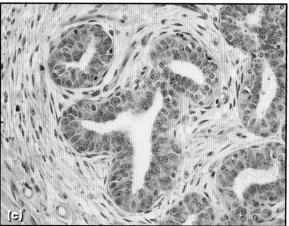

16.11 **(a)** Mammary fibroadenomatous hyperplasia in a 4-year-old DSH queen (after progestin treatment). Multiple hyperplastic glands are bilaterally significantly enlarged, with oedema and ulceration of the skin in the first two cranial glands. **(b)** Macroscopically, the tumour is multinodular and light yellow. **(c)** Histopathology shows a netlike pattern building up epithelial ducts. (H&E, orginal magnification X100) (b,c courtesy of Erika Karlstam, National Veterinary Institute, Uppsala, Sweden)

symptoms may take time to resolve. Other treatments with variable results are diuretics, corticosteroids, testosterone and aglepristone. In severe cases the skin may be ulcerated and localized or systemic infection may occur. In this case general supportive care and antibiotics should be given.

If the glands are still greatly enlarged, ovariohysterectomy through a flank incision should be performed instead of via a linea alba incision.

Clinical staging

Of specific importance when staging feline mammary tumour (see Chapter 3) is to describe the primary tumour (define T) and evaluate the presence of metastasis (define M). For the primary tumour, number of tumours, size (of prognostic significance on its own), location and signs of infiltrative growth (fixation to skin/underlying fascia) should be examined. Regional lymph nodes (define N) should be examined for signs of metastasis (Figure 16.12). Enlarged lymph nodes, especially the axillary nodes, should be aspirated prior to surgery to decide whether to include them in the mastectomy.

T – primary tumour size	
T1	<1 cm maximum diameter
T2	1–3 cm maximum diameter
T3	>3 cm maximum diameter
T4	Inflammatory carcinoma
N – regional lymph node status	
N0	No metastasis [a]
N1	Metastasis to ipsilateral node
N2	Metastasis to contralateral lymph node
M – distant metastasis	
M0	No distant metastasis
M1	Distant metastasis

(a) TNM classification. [a] Evidence of lymph node involvement based upon cytological or histological analysis.

I	T1	N0	M0
II	T0–1	N1	M0
	T2	N0–1	M0
III	T3	Nx	M0
	Tx	N2	M0
IV	Tx	Nx	M1
	T4	Nx	Mx

(b) Stage grouping.

16.12 Clinical staging of feline malignant mammary tumours. (Modified from Owen, 1980)

Although a minimum database of CBC, biochemistry profile and urinalysis is generally unremarkable in feline MT, it is necessary to rule out other concomitant disease. Thoracic radiographs, both right and left lateral and ventrodorsal views, should be obtained to look for metastasis. Signs of metastasis are small to large nodular opacities, but also miliary pleural lesions that may produce prominent malignant effusions. Both bronchial and sternal lymph node enlargement may be signs of metastatic spread. In the geriatric patient changes are normally present in the lungs and pleura. This alongside inactive inflammatory lesions may confuse in the evaluation of chest radiographs. Abdominal radiographs may be valuable for detection of iliac lymph node enlargement in caudal tumours. Abdominal ultrasonography may help in detecting abdominal metastasis, although thoracic metastasis is generally

the most commonly encountered. Vague signs of metastatic disease should not delay treatment, due to the disease's aggressive nature.

Because of the high rate of malignant tumours, an aggressive approach is mandatory to achieve diagnosis via histopathological examination at the time of mastectomy. A pre-surgical biopsy is not advisable. As in the dog, cytology is seldom recommended before surgery, but may of course be useful to rule out non-mammary malignancies or inflammatory conditions. If these are present, cytological examination should be performed from pleural effusion if the cat has a tumour in the mammary gland, to look for malignant cells.

Management and prognosis

Surgery is the preferred therapy for feline mammary gland tumours (see Figure 16.9). Since there is a high frequency of malignant tumours that significantly reduce time to progression and overall survival, adjuvant therapy (e.g. chemotherapy and radiation therapy) is suggested in defined cases. There are no major prospective trials to verify the superiority of certain chemotherapy protocols; thus there is a need for such studies to be conducted. Prognostic markers that may prove to be more frequently addressed in the future are HER2/neu, immunohistochemical expression of topoisomerase II-beta binding protein 1 (TopβP1), vascular endothelial growth factor (VEGF) and the expression of cyclo-oxygenase 2 (COX-2) receptors (Morris et al., 2008).

Surgery

As the time from first occurrence to veterinary examination may be excessively long, the surgeon often faces a large infiltrative tumour that will diminish the probability of tumour removal with clean margins. It is reported that unilateral mastectomy significantly decreases the degree of local recurrence compared with lumpectomy. Hence a more radical approach is recommended in feline mammary tumours compared with their canine counterparts. Cats with tumours <2 cm have been reported to survive >3 years, while cats with tumours >3 cm will survive <12 months despite surgery.

The cat has four pairs of mammary glands: the two cranial pairs drain to the axillary lymph node, while the two caudal pairs drain to the superficial inguinal node. Unlike in the dog, there is sometimes communication between the two mammary chains, across the midline. Thus, staged bilateral mastectomy is recommended, performed 3–4 weeks apart to allow healing and relaxation of stretched skin. Simultaneous bilateral mastectomy should be avoided, as most studies report no significant benefit in overall survival and the procedure will most likely cause unnecessary postoperative discomfort and increase the risk of wound dehiscence. Additionally, worries about closure of the wound often result in a compromised resection surgery. If the tumour has invaded the abdominal musculature the excision must include a portion of the abdominal wall and reconstruction with mesh may be necessary to prevent increasing intra-abdominal pressure too much.

The superficial inguinal lymph node is almost invariably excised along with the caudal gland. The axillary node should only be removed if proven to be metastatic by cytology preoperatively, as there is no evidence that prophylactic removal of this node will provide a better outcome.

It is crucial to stress that separate mammary masses on the same animal may be of different histological types, as in dogs. Therefore all masses should be excised (using separate instruments) and submitted for histopathological examination. It is important to ensure that each mass can be individually distinguished when the pathological report returns.

Simultaneous ovariohysterectomy has not been proven to decrease incidence of recurrence or promote overall survival benefits. It will prevent uterine disease (e.g. pyometra, metritis) and significantly decrease female hormonal influence on existing lesions. It is primarily performed in the case of feline fibroadenomatous hyperplasia, and is often followed by regression of hyperplastic tissue. It is important to remember that this benign condition often resolves spontaneously within a couple of weeks, whether an ovariohysterectomy is performed or not. The risk of relapse does, however, decrease following ovariohysterectomy.

Radiation therapy
There is no evidence that radiotherapy is beneficial in improving clinical outcome in feline mammary tumours compared with surgery alone, and it is seldom used in an adjuvant setting.

Chemotherapy
Because of the aggressive nature of feline mammary tumours with significantly reduced overall survival if tumour size exceeds 3 cm, there have been many attempts to use adjuvant chemotherapy (see Chapter 7) following surgery or sometimes as the only therapy in non-resectable cases. Drugs used alone or in combination are: doxorubicin, carboplatin, cyclophosphamide and mitoxantrone.

In smaller studies it has been reported that doxorubicin alone, or in combination with cyclophosphamide, has resulted in partial responses in cats with non-resectable local disease or distant metastasis, and it has efficacy against macroscopic feline mammary carcinomas (Stolwijk *et al.*, 1989).

In a larger retrospective multicentre study on 67 cats with histologically confirmed mammary gland adenocarcinomas treated with adjunctive doxorubicin at a dose of 1 mg/kg intravenously every 3 weeks for a maximum of five treatments, or until the cat developed progressive disease or concurrent illness, it was shown that cats that completed the adjunctive doxorubicin protocol had significantly improved survival (Novosad *et al.*, 2006). The median survival time of cats that received surgery and doxorubicin was 448 days, while the median disease-free interval (DFI) was 255 days. Prognostic factors for DFI apart from completion of chemotherapy were: tumour volume, histological subtype, development of metastatic disease and location of metastatic disease. Cats with lymph node metastasis had a median DFI of 1,122

days, while cats with pulmonary metastasis progressed at a median of 183 days. The worst prognosis was among cats with pleural metastasis and anaplastic high-grade histological subtype, staying free of disease 115 and 95 days, respectively, despite adjuvant chemotherapy. Almost half the group had a DFI of 4 years or longer (41.5%), clearly indicating a possibility for treating selected cases of feline mammary tumours with adjuvant doxorubicin. The most common reasons for discontinuing doxorubicin included progressive disease (7.5%) and the development of renal disease (4.5%).

The major side effects with these protocols have been anorexia and mild myelosuppression. Reducing the dose of doxorubicin or substituting with mitoxantrone may limit toxicity to an acceptable level. Doxorubicin can be nephrotoxic to the cat, though this is considered uncommon. Prospective studies using combined adjuvant chemotherapy and mastectomy in the cat have yet to be performed.

References and further reading

Antuofermo E, Miller MA, Pirino S *et al.* (2007) Spontaneous mammary intraepithelial lesions in dogs – a model of breast cancer. *Cancer Epidemiology Biomarkers and Prevention* **16**, 2247–2256

de las Mulas JM, van Niel M, Millan Y *et al.* (2000) Immunohistochemical analysis of estrogen receptors in feline mammary gland benign and malignant lesions: comparison with biochemical assay. *Domestic Animal Endocrinology* **18**, 111–125

Djupsjobacka A and Eksell P (2003) Frequency of radiographically detected pulmonary metastases in bitches with mammary gland neoplasia. *European Journal of Companion Animal Practice* **13**, 149–155

Dobson JM, Samuel S, Milstein H *et al.* (2002) Canine neoplasia in the UK: estimates of incidence rates from a population of insured dogs. *Journal of Small Animal Practice* **43**, 240–246

Egenvall A, Bonnett BN, Öhagen P *et al.* (2005) Incidence of and survival after mammary tumors in a population of over 80,000 insured female dogs in Sweden from 1995 to 2002. *Preventive Veterinary Medicine* **69**, 109–127

Gama A, Paredes J, Gartner F *et al.* (2008) Expression of E-cadherin, P-cadherin and beta-catenin in canine malignant mammary tumours in relation to clinicopathological parameters, proliferation and survival. *Veterinary Journal* **177**, 45–53

Karlsson EK, Baranowska I, Wade CM *et al.* (2007) Efficient mapping of mendelian traits in dogs through genome-wide association. *Nature Genetics* **39**, 1321–1328

Kumaraguruparan R, Prathiba D and Nagini S (2006) Of humans and canines: immunohistochemical analysis of PCNA, Bcl-2, p53, cytokeratin and ER in mammary tumours. *Research in Veterinary Science* **81**, 218–224

Lindblad-Toh K, Wade CM, Mikkelsen TS *et al.* (2005) Genome sequence, comparative analysis and haplotype structure of the domestic dog. *Nature* **438**, 803–819

Marconato L, Lorenzo RM, Abramo F *et al.* (2008) Adjuvant gemcitabine after surgical removal of aggressive malignant mammary tumours in dogs. *Veterinary and Comparative Oncology* **6**, 90–101

McAloose D, Munson L and Naydan DK (2007) Histologic features of mammary carcinomas in zoo felids treated with melengestrol acetate (MGA) contraceptives. *Veterinary Pathology* **44**, 320–326

Merlo DF, Rossi L, Pellegrino C *et al.* (2008) Cancer incidence in pet dogs: findings of the Animal Tumor Registry of Genoa, Italy. *Journal of Veterinary Internal Medicine* **22**, 976–984

Misdorp W, Else RW, Hellmen E *et al.* (1999). Histological classification of mammary tumors of the dog and cat. WHO International Histological Classification of Tumors in Domestic Animals. Armed Forces Institute of Pathology, Washington DC

Morris JS, Dobson JM and Bostock DE (1993) Use of tamoxifen in the control of canine mammary neoplasia. *Veterinary Record* **133**, 539–542

Morris JS, Nixon C, Bruck A *et al.* (2008) Immunohistochemical expression of TopBP1 in feline mammary neoplasia in relation to histological grade, Ki67, ERalpha and p53. *Veterinary Journal* **175**, 218–226

Novosad CA, Bergman PJ, O'Brien MG *et al.* (2006) Retrospective evaluation of adjunctive doxorubicin for the treatment of feline mammary gland adenocarcinoma: 67 cases. *Journal of the American Animal Hospital Association* **42**, 110–120

Nyman HT, Kristensen AT, Skovgaard IM *et al.* (2005) Characterization of normal and abnormal canine superficial lymph nodes using gray-scale B-mode, color flow mapping, power, and spectral Doppler ultrasonography: a multivariate study. *Veterinary Radiology and Ultrasound* **46**, 404–410

Overley B, Shofer FS, Goldschmidt MH *et al.* (2005) Association between ovariohysterectomy and feline mammary carcinoma. *Journal of Veterinary Internal Medicine* **19**, 560–563

Owen LN (1980) *TNM Classification of Tumours in Domestic Animals.* World Health Organization, Geneva

Philibert JC, Snyder PW, Glickman N *et al.* (2003) Influence of host factors on survival in dogs with malignant mammary gland tumors. *Journal of Veterinary Internal Medicine* **17**, 102–106

Rao NA, van Wolferen ME, van den Ham R *et al.* (2008) cDNA microarray profiles of canine mammary tumour cell lines reveal deregulated pathways pertaining to their phenotype. *Animal Genetics* **39**, 333–345

Seixas F, Palmeira C, Pires MA *et al.* (2008) Are complex carcinoma of the feline mammary gland and other invasive mammary carcinoma identical tumours? Comparison of clinicopathologic features, DNA ploidy and follow up. *Research in Veterinary Science* **84**, 428–433

Simon D, Schoenrock D, Baumgartner W *et al.* (2006) Postoperative adjuvant treatment of invasive malignant mammary gland tumors in dogs with doxorubicin and docetaxel. *Journal of Veterinary Internal Medicine* **20**, 1184–1190

Skorupski KA, Overley B, Shofer FS *et al.* (2005) Clinical characteristics of mammary carcinoma in male cats. *Journal of Veterinary Internal Medicine* **19**, 52–55

Sorenmo KU, Shofer FS and Goldschmidt MH (2000) Effect of spaying and timing of spaying on survival of dogs with mammary carcinoma. *Journal of Veterinary Internal Medicine* **14**, 266–270

Sorenmo KU, Kristiansen VM, Cofone MA *et al.* (2009) Canine mammary gland tumours; a histological continuum from benign to malignant; clinical and histopathological evidence. *Veterinary and Comparative Oncology* **7**(3), 162–172

Stolwijk JA, Minke JM, Rutteman GR *et al.* (1989) Feline mammary carcinomas as a model for human breast cancer. II. Comparison of in vivo and in vitro adriamycin sensitivity. *Anticancer Research* **9**, 1045–1048

van Garderen E and Schalken JA (2002) Morphogenic and tumorigenic potentials of the mammary growth hormone/growth hormone receptor system. *Molecular and Cellular Endocrinology* **197**, 153–165

von Euler H, Khoshnoud R, He Q *et al.* (2005) Time-dependent RNA degradation affecting cDNA array quality in spontaneous canine tumours sampled using standard surgical procedures. *International Journal of Molecular Medicine* **16**, 979–985

Wakui S, Muto T, Yokoo K *et al.* (2001) Prognostic status of p53 gene mutation in canine mammary carcinoma. *Anticancer Research* **21**, 611–616

17

Tumours of the urogenital system

Robert N. White and Malcolm Brearley

Tumours of the kidney

General considerations

Primary tumours of the kidney are listed in Figure 17.1. The kidneys are relatively common sites for development of metastases, but primary tumours of the kidney are uncommon in both the dog and cat. They account for only 1.7% and 2.5% of all dog and cat tumours, respectively (Crow, 1985). In the dog, adenocarcinoma is the most frequent primary tumour

Benign
• Adenoma • Fibroma • Haemangioma • Interstitial cell tumour • Leiomyoma • Transitional cell papilloma
Malignant
• Adenocarcinoma/carcinoma • Fibrosarcoma • Haemangiosarcoma • Leiomyosarcoma • Nephroblastoma • Transitional cell carcinoma • Lymphoma

17.1 Primary tumours of the kidney.

type and it is most commonly seen in middle-aged and older dogs. Males are more frequently affected than females. In the cat, lymphoma is the most common renal tumour; it may be primary or secondary. There is no sex predisposition for feline renal lymphoma; it is most frequently reported in individuals of 6–7 years of age. Although FeLV infection is considered a risk factor for the development of renal lymphoma in the cat, reports suggest that only 25–50% of affected individuals are FeLV-positive. As with the dog, renal carcinomas (tubular and tubulopapillary) are the most frequently diagnosed primary renal neoplasm in the cat (Henry *et al.*, 1999).

Nephroblastoma (Wilm's tumour; embryonal nephroma; Figure 17.2) is an embryoma and occurs most frequently in young dogs, often less than 1 year of age (mean age 4 years). The tumour may be present in only one pole of an affected kidney. Histologically, it may demonstrate primitive epithelial and mesenchymal tissues such as vestigial tubules,

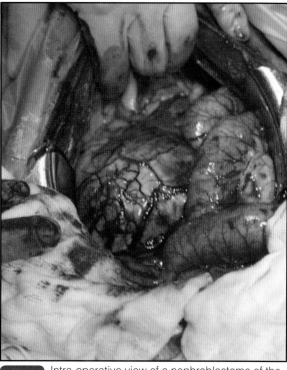

17.2 Intra-operative view of a nephroblastoma of the right kidney.

muscle, cartilage and bone at various stages of differentiation.

Presentation and clinical signs

Primary tumours of the kidney are usually solitary and unilateral, whereas metastatic tumours are commonly multiple and bilateral. Bilateral renal cystadenocarcinoma is a rare tumour reported in the German Shepherd Dog as part of a syndrome associated with nodular dermatofibrosis and uterine polyps (Moe and Lium, 1997).

Classically, specific clinical signs associated with renal tumours include:

• Palpable renal mass (there is often bilateral renal enlargement in a cat with renal lymphoma)
• Intermittent or persistent haematuria throughout urination
• Abdominal distension
• Abdominal discomfort
• Development of pelvic limb oedema when lymphatic drainage is compromised.

In many instances, the clinical signs are not so well defined and only vague signs of illness such as anorexia, depression, weight loss and lethargy may be present. Signs of overt renal failure are rarely present unless there is severe, bilateral involvement (e.g. in renal lymphoma in the cat) or the other kidney is compromised by a non-neoplastic process.

Clinical approach

Blood samples
Complete blood profiles will be unremarkable in many cases.

- In individuals with haematuria there may be evidence of a regenerative anaemia.
- Polycythaemia vera may occur as a paraneoplastic syndrome in some cases of renal carcinoma where the tumour autonomously produces erythropoietin.
- Renal serum biochemistry results will mostly be normal unless there is severe bilateral renal involvement.
- Hypercalcaemia may occasionally be seen as a paraneoplastic syndrome.
- All cats with suspected renal lymphoma should be tested for FeLV status.

Urinalysis
Neoplastic cells may occasionally be seen on cytological examination of urine sediment, but urinalysis is generally unrewarding when looking for the presence of tumour cells. Proteinuria is a common finding and haematuria may be observed in individuals suffering from invasive, destructive tumours such as haemangiosarcoma and renal carcinoma.

Imaging techniques
Renal tumours that demonstrate renomegaly may be detectable on plain survey abdominal radiographs. Assessment of renal function and intraparenchymal architecture may be enhanced by performing intravenous urography (IVU) or a renal angiography study. In most instances, the use of ultrasonography will complement or supersede these radiographic investigations. Renal ultrasonography allows renal architecture to be assessed in a non-invasive manner and it enables accurate percutaneous fine-needle aspiration (FNA) or needle biopsy of any abnormal structures to be undertaken safely. Ultrasonography will also allow the assessment of local tumour invasion into adjacent vascular structures such as the vena cava.

More advanced methods of investigation include magnetic resonance imaging (MRI) and computed tomography (CT) and the use of scintigraphy for assessment of renal function and glomerular filtration rate (GFR). These techniques are becoming more widely available and will often provide unparalleled information for the surgical planning of cases with local vascular invasion. Scintigraphy or excretion urography can be used preoperatively to confirm that a contralateral 'normal' kidney possesses adequate excretory function for an individual to function normally following an elective nephrectomy.

Management

Surgery
In the majority of animals with a unilateral renal tumour and no evidence of metastatic disease, the treatment of choice is ureteronephrectomy. The procedure is similar to that described for ureteronephrectomy for other conditions. When removing a neoplastic kidney it is important to minimize the handling of the affected structures, since handling may induce intravascular seeding of the tumour. Similarly, it is important to isolate the blood supply to and from the affected kidney as early as possible during the resection. Ideally, the renal capsule should be removed intact with the kidney to minimize the potential spread of tumour cells within the peritoneal cavity. Some embryonal tumours may achieve a massive size prior to detection and resection. The sheer volume of such tumours will make the use of a scrubbed surgical assistant imperative.

Many renal tumours are readily amenable to resection, but some carcinomas may demonstrate local invasion into neighbouring structures such as the infrarenal vena cava. These cases may prove to be surgically demanding and may require the placement of autologous venous or prosthetic vascular grafts.

Radiotherapy and chemotherapy
The consequences of local intraperitoneal organ radiation damage mean that radiotherapy is, in general, not used in the management of renal tumours in the dog and cat.

Combination chemotherapy is the treatment of choice in individuals with renal lymphoma as the condition is commonly bilateral and/or generalized. Standard protocols, as discussed in Chapter 19a, may be used. The response is often not as good as that seen with other forms of lymphoma. For animals with unilateral renal lymphoma there may be a role for nephrectomy. Unfortunately, it may not be possible to prove that only one kidney is affected; therefore most authorities would advocate the use of chemotherapy in all cases with renal lymphoma. Adjunctive chemotherapy may be considered in cases with non-resectable or resected non-lymphoid tumours, but objective evidence for a response is lacking.

Prognosis
The prognosis for the majority of renal tumours remains poor because of their invasive nature and high tendency for metastasis prior to detection and treatment. Survival times for renal carcinoma following ureteronephrectomy are considered to be 6–12 months on average. Nephroblastoma carries a better prognosis and, with adequate surgical excision, many cases may be cured. Renal lymphoma appears to respond less well to chemotherapy than do other forms of lymphoma; long-term remission and survival are rarely achieved.

Tumours of the ureter

General considerations
The primary tumours of the ureter are listed in Figure 17.3. Tumours of the ureters are extremely rare in the dog and cat. The ureter can be the site of a primary neoplasm or it may be invaded by local spread from an invasive tumour affecting its associated kidney.

Benign
• Leiomyoma

Malignant
• Leiomyosarcoma
• Transitional cell carcinoma

17.3 Primary tumours of the ureter.

Presentation and clinical signs
The narrow diameter of the ureter means that even a small tumour may result in obstruction to urine flow and the development of proximal hydroureter and hydronephrosis. These, along with unilateral renal compromise, may result in clinical signs. However, the functional capacity of the unaffected contralateral kidney means that signs of renal failure are often masked and not detected. Signs are, therefore, often non-specific and include lower back pain, stiffness and lethargy.

Clinical approach

Blood samples
A complete blood profile reveals no specific haematological or biochemical changes in individuals with a ureteral tumour.

Imaging techniques
Investigation of ureteral abnormalities should include contrast radiographic studies; plain survey radiographs rarely allow the ureters to be defined. Performing IVU will allow precise assessment of the intraluminal ureteral structure to be made (Figure 17.4). Both lateral and ventrodorsal views should be obtained at various time points following the administration of the intravenous contrast medium. If malignancy is suspected, thoracic radiographs should be obtained for staging.

Ultrasonography may also be used to assess the structure of the affected ureter and its associated

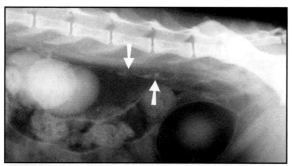

17.4 Intravenous urogram revealing the presence of filling defects in the ureter of a cat (arrowed). Excisional surgery (nephrectomy and ureterectomy) and histopathology confirmed the lesion to be a ureteral carcinoma.

kidney. Percutaneous ultrasound-assisted biopsy may be possible, but in many instances the ureteral tumour will prove too small for a biopsy to be performed safely and accurately by this technique.

Management
In general, the treatment of choice for tumours of the ureter that have not metastasized or invaded locally is ureteronephrectomy. The function of the contralateral kidney should be assessed prior to performing this surgery. In cases where contralateral kidney function is considered compromised, it may prove necessary to perform a local resection of the affected portion of the ureter followed by end-to-end ureteral anastomosis. In some instances the associated kidney must be transposed caudally, to ensure that no undue tension is placed on the anastomosis suture line.

There are no reports on the use of chemotherapy or radiotherapy in the management of ureteral tumours.

Prognosis
Most recognized ureteral tumours are malignant and so the presence of local invasion and/or metastasis makes the prognosis for this condition poor. The resection of a benign tumour carries the possibility of complete cure.

Tumours of the urinary bladder

General considerations
Tumours of the urinary bladder are listed in Figure 17.5. Tumours of the bladder are the most common form of cancer affecting the urinary tract in the dog. After renal lymphoma, bladder cancer is the second most common location for cancer of the urinary tract in the cat. In both species, however, the bladder is still an uncommon site for cancer development, with a frequency of less than 1% of all tumours in the dog and with an even lower frequency in the cat (Crow, 1985). In the dog, bladder cancer is more common in bitches and the mean age at presentation is approximately 10 years. Certain breeds, including the West Highland White Terrier, Jack Russell Terrier, Beagle and Scottish Terrier, may be more at risk. In the cat, the disease appears to have no breed predilection, but is seen with greatest frequency in aged males (mean 9–10 years).

Benign
• Leiomyoma
• Fibroma
• Haemangioma

Malignant
• Transitional cell carcinoma (commonest)
• Lymphoma
• Leiomyosarcoma
• Haemangiosarcoma
• Undifferentiated carcinoma
• Squamous cell carcinoma
• Rhabdomyosarcoma (embryonal)
• Fibrosarcoma
• Adenocarcinoma

17.5 Tumours of the urinary bladder.

The majority of bladder tumours in both the dog (97% of cases) and cat (80% of cases) are malignant and epithelial in origin, the most frequent being transitional cell carcinoma (TCC). Tumours most commonly arise from the trigone region of the bladder. TCC is usually locally invasive and may extend beyond the bladder wall into adjacent organs such as the prostate, vagina, uterus or rectum. This tumour is capable of both local (hypogastric and medial iliac lymph nodes) and distant (liver, lungs, spleen) metastasis and metastases may be present in up to 50% of cases at the time of diagnosis.

It has been hypothesized that the difference in prevalence of bladder neoplasia between the dog and the cat is related to differences in metabolism of tryptophan and its carcinogenic intermediary metabolites. Although dogs excrete appreciable quantities of tryptophan metabolites in their urine, cat urine is almost devoid of these substances. The prolonged exposure of the bladder mucosa to such carcinogenic substances may be important in the development of bladder neoplasia.

Presentation and clinical signs

All epithelial bladder tumours may be solitary or multiple and appear as papillary or non-papillary (Figure 17.6) growths. Mesenchymal tumours are most likely to be locally invasive, although some, such as haemangiosarcoma, are likely to exhibit metastasis.

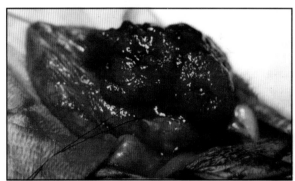

17.6 Cystotomy for partial excision of a large TCC. The presenting clinical signs were haematuria, dysuria and intermittent stranguria.

Bladder tumours often show clinical signs consistent with cystitis, including:

- Dysuria
- Haematuria
- Pollakiuria (increased frequency of micturition).

These clinical signs may show a temporary response to symptomatic therapy, but invariably return either whilst the animal is still being medicated or once therapy has been stopped. The recurrent nature of these signs should alert the clinician to the possibility of underlying bladder neoplasia.

Clinical approach

Blood samples

Complete blood profiles will, in many cases, be unremarkable. In individuals suffering from chronic haematuria, there may be evidence of a regenerative or non-regenerative anaemia.

Urinalysis

Urinalysis, urine culture and antibiotic sensitivity testing should be performed in all cases of suspected bladder tumour. To minimize the risk of seeding neoplastic cells, it is advisable to obtain a urine sample by 'free catch' rather than conventional cystocentesis. In some cases, cytological examination of urine sediment will reveal the presence of pleomorphic tumour cells. Unfortunately this is not always reliable, as some bladder tumours, especially sarcomas, do not exfoliate well, leading to a false-negative result. Care should be taken to avoid confusing neoplastic cells with those that are merely dysplastic and associated with a benign cystitis. A urine dipstick test is available for the detection of bladder tumour antigen in dogs, but care should be taken in interpreting the results in the face of haematuria and proteinuria, when false-positive results are not uncommon.

Cytology

FNA of bladder wall lesions may be attempted under ultrasound guidance and this method of diagnosis is advocated by some. However, in the case of TCC especially, there is a serious risk of seeding tumour cells along the needle tract (into the peritoneal cavity and the abdominal wall), and alternative methods of collecting tissue, via cystoscopy or using a blind catheter suction technique, may be safer.

Imaging techniques

Contrast radiography and ultrasonography are useful techniques for investigation of suspected bladder neoplasia. Ultrasonography lends itself particularly well to investigation of the bladder since the lumen generally contains urine, allowing for good transmission of sound and the generation of clear ultrasound images. Mucosal abnormalities at the interface between the intraluminal fluid and soft tissue structures of the wall will be most clearly visualized; the technique will also allow the extent of local invasion to be assessed (Figure 17.7). When bladder urine volume is low it may prove helpful to distend the structure with the administration of saline.

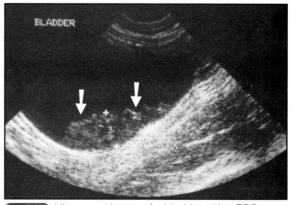

17.7 Ultrasound image of a bladder with a TCC (arrowed) at the level of the trigone.

Plain radiographs of the bladder will often be unremarkable, but in some circumstances they may indicate a change in bladder shape or position. Contrast radiography is considerably more informative. Negative contrast studies (pneumocystogram) will often indicate the presence of an intraluminal mass or an irregular mucosal surface consistent with a tumour. Most information can be gained by obtaining a double contrast cystogram. The addition of a small volume of positive contrast prior to inflation with air will often highlight the presence of an epithelial abnormality (Figure 17.8).

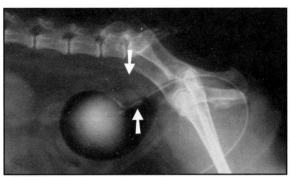

17.8 Double contrast cystogram demonstrating a mass (arrowed) associated with the dorsal bladder wall. The urothelium appears smooth, suggesting that the mass might be mesenchymal and not epithelial in origin. These findings may also be suggestive of a benign rather than a malignant tumour.

Management
Ideally, complete staging should be undertaken prior to any intervention. Both regional and distant metastases are not uncommon in individuals suffering from malignant bladder neoplasia and the finding of metastatic disease will significantly influence how the condition is managed and what the likely outcome of management will be. Treatment is unlikely to affect metastatic rate or alter disease progression or survival times once gross metastasis is detected.

Surgery
The aims of surgery should be clearly defined at the outset: is the procedure being undertaken in an attempt to cure the individual, or is the proposed surgery an attempt to achieve the palliative relief of urinary obstruction?

Partial cystectomy: Surgical therapy for the majority of TCCs is often unrewarding, since the most common site for these tumours is at the trigone. Although it may be possible to perform a partial cystectomy, including transection of the ureters and their re-implantation into the apex of the bladder, the removal of the trigone will typically result in urinary incontinence. The multiple and diffuse nature of many epithelial tumours makes margin assessment difficult, and local recurrence following apparently successful resection is common.

Submucosal resection: In select cases of extensive disease where partial cystectomy is not considered feasible, or in cases where the TCC involves the trigone and/or peri-ureteral regions, submucosal resection of the superficial tumour may be performed to reduce tumour load. The mucosa is approached via a cystotomy and the affected portion is undermined superficial to the submucosa, allowing the mucosa to be 'peeled' away. Ideally, the remaining mucosa should be used to close the mucosal defect that has been created. Alternatively, the defect can be left to close by second intention granulation, epithelialization and contraction. This palliative operation is not without potentially serious complications, but in certain cases may reduce clinical signs and increase the effectiveness of adjunctive chemotherapy by reducing tumour target volume.

Total cystectomy: There are a number of experimental and clinical reports describing total cystectomy in the dog. To perform such surgery requires the ureters to be implanted into a distant site that will allow unimpeded urine to flow from their associated kidneys. A number of implantation sites have been described; these include the colon, the urethra and the passage of the ureters through the abdominal wall with cutaneous stoma formation. The colon cannot be recommended as a site, because implantation results in the development of pyelonephritis and/or faecal incontinence. Both urethral and cutaneous implantation sites result in urinary incontinence and the possible development of an ascending pyelonephritis. Although in many instances the incontinence may be managed with the use of disposable children's nappies, the ethical implications and high patient morbidity of such procedures should not be underestimated.

Cutaneous cystostomy: The creation of a permanent cutaneous cystostomy has been described in dogs with stranguria associated with inoperable bladder tumours. The availability of one-way valves manufactured from biologically inert materials has allowed permanent cystotomy sites to be created without associated urinary incontinence. Experience would suggest that the development of ascending infections within a bladder is common following the placement of such a device and, again, it is advised that such surgical procedures should be undertaken with caution.

Tumour resection: Resection of mesenchymal tumours that can be completely excised (apex and body tumours) and benign tumours may prove more rewarding (Figure 17.9). Some two-thirds of the bladder body may be resected without significantly affecting bladder function.

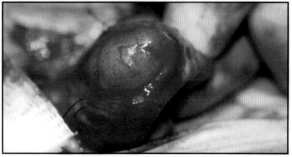

17.9 Intra-operative view of a smooth non-infiltrative mesenchymal mass associated with the dorsal bladder wall. The gross findings were considered consistent with a benign tumour. Histopathology confirmed the mass to be a leiomyoma.

Medical therapy
Non-resectable TCCs have been managed medically with the non-steroidal anti-inflammatory drug piroxicam (0.3 mg/kg orally q24h). It is thought that COX-2 inhibition is involved in tumour response, and other more potent COX-2 inhibitors may provide a similar effect. In one study, partial or complete remission was noted in 6 of 34 dogs; many other dogs subjectively had an improved quality of life, despite lack of tumour remission (Knapp *et al.*, 1994). Other non-selective COX-2 inhibitors appear as effective as piroxicam; this applies to meloxicam (personal observation) and firocoxib.

Improved remission rates and remission times may be achieved in a subset of patients by combining COX-2 inhibitors with platinum-based chemotherapy and, to a greater extent, mitoxantrone. However, there are conflicting reports in the literature and the benefit of these therapies is still under investigation.

There have been reports that locally applied interleukin-2 may be of value in the management of canine bladder tumours, but these have not yet been substantiated in published clinical trials.

Prognosis
The prognosis for most malignant tumours of epithelial origin is poor because of their diffuse, sometimes multiple and infiltrative nature. Also, their tendency to develop at the trigonal region of the bladder often makes them inoperable. Survival time following excision of bladder carcinomas is usually less than 6 months. Mesenchymal tumours carry a slightly better prognosis if they are diagnosed early and are amenable to surgical excision. The prognosis for benign tumours of the bladder depends on the site of growth; in many instances, surgical resection will prove curative.

Tumours of the urethra

General considerations
Tumours of the urethra are listed in Figure 17.10. Infiltrative urethral disease is uncommon in dogs and cats; neoplasia and granulomatous urethritis are the two conditions most frequently described (Matthiesen and Moroff, 1989). The commonest urethral tumours

Benign
• Adenoma
• Fibroma
• Leiomyoma
• Myxoma
• Papilloma

Malignant
• Transitional cell carcinoma (commonest)
• Adenocarcinoma
• Haemangiosarcoma
• Rhabdomyosarcoma
• Myxosarcoma
• Squamous cell carcinoma

17.10 Tumours of the urethra.

in the dog are of epithelial origin and include TCC and squamous cell carcinoma (SCC). In the dog, tumours of the urethra present less commonly than those of the bladder. Urethral tumours are considered extremely rare in cats.

The mean age of dogs with urethral tumours is 10 years and there is a predilection for urethral tumour development in the bitch. TCC most commonly affects the proximal third of the urethra, whereas SCC predominates in the distal portion of the urethra and urethral tubercle. Both tumours are highly malignant, showing local invasion through the urethral wall, urethral luminal obstruction and metastasis to both local lymph nodes and local pelvic organs.

Presentation and clinical signs
Clinical signs associated with urethral tumours include:

- Dysuria
- Haematuria
- Pollakiuria
- Stranguria (in advanced cases).

Signs may be very similar to those seen with bladder neck tumours. In early disease, signs may be less pronounced and are likely to be those of an unresponsive cystitis and/or urethritis.

Clinical approach

Physical examination
The majority of urethral tumours, especially those situated within the distal urethra, will be palpable either per vaginum or per rectum. They may be detected as a discrete mass or a more diffuse swelling within the urethral wall. Palpation per vaginum may also indicate the presence of local infiltration into the adjacent ventral vaginal wall.

Blood samples
A complete blood profile will reveal no abnormalities associated specifically with urethral neoplasia.

Urinalysis
Although urinalysis will commonly fail to reveal the presence of neoplastic cells, it may indicate the presence of proteinuria and haematuria. Urine should also be submitted for culture and sensitivity testing. The urine sample may be obtained by cystocentesis, but it would be safer to obtain the sample by 'free catch' if the diagnosis is in doubt and there is a possibility of the presence of bladder tumour.

Imaging techniques
Further investigations of an animal with clinical signs indicative of lower urinary tract disease should include a lower urinary tract radiographic study. The most valuable information regarding the presence and size of a urethral tumour will often be obtained by performing retrograde positive contrast urethrography or vaginourethrography (Figure 17.11).

253

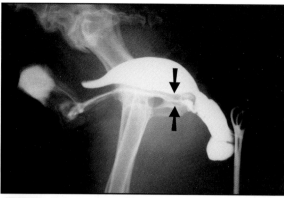

17.11 Retrograde positive contrast vaginourethrogram of a bitch with haematuria and dysuria. There is a filling defect within the distal urethra (arrowed) consistent with a urethral tumour. Exfoliative histopathology confirmed the lesion to be a TCC. The bitch subsequently underwent successful tumour resection and reconstructive vaginourethroplasty.

Enlarged regional lymph nodes (medial iliac, sacral and hypogastric nodes) may indicate the presence of local metastasis. Thoracic radiographs should be obtained to rule out the presence of distant lung metastasis. The lower urinary tract radiographic study will require the urethra in both the dog and the bitch to be catheterized. This will provide information regarding the site and degree of urethral constriction. A urethral lesion may cause complete obstruction of the lumen and so make it impossible to pass a urethral catheter safely. In such cases, urine can be removed from the bladder by intermittent cystocentesis or a urinary diversion procedure such as a tube cystostomy.

In the bitch, the vestibule, urethral tubercle, vestibulovaginal junction and vagina should be examined visually with the aid of a scope (Figure 17.12) or speculum (in many instances, the use of a simple otoscope will provide a satisfactory view). This procedure may well be performed at the same time as the placement of a urethral catheter.

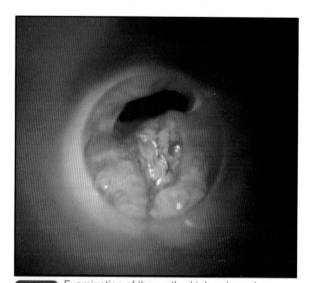

17.12 Examination of the urethral tubercle and vestibulovaginal junction with the aid of a rigid endoscope. A soft fleshy mass can be seen protruding from the urethral orifice. Pinch biopsies confirmed the mass to be a urethral TCC.

Biopsy

It is important to obtain biopsy material from an infiltrative urethral lesion for histological diagnosis of tumour type and distinction from the non-neoplastic condition of granulomatous urethritis. Adequate biopsy material can often be obtained by applying negative pressure with a syringe to a urinary catheter that has been placed within the vicinity of the urethral lesion. The samples obtained will often be large enough to be submitted for histopathological examination.

Management

Surgery

In animals with urethral tumours that show no evidence of local or distant metastasis, it may be possible to resect the tumour surgically. In the male dog, distal urethral tumours may be removed by performing a penile amputation and scrotal or perineal urethrostomy. Small, proximal tumours may be amenable to local urethral excision and end-to-end anastomosis. In the bitch, successful management of both benign and malignant tumours affecting the distal urethra and urethral tubercle has been described (White *et al.*, 1996). Up to 50% of the distal urethra can be removed and repaired by performing a vaginourethroplasty whilst maintaining urinary continence postoperatively. In both the dog and the bitch, access to the intrapelvic urethra requires either pubic symphysectomy or sagittal pubic osteotomy. Proximal tumours close to the bladder neck are often more difficult to remove. In the dog, intraprostatic urethral tumours will require prostatectomy, resulting almost invariably in postoperative urinary incontinence.

As with certain inoperable bladder tumours, the creation of a permanent cutaneous cystotomy utilizing some form of biologically inert one-way valve can be considered in individuals with urethral tumours showing signs of severe dysuria or stranguria. Chronic ascending infections of the bladder are common following this type of surgery and the implications for the welfare of the patient should be considered before such surgery is embarked upon. Alternatively, the recent availability of suitably sized metallic stents has led to their palliative use in the management of malignant urethral obstructions in dogs (Weisse *et al.*, 2006). Their use remains controversial as the treatment is only palliative and may be associated with significant complications such as severe incontinence and stent migration.

Radiotherapy and chemotherapy

Urethral tumours are, in general, not responsive to either radiotherapy or chemotherapy. Side effects associated with radiation of the intrapelvic structures and bladder are generally unacceptable. The use of COX-2 inhibitors plus chemotherapy may have a role in the short-term management of urethral tumours, but evidence of efficacy is lacking at present.

Prognosis

The prognosis for the majority of malignant urethral tumours is poor, since most will not be amenable to surgical resection by the time they are recognized. In contrast, the prognosis for excisable benign tumours such as the leiomyoma is very favourable.

Tumours of the ovary

General considerations

Tumours of the ovary are listed in Figure 17.13 and are rare in both the dog and cat. They account for less than 1.2% and 3.6% of all neoplasms in the dog and cat, respectively. A reason for their infrequent recognition is that many bitches and queens undergo ovariohysterectomy at a young age. Affected individuals are most frequently older, nulliparous individuals, but teratoma will often occur in younger animals. Reported tumour types relate to the tissue types found in the normal ovary.

Tumour site	Benign	Malignant
Surface epithelial tumours (40–50% of cases)	Cystadenoma Papillary adenoma	Cystadenocarcinoma Papillary adenocarcinoma Undifferentiated carcinoma
Gonadostromal tissue tumours (35–50% of cases)	Thecoma Luteoma	Granulosa cell tumour
Germ cell tumours (6–20% of cases)	Teratoma	Dysgerminoma Teratoma Carcinoma

17.13 Tumours of the ovary.

Surface epithelial tumours

Surface epithelial tumours include cystadenoma/adenocarcinoma and papillary adenoma/adenocarcinoma. These tumours are very rare in queens, but account for approximately half of ovarian tumours seen in bitches. They may be unilateral or bilateral and can vary considerably in size. Capillary or cystic (Figure 17.14) forms of both benign and malignant surface epithelial neoplasms are recognized.

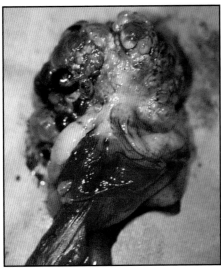

17.14 A cystic adenocarcinoma of an ovary following ovariohysterectomy in a bitch.

Malignant surface epithelial tumours often metastasize to both the lungs and neighbouring abdominal organs such as the kidneys, omentum, liver and para-aortic lymph nodes. They can seed cancer cells throughout the peritoneal and, sometimes, the pleural cavities, resulting in the condition of carcinomatosis. Lymphatic obstruction may result in the development of a peritoneal and/or pleural effusion.

Gonadostromal tumours

Gonadostromal tumours include the benign thecoma and luteoma and the mostly malignant granulosa cell tumour. Granulosa cell tumour is the most common ovarian tumour in queens. In bitches, it is seen with a similar frequency to surface epithelial tumours. Granulosa cell tumours are most commonly unilateral and spherical, with a smooth surface. They may contain both solid and polycystic areas. Although some may be benign, it is best to consider that all are malignant until proven otherwise. Malignant forms may metastasize to local (kidney, omentum, liver and abdominal lymph nodes) and distant (lungs) sites. Peritoneal seeding (carcinomatosis) is also possible. Granulosa cell tumours can be hormonally active, producing oestrogen.

Thecoma and luteoma are extremely rare in both bitches and queens.

Germ cell tumours

Germ cell tumours include dysgerminoma and teratoma; both tumours are uncommon. Dysgerminoma is analogous to testicular seminoma in the male dog arising from undifferentiated germ cells. This tumour often attains a large size and has a smooth, lobulated surface. Metastasis to regional lymph nodes and adjacent abdominal structures occurs in up to 30% of cases.

Teratoma is commonly well differentiated and benign, though malignant forms have been reported in both bitches and queens. Teratoma is often composed of tissues from two or three germinal layers including bone, cartilage, glandular epithelium or brain.

Presentation and clinical signs

The clinical signs of ovarian tumours in entire bitches are extremely variable, but they can include:

- Pyometra
- Abnormal oestrus
- Vaginal discharge
- Secondary sex organ change
- Lumbar pain
- The presence of an abdominal mass
- An enlarged abdomen (from mass and/or effusion)
- Lethargy
- Weight loss or weight gain.

Many tumours are clinically silent and are discovered as an incidental finding at the time of coeliotomy for what was thought to be a routine ovariohysterectomy. An ovarian tumour should be suspected in any sexually intact female dog or cat with a history of abnormal oestrus.

Animals with granulosa cell tumour may show clinical signs related to oestrogen secretion:

- Abnormal oestrus (often prolonged)
- Bilateral alopecia
- Mammary hyperplasia
- Cystic endometrial hyperplasia/pyometra
- Vaginal discharge
- Swollen vulva
- Attractiveness to male dogs
- Myelosuppression (rare).

Clinical approach

Physical examination
Abdominal palpation may suggest the presence of a mass in the region of the kidneys. Ovarian tumours will often be more mobile on palpation than tumours of the kidney.

Blood samples
No specific changes on a complete blood profile are reported in bitches or queens with ovarian tumours. In rare cases where hyperoestrogenism leads to myelosuppression, haematological abnormalities may include anaemia, thrombocytopenia and neutropenia.

Imaging techniques
Plain abdominal radiographs may suggest the presence of a soft tissue mass adjacent to either the right or left kidney. Radiography may also indicate the presence of a peritoneal effusion, which will complicate the assessment of abdominal soft tissue structures. Teratomas may demonstrate areas of mineralization and/or odontogenesis. Thoracic radiographs should be obtained for assessment of pulmonary metastasis.

Abdominal ultrasonography is useful in the assessment of the primary ovarian mass and it can also be used in the assessment of peritoneal effusion, local metastasis and the presence of diffuse carcinomatosis.

Cytology
In cases with peritoneal effusion, abdominocentesis will allow samples of fluid to be obtained for cytological interpretation. In most instances, analysis reveals only the presence of a modified transudate, but sediment examination may confirm the presence of tumour cells in individuals with metastatic spread.

Biopsy
When a large primary tumour is detected, it may prove possible to perform either a direct FNA or a direct core biopsy. With smaller tumours, it is easier and safer to perform similar biopsies with the aid of ultrasound guidance. In some instances (for example, when the tumour is discovered as an incidental finding at coeliotomy) diagnosis will be made on excisional (ovariectomy) biopsy.

Management

Surgery
In cases of benign ovarian tumours, or in those with no evidence of metastasis, the surgical removal of the affected ovary is the treatment of choice. In most instances, this means performing an ovariohysterectomy, but leaving a single ovary and uterus for the purposes of future breeding is a possibility in some cases. In individuals demonstrating cystic endometrial hyperplasia or pyometra, it is advisable to perform a complete ovariohysterectomy.

Radiotherapy and chemotherapy
Radiotherapy is rarely indicated in the management of ovarian neoplasia. Primary tumours are best managed surgically and radiation therapy for metastatic spread is rarely safe or feasible.

Similarly, there does not appear to be a role for chemotherapy in the management of primary ovarian neoplasia. In cases with metastatic spread and peritoneal carcinomatosis, however, there may be a role for peritoneal lavage or systemic therapy with platinum-based chemotherapeutic agents. The efficacy of these treatments has not been confirmed.

Prognosis
Following ovariectomy or ovariohysterectomy, the prognosis for benign ovarian tumours is extremely good. Malignant tumours carry a guarded prognosis and the prognosis for individuals with significant metastasis or carcinomatosis is grave.

Tumours of the uterus and cervix

General considerations
Tumours of the uterus (Figure 17.15) are rare in both the dog and cat. They have no known aetiology and they most commonly occur in the older individual. In the bitch, benign tumours occur with greatest frequency. Malignant tumours, although still very uncommon, are seen more frequently in queens.

The leiomyoma is the most common benign uterine tumour in both bitches (Figure 17.16) and queens. Benign tumours often develop as multiple nodules in the uterine wall. Benign mesenchymal tumours are non-invasive and slow growing. An association between benign uterine tumour development and both nodular dermatofibrosis and renal

Benign
- Fibroma
- Fibroleiomyoma
- Leiomyoma
- Adenoma

Malignant
- Fibrosarcoma
- Leiomyosarcoma
- Adenocarcinoma
- Lymphoma

17.15 Tumours of the mesosalpinx, uterus and cervix.

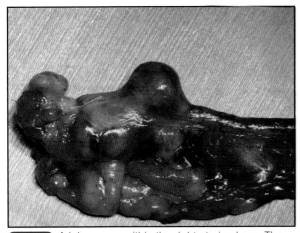

17.16 A leiomyoma within the right uterine horn. The tumour was found as an incidental finding in a 10-year-old bitch undergoing ovariohysterectomy.

cystadenocarcinoma appears to exist in the German Shepherd Dog (Moe and Lium, 1997). A recent report has described a leiomyoma in the mesosalpinx of a terrier bitch (Eker *et al.*, 2006).

Of the malignant uterine tumours, the most frequently reported is the adenocarcinoma arising from the endometrium. This tumour is more common in queens than in bitches. It demonstrates both local invasion and metastasis. Metastasis can be widespread and has been reported in local lymph nodes, other abdominal organs, the lung, the eye and the brain. Malignant mesenchymal tumours of the uterus are occasionally reported, especially in queens, but in both species they are considered very rare.

Presentation and clinical signs

The clinical signs associated with uterine tumours are often non-specific and in fact, in many instances, the tumour is identified as an incidental finding at the time of exploratory coeliotomy. An abdominal mass may be palpable and occasionally a vaginal discharge may be noted. There may be signs of lumbar and/or abdominal discomfort. Inconsistent signs such as lethargy, malaise, anorexia and cachexia may also be present.

Clinical approach

Physical examination

Abdominal palpation may detect the presence of a mass within the mid to caudal abdomen.

Blood samples

No specific changes on a complete blood profile are reported in bitches or queens with ovarian tumours. A neutrophilia with left shift may be seen in individuals with a concurrent pyometra.

Imaging techniques

Plain abdominal radiographs may confirm the presence of a soft tissue mass consistent with an enlargement of the uterus. In individuals with a concurrent pyometra, there may be evidence of generalized uterine enlargement. Thoracic radiographs should be obtained to assess the presence of pulmonary metastasis.

Abdominal ultrasonography is useful in the assessment of uterine tumours. The technique will also allow for the assessment of pyometra and abdominal metastatic spread. Ultrasound-guided fine-needle aspirates may be obtained, but in the majority of cases further assessment is best made at the time of exploratory coeliotomy.

Management

The treatment of choice for the majority of uterine or cervical tumours which demonstrate no evidence of metastasis is ovariohysterectomy. At present, there appears to be no role for radiotherapy in the management of uterine tumours. Similarly, the role of chemotherapy in the management of both primary and secondary tumours of the uterus has yet to be established.

Prognosis

Following ovariohysterectomy, the prognosis for the majority of uterine tumours in the dog is good, since most tumours prove to be benign. In the cat, the prognosis is worse, because adenocarcinoma is the most frequently encountered tumour and metastasis is likely to have occurred by the time of diagnosis.

Tumours of the vagina and vulva

General considerations

Tumours of the vagina and vulva are listed in Figure 17.17. Excluding mammary gland neoplasia, vaginal, vestibular and vulval tumours are the most common tumours of the reproductive tract in the bitch. Tumours at these sites are rare in queens. In general, benign mesenchymal vaginal tumours, such as leiomyoma, affect entire, aged bitches (mean age 10–11 years), whereas the lipoma affects slightly younger individuals (mean age 6 years). The majority of tumours are seen in nulliparous individuals.

Benign smooth muscle tumours account for approximately 80–90% of vaginal and vulval tumours reported in bitches. The growth of many of these benign smooth muscle tumours is associated with the ovarian secretion of oestrogen. Therefore, unless the

Benign
• Leiomyoma
• Fibroma
• Fibroleiomyoma
• Lipoma

Malignant
• Leiomyosarcoma
• Adenocarcinoma
• Transmissible venereal tumour
• Squamous cell carcinoma
• Haemangiosarcoma
• Osteosarcoma
• Mast cell tumour

17.17 Tumours of the vagina and vulva.

bitch is receiving exogenous oestrogens, it is very unusual to find such tumours in an animal that has undergone ovariectomy or ovariohysterectomy.

The most commonly reported malignant tumour of the vagina and vulva is the leiomyosarcoma. These tumours are locally invasive and also show local and distant metastasis. Similar to the male dog, transmissible venereal tumour (TVT) tends to affect younger sexually active breeding bitches. TVT is seen more commonly in females than in males.

In addition to the tumours listed in Figure 17.17, the vulval labia can be associated with any form of cutaneous tumour, particularly SCC and mast cell tumours (MCT).

Presentation and clinical signs

Benign smooth muscle tumours may present as either extraluminal or intraluminal forms. Extraluminal tumours are mostly well encapsulated and their growth results in a noticeable perineal swelling (Figure 17.18). Intraluminal tumours tend to be attached to the wall of the vestibule or vagina by a thin pedicle. They are often ovoid and firm, and their pedicle attachment allows them to protrude from the vulva. Large intraluminal tumours may become traumatized, oedematous and infected. Their appearance may be similar to that of vaginal oedema (hyperplasia), although this is a condition of younger, entire females and is associated with oestrus. It is not unusual for mammary gland tumours, ovarian cysts and cystic endometrial hyperplasia to be seen concurrently with the development of smooth muscle tumours of the vagina.

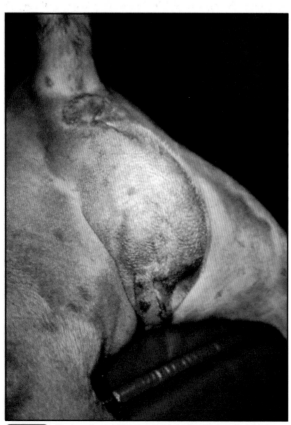

17.18 Perineal swelling associated with benign vaginal leiomyoma in a bitch.

Clinical signs associated with vaginal tumours are variable, but are mostly related to the size and position of the mass:

- Bulging of the perineum
- Prolapse of tumour tissue from the vulva
- Dysuria
- Stranguria
- Haematuria
- Vulval bleeding and/or discharge
- Faecal tenesmus
- Constipation
- Obstruction to copulation in entire females.

Clinical approach

Physical examination
Clinical history and clinical signs at presentation will often suggest the presence of a vaginal/vestibular mass. Preliminary examination of the vagina can be achieved with digital palpation via the rectum or the vagina.

Blood samples
No specific changes on a complete blood profile are reported in dogs or cats with vaginal/vestibular tumours. A neutrophilia with left shift may be seen in individuals with a concurrent secondary vaginitis or pyometra.

Imaging techniques
Plain caudal abdominal radiographs may suggest the presence of an intrapelvic soft tissue mass, but they will rarely confirm the true extent or position of the lesion. Findings suggestive of a vaginal mass include elevation or compression of the rectum, cranioventral displacement of the bladder, and faecal or urinary retention. Plain films can be used to assess possible metastasis to regional lymph nodes (medial iliac, sacral and hypogastric nodes). Contrast radiographic studies (including positive contrast retrograde vaginourethrography) and MRI or CT imaging will provide the most information regarding the position and extent of the primary tumour. In the case of malignant tumours, thoracic films should be obtained to investigate the presence of pulmonary metastasis.

The intrapelvic position of most vaginal tumours makes meaningful ultrasonographic assessment difficult.

Endoscopy
Endoscopic examination of the vagina will allow the extent of the tumour to be assessed and may aid in the retrieval of fine-needle aspirate or core biopsy material.

Histology
Definitive diagnosis can only be made on histological examination of excised tissue samples. Since the majority of vaginal tumours in the dog are benign, many authorities suggest that definitive diagnosis can be made by examination of material removed during surgical excision of the tumour.

Management

Surgery

For benign and malignant tumours with no evidence of metastasis, the treatment of choice is surgical excision. Surgery often involves a dorsal episiotomy and care should always be taken to recognize and preserve the urethral tubercle (catheterization of this structure prior to surgery is recommended). The strong association of most vaginal tumours with the secretion of oestrogen suggests that tumour resection should be combined with ovariectomy or ovariohysterectomy. Removal of the source of oestrogen production should minimize the recurrence of these oestrogen-influenced tumours. Malignant vaginal carcinomas will often prove very challenging to remove, since they are rarely well circumscribed.

Radiotherapy and chemotherapy

Radiotherapy is rarely indicated in the management of vaginal tumours, but may be useful in the management of SCC or MCTs involving the vulva. In most instances, radiation therapy is utilized where complete surgical excision cannot be achieved. TVTs are also very sensitive to radiation therapy and can often be treated successfully with low-dosage radiation (15 Gy).

There is little information available regarding the use of chemotherapy in the management of malignant vaginal or vulval tumours. It does not appear to be indicated in the management of benign tumours, where surgical excision can be most effective. An exception to this is TVT. Weekly administration of vincristine sulphate at a dosage of 0.5 mg/m^2 will often result in a complete cure after 4–6 weeks of treatment.

Prognosis

Following surgical resection combined with ovariohysterectomy, the prognosis for benign vaginal and vulval tumours is good. In contrast, the high likelihood of local recurrence and metastasis for malignant tumours such as adenocarcinoma and SCC makes their prognosis guarded to poor.

Tumours of the testicle

General considerations

Testicular tumours are common in the male dog and represent approximately 75% of all tumours involving the reproductive tract of the male dog. No breed predisposition for the development of testicular tumours has been recognized. Tumours are usually seen in dogs older than 10 years, but the development of tumours in cryptorchid animals is likely to occur earlier. Cryptorchid dogs are stated to have up to 20-fold increased risk of testicular neoplasia.

The three most common tumour types seen in the dog are the interstitial cell tumour, seminoma and Sertoli cell tumours (Figure 17.19). Recent studies suggest that the interstitial cell tumour and seminoma occur with the same frequency, though the Sertoli cell

Tumour site	Benign	Malignant
Gonadostromal tissue tumours	Interstitial cell (Leydig) tumour	Sertoli cell tumour
Germ cell tumours	Teratoma	Seminoma

17.19 Tumours of the testicle.

tumour may be less prevalent (Grieco *et al.*, 2008). It has also been suggested that, as reported in humans, testicular tumours in dogs have increased in prevalence during the last 40 years. The cause for such an increase remains unclear but the role of environmental pollutants has been implicated in humans. Many older dogs demonstrate the presence of multiple tumours in one or both of the testicles.

In the normal animal, interstitial (Leydig) cells are responsible for the production of testosterone. It has been suggested that interstitial cell tumours result in the production of excess testosterone leading to the development of perianal adenomas, perineal herniation and benign prostatic hyperplasia. In fact, tumours derived from this cell line do not show autonomous secretion of testosterone and many authorities believe that these conditions are encountered with equal frequency in the normal male dog. Sertoli cell tumours will often produce excess oestrogen, causing the development of feminization syndrome and squamous metaplasia of the prostate. Seminomas of the testicle may also occasionally be associated with the development of feminization syndrome.

Testicular neoplasms are rarely seen in the cat and this, in part, is related to the practice of elective castration of any male that is not to be used as a stud cat. Although cryptorchidism does occur in tom cats, it does not appear to be a risk factor for the development of testicular tumours.

Cryptorchidism predisposes to the development of Sertoli cell tumours and seminomas. The abdominal or inguinal positioning of the testis in such individuals maintains the structure at an abnormally high temperature, leading to damage to spermatogenic cells and possible neoplastic transformation.

The scrotum may be affected by any type of skin tumour. Tumours most commonly associated with this site are MCTs and melanomas.

Presentation and clinical signs

Sertoli cell tumours and, occasionally, seminomas may cause the development of feminization syndrome. The clinical signs associated with feminization syndrome due to oestrogen secretion are:

- Bilaterally symmetrical alopecia
- Reduced libido
- Attractiveness to other male dogs
- Pendulous prepuce
- Gynaecomastia (mammary enlargement, nipple elongation)
- Atrophy of unaffected testicle
- Myelosuppression (anaemia, neutropenia and thrombocytopenia).

Clinical approach

In the majority of animals, the presence of a testicular tumour will be discovered on palpation of an enlarged testicle or testicular mass on routine examination. In some animals, signs of feminization syndrome will suggest the presence of an oestrogen-producing testicular tumour. In an apparently castrated dog showing signs of feminization, careful examination of the animal's records should be made to ensure that the possibility of cryptorchidism can be excluded definitively. If there is any doubt about the dog's castration history, cryptorchidism should be considered a likely possibility.

Management

Surgery

The treatment of choice in the majority of animals with testicular tumours is castration (orchiectomy). Since the majority of canine testicular tumours demonstrate a low metastatic potential, removal of the testicles will often prove curative. It is suggested that the castration procedure should be performed using a 'closed' rather than an 'open' technique since this will minimize the chance of tumour cell contamination of the vaginal tunic and local tissues. Undoubtedly, it is sensible to excise as long a length of spermatic cord and associated spermatic vessels as possible, to minimize the potential of local tumour extension.

Similarly, the treatment of choice for the majority of individuals with testicular tumours associated with abdominal cryptorchidism is orchiectomy via a midline coeliotomy (Figure 17.20). In these animals the surgical procedure will be less straightforward than a scrotal castration and both inguinal and abdominal exploration may be required. In animals demonstrating feminization syndrome, resolution of most of the associated signs will occur within 6 weeks of the removal of the primary tumour; bone marrow recovery may take longer (see below). In some instances, persistence of feminization signs may indicate the presence of secondary growths that are actively secreting oestrogen.

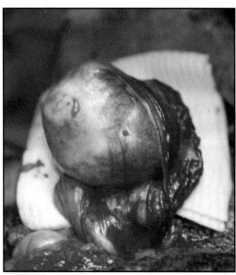

17.20 A Sertoli cell tumour associated with a cryptorchid testicle in a dog.

Radiotherapy and chemotherapy

There is only limited information available on the use of radiotherapy or chemotherapy in the management of testicular tumours. Reasons include the fact that primary tumours can be so effectively managed surgically, secondary tumours will rarely be situated at a site amenable to radiation therapy and reported chemotherapy for the management of secondary testicular tumours has demonstrated little beneficial effect. Interestingly, in humans, platinum-based (cisplatin) chemotherapy protocols have proved to be very effective in the management of germ cell testicular tumours and the use of these agents for the management of testicular tumours in the dog and cat might warrant further investigation.

Prognosis

The prognosis for the majority of testicular tumours is considered good following their removal by castration. In individuals with metastatic disease the prognosis is less favourable. The worst prognosis is often seen in individuals demonstrating myelosuppression associated with feminization syndrome. Following removal of Sertoli cell tumours in animals with myelosuppression, the rate of recovery of bone marrow function can be very slow, and take up to 6 months.

Tumours of the penis

General considerations

Tumours of the penis (Figure 17.21) are, in general, rare in both the dog and cat. However, transmissible venereal tumour (TVT) is recognized as a relatively common condition in certain parts of the world. Areas where this tumour is enzootic include the Mediterranean countries, the south-eastern USA and the Caribbean. Apart from TVT, which occurs in sexually active, younger dogs, the majority of penile tumours occur in the older dog. There does not appear to be any breed predisposition for tumour development at this site. TVT is transmitted by transplantation of cells at coitus. TVT does not commonly metastasize, but may be transplanted to other parts of the body, such as the face and nose, by grooming, licking and trauma. An affected individual will mount an immune response to the tumour and this may result in the slowing of its development and its eventual regression.

In areas of the world where TVT is not enzootic, SCC is the most common tumour of the penis in the dog.

Benign
• Papilloma
Malignant
• Squamous cell carcinoma • Transmissible venereal tumour • Haemangiosarcoma

17.21 Tumours of the penis.

The prepuce may be affected by any type of skin tumour. Tumours commonly associated with this structure include MCTs, melanomas and perianal gland adenoma.

Presentation and clinical signs

TVT often affects the glans or more caudal penis, and the tumour can be vegetative, pedunculated, papillary or nodular in appearance. Metastasis to local inguinal lymph nodes and abdominal organs has been reported in some cases, but this finding is considered unusual.

SCC of the penis presents as an ulcerated sessile lesion, most commonly affecting the glans penis, though it can also affect the lining of the prepuce. In some instances it may have the appearance of a cauliflower-like growth. SCC is locally invasive and may spread to the local inguinal lymph nodes. Distant metastasis is also possible in the more aggressive or advanced case.

Clinical signs associated with penile tumours are related to local tissue irritation, infection and bleeding:

- Licking of prepuce and penis
- Haemorrhagic and/or purulent discharge from the prepuce
- Haematuria (may be frank blood at beginning or end of micturition)
- Dysuria
- Increased frequency of urination
- Phimosis
- Paraphimosis (occasionally).

The majority of penile tumours will not be discernible whilst the penis lies within the prepuce.

Skin tumours of the prepuce are often obvious as discrete masses, but the presence of local swelling and oedema may mask the location of a mast cell tumour.

Clinical approach

Obtaining a clinical history that includes one or more of the signs listed above should alert the clinician to the possible presence of a penile tumour.

Physical examination

In most instances, the presence of a tumour will be obvious once the penis has been fully extruded from the prepuce (Figure 17.22). This can usually be performed in the conscious animal, but a more comprehensive examination will be achieved in the sedated or anaesthetized animal. A careful examination of local inguinal lymph nodes should be undertaken and the presence of nodal enlargement should prompt an assessment for local metastasis. Thoracic radiography can be used to assess distant metastasis.

Blood samples

A complete blood profile will not demonstrate any changes indicative of the presence of a tumour of the penis.

Cytology

Cytological samples may be obtained from any lesion using either direct impression smears or fine-needle aspirates.

Biopsy

Where necessary, histological samples may be obtained by grab, punch or incisional biopsy.

A diagnosis of TVT can be made either on histopathology or by chromosome karyotypic analysis. The tumour is characterized by a modal chromosome number of 59 ± 5, instead of the usual 78 found in normal canine cells (Murray *et al.*, 1969). In most instances, histopathology investigation will be sufficient for clinical diagnostic purposes.

Management

Surgery

The treatment of choice for the majority of penile tumours (apart from TVT) is surgical excision. In most instances, this will involve either a partial or a total penile amputation with castration and the construction of a scrotal urethrostomy (Figure 17.23). Adjunctive radiotherapy for SCC may be considered postoperatively.

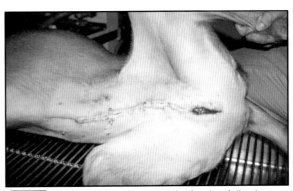

17.23 Postoperative photograph of a dog following total penile amputation with castration and the construction of a scrotal urethrostomy.

Radiotherapy and chemotherapy

TVT can be treated using either chemotherapy or radiotherapy. Complete regression (including metastatic disease in most cases) will occur with weekly doses of vincristine sulphate at 0.5 mg/m² every 7 days for a course of 4–6 weeks. Alternatively, regression can be achieved using low-dose radiotherapy (15 Gy).

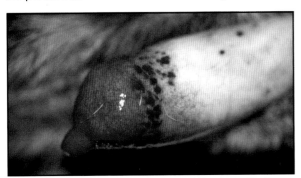

17.22 Multiple petechial lesions within the epithelium of the glans penis. Full-thickness biopsy samples confirmed the lesions to be haemangiosarcoma, necessitating total penile amputation.

Prognosis

Following wide-margin excision for SCC of the penis, the prognosis is favourable in those animals with no evidence of either local or distant metastasis. Local or distant metastasis always remains a possibility. The prognosis for TVT following either chemotherapy or radiotherapy is excellent in the majority of individuals.

Tumours of the prostate gland

General considerations

Tumours of the prostate gland are listed in Figure 17.24. Prostatic neoplasia occurs most commonly in old (mean age 10 years), medium or large breed dogs. Prostatic tumours in the dog are almost invariably malignant, though there are occasional reports of benign primary tumours of the gland. The prostate may also be the site of secondary, metastatic tumours such as lymphoma and perianal adenocarcinoma. Prostatic neoplasia is an extremely rare finding in the cat.

Benign
• Fibroma
• Leiomyoma
• Benign prostatic hyperplasia
Malignant
• Adenocarcinoma (commonest)
• Leiomyosarcoma
• Squamous cell carcinoma
• Transitional cell carcinoma
• Undifferentiated carcinoma

17.24 Tumours and tumour-like enlargements of the prostate gland.

The malignant tumour arising from prostatic glandular tissue is an adenocarcinoma; however, TCC from the prostatic urethra can invade into the prostate. Differentiation between these tumour types can be very difficult on clinical grounds; it may be possible by detailed histopathological assessment but immunohistochemical techniques may be required.

In the entire male dog, the commonest cause of an enlarged prostate (prostatomegaly) is benign prostatic hyperplasia. In the castrated individual, hyperplasia will regress; prostatomegaly may signal the presence of a more serious neoplastic condition. The relationship between the presence of benign prostatic hyperplasia and the subsequent development of a prostatic tumour remains unclear, but most authorities would agree that the development of prostatic tumours is not influenced by the sexual integrity of the dog; indeed, prostatic carcinoma may be more common in castrated dogs (Bryan *et al.*, 2007).

Presentation and clinical signs

Prostatic tumours often cause clinical signs consistent with lower urinary tract disease, including haematuria, dysuria and a purulent penile discharge. In individuals with a significant prostatomegaly, the clinical signs may include constipation and faecal tenesmus.

The neoplastic prostate gland is usually painful on both palpation of the caudal abdomen and palpation of the gland per rectum. Animals with benign prostatic hyperplasia rarely show such discomfort on prostatic palpation. In animals with a prostatic tumour, palpation also reveals gland asymmetry and a nodular consistency. It may also be possible to palpate enlarged sublumbar (hypogastric and medial iliac) and pelvic (sacral) lymph nodes that are suggestive of local metastasis. In animals with metastatic lesions within the pelvic bones or spine there may be clinical signs of pelvic limb weakness, lameness and/or neurological deficits. Bones containing metastatic lesions will be painful on manipulation.

By far the commonest prostatic tumour type in the dog is the adenocarcinoma. This tumour is very malignant and shows local invasion and early metastasis. Approximately 70% of cases will have metastasized by the time the tumour is diagnosed.

Clinical approach

Blood samples

A complete blood profile will not demonstrate any findings that are specifically consistent with a tumour of the prostate, although many individuals will show a regenerative or non-regenerative anaemia, elevations in both alkaline phosphatase and alanine transferase, hypoalbuminaemia, and hypercalcaemia. In individuals with intraprostatic urethral obstruction there may be evidence of an obstructive renal failure.

In humans, the early detection of prostatic cancer has been enhanced by the measurement of serum prostatic specific antigen (PSA). This has allowed the early diagnosis of organ-confined disease which can be surgically managed, resulting in an excellent prognosis for a cure. In the dog, prostatic adenocarcinoma does not appear to be associated with significant increases in PSA and reliable serum or seminal plasma markers have as yet to be found.

Physical examination

The digital rectal examination of the prostate gland is one of the most useful techniques for detecting prostatic abnormalities. In the male dog, the yearly check-up examination performed at booster vaccination should always include per rectum palpation of the prostate to screen for the presence of early prostatic disease.

Imaging techniques

In general, plain radiography is not sensitive in detecting the presence of prostatic neoplasia. Prostatic enlargement will often be detectable on a survey lateral abdominal film, but many prostatic tumours do not demonstrate significant prostatomegaly. Plain radiographs may be useful in assessment of tumour metastasis. Enlarged regional lymph nodes (medial iliac, sacral and hypogastric nodes), lytic or sclerotic bone lesions in the vertebrae or pelvis and/or pulmonary lesions on thoracic films may indicate the presence of tumour metastasis.

The use of negative (pneumourethrocystogram)

and positive (retrograde urethrogram) contrast radiographic studies will often provide information that supports a diagnosis of prostatic tumour. The invasive nature of prostatic carcinoma often results in the presence of mucosal irregularity within the intraprostatic urethra. The mucosa may be damaged to such a degree that contrast agent can be seen to leak (extravasation) into the prostatic parenchyma (Figure 17.25).

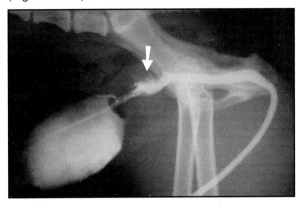

17.25 Retrograde positive contrast urethrogram demonstrating an irregular intraprostatic urethral margin and leakage of contrast agent into the prostatic parenchyma (arrowed) in a dog with prostatic adenocarcinoma.

The use of ultrasonography is indicated in any individual with prostatic disease. Clear information regarding the internal structure of the gland can be gained non-invasively, and biopsy samples taken percutaneously from any relevant abnormalities. Ultrasonography will aid the differentiation of other types of prostatic pathology such as prostatitis, benign hyperplasia, prostatic cystic disease and abscessation.

Magnetic resonance imaging and computed tomography may be considered in the investigation of prostatic disease and the assessment of local metastatic spread. In general, however, since surgical intervention is rarely indicated in the management of canine prostatic cancer, the expense of such an investigation is not warranted.

Biopsy
Although the investigative tests described will often be highly suggestive of a specific prostatic condition, confirmation requires the microscopic examination of either a biopsy specimen or an aspirate of the lesion. These are best obtained with the aid of ultrasound guidance, though direct palpation of the gland can be achieved in individuals with marked prostatomegaly. In most instances, core biopsies can be performed via the inguinal region, but it may prove necessary to use a perineal approach if the prostate is positioned within the pelvic canal.

Cytological material may be obtained by performing a urethral wash in conjunction with transrectal prostatic massage. This technique, although easy to perform, may not provide confirmation of a diagnosis because representative cells may fail to exfoliate into the urethral aspirate. If clinical signs suggest a prostatic tumour, a negative result on cytological examination should always be treated with some scepticism.

Management

Surgery
Although many of the currently available veterinary surgical textbooks still carry information regarding the technique of total prostatectomy for the management of prostatic neoplasia, most authorities would now agree that very few canine prostatic carcinomas are amenable to surgical resection. Total prostatectomy for the management of carcinoma will almost invariably result in unmanageable urinary incontinence; therefore the technique cannot be recommended in the majority of cases.

Radiotherapy and chemotherapy
The intraoperative administration of external beam radiotherapy has been used as a palliative treatment for localized prostatic tumours, but this approach has proved to be of limited benefit (Turrel, 1987).

Prostatic adenocarcinoma responds poorly to chemotherapy. Castration or administration of antiandrogens is not considered effective in the management of canine prostatic tumours since most develop independently of hormonal stimulation. Although the use of COX-2 inhibiting drugs such as piroxicam or meloxicam does not appear to have any effect on tumour growth, their administration is often helpful in controlling the discomfort associated with this form of tumour. In that TCC from the prostatic urethra can be difficult to exclude, it is often worth trying COX-2 inhibitors and platinum-based therapy but with a very guarded prognosis.

Prognosis
The highly malignant nature of most prostatic tumours and their high tendency to metastasize make the prognosis for this condition extremely grave. When dealing with an individual with prostatic disease it is imperative that the possibility of a prostatic tumour is excluded early in the management of the case.

References and further reading

Bryan JN, Keeler MR, Henry CJ et al. (2007) A population study of neutering status as a risk factor for canine prostate cancer. *Prostate* **67**, 1174–1181

Crow SE (1985) Urinary tract neoplasms in dogs and cats. *Compendium on Continuing Education for the Practicing Veterinarian* **7**, 607–618

Eker K, Salmanoglu MR and Vursal SA (2006) Unilateral leiomyoma in the mesosalpinx of a dog. *Journal of the American Animal Hospital Association* **42**, 392–394

Grieco V, Riccardi E, Greppi GF et al. (2008) Canine testicular tumours: a study on 232 dogs. *Journal of Comparative Pathology* **138**, 86–89

Henry CJ, Turnquist SE, Smith A et al. (1999) Primary renal tumours in cats: 19 cases (1992–1998). *Journal of Feline Medicine and Surgery* **1**, 165–170

Knapp DW, Richardson RC and Chan TCK (1994) Piroxicam therapy in 34 dogs with transitional cell carcinoma of the urinary bladder. *Journal of Veterinary Internal Medicine* **8**, 273–278

Matthiesen DT and Moroff SD (1989) Infiltrative urethral diseases in the dog. In: *Current Veterinary Therapy, 10th edn – Small Animal Practice*, ed. RW Kirk, pp. 1161–1163. WB Saunders, Philadelphia

Moe L and Lium B (1997) Hereditary multifocal cystadenocarcinomas and nodular dermatofibrosis in 51 German Shepherd Dogs. *Journal of Small Animal Practice* **38**, 498–505

Murray M, James H and Martin WJ (1969) A study of the cytology and karyotype of the canine transmissible venereal tumour. *Research in Veterinary Science* **10**, 565–568

Obradovich J, Walshaw R and Goullaud E (1987) The influence of castration on the development of prostatic carcinoma in the dog: 43 cases (1978–1985). *Journal of Veterinary Internal Medicine* **1**, 183–187

Turrel JM (1987) Intraoperative radiotherapy of carcinoma of the prostate gland in ten dogs. *Journal of the American Veterinary Medical Association* **190**, 48–52

Weisse C, Berent A, Todd K, Clifford C and Solomon J (2006) Evaluation of palliative stenting for management of malignant urethral obstructions in dogs. *Journal of the American Veterinary Medical Association* **229**, 226–234

White RN, Davies JV and Gregory SP (1996) Vaginourethropexy for treatment of urethral obstruction in the bitch. *Veterinary Surgery* **25**, 503–510

Tumours of the respiratory system and thoracic cavity

B. Duncan X. Lascelles and Robert N. White

Tumours of the nasal planum

Tumours of the nasal planum are summarized in Figure 18.1.

Benign
• Fibroma • Eosinophilic granuloma • Haemangioma
Malignant
• Squamous cell carcinoma (SCC) • Lymphoma • Fibrosarcoma • Melanoma • Mast cell tumour

18.1 Tumours of the nasal planum. SCC is by far the most common cancer at this site.

Presentation and clinical signs

Cancer of the nasal planum is rare in the dog but is fairly common in the cat. The most common cancer of the nasal planum is the squamous cell carcinoma (SCC). In the cat, invasive SCC is usually preceded by a protracted disease course (several months to years) progressing from solar dermatitis, through carcinoma *in situ*, to superficial SCC and then invasive SCC.

Clinically, crusting and erythema are seen first, then superficial erosions and ulcers and, finally, deeply erosive lesions. The development of SCC has been correlated with exposure to ultraviolet light (sunlight) and a lack of pigment protection (white hair and non-pigmented nasal planum). Often in cats, eyelid, pre-auricular skin and ear pinna lesions will also be seen if these areas have white hair and are not protected with pigment (see also Chapter 12).

Clinical approach

Biopsy

SCC is a local disease. A wedge biopsy should be performed on erosive lesions. Care must be taken to locate the biopsy in such a position that any subsequent surgical resection is not compromised, i.e. the biopsy should not be placed in a position where resection of the biopsy tract and the tumour would result in larger margins than if the biopsy tract were not present. Cytological examination (such as of skin

scrapings) is of little use, tending to reflect the inflammation that is invariably present. During a biopsy of the nasal planum, haemorrhage can be brisk but it is rarely of concern; the site should be closed with two or three sutures and pressure applied.

Metastasis to lymph nodes is rare, but all lymph nodes should be palpated and aspirated. Regional radiography is not indicated and metastasis to lung tissue is very rare.

Imaging

Once a diagnosis of SCC of the nasal planum has been made, the priority is to establish how far the disease extends caudally. Direct visualization inside the nares (with an otoscope or arthroscope) is rarely informative and palpation is often misleading. Computed tomography (CT) or, better, magnetic resonance imaging (MRI) is a valuable diagnostic tool to help define the extent of the disease, but invasive SCC is often so diffuse that CT or MRI does not always accurately define the true extent of disease. Additionally, even using intravenous contrast with these techniques does not always indicate the full extent of the disease. When defining the required extent of therapy (e.g. local radiation therapy or surgery) it is better to err on the side of overestimating the extent of disease.

Management and prognosis

Preventive measures are listed in Figure 18.2.

Therapy	Notes
Prevent exposure to sunlight	Limiting exposure to sunlight may arrest the course of the preneoplastic process, and is the most effective prevention for SCC
Tattooing	If inflammation and ulceration are present, it is difficult to maintain the tattoo
Topical sunscreen	These are often licked off
Synthetic vitamin A derivatives	These may be of help in reversing or limiting the growth of preneoplastic lesions

18.2 Measures for prevention of UV-induced squamous cell carcinoma of nasal planum.

SCC of the nasal planum in cats falls into two categories for treatment: superficial and invasive. Canine nasal planum SCC is invariably invasive. Treatment options for nasal planum SCC are:

- Cryosurgery (cats)
- Intralesional chemotherapy (cats)
- Photodynamic therapy (cats)
- Radiation therapy (cats and dogs)
- Strontium-90 plesiotherapy (cats)
- Surgical resection (cats and dogs).

Superficial nasal planum SCC in the cat can be managed using any of the options listed above. The optimal treatment for invasive SCC of the nasal planum in cats and dogs has not been systematically evaluated but the disease is probably best managed using surgery in both species.

Cryosurgery
Cryosurgery is the destruction of tissue by the controlled use of freezing and thawing. In one study of 90 cats with nasal planum SCC, 84% were tumour free at 12 months and 81% were tumour free at 36 months, though many required multiple treatments (Clarke, 1991). A later study in cats indicated a 73% recurrence rate after cryosurgery (Lana et al., 1997).

Intralesional chemotherapy
Intralesional chemotherapy using carboplatin has been described, and early work suggested a 70% response rate with a 30% recurrence rate. No further work has been performed, suggesting that this approach is not practical on a routine basis.

Photodynamic therapy
Several studies have described the use of photodynamic therapy (PDT) for the treatment of feline SCC. A topical photosensitizer, 5-aminolaevulinic acid (5-ALA), is widely used in human SCC treatment and has recently been evaluated in cats as a single topical treatment using high-intensity light-emitting diodes as the light source (Bexfield et al., 2008). The results indicated that 96% of superficial nasal planum SCCs treated with PDT using topical 5-ALA responded to therapy, with a complete response rate of 85%. Although initial response rates were encouraging, PDT did not lead to durable remission or cure in all cases, with a recurrence rate of 51% at a median of 157 days.

Radiation therapy
In cats, overall, the literature suggests that patients with small volumes of tumour have longer disease-free intervals and survival times. The disadvantage of radiation therapy is the requirement for multiple treatments. In dogs, radiation therapy did not seem to be effective (Lascelles et al., 2000).

Strontium-90 plesiotherapy
This involves the direct application of radioactive strontium (^{90}Sr) to the surface of a lesion. The maximal radiation dose is delivered to the surface of the skin with a rapid decrease in dose with depth below the surface, such that <10% of the surface dose penetrates to a depth of 3 mm. Of 49 cats that underwent strontium plesiotherapy, using 1–6 applications at a single treatment time point, 98% had a response to treatment and 88% had a complete response

(Hammond et al., 2007). The histological diagnosis was SCC in 37 cats, and SCC in situ in 14 cats. More applications were used in larger tumours, and although there was no significant association between number of applications and overall survival times, it did appear that the more applications that were required, the greater was the chance of recurrence, suggesting that this therapy may work best for superficial SCC.

Surgical resection
In many cases surgery is the treatment of choice. Surgical resection of the nasal planum can be performed, with good cosmetic results. The attainment of tumour-free margins in both cats and dogs is correlated to prolonged survival and cure (Lana et al., 1997; Lascelles et al., 2000, 2004). The line of excision is marked out (Figure 18.3a) and the affected area removed with a 360 degree incision, which extends down through the skin and the underlying rostral turbinates (Figure 18.3b). In dogs, a 1 cm margin should be obtained. In cats, a 0.5 cm margin is needed for superficial lesions; for deeper or more diffuse lesions, a 1 cm margin should be obtained.

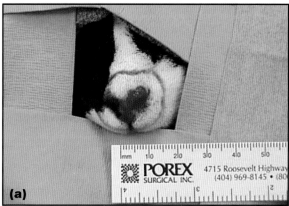

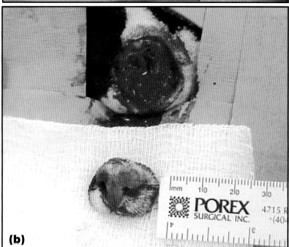

18.3 Surgical resection of SCC of the nasal planum. **(a)** For superficial lesions in the cat, a margin of 0.5 cm of grossly normal tissue should be resected; for deeper lesions, a 1 cm margin of normal tissue should be resected. This should be marked out on the animal prior to cutting. **(b)** In both cats and dogs, the line of excision is marked out, and the affected area removed with a 360 degree incision that extends down through the skin and the underlying rostral turbinates. (continues) ▶

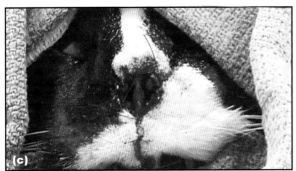

18.3 (continued) Surgical resection of SCC of the nasal planum. **(c)** A new nasal orifice is created using a purse-string suture, or, as in this case, reconstructing the area with simple interrupted sutures.

Bleeding can only be controlled once the affected tissue is removed, and a combination of direct pressure and electrocautery is used. The nasal orifice can be reconstructed with either a single purse-string suture, not pulled too tight, or using simple interrupted sutures of nylon (Figure 18.3c). In the authors' experience, a single purse-string suture results in stricture formation more often than using simple interrupted sutures of 1.5 metric (4/0 USP) or 1 metric (5/0 USP) nylon to suture the haired skin to the nasal mucosa. The area will crust and scab over and needs to be kept clean by gentle debridement using cotton-tipped applicators ('cotton buds') by the owners during the healing process. Healing is usually complete by 4–6 weeks postoperatively and the cosmetic result is acceptable (Figure 18.4). Occasionally, progressive stricture formation develops and may require further surgery. If margins contain tumour tissue, further resection can be carried out, or radiation therapy tried.

For more invasive SCC and for other invasive or extensive cancers involving the nasal plate and rostral maxilla, radical resection of the nasal plate and rostral maxilla has been described and is tolerated well by dogs (Figure 18.5) and probably cats (Figure 18.6) (Kirpensteijn *et al.*, 1994).

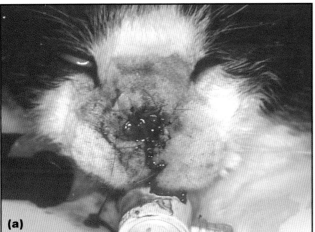
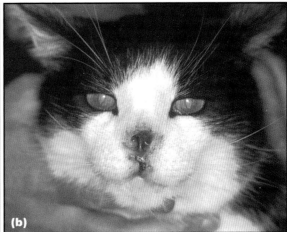

18.4 Appearance of a cat **(a)** immediately following nosectomy for SCC and **(b)** 14 weeks after surgery, showing the good cosmetic result obtained.

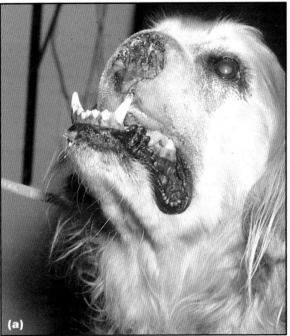
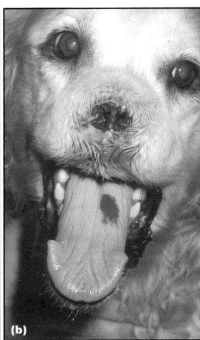

18.5 Appearance of a dog **(a)** 2 weeks after combined resection of the nasal planum and rostral maxilla to the level of the 2nd/3rd premolar as treatment for a fibrosarcoma of the rostral nasal area and **(b)** 14 weeks after surgery. The site of surgery has healed, and the cosmetic appearance is acceptable, even after such radical surgery.

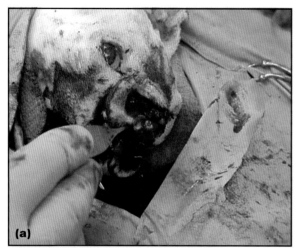

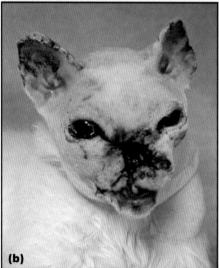

18.6 **(a)** A cat with an invasive SCC of the nasal planum undergoing radical nosectomy (all of the tissue rostral to the 2nd premolar). **(b)** Appearance of the same cat the day after surgery. Note the crusting around the new nasal orifice. This needs to be gently cleaned for several weeks as healing progresses. This cat also had actinic changes on the tips of its ears and these were also removed.

Prognosis

The prognosis for early non-invasive disease is very good, though subsequent development of SCC at other sites on the nasal planum is not uncommon. Invasive disease can be cured by appropriately aggressive surgery. With surgery ('nosectomy'), >80% of cats will be alive and free of disease at 1 year, and median survival times (MSTs) of 22 months have been reported (Lana *et al.*, 1997). With nosectomy in dogs, where tumour-free margins are obtained, median follow-up times (at which point no tumour recurrence was seen) have been reported as 24 and 32 months; but when tumour-free margins are not obtained SCC invariably recurs, in one study at about 6 weeks. In cats, the literature would suggest that although recurrence is more likely when clean resections are not obtained, it does not always happen, but this may be simply due to insufficient follow-up times. Radiation therapy is relatively ineffective, and active growth or recurrence of tumours tends to occur 8–12 weeks after treatment.

Tumours of the nasal cavity

Tumours of the nasal cavity are summarized in Figure 18.7.

Benign
• Occasionally benign sarcomas occur (e.g. chondrosarcoma) • Fibromas • Polyps

Malignant
• Carcinomas (adenocarcinoma, squamous cell carcinoma, undifferentiated carcinoma) • Sarcomas (fibrosarcomas, chondrosarcoma, osteosarcoma, undifferentiated sarcoma) • Lymphoma

18.7 Tumours of the nasal cavity. Carcinomas make up about two-thirds of nasal tumours; sarcomas comprise the majority of the rest.

Presentation and clinical signs

In dogs, two-thirds of intranasal tumours are carcinomas, with approximately one-third being sarcomas. Nasal tumours are relatively rare in dogs, accounting for about 1% of all tumours. In cats, the most common form of intranasal neoplasia is lymphoma, with carcinomas being the second most common. Despite the fact that nasal lymphoma is the most common nasal tumour in cats, it is relatively rare, accounting for <1% of all feline tumours. In both species, carcinomas and sarcomas occur in older animals.

The average duration of clinical signs in dogs with nasal tumours is 3 months and in cats this time period is more variable – weeks to years. In an older dog, a history of progressive but intermittent signs of sneezing and snorting, unilateral nasal discharge and/or epistaxis, progressing to bilateral signs, increased difficulty in breathing and sometimes facial deformity, is strongly suggestive of cancer. Epiphora, dullness and neurological signs may also be seen. Unlike nasal neoplasms in the dog, nasal discharge and epistaxis are less common signs in cats, occurring in only about one-third of those affected. Seizures can be an associated sign in both species if the neoplasm has extended beyond the cribriform plate. In both species, there has been a suggestion that animals with longer nasal passages may have a predisposition for developing nasal malignancies.

Differential diagnoses include bleeding disorders, hypertension, fungal rhinitis, bacterial rhinitis, immune-mediated rhinitis and foreign body. In cats, nasopharyngeal polyp should also be a differential, depending on the age of the cat.

Clinical approach

A thorough clinical examination should be performed, including an intraoral examination (looking for distortion or destruction of the hard palate). If epistaxis is present, bleeding disorders should be ruled out with appropriate laboratory tests. Further diagnostic evaluation is then carried out under general anaesthesia.

Imaging

Definitive diagnosis requires a biopsy but radiographs should be taken prior to this (bleeding after the biopsy procedure can obscure intranasal detail). The most useful radiographic views are:

- Ventrodorsal open-mouth 20 degrees angled view to image the nasal cavity and cribriform plate (or the intranasal view with radiographic film placed within the mouth and the image taken in the DV position)
- Skyline view of the frontal sinus.

Turbinate destruction and replacement by material of soft tissue radiodensity suggests a tumour, but a biopsy is required to make the definitive diagnosis.

MRI is a very useful tool, both to help to decide whether there is tumour present and to delineate its extent (Figure 18.8). CT is probably the imaging modality of choice because of the high definition of soft tissue within the nasal and frontal sinuses and adjacent orbit and brain (Figure 18.9).

Biopsy

While the patient is still under anaesthesia from its imaging procedures, rhinoscopy can be used to visualize the tumour before a biopsy procedure. Although tissue samples are relatively easy to obtain through most endoscopes, this method is not a recommended sampling procedure as samples procured are generally limited to the superficial layer of tissue, due to the small size of the instrument. A nasal biopsy should be collected using a closed nasal biopsy technique – a closed suction technique, a bone curette, alligator forceps or 'melon-baller' forceps. It does not matter which instrument is used to procure a sample but, whatever the method, care must be taken to ensure that the cribriform plate is not punctured and the brain is not entered, and that a large enough sample from the correct location is obtained.

The location of the suspected tumour is read from radiographs or CT/MRI images and either a plastic cannula or 'melon baller' cup forceps (such as mare uterine biopsy forceps) can be advanced via the nostril towards the lesion. Prior to this, the biopsy instrument should be marked off with tape so that it is not advanced further than the distance from the tip of the nares (*not* the rostral edge of the nasal bone) to the medial canthus. Tumour tissue is usually very soft (not 'crunchy' like turbinates) and a white or yellow colour.

Haemorrhage can be profuse, but usually subsides after a few minutes. The following methods to deal with significant haemorrhage may be used:

- Keep the animal anaesthetized, or sedated and quiet, until bleeding subsides
- Pack the pharynx and the rostral nares (in anaesthetized animals) and let clots form
- If blood pressure is adequate, small amounts of acepromazine can be administered
- Use gauze swabs with a small amount of adrenaline (epinephrine)

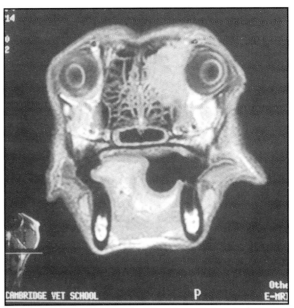

18.8 Transverse MRI section through the skull of a dog, at the level of the eyes, showing a tumour in the left nasal cavity and invading the orbit.

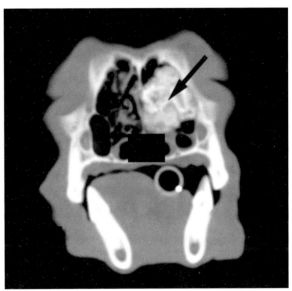

18.9 CT scan of the mid-nose area of an 11-year-old crossbred dog with an intranasal chondroblastic osteosarcoma (arrowed). The CT enables the extent of the tumour to be defined and also allows planning for radiation therapy.

- Adrenaline can be placed in the external nares
- In the event of significant bleeding, the unilateral carotid artery could be permanently ligated. The authors have never had to resort to this method.

Other considerations

Nasal washing and brush cytology are of limited value and not recommended as the sole method of diagnosis.

Lymph node metastasis is usually present in 10% of cases at the time of diagnosis, but later in the disease up to 40% of nasal tumours may metastasize to lymph node and lung.

Management and prognosis

Dogs

The therapy of choice in dogs is radiation therapy, with or without a radiosensitizer (e.g. low-dose cisplatin). Most of these tumours present late in the disease process and cannot be completely removed by surgery. Surgical cytoreduction is usually of no benefit prior to radiation therapy (but is necessary when low-energy orthovoltage radiation is used) and surgery makes no difference to survival when used on its own. However, a benefit of pre-radiation surgical cytoreduction of chondrosarcomas has been shown, presumably because these are slow-growing tumours.

Computerized planning of radiation therapy helps to maximize the dose to the tumour, whilst sparing normal tissue (such as eyes and brain) as much as possible. Total doses of 40–57 Gy are usually administered in 12–19 fractions over 3–4 weeks. Hypofractionated radiotherapy (4 × 8–9 Gy fractions) has also been reported to provide good palliation (Mellanby *et al.*, 2002a).

Mucositis (reaction of the mucous membranes) and rhinitis are often severe in animals treated with the high-dose fractionated regimens, although this is not the case for palliative protocols. Analgesia is very important over the 3–4 weeks of these symptoms. Keratoconjunctivitis sicca, corneal ulcers and cataract formation can all occur if an eye receives sufficient radiation.

Cats

Supportive care is particularly important in cats. Cats with nasal tumours have a reduced ability to smell and should be treated with appetite stimulants and have their food heated to entice them to eat. If oral nutrition is not of an adequate amount, placement of an enteral feeding tube should be considered

Lymphoma: In cats without systemic involvement, radiation therapy can result in extended survival times or may be curative. An important prognostic factor may be the patient's FeLV status, with FeLV-positive status being associated with poor survival rates. A recent retrospective study found no difference in survival between cats treated with radiotherapy alone, chemotherapy alone, or a combination of the two; however, there was a suggestion that higher doses of radiotherapy may be associated with longer survival. When looking at deaths caused by progressive disease, overall survival times were about 16 months, but when looking at deaths regardless of cause, overall survival was 6 months. Anaemia was a negative prognostic variable (Haney *et al.,* 2009). Patients with systemic disease require chemotherapy.

Intranasal carcinomas and sarcomas: Surgery alone results in relatively fast tumour recurrence. The use of radiation therapy (48 Gy and varying protocols in a small number of cats) resulted in 1- and 2-year survival rates of 44% and 17%, with the side effects of radiation therapy in cats being less than in dogs.

Prognosis

Overall, the prognosis for canine nasal tumours is very poor. The mean survival time without treatment, or with surgery or chemotherapy, is 2–5 months. This is improved to between 8 and 25 months with radiation therapy, depending on the protocol used, with 1- and 2-year survivals of about 40–80% and 20–40%, respectively (Lana and Withrow, 2001).

The prognosis for sarcomas is thought to be slightly better than for carcinomas; of the latter, the adenocarcinomas respond slightly better than SCC or undifferentiated carcinoma. However, even if clinical signs resolve, few dogs are considered cured and metastasis is more likely to be seen in longer-surviving patients. The use of platinum agents as radiation sensitizers improves survival times. The combination of radiation therapy followed by surgery has resulted in longer disease-free intervals, but not significantly so.

Using surgery followed by radiation therapy, it was found that dogs that underwent both were significantly more likely to develop rhinitis or osteomyelitis than dogs treated with radiation therapy alone (Adams *et al.*, 2005). Also noted in the same study was that the rate of local recurrence of neoplasia was not significantly different between the two groups. However, the 2-year survival rate for dogs in the surgery group was 69%, compared with 44% for the radiation therapy group.

The prognosis for cats with lymphoma is better, with one study reporting a median survival of 4 years in cats with nasal lymphoma treated by radiation alone. Non-lymphoid neoplasia survival rates in the cat following radiation therapy appear similar to those in the dog (Theon *et al.*, 1994; Mellanby *et al.*, 2002b).

Tumours of the larynx and trachea

Cancer of the larynx or trachea is rare in the dog and cat, though both malignant and benign tumours are recognized at each site (Figures 18.10 and 18.11). Malignant tumours are more common than benign tumours. There is some confusion over the true nature of the rhabdomyoma and the oncocytoma.

Benign
<ul><li>Leiomyoma</li><li>Lipoma</li><li>Osteochondroma</li><li>Rhabdomyoma</li><li>Oncocytoma</li><li>Fibropapilloma</li></ul>
Malignant
<ul><li>Squamous cell carcinoma</li><li>Adenocarcinoma</li><li>Poorly differentiated carcinoma</li><li>Chondrosarcoma</li><li>Lymphoma</li><li>Malignant melanoma</li><li>Mast cell tumour</li><li>Osteosarcoma</li><li>Rhabdomyosarcoma</li><li>Plasma cell tumour</li></ul>

18.10 Tumours of the larynx.

Benign
• Leiomyoma
• Osteochondroma
• Osteochondral dysplasia
• Polyp

Malignant
• Adenocarcinoma
• Squamous cell carcinoma
• Poorly differentiated carcinoma
• Chondrosarcoma
• Lymphoma
• Osteosarcoma
• Plasma cell tumour
• Mast cell tumour
• Rhabdomyosarcoma

18.11 Tumours of the trachea.

Although these tumours arise from different cell lines (rhabdomyoma arises from striated muscle cells, whereas oncocytoma arises from epithelial cells called oncocytes), they can prove hard to differentiate histologically and immunohistochemistry may be required to differentiate the two.

Presentation and clinical signs

Laryngeal tumours
In the dog, the clinical signs of a laryngeal tumour are most commonly associated with distortion of the laryngeal cartilages and with progressive stenosis of the laryngeal lumen (rima glottidis). The signs will include changes in voice or bark and, in those individuals with stenosis of the rima glottidis, the presence of stridorous respiratory function. As with the condition of idiopathic bilateral laryngeal paralysis, the laryngeal stridor will be worsened by anything causing an increase in respiratory rate, such as excitement, panting and exercise; therefore, individuals will often suffer from exercise intolerance.

In the cat, the presence of a laryngeal tumour will commonly result in an inability to purr as well as a change of voice. Laryngeal stridor and expiratory dyspnoea localized to the larynx will also occur, but the sedentary nature of many cats often allows these individuals to hide the obstructive clinical signs until they become severe.

In both species, advanced laryngeal tumours may cause pharyngeal signs. This will result in dysphagia, caused either by infiltration of an aggressive tumour type into the local pharyngeal tissues or, more commonly, by the sheer size of the laryngeal mass.

Tracheal tumours
In both the dog and the cat, the clinical signs of tracheal tumours are in general associated with the space-occupying nature of the tumour within the tracheal lumen. It is, therefore, not surprising that the clinical signs seen with tracheal tumours include coughing, dyspnoea and exercise intolerance. Clinical signs are often insidious and in most instances their severity will be related to the size of the mass in relation to the size of the tracheal lumen. Early in development, small tracheal masses will often produce no clinical signs whatsoever. These masses are mostly covered with normal tracheal mucosa and will rarely lead to the initiation of a cough reflex.

Clinical approach

Imaging and biopsy
Under general anaesthesia the majority of laryngeal tumours can be visualized, and biopsy performed, through the mouth (Figure 18.12). Endoscopy may also be used.

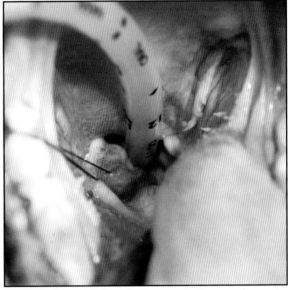

18.12 Intraoral view of a laryngeal adenocarcinoma in a dog.

Tracheal tumours are best visualized intraluminally with the aid of either a rigid or a flexible endoscope (Figure 18.13). Certain tracheal tumours fail to demonstrate any significant degree of intraluminal protrusion, making endoscopic biopsy procedures impossible, and in such cases an incisional or excisional biopsy may have to be performed as part of surgical exploration.

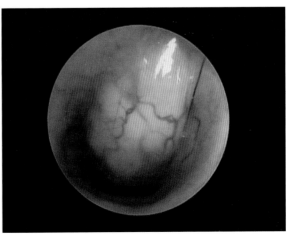

18.13 Endoscopic view of a tracheal lymphoma in a cat.

Radiography of the larynx is generally unhelpful, though it may be used to assess local lymph node (retropharyngeal) enlargement and the extent of displacement of local structures in the neck and pharyngeal region. Plain radiographs of the cervical and thoracic regions may demonstrate the presence of intraluminal tracheal narrowing, which is often associated with the presence of a tracheal tumour (Figure 18.14). In many instances, appropriate radiographic interpretation can prove difficult even when good quality radiographs have been obtained.

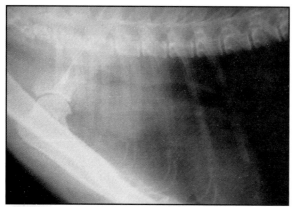

18.14 Lateral thoracic radiograph of a cat with a tracheal chondrosarcoma. Note the discrete narrowing of the tracheal lumen at the site of the tumour.

Staging

Tumour staging should be undertaken for both lymphoid and non-lymphoid tumours. Staging for non-lymphoid tumours should include evaluation of regional lymph nodes and lungs for metastasis. Lymphoid tumour staging should also include thoracic lymph node, abdominal organ and bone marrow evaluation for evidence of metastasis. Cats with laryngeal or tracheal lymphoma should also have evaluation of their FeLV and FIV status performed. CT/MRI imaging may be used to assess the extent and invasiveness of the primary tumour and also can be part of the assessment for local/distant metastatic disease.

Management and prognosis

Surgery

Laryngeal tumours: There are a number of reports describing the successful resection of benign laryngeal tumours such as rhabdomyomas (oncocytomas) whilst preserving relatively normal laryngeal function. Unfortunately, the majority of malignant laryngeal tumours are not amenable to local laryngeal resection. In such cases, total laryngectomy is required to achieve complete tumour resection. Although this technique can technically be accomplished in both the dog and the cat, it represents an extreme form of treatment which is associated with many potential complications. Such surgery involves the formation of a permanent tracheostomy and may result in varying degrees of pharyngeal dysphagia. Therefore, although the technique is described in many surgical textbooks, the authors consider it is rarely indicated in the management of laryngeal tumours in the dog and cat. The

implications for the animal's welfare and its long-term care should be discussed carefully with the owner.

Tracheal tumours: Tracheal tumours may be amenable to surgical resection (Figure 18.15). In most instances this will require resection of the affected tracheal rings followed by subsequent end-to-end anastomosis of the separated tracheal ends. Although reports suggest that up to 30–40% of the trachea can be resected with successful re-anastomosis, tension-free and therefore complication-free repair is more likely to be accomplished if no more than five or six rings are resected. This surgery will be performed more readily when the tumour affects the cervical trachea as opposed to the thoracic trachea. Resection and repair of the tracheal bifurcation can be accomplished but is technically demanding and associated with a high incidence of complications, such as air leakage caused by dehiscence of the anastomosis.

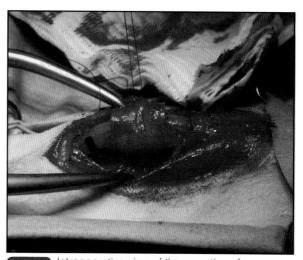

18.15 Intraoperative view of the resection of a chondrosarcoma involving four to five rings of the proximal cervical trachea in a cat.

Radiation therapy

In cases with radiosensitive tumours such as lymphoma, the treatment of choice may be radiotherapy. This would certainly be the case in individuals with either non-resectable radiosensitive tumours or in cases where the resection of such a tumour was likely to result in life-threatening complications. As such, the potential importance of obtaining a diagnosis on biopsy is clear. It is important to note that, although it may be tempting to administer corticosteroids in an attempt to relieve the respiratory signs, this will often mask the diagnosis of lymphoma and so result in a potentially unnecessary intervention.

Chemotherapy

Feline laryngeal lymphoma may also be treated by chemotherapy, using protocols described in Chapter 19a. Response is often favourable.

Prognosis

Benign tumours of the larynx and trachea carry a good prognosis if they can be completely excised surgically. Although there are few reports describing the management of malignant tumours affecting the larynx and trachea, the site of development of such tumours makes their prognosis very poor, regardless of treatment.

Tumours of the lungs

Primary tumours of the lungs are summarized in Figure 18.16 and differential diagnoses for lung masses are given in Figure 18.17.

- Adenocarcinoma/carcinoma
  - o Bronchial gland
  - o Bronchogenic
  - o Bronchiolar–alveolar (commonest in both dog and cat)
- Anaplastic carcinoma
  - o Small cell
  - o Large cell
- Squamous cell (epidermoid) carcinoma
- Sarcomas
- Pulmonary lymphomatoid granulomatosis (dog)
- Benign tumours (very rare)

18.16 Primary tumours of the lungs.

- Pulmonary neoplasia
- Mediastinal neoplasia
- Pulmonary abscess
- Mediastinal abscess
- Pulmonary granuloma
- Lung lobe torsion
- Focal pneumonia/consolidation

18.17 Differential diagnoses for lung masses.

The lung represents a very common site for the development of secondary metastatic tumours in the dog and the cat. Development of primary lung tumours in both species is much less common, accounting for approximately 1% of all tumours in the dog and <0.5% in the cat. Most primary lung tumours are malignant; sites of metastasis include regional (tracheobronchial and sternal) lymph nodes, lung and bone. The rate of metastasis of primary lung tumours should be considered moderate at the time of diagnosis and high late in the course of the disease.

The most common type of primary lung tumour in both cats and dogs is the adenocarcinoma. This tumour type may be classified as differentiated or undifferentiated (carcinoma) and it may also be classified by its location, with bronchial gland, bronchogenic and bronchiolar–alveolar forms being recognized. Bronchiolar–alveolar carcinoma is the commonest form, whereas bronchogenic carcinoma is considered very rare in the dog and cat.

Other forms of primary tumour, such as SCC and anaplastic carcinoma (small and large cell), are less common. Sarcomas and benign tumours are considered extremely rare.

Presentation and clinical signs

In many individuals the clinical signs associated with a primary lung tumour are related to its size. When the mass is small (<2 cm diameter in the dog,

<0.5 cm diameter in the cat), it will often produce no clinical signs at all. In these individuals the mass may be detected as an incidental finding on a survey thoracic radiograph that was obtained, for example, for an unrelated condition. In an individual with a larger mass, clinical signs including coughing, lethargy, haemoptysis and dyspnoea may be seen. Non-specific signs such as anorexia, pyrexia, weight loss and exercise intolerance may also be noted. Under certain circumstances the lung mass may lead to the production of a pleural effusion and, depending on the tumour size and position, regurgitation may also occur.

In approximately 15% of dogs, and more rarely in the cat, the paraneoplastic syndrome hypertrophic osteopathy (Marie's disease) may occur. The underlying mechanism for this condition remains unclear, but it is characterized by painful, proliferative periosteal new bone growth on the distal limbs associated with a rapid increase in peripheral blood flow to the distal extremities. The presence of lameness and painful, non-pitting warm swelling on the distal limbs should alert the clinician to the possibility of hypertrophic osteopathy. It is important to note that this condition may result from a space-occupying mass in either the thoracic or the abdominal cavities (see also Chapter 4).

Clinical approach

Ideally, a definitive diagnosis should be made in all cases. Despite the rationale that the treatment of choice for any well circumscribed consolidated lung lesion is its removal by total or partial lobectomy, there is no reason to consider lung tumours any different than any other form of cancer; that is, an attempt to make a definitive diagnosis should always be made so that an informed decision can be taken with regard to the appropriate treatment of the condition. Similarly, tumour staging should be considered mandatory, as the results of this may have a dramatic effect on both prognosis and any requirements for adjunctive therapy. Tumour staging involves determining the size of the primary tumour, the presence or absence of local (generally tracheobronchial) lymph node metastasis and/or distant (lung or bone) metastasis.

Blood testing
Complete blood profiles will often be unremarkable, though hypercalcaemia has been reported in some cases.

Imaging
Survey thoracic radiographs are still considered the most reliable form of investigation (Figure 18.18). Most authorities would consider that three views are required: both lateral views and the ventrodorsal view. Good quality thoracic radiographs are important and can best be achieved in the anaesthetized intubated individual, where inflated views may be obtained. In cases with suspected hypertrophic osteopathy, or those with suspected distant bone metastasis, radiography of the abdomen, spine and peripheral appendicular skeleton (Figure 18.19) should be performed.

CT may be used to great effect for the assessment of metastatic lung tumours in the dog (Figure 18.20) and cat. In fact, CT offers the most sensitive method for the detection of lung metastasis and the presence or absence of local tracheobronchial lymph node enlargement. It should be considered superior to plain radiography and the imaging investigation of choice, if costs and availability allow.

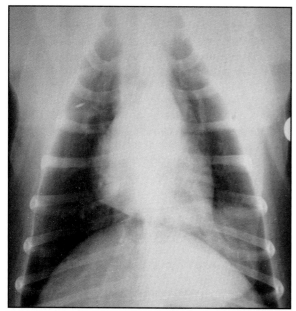

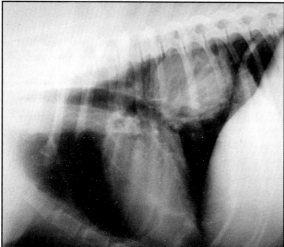

18.18 Ventrodorsal and lateral thoracic radiographs of a dog with a well circumscribed mass in the left caudal lung lobe.

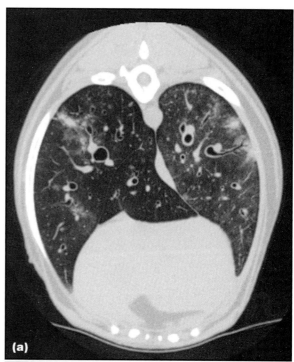

(a)

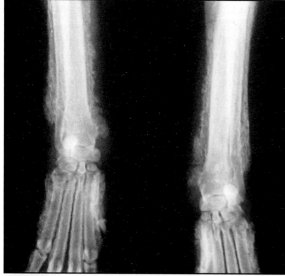

18.19 Radiograph of the distal forelimbs, demonstrating periosteal new bone characteristic of hypertrophic osteopathy.

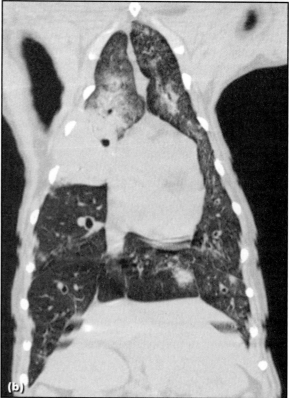

(b)

18.20 **(a)** Axial CT scan of a dog showing multiple metastatic lung tumours. **(b)** Coronal CT scan of the thorax of the same dog showing a primary lung tumour and multiple metastatic lung tumours.

In cases with metastatic lung tumours, the location of the primary tumour may require further survey radiography or advanced imaging of other parts of the animal's body. Diagnosis of diffuse pulmonary metastasis is often presumed by the presence of multiple consistent lung lesions on survey thoracic radiographs, especially in individuals with a concurrent or previous diagnosis of a malignant tumour with metastatic potential.

Ultrasonography of pulmonary masses may prove difficult unless the tumour is large and there is no overlying air-filled lung. In cases where the lesion is adjacent to the thoracic wall, fine-needle aspirates or core biopsy samples may be obtained with the aid of ultrasound guidance. Obtaining percutaneous biopsy samples can be associated with potentially life-threatening complications, including pneumothorax and interpleural haemorrhage. At worst, these techniques may actually lead to inappropriate tumour spread by seeding. The pros and cons of obtaining such biopsy samples should be carefully explained to the owner before such procedures are embarked upon.

Enlarged regional lymph nodes may also be detectable with ultrasound. Although it may prove difficult or impossible to perform a biopsy (tracheobronchial) in these cases, the presence of node enlargement is still prognostically significant and in the majority of cases suggests a less favourable outcome.

Bronchoscopy

Bronchoscopy may be performed to investigate the presence of lower airway disease but it will commonly be less rewarding in the confirmation of a primary lung tumour. It sometimes proves possible to obtain aspirate and/or grab biopsy material via bronchoscopy. This procedure is associated with similar complications to those described for ultrasonography and in a similar way should not be undertaken without careful consideration and a fully informed owner.

Cytology

Cytological examination of tracheobronchial washes will often fail to detect the presence of neoplastic cells. Similarly, obtaining pleural fluid samples in individuals with an effusion will often confirm the presence of a modified transudate without revealing the presence of neoplastic cells.

Thoracoscopy

Recent developments and the greater availability of minimally invasive techniques have confirmed that thoracoscopy can now be considered a safe means for both visualization and safe biopsy of primary lung tumours, regional lymph nodes and lung metastatic lesions. As these techniques become more widely available, it is likely that their role in the assessment and treatment of lung tumours will develop further, with the possibility that thoracoscopic assessment will become the primary means of staging primary lung tumours in both the dog and the cat.

Management and prognosis

Treatment is based on clinical stage of the disease and, ideally, on a lesion that has been confirmed to be a primary lung tumour by histology rather than on one with only a presumed diagnosis.

Surgery

The treatment of choice for solitary primary lung tumours with no evidence of distant metastasis is the resection of the affected lung lobe with concurrent visual inspection of the regional tracheobronchial lymph nodes. In individuals with preoperative staging suggestive of regional lymph node enlargement, or in individuals proving to have lymph node enlargement at the time of surgery, biopsy samples of the offending lymph node or nodes should be submitted for histopathology.

In most cases the surgery can be performed via lateral intercostal thoracotomy. In some instances, for example when contemplating removal of a very large lung tumour or where there is uncertainty as to which lobe is affected, it may be tempting to consider entering the thoracic cavity via a median sternotomy. Although all lung lobes can be removed via this approach, their resection is made more difficult by the position of the dorsally situated hilar vessels and bronchi. In rare cases, a tumour within the peripheral aspect of the right accessory lobe may appear, radiographically, to be within the left caudal lung lobe. Although not an ideal approach for such a resection, it is feasible to remove the right caudal lung lobe via a left lateral thoracotomy. Many primary lung tumours prove readily resectable and the prospect of thoracic surgery may seem appealing, but it should be clearly understood that surgery is best performed by a specialist with adequate expertise, equipment and instrumentation.

There is little doubt that, with the advent of surgical stapling equipment, the partial or full lobectomy procedure can be performed both more quickly and more safely than by conventional techniques. The thoracoabdominal (TA) stapler that is used fires a double or triple row of B-shaped staples (Figure 18.21).

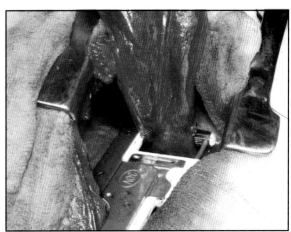

18.21 Intraoperative use of a thoracoabdominal stapler to close the bronchus of the right caudal lung lobe in a dog prior to its excision for the management of a primary lung tumour.

Pneumonectomy may be considered but a lung mass showing this degree of involvement carries a significantly worse prognosis.

Local lymph nodes should always be inspected (Figure 18.22). If there is evidence of enlargement, samples should be submitted for diagnostic histopathology.

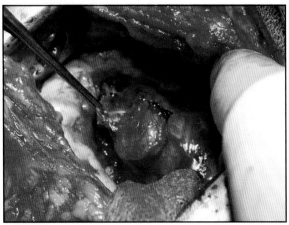

18.22 Enlarged hilar lymph node which can be visualized following the resection of a caudal lung lobe in a dog for the management of lung neoplasia. Node enlargement may represent reactive hypertrophy or metastatic spread of the tumour.

Metastatic tumours are usually multiple and rarely amenable to surgery, though the resection of solitary slow-growing metastases has been attempted. The resection of osteosarcoma lung metastases has been performed in the dog, but this has not been shown to produce any significant improvement in lifespan.

Histopathology should be performed on all resected lesions, as this information can be used to type and grade the tumour.

Radiation therapy
Radiotherapy is not undertaken in animals with either primary or metastatic lung tumours, since the lungs are particularly radiosensitive tissues and are susceptible to radiation side effects.

Chemotherapy
The majority of primary lung tumours (carcinomas) are not particularly sensitive to chemotherapy and efficacy is considered to be minimal, except for lymphoma. The use of adjunctive chemotherapy is dependent on the presence or absence of regional and/ or distant metastatic disease. The choice of agent is based on the tumour type; for example, carcinoma may show a positive response to the administration of platinum drugs such as carboplatin, whereas a short-lived partial or complete remission is possible for histiocytic sarcoma following the administration of lomustine (CCNU).

Prognosis
Adenocarcinoma and papillary carcinoma of the lung tend to have a slightly better prognosis (mean survival time of 19 months) than SCC (mean survival time 8 months) (Mehlaff *et al.*, 1983).

In the dog, there are several factors associated with a poorer prognosis. These include a larger tumour size (>5 cm diameter), the presence of clinical signs, and metastasis to regional lymph nodes. Well differentiated (low-grade) tumours have a better survival time and disease-free interval when compared with tumours that are moderately or poorly differentiated (high-grade). Tumours located centrally or in the perihilar region generally carry a worse prognosis than those located in the periphery on the lung. The presence of pleural effusion should also be considered a negative prognostic indicator.

In general, postoperative mean survival times for solitary primary lung tumours that demonstrate no evidence of metastases can extend to >12 months and can be >2 years in some cases. On the contrary, in individuals demonstrating one or more of the negative prognostic indicators described above, the median survival following primary tumour resection may be only 1–8 months. MST for dogs with unresectable primary tumours is several weeks to a few months.

Lung tumours in cats
In general, the clinical signs, investigations and management of primary lung tumours are similar for both dogs and cats, but there are some interesting and specific clinical differences in the cat that warrant further discussion.

Primary lung tumours are less common in the cat than in the dog, but, as in the dog, epithelial tumours (carcinoma) predominate. The rate of metastasis of primary tumours is similar or possibly slightly greater than in the dog; it should be considered moderate to high at the time of diagnosis (unless the tumour was detected as an incidental finding). The sites of metastasis are similar to those for the dog (regional lymph node, lung and bone) but, specifically, cats suffering from pulmonary epithelial tumours not uncommonly show metastatic spread to multiple digits (lung–digit syndrome).

Like the dog, treatment in cats is based on biopsy diagnosis and the clinical stage of the disease. Surgical excision is the treatment of choice for solitary lung tumours with no metastasis. Overall MST for cats with resectable primary lung tumours is approximately 4 months after surgery; however, individual cats can survive for much longer (2–3 years or more). Like the dog, a positive prognostic indicator would be the resection of a small lesion in a cat showing no clinical signs in which the tumour was found as an incidental finding. Not surprisingly, poorly differentiated tumours are associated with a much worse prognosis. The benefit of chemotherapy for the adjunctive management of gross primary or metastatic disease is not clearly defined and in the majority of cases is likely to have minimal positive effect.

Tumours of the chest wall

Primary mesenchymal tumours of the chest wall and differential diagnoses for chest wall masses are listed in Figures 18.23 and 18.24.

- Osteosarcoma (most common)
- Chondrosarcoma (second most common)
- Undifferentiated sarcoma
- Fibrosarcoma
- Haemangiosarcoma
- Haemangiopericytoma
- Myxosarcoma
- Chondroma

18.23 Primary mesenchymal tumours of the chest wall.

- Abscess (most common?)
- Neoplasia (benign or malignant)
- Osteomyelitis
- Fungal infection

18.24 Differential diagnoses for chest wall masses.

Tumours of the thoracic wall most commonly involve the ribs, but can also occur in the sternum. Tumours of the thoracic wall are rare in the dog and even rarer in the cat. There does not appear to be a sex predilection and most cases are seen in middle-aged to old individuals. Large-breed dogs are over-represented. Most thoracic wall tumours are mesenchymal in origin and nearly all are malignant.

Presentation and clinical signs
The most common clinical sign is a visible mass on the thoracic wall. Tumours most frequently occur at the costochondral junction, affecting the sixth, seventh and eighth ribs. Right- and left-sided masses appear to occur with equal frequency.

Other clinical signs include lethargy, weight loss, coughing, dyspnoea and lameness (most associated with hypertrophic osteopathy). Although not proven, there is some suggestion that the development of a proportion of thoracic wall sarcomas is associated with a previous traumatic episode to the thoracic wall.

Clinical approach

Haematology
Complete blood profiles in general provide little information of diagnostic value, but an infectious process such as an abscess may commonly be associated with a neutrophilia with or without a regenerative left shift.

Imaging
Good quality survey thoracic radiographs (at least two orthogonal views) should be obtained. These will often confirm the rib with primary involvement and may also provide information on local invasion into adjacent ribs. Many mesenchymal tumours of the rib will demonstrate the so-called 'iceberg' effect, i.e. the size of the mass on its intrapleural aspect will be significantly larger than the size of the external, lateral aspect of the growth. In some instances, the mass will be associated with the presence of a pleural effusion. The effusion may require drainage to allow clear radiographic interpretation.

Advanced scanning modalities such as CT will often provide greater information than that obtained with survey radiographs. CT scans will also provide

the clearest information regarding metastasis to the lungs and local lymph nodes.

Ultrasonography may be used in certain circumstances, but will often provide little further information than that obtained from survey radiographs.

Biopsy
A biopsy should be performed on any chest wall mass prior to treatment. Cells may be collected using fine-needle aspiration, but many mesenchymal tumours do not exfoliate well and so it is often better to perform a core biopsy. Survey radiographs may be used to decide the site of biopsy. Samples should be taken in a manner that ensures that they are within tissues which will be removed should surgical intervention be undertaken.

Despite obtaining core biopsy samples, the differentiation between chondrosarcoma and chondroblastic osteosarcoma remains difficult in many cases. In some instances, the true nature of the tumour can only be ascertained following open biopsy.

Pleural fluid samples
In cases with pleural effusion, samples of the effusion may be submitted for cytology, but these will often only reveal the presence of a modified transudate.

Management and prognosis

Surgery
The definitive therapy for chest wall tumours is *en bloc* surgical resection (Figure 18.25). Intercostal thoracotomies should be performed cranial and caudal to the rib mass, and the intrathoracic extent of the mass can then be ascertained. Ideally, at least one normal rib both cranial and caudal to the mass should be removed. All structures in contact with the mass should be resected with at least a 3 cm margin of grossly normal tissue. At no time should the tumour be incised, because this will result in contamination of the surgical bed and, potentially, the thoracic cavity.

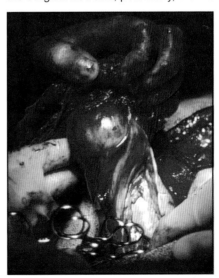

18.25 *En bloc* surgical resection of a chest wall chondrosarcoma. Ideally, at least one normal rib both cranial and caudal to the mass should be removed. The tumour should not be incised during the excision surgery as this might result in neoplastic contamination of the surgical site.

After resection, margins should be marked with ink or sutures for evaluation by the histopathologist. Alternatively, further small samples may be obtained from sites within the surgical field that warrant histological assessment. It is the authors' opinion that, when dealing with large tumours, this method of assessment is often preferable and easier to perform than that of marking the main mass.

When no more than three ribs have been removed, closure can often be accomplished locally. The removal of more than three ribs will often require more complicated closure techniques, such as the use of local muscle flaps (e.g. latissimus dorsi or diaphragm) or synthetic mesh. Complications of healing associated with the use of synthetic mesh suggest that its use is best avoided if possible. The caudal position of the majority of thoracic masses means that synthetic mesh is rarely required and surrounding soft tissues can be used to close the majority of defects. Although resection may be relatively straightforward, the techniques required for complication-free thoracic closure will often require considerable expertise, and surgical cases are then better managed by a surgeon who specializes in such techniques.

Radiation therapy

The site and poor response of most tumours make radiation therapy of little use in the adjunctive management of thoracic chest wall tumours, but the increasing availability of linear accelerators with electron beam facilities makes the use of radiation to treat chest wall tumours more feasible.

Chemotherapy

Little information is available regarding the effects of adjunctive chemotherapy. It is likely that the administration of drugs such as carboplatin, cisplatin (do NOT use in cats) and/or doxorubicin will provide an increase in disease-free intervals for tumours such as osteosarcoma, chondrosarcoma and haemangiosarcoma.

Prognosis

The prognosis following surgical resection of a chest wall mass depends on histological diagnosis and the completeness of clean surgical margins. Resection of benign tumours such as the chondroma will carry a favourable long-term prognosis and surgery in such cases will be curative. Conversely, the prognosis for the majority of malignant tumours is poor. A recent study suggested that the MST for animals with osteosarcoma was 17 weeks and for fibrosarcoma was 26 weeks (Baines *et al.*, 2002). A better long-term outcome was achieved following the resection of chondrosarcoma, with 50% of animals still alive 2 years postoperatively.

Tumours of the heart

Primary and secondary heart tumours are summarized in Figures 18.26 and 18.27.

- Haemangiosarcoma (most common)
- Chemodectoma (second most common)
- Chondroma
- Chondrosarcoma
- Fibroma
- Fibrosarcoma
- Granular cell tumour
- Haemangioma
- Myxoma
- Rhabdomyosarcoma
- Teratoma

18.26 Primary cardiac tumours reported in the dog.

- Haemangiosarcoma (most common in dogs)
- Lymphoma (most common in cats)
- Malignant melanoma
- Mammary carcinoma
- Mast cell tumour
- Pulmonary adenocarcinoma
- Salivary adenocarcinoma

18.27 Secondary cardiac tumours reported in the dog and cat.

Presentation and clinical signs

Cardiac tumours are considered uncommon in the dog and even more rare in the cat. Tumours may be primary or secondary in nature and may occur in intracavitary, intramural or pericardial locations. The most common cardiac tumour in the dog is haemangiosarcoma, to which the German Shepherd Dog appears to be predisposed. Aortic body tumours (chemodectomas) represent the second most common cardiac tumour in the dog and these appear to have a predisposition in older individuals of the brachycephalic breeds.

Secondary lymphoma represents the most common tumour affecting the heart in cats. Primary heart tumours are extremely rare in this species, with only two cases of chemodectoma having been reported (Tilley *et al.*, 1981).

The pericardium may be a site for the development of both primary (e.g. mesothelioma) and secondary (e.g. lymphoma) tumours; these are not strictly tumours of the heart.

The nature of the clinical signs associated with cardiac tumours will depend to a large degree on the site of their development. For example, tumours such as the chemodectoma, which commonly develop at the base of the aorta, will generally not affect cardiac rhythm, but may result in the production of a pericardial effusion leading to signs of cardiac tamponade and right-sided heart failure. Tumours developing within the cardiac muscle may well interfere with the electrical activity of the heart, leading to the development of life-threatening dysrhythmias. Intracavitary tumours may result in obstruction to blood flow and the development of peripheral or pulmonary oedema.

Animals suffering from heart tumours will in general present with clinical signs associated with cardiac dysfunction. In its most extreme form this may mean the sudden death of an individual from either rupture of the tumour or development of a fatal cardiac dysrhythmia. Tumours that result in the formation of a pericardial effusion (chemodectoma) or pericardial haemorrhage (right atrial haemangiosarcoma) will induce clinical signs of right-sided heart failure including exercise intolerance, dyspnoea, syncope, ascites, dysrhythmias and weight loss. Examination of these cases may reveal muffled heart sounds and the presence of pulse deficits.

Haemangiosarcoma, being a highly malignant tumour, will commonly demonstrate widespread dissemination by the time of clinical presentation. This may result in the development of haemorrhagic diathesis due to disseminated intravascular coagulation.

Clinical approach

Clinical signs are often non-specific, since they are related to either cardiac rhythm disturbance or right- or left-sided heart failure. Haemangiosarcoma is most commonly associated with haemorrhagic pericardial effusion and cardiac tamponade. Tumours causing obstruction to blood flow within the right or left sides of the heart may lead to clinical signs such as the presence of a murmur, jugular distension, cranial vena cava syndrome, ascites, pleural effusion and/or pulmonary oedema.

Haematology

Complete blood profiles will often be uninformative but schistocytes or acanthocytes may be seen in cases of haemangiosarcoma (see Chapter 19b). Clotting profiles should be performed in cases where haemangiosarcoma is suspected.

Imaging

Survey thoracic radiographs may be unrewarding, but with certain tumours they may indicate the presence of cardiomegaly and/or pericardial effusion. Radiographic signs associated with right- or left-sided heart failure may also be present, such as pulmonary oedema in cases with left-sided heart failure. Thoracic CT may provide valuable information on the site and size of a tumour associated with the heart or pericardium.

In most instances, the use of cardiac ultrasonography represents the most useful and least invasive form of investigation. Echocardiography will allow the accurate interpretation of most intracavitary, intramural or pericardial lesions. Ultrasound examinations will also provide information regarding the feasibility of surgical excision of certain tumours. Of greater significance, considering that the majority of cardiac tumours cannot be resected, is that echocardiography can provide considerable information regarding the effects of the tumour on haemodynamic function of the heart. This can be used to monitor the progression of the tumour, with or without treatment into the longer term.

Numerous contrast techniques such as angiography and pericardiography have been described for the investigation of heart tumours. In most circumstances, these techniques have been superseded by the use of ultrasound examinations.

Electrocardiography

A complete cardiac examination should include an ECG. This may be used to demonstrate the presence of altered complex amplitudes suggestive of chamber enlargement and also the presence of rhythm abnormalities suggestive of a focal disease. For example, the presence of a pericardial effusion may result in the formation of electrical alternans, whereas the presence of an intramural lesion may result in the development of ventricular premature complexes (see *BSAVA Manual of Canine and Feline Cardiorespiratory Medicine*).

Cytology

Cytological analysis of an effusion associated with a cardiac tumour (pleural or pericardial) will commonly fail to identify the presence of neoplastic cells, but such analysis may be useful in ruling out other causes of effusion such as infection.

Management and prognosis

Surgery

The majority of cardiac tumours are not amenable to surgical resection. However, there are a number of cardiac tumours for which surgical intervention should be considered. These include chemodectomas, haemangiosarcomas confined to the right atrial appendage (Figure 18.28) and certain benign intracavitary tumours.

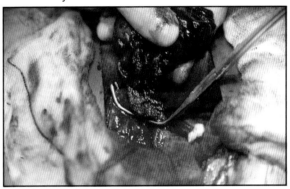

18.28 Intraoperative view of a right atrial haemangiosarcoma in a dog.

Surgical intervention for the management of chemodectomas often involves the complete excision of the tumour from its position at the origin of the great vessels. Under certain circumstances (for tumours demonstrating local invasion and infiltration), it is not possible to resect the tumour. In these circumstances an effective long-term management of this tumour type can often be achieved by performing a subtotal pericardiectomy (Ehrhart *et al.*, 2002).

The resection of a primary haemangiosarcoma associated with the right atrium often proves less satisfactory. Although assessment may indicate that the tumour is confined to its primary atrial site, undiagnosed metastasis prior to surgical resection often means that postoperative survival prior to fatal metastatic growth may be measured only in months.

With the advent of open heart surgery using cardiopulmonary bypass, it is now possible to consider the removal of slow-growing intracavitary tumours. All forms of cardiac surgery require considerable expertise and equipment, and referral of such cases to a specialist should be considered mandatory.

Radiation therapy
Little information is available regarding the use of radiotherapy in the treatment of cardiac tumours. Radiation may be considered as a palliative measure in the management of inoperable chemodectomas (Turrel, 1987), but further studies are required to ascertain the true efficacy of this technique in small animals.

Chemotherapy
There is no evidence that chemodectoma is sensitive to chemotherapy. There are a number of reports regarding the use of chemotherapy in the management of haemangiosarcoma. Combination therapy with vincristine, doxorubicin and cyclophosphamide appears to be most effective (de Madron *et al.*, 1987). As with other forms of haemangiosarcoma, the prognosis for long-term resolution of the disease remains guarded, regardless of how aggressively the condition is managed. In many individuals, management is aimed at controlling the secondary clinical signs associated with heart failure and/or dysrhythmia.

Prognosis
In general the prognosis for cardiac tumours in small animals is poor. This is particularly the case with cardiac haemangiosarcomas, where the mean survival time following surgery (without chemotherapy) is reported to be only 4 months (Aronsohn, 1985). In cases undergoing surgical resection of the primary tumour with pericardiectomy and combined chemotherapy, the MST may be extended to between 5 and 8 months.

While the prognosis for chemodectomas and mesotheliomas of the pericardium is guarded, in some cases direct surgical resection or palliative pericardiectomy may produce a significant disease-free interval of many months.

Tumours of the thymus

Thymomas are uncommon tumours in both the dog and the cat. Although the thymus gland is most active in the younger individual under 6 months of age, tumour development is most commonly diagnosed in older dogs and cats over 9 years of age. Most studies show no sex or breed predilection, but medium- and large-breed dogs may be over-represented.

All thymomas originate from thymic epithelium, but many of the tumours are infiltrated to a greater or lesser extent by mature lymphocytes. While different histological cell types are recognized, there does not appear to be any prognostic value in this information. Distant metastasis is rare but may occur.

Differential diagnoses for a mass in the cranial mediastinum are listed in Figure 18.29.

- Mediastinal lymphoma (most common)
- Thymoma
- Tumours of the cranial lung lobes
- Thyroid haemorrhage associated with involution
- Other tumours of the thyroid, e.g. thyroid melanoma

18.29 Differential diagnoses in the dog and cat for a mass within the cranial mediastinum.

Presentation and clinical signs
In the majority of individuals, clinical signs are associated with the presence of a large space-occupying mass in the cranial mediastinum. Signs of respiratory distress, including coughing, dyspnoea and tachypnoea, are common. In some instances the size of the mass will obstruct the great veins and lymphatic system within the cranial mediastinal space, leading to the formation of precaval syndrome. This manifests itself with the development of swelling and oedema to the head, neck and front legs.

Thymomas are also associated with the paraneoplastic syndrome of myasthenia gravis. This condition may be seen in up to 40% of dogs affected by the tumour but appears to be much rarer in the cat. Myasthenia gravis is characterized by a general muscle weakness and, in some individuals, the presence of megaoesophagus. There also appears to be an association between various autoimmune diseases, such as immune-mediated anaemia and polymyositis, and the presence of thymoma. In the cat, an association has been reported between exfoliative dermatitis and the presence of thymoma (Scott *et al.*, 1995).

Clinical approach
Small thymic masses will often produce no clinical signs and may go unnoticed. In individuals with a suspected thymoma, a full clinical examination should include thoracic auscultation and an assessment for the development of precaval syndrome. Evidence of pitting oedema of the head, neck or front legs, with or without jugular vein distension, may indicate the presence of a large cranial mediastinal mass. Decreased lung sounds over the cranial mediastinum may also indicate a cranial mediastinal mass. In some instances the presence of a mass at this site may alter the cardiac axis, resulting in the unusual positioning of heart sounds on auscultation. Thoracic percussion of the cranial thorax may indicate a dullness consistent with the presence of a soft tissue mass.

Haematology
Blood profiles will generally be unremarkable, though both leucocytosis and, more rarely, hypercalcaemia have been reported.

Imaging
Survey thoracic radiography will, in most instances, reveal the presence of a variably sized mass within the cranial mediastinum (Figure 18.30).

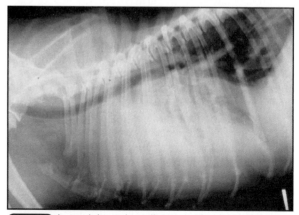

18.30 Lateral thoracic radiograph of a dog with a cranial mediastinal mass.

Radiographic diagnosis may be confused by a pleural effusion; and definition of the cardiac silhouette may be obscured by the presence of the adjacent mass and also by its ability to induce displacement of local structures. In any individual that demonstrates possible myasthenia gravis and/or oesophageal dysfunction, a lateral thoracic radiograph should be obtained of the conscious patient to rule out the presence of megaoesophagus. Myasthenia gravis may be further investigated by assessment of anti-acetylcholine receptor autoantibody concentrations. Thoracic CT may provide valuable further information and, if available, may be considered the radiographic imaging technique of choice (Figure 18.31).

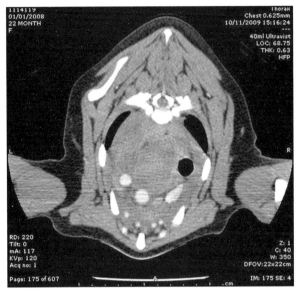

18.31 Post-contrast axial CT scan of the thymoma within the cranial thorax of a dog. The great vessels (white) are displaced ventrally, whereas the trachea (black) has been displaced to the right side.

In most cases, the craniomediastinal mass will have obtained such a size that the cranial lung lobes will be displaced in a caudal direction. This will allow ultrasonographic assessment of the mass via either a cranial intercostal or a thoracic inlet window. Although some thymomas may contain cystic cavities as opposed to the more homogenous appearance of lymphoma, the considerable variety of textures observed means that ultrasonography cannot be used as a definitive guide to the histology of the mass. Ultrasonography may be best used to assess the development of pleural effusion, to investigate the development of local invasion, and to aid in the collection of biopsy or aspirate material.

Biopsy

The definitive diagnosis of thymoma requires biopsy. Fine-needle aspiration is considered a safe (with the aid of ultrasound guidance) and non-invasive method for obtaining cytological material, but results are often very unreliable. The major differential diagnosis for thymoma, especially in the cat, is mediastinal lymphoma. The epithelial component of the thymoma rarely exfoliates well and samples tend to contain large numbers of lymphocytes, making their differentiation from a lymphoma difficult. It is often easier to establish a positive diagnosis of mediastinal lymphoma following the observation of large numbers of lymphoblasts.

Staging

The canine thymoma can be clinically staged, but this can prove difficult to accomplish prior to exploratory surgery since it requires assessment of the tumour capsule, the assessment of tumour invasion into adjacent tissues and the presence of metastasis (Figure 18.32).

Stage	Description
I	Growth completely within intact thymic capsule
II	Pericapsular growth into mediastinal fat tissue, adjacent pleura and/or pericardium
III	Invasion into surrounding organs and/or intrathoracic metastases
IV	Extrathoracic metastases

18.32 Clinical staging of thymoma in the dog.

Management and prognosis

Surgery

The definitive therapy for thymoma is surgical resection (thymectomy). The surgical approach for thymectomy depends on the relative size of the mass. Small masses may be approached via an intercostal thoracotomy (most commonly from the left side) whilst larger masses may require an anterior sternotomy (Figure 18.33).

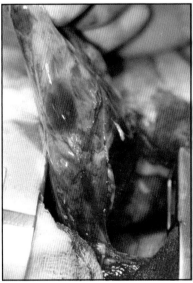

18.33 Intraoperative appearance of a thymoma in a crossbred dog.

The so-called 'benign' thymomas are non-invasive and well encapsulated, whereas 'malignant' thymomas will be found to be invading adjacent structures. Metastasis is rare. It is important to remember, from a surgical standpoint, that the size of the thymoma on radiography and/or ultrasound examination imparts little information regarding whether the tumour can be successfully resected or not. Approximately 70% of thymomas are resectable, regardless of their size at surgery. Surgical debulking of the unresectable invasive form of thymoma is often not very successful and may lead to considerable intraoperative haemorrhage and postoperative morbidity. As the feasibility of complete tumour resection can often only be assessed at the time of surgery, it is prudent to discuss the possibility of intraoperative euthanasia prior to performing the procedure.

In the cat, thymoma is much less common than mediastinal lymphoma. This, and the problems associated with cytological diagnosis, has led to the practice of treating all cranial mediastinal masses in the cat with chemotherapy effective against lymphoma. Unfortunately, in the cases where this treatment proves ineffective, further surgical investigation and possible removal of a thymoma may be compromised due to prolonged wound healing associated with the use of chemotherapy drugs. This group of animals presents the general practitioner with a serious dilemma and it is highly recommended that advice from, or referral to, a specialist is sought in such cases.

Radiation therapy
There is little information available regarding the use of radiotherapy in the treatment of thymoma. Theoretically, radiation therapy might be expected to decrease the lymphoid component of the mass. In very large 'unresectable' tumours it may be possible to downstage (shrink) the tumour using radiation so that it becomes amenable to surgical excision.

Chemotherapy
The use of chemotherapy in the treatment of thymoma in the dog and cat is unrewarding. As stated above, a chemotherapy regime that is effective against mediastinal lymphoma has been used as a means to differentiate the two tumour types. Unless it is absolutely clear that the individual is not to undergo thymectomy, the consequences of this approach to the successful outcome of possible future surgery should be clearly explained to the owner. Similarly to radiation, chemotherapy (cyclophosphamide) may be used to shrink a large 'unresectable' tumour so that it becomes significantly smaller and amenable to surgical resection.

Prognosis
The prognosis for thymoma depends on the feasibility of surgical resection and also the presence of paraneoplastic myasthenia gravis. In individuals without myasthenia gravis and/or megaoesophagus, the prognosis is good if the tumour can be removed. Dogs without megaoesophagus and with a resectable tumour have been reported to have an 83% 1-year survival rate. With surgery, long-term remissions can therefore be expected in individuals in this group.

Conversely, the prognosis is poor in individuals with either a non-resectable thymoma or with evidence of megaoesophagus and myasthenia gravis. Although a number of reports describe the resolution of myasthenia gravis following thymectomy, this improvement is by no means certain and in many instances may take months. Therefore, if the myasthenia gravis is complicated by the presence of megaoesophagus it is unlikely that the dog will survive long enough following surgery to allow an improvement to be seen. On rare occasions, myasthenia gravis may develop following thymectomy.

The surgical resection of thymoma in cats appears to have a favourable prognosis. One study reported a median survival approaching 2 years (Gores *et al.*, 1994).

Mesothelioma

Mesothelioma is a rare tumour in dogs and cats. It arises from the serosal lining of the body cavities and so any part of the body possessing a serosal lining may be affected. In both the dog and cat, forms affecting the pleural, pericardial and peritoneal cavities are the most common.

In general, the aetiology of mesothelioma is unknown, but dogs with the pleural form of the disease have been shown to have higher levels of asbestos in their lungs than normal controls. Affected dogs often have owners who have occupations or hobbies in which exposure to asbestos is a known risk; therefore, exposure to airborne asbestos fibres has been implicated in the aetiology of pleural mesothelioma (Glickman *et al.*, 1983).

Presentation and clinical signs
Mesothelioma classically occurs as a diffuse nodular mass covering the surfaces of the affected body cavity. It is a highly effusive tumour and the clinical signs are most commonly associated with the effusion. For example: dyspnoea will be seen in individuals with a pleural effusion; cardiac tamponade and signs of right-sided heart failure will be seen in individuals with a pericardial effusion; and abdominal distension will be seen in individuals with a peritoneal effusion.

Clinical approach
A diagnosis of mesothelioma should be considered in adult dogs with evidence of a chronic effusive disease. The major differential diagnoses for mesothelioma are listed in Figure 18.34. Establishing a definitive diagnosis of mesothelioma may prove difficult, since mesothelial cells can be expected to proliferate under any circumstance that leads to the

Diseases causing pleural effusion
• Haemangiosarcoma • Pyothorax • Primary pulmonary neoplasms • Metastatic carcinoma • Feline infectious peritonitis
Diseases causing pericardial effusion
• Idiopathic pericardial effusion • Haemangiosarcoma • Coagulopathy • Pericardial cyst

18.34 Differential diagnoses for mesothelioma.

production of an effusion. Therefore, the cytological differentiation between physiological mesothelial cell proliferation and a malignant mesothelioma is often not possible. In general, large samples of affected serosal tissues obtained via thoracotomy or an open biopsy are required for definitive diagnosis.

Haematology
The interpretation of a complete blood profile is often unrewarding in establishing a diagnosis of mesothelioma but may be helpful in ruling out other causes of effusions.

Imaging
Survey radiographs of affected cavities will often only indicate the presence of fluid within the cavity. Films taken after fluid drainage may provide further information but are still unlikely to demonstrate clearly the presence of the tumour. Similarly, ultrasound investigation can commonly be unrewarding. The diffuse nature of the tumour makes establishing a definitive ultrasonographic diagnosis difficult.

Endoscopy and biopsy
The increasing availability of thoracoscopy and laparoscopy in small animals may allow for a less invasive way of patient evaluation than undertaking an open biopsy.

It should be remembered that this is a disease that can prove difficult to diagnose by conventional means. Obtaining a negative result on biopsy does not always rule out the presence of mesothelioma. The authors can remember a number of cases where a definitive diagnosis was only confirmed at open surgical investigation, or, of more concern, on post-mortem examination.

Management and prognosis

Surgery
There is at present no effective method of treatment for mesothelioma. The diffuse and effusive nature of the disease means that the whole of an affected body cavity is considered contaminated with the tumour. Therefore, in most instances the surgical excision of grossly affected serosal surfaces is of little benefit. Performing a pericardiectomy may prove palliative in individuals with clinical signs such as cardiac tamponade associated with the pericardial form of the disease (Closa *et al.*, 1999).

Radiation therapy
The diffuse and widespread nature of the disease prevents the use of radiotherapy as a treatment option.

Chemotherapy
In humans, the administration of intracavitary cisplatin is sometimes used to manage and slow the progression of the disease. The drug appears to be well tolerated and its administration has been shown to decrease the production of the malignant effusion. This technique may have a role in the management of canine mesothelioma. In the dog, it has been suggested that cisplatin may retard the progression of the tumour itself (Moore *et al.*, 1991). There are few data available regarding the consequences of intracavitary administration of cisplatin in the management of mesothelioma. Further studies are required before the true role of this drug can be delineated. **Cisplatin must not be administered to cats.**

Prognosis
Survival figures for mesothelioma are sparse as the majority of animals are euthanized on diagnosis.

The lack of an effective method of treatment means that the prognosis in most instances is poor. Individuals with the pericardial form of the disease may benefit from a palliative pericardiectomy, since this will prevent the occurrence of clinical signs associated with pericardial effusion.

References and further reading

Adams WM, Bjorling DE, McAnlty JF *et al.* (2005) Outcome of accelerated radiotherapy alone or accelerated radiotherapy followed by exenteration of the nasal cavity in dogs with intranasal neoplasia: 53 cases (1990–2002). *Journal of the American Veterinary Medical Association* **227**, 936–941

Aronsohn MG (1985) Cardiac haemangiosarcoma in the dog: a review of 38 cases. *Journal of the American Veterinary Medical Association* **187**, 922–926

Baines SJ, Lewis S and White RAS (2002) Primary thoracic wall tumours of mesenchymal origin in dogs: a retrospective study of 46 cases. *Veterinary Record* **150**, 335–339

Bexfield NH, Stell AJ, Gear RN and Dobson JM (2008) Photodynamic therapy of superficial nasal planum squamous cell carcinomas in cats: 55 cases. *Journal of Veterinary Internal Medicine* **22**, 1385–1389

Clarke RE (1991) Cryosurgical treatment of cutaneous squamous cell carcinoma. *Australian Veterinary Practice* **21**, 148–153

Closa JM, Font A and Mascort J (1999) Pericardial mesothelioma in a dog: long-term survival after pericardiectomy in combination with chemotherapy. *Journal of Small Animal Practice* **40**, 383–386

de Madron E, Helfand SC and Stebbins KE (1987) Use of chemotherapy for the treatment of cardiac haemangiosarcoma in the dog. *Journal of the American Veterinary Medical Association* **190**, 887–891

Ehrhart N, Ehrhart EJ, Willis J *et al.* (2002) Analysis of factors affecting survival in dogs with aortic body tumours. *Veterinary Surgery* **31**, 44–48

Glickman LT, Domanski LM, Maguire TG, Dubielzig RR and Churg A (1983) Mesothelioma in pet dogs associated with exposure of their owners to asbestos. *Environmental Research* **32**, 305–313

Gores BR, Berg J, Carpenter JL and Aronsohn MG (1994) Surgical treatment of thymoma in cats: 12 cases (1987–1992). *Journal of the American Veterinary Medical Association* **204**, 1782–1785

Hammond GM, Gordon IK, Theon AP and Kent MS (2007) Evaluation of strontium Sr 90 for the treatment of superficial squamous cell carcinoma of the nasal planum in cats: 49 cases (1990–2006). *Journal of the American Veterinary Medical Association* **231**, 736–741

Haney SM, Beaver L, Turrel J *et al.* (2009) Survival analysis of 97 cats with nasal lymphoma: a multi-institutional retrospective study (1986–2006). *Journal of Veterinary Internal Medicine* **23**, 287–294

Kirpensteijn J, Withrow SJ and Straw RC (1994) Combined resection of the nasal planum and premaxilla in three dogs. *Veterinary Surgery* **23**, 341–346

Lana SE, Ogilvie GK, Withrow SJ, Straw RC and Rogers KS (1997) Feline cutaneous squamous cell carcinoma of the nasal planum and the pinnae: 61 cases. *Journal of the American Animal Hospital Association* **33**, 329–332

Lana SE and Withrow SJ (2001) Nasal tumors. In: *Small Animal Clinical Oncology*, ed. SJ Withrow and EG MacEwen, pp. 370–377. WB Saunders, Philadelphia

Lascelles BD, Henderson RA, Seguin B, Liptak JM and Withrow SJ (2004) Bilateral rostral maxillectomy and nasal planectomy for large rostral maxillofacial neoplasms in six dogs and one cat. *Journal of the American Animal Hospital Association* **40**, 137–146

Lascelles BDX, Parry A, Stidworthy MF, Dobson JM and White RAS (2000) Squamous cell carcinoma of the canine nasal plate: 17 cases (1986–1997). *Veterinary Record* **147**, 473–476

Mehlaff CJ, Leifer CE, Patnaik AK and Schwarz PD (1983) Surgical treatment of primary pulmonary neoplasia in 15 dogs. *Journal of* the *American Veterinary Medical Association* **20**, 799–803

Mellanby RJ, Herrtage ME and Dobson JM (2002b) Long-term outcome of eight cats with non-lymphoproliferative nasal tumours treated by megavoltage radiotherapy. *Journal of Feline Medicine and Surgery* **4**, 77–81

Mellanby RJ, Stevenson RK, Herrtage ME, White RAS and Dobson JM (2002a) Long-term outcome of 56 dogs with nasal tumours treated with four doses of radiation at intervals of 7 days. *Veterinary Record* **151**, 253–257

Moore AS, Kirk C and Cardona A (1991) Intracavitary cisplatin chemotherapy experience in six dogs. *Journal of Veterinary Internal Medicine* **5**, 227–231

Scott DW, Yager JA and Johnson KM (1995) Exfoliative dermatitis in association with thymoma in three cats. *Feline Practice* **23**, 8–13

Theon AP, Peaston AE, Madewell BR and Dungworth DL (1994) Irradiation of non-lymphoproliferative neoplasms of the nasal cavity and paranasal sinuses in 16 cats. *Journal of the American Veterinary Medical Association* **204**, 78–83

Tilley LP, Band B, Patnaik AK and Liu SK (1981) Cardiovascular tumours in the cat. *Journal of the American Animal Hospital Association* **17**, 1009–1021

Turrel JM (1987) Principles of radiation therapy. II. Clinical applications. In: *Veterinary Cancer Medicine*, ed. GH Theilen and BR Madewell, pp. 148–156. Lea & Febiger, Philadelphia

Withrow SJ (2001) Tumors of the respiratory system, In: *Small Animal Clinical Oncology*, ed. SJ Withrow and EG MacEwen, pp. 354–377. WB Saunders, Philadelphia

Tumours of the haemopoietic system

David M. Vail

Canine lymphoma

The lymphomas (malignant lymphoma or lympho-sarcoma) are a diverse group of neoplasms that have in common their origin from lymphoreticular cells. They are one of the most common neoplasms seen in the dog and usually arise in lymphoid tissues such as lymph nodes, spleen and bone marrow. However, they may arise in almost any tissue in the body, including non-lymphoid sites. The annual incidence has been estimated to range between 13 and 24 per 100,000 dogs at risk (Backgren, 1965; Kaiser, 1981), but, as in people, this rate is increasing annually and these older data likely greatly underestimate the true incidence. A more recent study from the UK showed an incidence rate of 114 per 100,000 dogs per year (Dobson *et al.*, 2002). Middle-aged to older dogs (median age 6–9 years) are primarily affected and gender is not an important risk factor. Breeds reported to have a higher incidence include Boxer, Bull Mastiff, Basset Hound, St Bernard, Scottish Terrier, Airedale Terrier and Bulldog, but lymphoma can occur in any breed.

Aetiology

The aetiology of canine lymphoma is likely multi-factorial. Retrovirus involvement has been suggested but has not been confirmed in dogs. Several cyto-genetic abnormalities have been characterized in dogs with lymphoma (Breen and Modiano, 2008). Additional suggested aetiologies, albeit weakly linked to this disease, include:

- Phenoxyacetic acid herbicides (e.g. 2,4-dichlorophenoxyacetic acid)
- Exposure to strong magnetic fields (observed in a preliminary epidemiological study (Reif *et al.*, 1995))
- Impaired immune function and immune system alterations such as immune-mediated thrombocytopenia
- Living in industrial areas
- Atopy and cutaneous lymphoma.

Classification

Lymphoma in dogs can be classified on the basis of anatomical location or by histological, cytological and immunophenotypic criteria.

Anatomical classification

The relative frequency of anatomical sites and clinical characteristics are shown in Figure 19.1. The most common anatomical forms of lymphoma in dogs include the multicentric (approximately 80%) (Figure 19.2), cranial mediastinal (Figure 19.3), cutaneous (Figure 19.4) and gastrointestinal forms. Primary extranodal forms, such as those occurring in the eye, central nervous system, bone, testis and nasal cavity, are less commonly observed.

Anatomical location	Approximate frequency of cases	Clinical signs	Site-specific diagnostics	Differential diagnosis
Multicentric (nodal)	80%	Painless lymphadenopathy. PU/PD if accompanying hypercalcaemia. Non-specific signs (lethargy, weight loss, anorexia) may be present in approximately 20% of cases. ± Splenic and hepatic enlargement	Biopsy of affected node: FNA or surgical. Staging (see text)	Disseminated infections (e.g. bacterial, viral, rickettsial, parasitic, fungal). Immune-mediated disorders (e.g. dermatopathies, vasculitis, polyarthritis, lupus). Tumours metastatic to nodes. Other haemopoietic tumours: (e.g. leukaemia, multiple myeloma, malignant or systemic histiocytosis)
Alimentary tract	7%	Non-specific signs related to the GI tract (vomiting, diarrhoea, weight loss). Abdominal mass possibly palpable. Thickened intestinal loops possibly palpable	Abdominal imaging (radiography, ultrasonography). Biopsy: ultrasound-guided FNA; endoscopic; surgical full-thickness. Staging (see text)	Several primary and secondary enteritides. Infiltrative enteritis (lymphocytic and plasmacytic enteritis). Other GI tumours

19.1 Characteristics of canine lymphoma in various anatomical locations. (continues) ▶

Anatomical location	Approximate frequency of cases	Clinical signs	Site-specific diagnostics	Differential diagnosis
Cutaneous	6%	Usually generalized but can be solitary. Non-specific skin changes. May have a progression from scaly alopecia to thickened erythematous ulcerative form, to plaque-like lesions (see Figure 19.4). Approximately half are pruritic	Biopsy: multiple dermal punch. Staging (see text)	Infectious dermatitis (e.g. advanced pyoderma). Immune-mediated dermatitis (e.g. pemphigus). Other cutaneous neoplasms
Mediastinal	3%	Dyspnoea/tachypnoea due to space-occupying mass or pleural effusion. Precaval syndrome (pitting oedema of head, neck and forelimbs). PU/PD secondary to hypercalcaemia	Thoracic radiography. Biopsy: ultrasound or CT-guided FNA or surgical (if not generalized disease). Analysis of pleural fluid if present. Staging (see text)	Other tumours: thymoma, chemodectoma, ultimobranchial cyst, ectopic thyroid carcinoma, pleural carcinomatosis, pulmonary lymphomatoid granulomatosis. Infectious disease: granulomatous disease, pyothorax. Miscellaneous: congestive heart failure, chylothorax, haemothorax
Extranodal	3%	Site-dependent. Includes CNS, bone, heart, nasal cavity, ocular and others	Imaging of affected site. Biopsy: tissue or fluid from affected site. Staging (see text)	Variable, depending on organ/system involved

19.1 (continued) Characteristics of canine lymphoma in various anatomical locations.

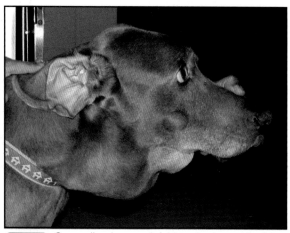

19.2 Generalized non-painful lymphadenopathy is the typical presentation for lymphoma in dogs.

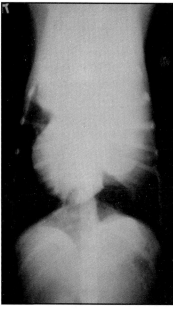

19.3 Ventrodorsal thoracic radiograph of a dog with cranial mediastinal lymphoma.

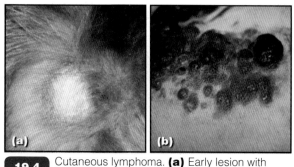

19.4 Cutaneous lymphoma. **(a)** Early lesion with scaly alopecia in a Golden Retriever. **(b)** Progressive late lesion in a Bulldog showing nodular disease.

Histological/immunophenotypical classification

Lymphomas arise from a clonal expansion of lymphoid cells with distinctive morphological and immunophenotypical features. Many histological systems have been used to classify non-Hodgkin's lymphoma in human patients and some of these systems have been applied to lymphoma in the dog (e.g. WHO, REAL, Kiel, NCI-Working Formulation). The newest World Health Organization (WHO) system (Valli *et al.*, 2002) is the most up to date for canine tumours. In these systems, tumours are categorized as low, intermediate or high grade. The low-grade lymphomas, composed of small cells with low mitotic rate, typically progress slowly; while they are less chemoresponsive than higher-grade tumours, they are associated with long survival times. In contrast, intermediate- and high-grade lymphomas with a high mitotic rate progress rapidly but are more likely to respond to chemotherapy.

Lymphoma can further be classified as being of B-cell, T-cell or null cell (neither B or T) lineage and this subclassification is prognostically important. In general, most canine lymphoma is of the B-cell immunophenotype, with approximately 25–30%

being of T-cell derivation (Modiano *et al.*, 2005). Furthermore, T-cell lymphomas tend to be associated with hypercalcaemia and cranial mediastinal involvement. Cutaneous lymphomas are mostly of T-cell origin and are termed mycosis fungoides if they are epitheliotrophic. The development of monoclonal antibodies to detect specific markers on canine lymphocytes has made immunophenotyping of tumours in dogs available in many commercial laboratories.

An updated morphological classification, combined with immunohistochemistry, has been shown to provide a clinically relevant classification, identifying six subsets of canine lymphoma that correlate not only with clinical presentation but also with response to treatment and prognosis. Most B-cell tumours were classified as centroblastic and polymorphic, but of note was a small subset of 'Burkitt-type' lymphomas which carried a very poor prognosis. The two main types of T-cell lymphoma were pleomorphic mixed and lymphoblastic, both of which were diffuse, but also of note was a small group of small clear-cell T lymphomas, showing a T-zone pattern and with the longest survival time of all (Ponce *et al.*, 2004). This classification system is based on a relatively small number of cases (*n* = 54) and will require larger numbers to confirm its relevance.

Presentation and clinical signs

Clinical signs are variable and depend on the extent and location of the tumour (see Figure 19.1), but the typical presentation is that of generalized lymphadenopathy as shown in Figure 19.2. Less common presentations include cases confined solely to the spleen, or spleen and liver.

Canine lymphoma may also be associated with paraneoplastic syndromes, the most clinically significant being hypercalcaemia. Approximately 15% of all dogs with lymphoma and nearly 50% of dogs with mediastinal involvement and/or T-cell immunophenotypes present with hypercalcaemia, characterized clinically by anorexia, weight loss, muscle weakness, lethargy, polyuria, polydipsia and, rarely, central nervous system depression and coma. Hypercalcaemia is usually related to the production of a hormone-like substance, parathyroid hormone-related peptide (PTH-rP), which is produced by the neoplastic cells; it is most commonly associated with T-cell lymphoma (Rosol *et al.*, 1992). Other paraneoplastic syndromes that may be encountered include monoclonal gammopathies, neuropathies and cancer cachexia (see Chapter 4). Lymphocytosis is uncommon and occurs in approximately 20% of affected dogs. Thrombocytopenia may be seen in 30–50% of cases, but spontaneous bleeding is seldom a clinical problem.

Clinical approach

For all dogs suspected of having lymphoma, irrespective of the anatomical site, the diagnostic evaluation should include a complete blood count (CBC with a differential cell count), platelet count and a serum biochemistry profile (including serum total or ionized calcium). Bone marrow fine-needle aspiration (FNA) or biopsy is indicated for complete staging and in dogs with anaemia, lymphocytosis, peripheral lymphocyte atypia or other peripheral cytopenias. While cytological assessment of a fine-needle aspirate (Figure 19.5) by a trained clinical pathologist is successful in making a definitive diagnosis of lymphoma in most cases, lymph node biopsy is preferred for histological classification and immunophenotyping. Care should be taken to avoid lymph nodes from reactive areas, such as the mandibular lymph nodes; the prescapular or popliteal lymph nodes are preferable sampling sites if also involved in the disease process. If possible, the diagnosis should be made by sampling peripheral nodes, avoiding percutaneous biopsy of liver and/or spleen. However, if there is no peripheral node involvement, it is appropriate to take biopsy samples of affected tissues in the abdominal cavity. Figure 19.1 gives further diagnostic procedures that are specific to the anatomical site involved.

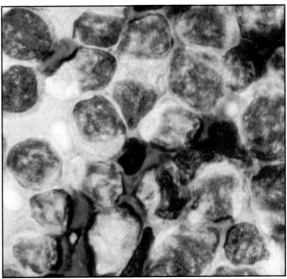

19.5 Fine-needle aspirate from a peripheral lymph node of a dog with high-grade lymphoma. The normal nodal cells have been replaced by a monotonous population of immature lymphoid cells. (Wright's–Giemsa stain; original magnification X1000)

Staging

After a diagnosis has been established, the extent of disease should be determined. A WHO staging system is routinely used to stage dogs with lymphoma (Figure 19.6). Most dogs (>80%) are presented in advanced stages (III–IV).

Bone marrow FNA or biopsy is important in clinical staging of the patient with lymphoma, as it may provide diagnostic and prognostic information. Thoracic and abdominal radiographs may be important in determining the extent of internal involvement. Diagnostic ultrasonography, including ultrasound-guided FNA or needle biopsy, can be useful for evaluation of involvement of the liver, spleen or mesenteric lymph nodes. However, if the client is intent on having their dog treated irrespective of stage or prognosis, some or all of the staging tests may not be essential and treatment can be initiated once confirmation of diagnosis is established.

Stage	Criteria
I	Single lymph node a. Without clinical signs of disease b. With clinical signs of disease
II	Multiple lymph nodes in a regional area a. Without clinical signs of disease b. With clinical signs of disease
III	Generalized lymphadenopathy a. Without clinical signs of disease b. With clinical signs of disease
IV	Liver and/or spleen involvement (with or without stage III) a. Without clinical signs of disease b. With clinical signs of disease
V	Bone marrow or blood involvement and/or any non-lymphoid organ (with or without stages I–IV) a. Without clinical signs of disease b. With clinical signs of disease

19.6 WHO clinical staging for domestic animals with lymphoma.

Advanced diagnostic techniques

In uncommon circumstances, routine cytological and histological assessments of tissues or cellular fluids are inadequate to confirm a diagnosis of lymphoma. When suspicious solid tissues, circulating lymphocytes and effusive samples include a mixed cell population or do not entirely discriminate malignant from benign reactive proliferations, immunophenotypic characterizations by flow cytometric methods (Lana et al., 2006) or assays of cellular clonality may be helpful (Avery and Avery, 2004). Clonality is the hallmark of malignancy: the malignant cell population theoretically should be derived from expansion of a single malignant clone characterized by a particular DNA region unique to that tumour. For example, in a dog with T-cell lymphoma all the malignant cells should contain the same DNA sequence for the variable region of the T-cell receptor gene; likewise, in a dog with B-cell lymphoma the malignant lymphocytes should have identical DNA sequences in the variable region of the immunoglobulin receptor gene. Conversely, in benign reactive lymphocytosis the cells are polyclonal for their antigen receptors. Currently, polymerase chain reaction (PCR) technology can be used to amplify the variable regions of the T-cell and immunoglobulin receptor genes to detect the presence of clonal lymphocyte populations in dogs. Such assays of clonality are approximately 70–90% sensitive. False-negative rates of approximately 5% can occur. In these cases, a diagnosis should be made only after considering the results of all diagnostic evaluations, including histological/cytological evaluation, immunophenotyping and clonality studies in conjunction with the signalment and physical findings.

Management and prognosis

Once a diagnosis is established, untreated dogs will generally live an average of 4–6 weeks, but several exceptions to this exist, including dogs with low-grade tumours. Initially the management of lymphoma is quite gratifying, as response rates approach 90% in dogs treated with multi-agent chemotherapeutic approaches. Importantly, client perception of their pet's experiences during chemotherapy are generally positive and the vast majority of clients feel that treatment is worthwhile and results in improvements in their companion's wellbeing and overall quality of life (Bronden et al., 2003; Mellanby et al., 2003). Unfortunately, most animals eventually succumb to relapse of chemotherapy-resistant, disseminated disease. Lymphoma, typically a systemic disease, requires a systemic approach to therapy (i.e. chemotherapy). Exceptions to this include cases of solitary nodal or solitary extranodal lymphoma, where local therapy (surgery or radiation therapy) may be initially indicated. In these latter cases, due diligence to the possibility of systemic spread in the future is essential and systemic chemotherapy may eventually be required.

Systemic chemotherapy

A variety of chemotherapeutic protocols have been reported in the veterinary literature. This probably reflects the inability to achieve a cure in the majority of cases. While remission rates approach 80–90% with available combination chemotherapy protocols and the quality of life of patients is generally very good during the period of remission, the majority of dogs will eventually succumb to relapse of their disease and often in a more drug-resistant form.

Prior to initiating therapy, caregivers should be informed about the advantages and disadvantages of several chemotherapy options as well as overall prognosis and expectations. Several factors should be considered and discussed, including the cost of treatment, the time commitment required, efficacy, toxicity and the experience of the clinician with the protocols in question.

The availability of generic drugs has allowed chemotherapy protocols to become affordable to more clients than before. In general, combination chemotherapy protocols represent a greater expense, are more time-consuming (repeated visits, closer monitoring) and are more likely to result in toxicity than simpler single-agent protocols. That being said, as a general rule, the more complex combination protocols will result in longer remission and survival durations.

A complete listing of all available protocols for dogs with lymphoma is beyond the scope of this discussion and the reader is referred to a recent review (Vail and Young, 2007). An example of the combination protocol used by the author, a protocol commonly used in Europe, and the most widely used single-agent protocols are presented below.

Combination protocols: Nearly all combination protocols used in veterinary practice are modifications of 'CHOP' protocols initially designed for treating human lymphoma. CHOP represents combinations of cyclophosphamide, doxorubicin (H, hydroxydaunarubicin), vincristine (O, Oncovin) and prednisone or prednisolone (P). Regardless of which CHOP-based protocol is used, response rates of 80–90% can be expected with overall median remission and survival times of approximately 8 and 12 months, respectively.

Approximately 25% of treated dogs will be alive 2 years or more after initiation of therapy. Response rates and length of response can be more individually predicted based on the presence or absence of prognostic factors presented in Figure 19.7.

Historically, following an induction period during which drugs are given weekly, treatment intervals are slowly spread out and drugs are given less frequently in what is termed the 'maintenance' phase of the protocol. Currently, the use of maintenance chemotherapy is no longer thought to be beneficial and

shorter protocols without long-term maintenance are the norm (Vail and Young, 2007; Simon *et al.*, 2008).

The author currently prefers a modified CHOP protocol, as outlined in Figure 19.8 (UW–Madison–Short). Chemotherapy is discontinued at 19 weeks if the dog is in complete remission at that time. After therapy is discontinued, dogs are re-evaluated monthly by physical examination, with special attention being paid to lymph node size or, in those cases not involving peripheral nodal disease, attention to the original anatomical site involved.

Factor	Strength of association with prognosis	Comments
WHO clinical stage	Modest	Stage I/II – favourable Stage V with significant bone marrow involvement – unfavourable
WHO clinical substage	Strong	Substage b (clinically ill) – associated with decreased survival
Histopathology	Moderate	High/medium-grade – associated with high response rate but reduced survival Low-grade tumours associated with lower response to chemotherapy but longer-term survival
Immunophenotype	Strong	T-cell phenotype usually associated with reduced survival
Hypercalcaemia	Moderate	Negative factor if associated with T-cell subtype and reduced renal function
Measures of proliferation	Weak	Contradictory reports exist
Prolonged steroid pre-treatment	Moderate	Most reports suggest previous steroid use shortens response durations, but length of exposure necessary is unknown
Presence of anaemia	Moderate	Dogs with anaemia are less likely to respond and duration of response is short
Molecular level alterations	Investigations continue	Examples include P glycoprotein expression, serum VEGF expression, survivin expression, plasma DNA, circulating glutathione-S-transferase, circulating thymidine kinase
Cranial mediastinal lymphadenopathy	Moderate	Large compilation of cases reports shorter remission and survival durations
Anatomical location	Moderate	Diffuse cutaneous and alimentary, and hepatosplenic forms associated with unfavourable prognosis

19.7 Factors known or suspected to affect the prognosis in dogs with lymphoma.

Treatment week	Drugs, dosage, route
1	Vincristine: 0.5–0.7 mg/m^2 i.v Prednisone: 2 mg/kg orally
2	Cyclophosphamide: 250 mg/m^2 i.v. Furosemide: 1 mg/kg i.v. [a] Prednisone: 1.5 mg/kg orally
3	Vincristine: 0.5–0.7 mg/m^2 i.v. Prednisone: 1 mg/kg orally
4	Doxorubicin: 30 mg/m^2 i.v. Prednisone: 0.5 mg/kg orally
5	*No treatment*
6	Vincristine: 0.5–0.7 mg/m^2 i.v.
7	Cyclophosphamide: 250 mg/m^2 i.v. Furosemide: 1 mg/kg i.v.
8	Vincristine: 0.5–0.7 mg/m^2 i.v.
9 [b]	Doxorubicin: 30 mg/m^2 i.v.
10	*No treatment*
11	Vincristine: 0.5–0.7 mg/m^2 i.v.
12	Cyclophosphamide: 250 mg/m^2 i.v. Furosemide: 1 mg/kg i.v.
13	Vincristine: 0.5–0.7 mg/m^2 i.v.
14	Doxorubicin: 30 mg/m^2 i.v.
15	*No treatment*
16	Vincristine: 0.5–0.7 mg/m^2 i.v.
17	Cyclophosphamide: 250 mg/m^2 i.v. Furosemide: 1 mg/kg i.v.
18	Vincristine: 0.5–0.7 mg/m^2 i.v.
19 [c]	Doxorubicin: 30 mg/m^2 i.v.

19.8 University of Wisconsin–Madison–Short combination chemotherapy protocol for dogs with lymphoma. [a] Furosemide is given concurrently with cyclophosphamide to decrease the incidence of sterile haemorrhagic cystitis. [b] If the patient is in complete remission at week 9, treatment continues to week 11. [c] If the patient is in complete remission at week 19, therapy is discontinued and the dog is rechecked monthly for recurrence. **Note:** A CBC should be performed before each chemotherapy treatment. If the neutrophil count is <1500 cells/μl, the clinician should wait 5–7 days and then repeat the CBC; the drug is administered if the neutrophil count has risen above the 1500 cells/μl cutoff.

Alternatives should be offered to caregivers who decline more aggressive systemic chemotherapy. These include modification of the original COP protocols, outlined in Figure 19.9, as well as single-agent doxorubicin (see below). These less aggressive protocols generally do not result in such high response rates or as durable remission lengths as CHOP-based protocols.

Protocol	Frequency of drug delivery
COP high dose for dogs	
Cyclophosphamide (250–300 mg/m² i.v. or orally)	Give once every 3 weeks for 1 year. If dog is in complete remission at 1 year, decrease to once every 4 weeks for 6 additional months. Discontinue if animal is in complete remission at 1.5 years
Vincristine (0.75 mg/m² i.v.)	Give once a week for 4 doses, then once every 3 weeks for a year on the same day as cyclophosphamide. If dog is in complete remission at 1 year, decrease to once every 4 weeks for 6 additional months. Discontinue if animal is in complete remission at 1.5 years
Prednisone/prednisolone (1 mg/kg orally)	Give daily for 22 days, then every other day for 1.5 years. Discontinue by gradual tapering over 3 weeks if animal is in complete remission at 1.5 years
COP low dose for dogs	
Cyclophosphamide (50 mg/m² orally)	Give q48h or for the first 4 days of each week
Vincristine (0.5 mg/m² i.v.)	Give q7d
Prednisone/prednisolone	Give at 40 mg/m² orally q24h for 7 days, then at 20 mg/m² orally q48h
Maintenance	After 8 weeks of induction, continue COP alternate-week treatment for 4 months, then 1 week in 3 for 6 months, and reduce to 1 week in 4 after 1 year
COP for cats	
Cyclophosphamide (300 mg/m² i.v.)	Give every 3 weeks on the day after vincristine. Discontinue if animal is in complete remission at 1 year
Vincristine (0.75 mg/m² i.v.)	Give q7d on weeks 1, 2, 3 and 4, then every 3 weeks thereafter, on the day before cyclophosphamide. Discontinue if animal is in complete remission at 1 year
Prednisone/prednisolone (50 mg/m² orally)	Give q24h for 1 year

19.9 COP protocols for lymphoma in dogs and cats. [a] For high-dose protocols, a CBC should be performed prior to each cyclophosphamide treatment. If the neutrophil count is <1500 cells/μl, the clinician should wait 5–7 days and then repeat the CBC. Treatment is given if neutrophils are ≥1.5 × 10⁹/l. For low-dose continuous protocols, a CBC should be performed every 2–4 weeks, depending on the neutrophil count.

Doxorubicin single-agent protocol: Doxorubicin therapy represents the most effective and commonly used single-agent chemotherapy protocol available for dogs with lymphoma. It is less expensive and time-consuming than CHOP or COP protocols, and is preferred by the author over COP when clients decline full CHOP-based protocols. Doxorubicin (30 mg/m², i.v.) is given every 3 weeks for a total of five treatments. This protocol results in response rates of approximately 70% and median remission and survival times of 5 and 7 months, respectively. Advantages of this protocol include a shorter time commitment, fewer hospital visits, and side effects that are only attributable to one drug.

If a situation arises where clients opt for only oral medications, then lomustine (CCNU; 70 mg/m² orally every 3 weeks) and prednisone therapy can be used, though response rates and durations are generally less than those achieved with single-agent doxorubicin (Sauerbrey et al., 2007).

In cases where clients decline 'chemotherapy', prednisone/prednisolone alone (2 mg/kg orally every day) will result in a short remission of approximately 1–2 months. It is important to educate clients that dogs receiving such therapy are more likely to develop multiple drug resistance over time and experience shorter remission and survival durations with combination protocols, should more aggressive therapy be pursued at a later date. The earlier that clients opt for more aggressive therapy, the more likely is a longer-lasting response.

Re-induction or rescue therapy: Most dogs experience a relapse of their disease following initially successful chemotherapy; the recurrent disease is typically more resistant to treatment with chemotherapeutic agents than on initial presentation. At the first recurrence, if the patient is a month or more out from discontinuation of initial induction therapy, it is recommended that re-induction be attempted by restarting the induction protocol that was initially successful. In this scenario, the likelihood of a second remission is still high (80–90%); however, the length of the second remission is typically half that of the initial remission, though a subset of animals will enjoy long-term re-induction.

If re-induction fails (or if the initial induction was not successful), the use of 'rescue' agents or protocols may be attempted. Rescue agents are drugs or drug combinations that are not found in standard CHOP protocols and are specifically used in cases of drug resistance. Various rescue protocols have been described (Vail and Young, 2007). These include single-agent or combination use of lomustine (CCNU), dactinomycin, mitoxantrone, doxorubicin (if doxorubicin was not part of the original induction protocol), dacarbazine, vinblastine, procarbazine and methclorethamine. The author's preferred first-line rescue protocol is a combination of lomustine (70 mg/m² orally) and crisantaspase (L-asparginase) (10,000 units/m² s.c.), given at 3-week intervals. Overall rescue response rates of 70–80% are expected, but most responses are not durable, with median durations of 1.5–3 months. Contact with an oncology specialist should be routine in these situations, as novel and investigational protocols are often available.

Treatment of extranodal lymphoma

If extranodal involvement is part of a multicentric disease process, systemic therapies previously discussed should be instituted. However, if the extranodal site is solitary and not part of a multicentric presentation, local therapy may be performed without institution of chemotherapy. In these cases, strict adherence to staging diagnostics, including bone marrow evaluation and radiographic or ultrasound imaging of the thorax and abdomen, are warranted to ensure that the process is localized. If the disease is confined to a single site, local surgery and/or radiation therapy is often effective. Clients should be forewarned that, in these cases, systemic disease is likely to occur months to years later and a regular recheck schedule should be instituted. It is the author's opinion that systemic therapy should be withheld until systemic disease is documented.

Treatment of cutaneous lymphoma

Cutaneous lymphoma can be solitary or generalized (see Figure 19.4). Generalized cutaneous epitheliotrophic lymphoma can have a waxing and waning course and is often not as chemoresponsive as is multicentric lymphoma. Solitary lesions can be dealt with by local therapy (see above), but generalized cases require systemic therapy. The current standard of care for generalized cutaneous lymphoma is oral lomustine (70 mg/m^2 orally q3wk) with or without prednisone or prednisolone. Approximately 70% of cases will respond, but remission lengths of only a few months are expected (Risbon *et al.*, 2006; Williams *et al.*, 2006). If this protocol is ineffective, CHOP-based protocols can be attempted. Other chemotherapeutics with reported activity against cutaneous lymphoma include *cis*-retinoic acid therapy (Accutane®, 1–3 mg/kg orally q12h), Doxil® (a liposome encapsulated form of doxorubicin), crisantaspase and dacarbazine.

Prognosis

The prognosis for dogs with lymphoma is variable and depends on a number of factors (see Figure 19.7). The two factors that currently are most consistently identified as having significant prognostic importance are immunophenotype and WHO substage. Many reports have confirmed that dogs with T-cell derived tumours are associated with significantly shorter remission and survival durations, but it is becoming apparent that there are subsets of B- and T-cell tumours that differ in their response to chemotherapy. Dogs presenting with WHO substage b disease (i.e. clinically ill) also tend to do poorly when compared with dogs with substage a disease. Dogs with stage I and stage II disease also have a better prognosis than those dogs in more advanced stages (III, IV and V).

Treating canine lymphoma can initially be a very rewarding experience for the dog, owner and veterinary surgeon. In most dogs with lymphoma, CHOP-based chemotherapy can induce an 80–90% clinical remission rate and a median survival time of approximately 12 months, with 25% of patients surviving for 2 years. The advances made in the past 20 years have greatly improved the management of this disease. However, newer drugs, drug delivery systems and novel therapy approaches are now needed to continue these advances.

The future of canine lymphoma therapy

Based on the similarity of results reported with the many varied combination chemotherapy protocols currently in use, it appears that the veterinary profession has gone as far as possible using available chemotherapeutic agents for lymphoma. All combination protocols reported to date are hitting the same 'brick wall': a 10–12-month median survival time. Advances in remission and survival durations await the development of new chemotherapeutic drugs, novel targeted therapies such as tyrosine kinase inhibitors, and affordable and practical marrow or stem cell transplant therapies. In human medicine, the past 10 years have heralded a new standard of care for B-cell lymphoma with the advent of rituximab, a commercially available monoclonal antibody that recognizes a B-lymphocyte extracytoplasmic surface antigen (CD20), that is now used in combination with standard chemotherapy. This particular antibody does not recognize an external antigen on canine lymphoma cells and therefore is ineffective for therapy. The veterinary profession awaits the characterization and development of effective monoclonal antibody therapies for use in dogs and cats.

Feline lymphoma

Lymphoma accounts for the majority of haemopoietic tumours in cats. As in humans and dogs, the annual incidence of lymphoma in the species appears to be increasing in North America, primarily due to a rise in the alimentary form in older cats (Louwerens *et al.*, 2005). Since the implementation of feline leukaemia virus (FeLV) containment and vaccination protocols, there has been a profound change in the presentation, signalment and frequency of anatomical sites in cats. In general, cats are at risk for a wider range of anatomical and histological forms of lymphoma than are dogs and, with the exception of low-grade small cell varieties (which are common, particularly in the alimentary form), tend not to respond as well to treatment. That being said, most cat owners who elect to pursue chemotherapy in their pets report a positive experience (Bronden *et al.*, 2003; Tzannes *et al.*, 2008).

Aetiology

The feline leukaemia virus was the most common cause of haemopoietic tumours in cats prior to widespread use of FeLV vaccines. However, only 25% or less of cases are associated with FeLV antigenaemia (Vail *et al.*, 1998; Louwerens *et al.*, 2005), compared with 60–70% of cases published prior to vaccine availability. Other aetiologies that have been suggested for feline lymphoma include gastric *Helicobacter* infection (Bridgeford *et al.*, 2008) and diet for feline gastric lymphoma, and environmental tobacco smoke ('second-hand' smoke) (Bertone *et al.*, 2002).

As would be predicted, along with a shift away from FeLV antigen-associated tumours came a shift away from traditional signalments and the relative frequency of various anatomical sites (Figure 19.10). The mediastinal form that occurs in younger, FeLV-antigenaemic cats used to be the most common anatomical presentation, but the alimentary form in older, FeLV-negative cats has now become the most common presentation. There is evidence that feline immunodeficiency virus (FIV) infection can increase the incidence of lymphoma in cats, though it appears to have an indirect role in tumorigenesis.

Classification

The classification of feline lymphoma involves both the anatomical location (Figure 19.10) and histological and immunophenotypic criteria. The morphological criterion of the NIH working formulation has been used to classify more than 600 cases of lymphoma in cats in North America (Valli et al., 2000). Low-grade lymphoma was found in 8.6%, intermediate in 35.1% and high-grade in 55.2% of the cases. In a large group compiled in Australia, 90% of cases were of medium to high grade when classified in a similar way (Gabor et al., 1999). More recently,

Anatomical site	Relative frequency	Age class	Clinical signs	Site-specific diagnostic tests	Differential diagnosis	Immunophenotype	FeLV status
Alimentary tract	50–70%	Late middle age to aged	Abdominal mass or thickened bowel loops. Weight loss, anorexia, vomiting. Abdominal distension. Haematochezia. Sepsis if bowel is perforated	Abdominal radiography, ultrasonography. Mass or mesenteric lymph node FNA. Biopsy: endoscopic or full thickness (intestine)	Inflammatory bowel disease. Feline infectious peritonitis (FIP). Other intestinal tumours. Primary and secondary enteritis. Hyperthyroidism	High-grade intestinal lymphomas either T- or B-cell in the literature. Small-cell low-grade intestinal forms are more likely to be T-cell	Usually negative
Multicentric (nodal)	20–30%	Depends on FeLV status [a]	Peripheral lymph node enlargement. Often liver or spleen involved (except Hodgkin's-like). Lethargy and depression (except Hodgkin's-like)	Lymph node excision preferred	Reactive or hyperplastic node syndromes. Systemic infection. FIV infection. Hodgkin's variant	T-cell if FeLV-associated. B-cell more likely if FeLV-negative. T-cell rich, B-cell if Hodgkin's-like	About one-third are positive
Mediastinal	10–20%	Young	Dyspnoea, tachypnoea. Non-compressible thorax. Dull heart and lung sounds. Rare Horner's syndrome	Thoracic radiographs/CT. Thoracocentesis and pleural fluid analysis. FNA cytology or needle biopsy of mediastinal mass	Thymoma. Chylothorax. Cardiomyopathy. Pyothorax. FIP. Mesothelioma. Diaphragmatic hernia	Generally T-cell	Usually positive
Nasal	5–10%	Late middle age to aged	Nasal discharge, sneezing. Dyspnoea. Epistaxis. Facial deformity. Epiphora. Exophthalmos	Nasal CT scan. Nasal biopsy or flush	Rhinitis (bacterial or fungal). Inflammatory polyps. Other tumour types. Bleeding diathesis	Generally B-cell	Usually negative
Renal	5%	Middle aged	Lethargy, depression, weight loss. Bilateral renal enlargement. PU/PD. Neurological signs (high percentage have CNS involvement)	Abdominal imaging. Transabdominal needle aspiration	Polycystic renal disease. FIP. Acute renal failure. Other renal tumours	Usually B-cell, however T-cell not uncommon	30–50%
Spine or central nervous system	1–3%	Mixed	Thoracolumbar myelopathy. Hindlimb weakness, ataxia. Bladder atonia. Tail flaccidity. Central signs if brain involvement	Spinal radiography, CT, MRI. CSF tap. CT-guided or surgical biopsy	Trauma. Other tumours. Feline infectious peritonitis. Disc disease. Mycosis. Aortic embolism	Equally divided between B- and T-cell lineages	About 50% are positive

19.10 Characteristics of feline lymphoma in the more common anatomical sites. [a] FeLV-positive cats tend to be younger, and the cancer is more commonly of T-cell derivation.

small-cell low-grade intestinal lymphoma in cats (a distinct form of alimentary lymphoma) was reported to make up approximately 13% of all cases of lymphoma in cats (Kiselow *et al.*, 2008).

Immunophenotypes

In most studies, the majority of lymphoma in cats is of the B-cell immunophenotype (approximately 75%). However, the mediastinal, leukaemic and small-cell low-grade intestinal forms are more likely to be of T-cell derivation. Controversy exists regarding the immunophenotype of cats with high-grade alimentary tract lymphoma. Two large compilations of cases found that most are derived from B-lymphocytes in gut-associated lymphoid tissue (Vail *et al.*, 1998; Gabor *et al.*, 1999). In conflict with this, others reported that the majority of alimentary cases sampled were composed primarily of T cells (Zwahlen *et al.*, 1998). This may represent geographical variations and will require further investigations.

Clinical approach

The diagnostic evaluation should include a complete blood count (CBC with differential cell count), platelet count, a serum chemistry profile and a test for FeLV and FIV. Bone marrow FNA or biopsy is indicated to assess the possible involvement and staging of the extent of disease. Bone marrow evaluation is particularly indicated if anaemia, cellular atypia or leucopenia is present. Furthermore, lymph node or organ biopsy, via surgical incision, endoscopy or needle-core biopsy to obtain tissue for histopathological evaluation is essential for definitive diagnosis.

Unlike with its canine counterpart, FNA alone of a lymph node is not generally sufficient in most cases of feline lymphoma, owing to difficulties encountered in distinguishing lymphoma from benign hyperplastic lymph node syndromes unique to the species. These include idiopathic peripheral lymphadenopathy, plexiform vascularization of lymph nodes, and peripheral lymph node hyperplasia of young cats. In these cases, whole lymph node excision is preferred, as the orientation, invasiveness and architectural abnormalities may be necessary for diagnosis. Additional site-specific diagnostic procedures are noted in Figure 19.10. Histochemical and immunohistochemical techniques can also be used to determine immunophenotype, tumour proliferation rates and clonality. The availability of such analysis is increasing, but none has proved to be consistently indicative of outcome.

Chemotherapy

As for the dog, most current combination protocols for intermediate or high-grade lymphoma in cats are modifications of 'CHOP' protocols initially designed for human oncological use (see below for low-grade lymphoma treatment protocols). The current protocol in use at the author's practice is shown in Figure 19.11. This protocol is generally well tolerated and gastrointestinal toxicity is less common than in the dog. As long-term maintenance protocols have not been shown to be superior in dogs and humans with lymphoma, it is likely that the same is true in the cat although there are currently no data to document this.

Treatment week	Drug, dosage, route
1	Vincristine: 0.5–0.7 mg/m^2 i.v. Crisantaspase: 400 U/kg s.c. Prednisone: 2 mg/kg orally
2	Cyclophosphamide: 200 mg/m^2 i.v. Prednisone: 2 mg/kg, orally
3	Vincristine: 0.5–0.7 mg/m^2 i.v. Prednisone: 1 mg/kg orally
4	Doxorubicin: 25 mg/m^2 i.v. Prednisone: 1 mg/kg, orally [a]
6	Vincristine: 0.5–0.7 mg/m^2 i.v.
7 [b]	Cyclophosphamide: 200 mg/m^2 i.v.
8	Vincristine: 0.5–0.7 mg/m^2 i.v.
9 [c]	Doxorubicin: 25 mg/m^2 i.v.
11	Vincristine: 0.5–0.7 mg/m^2 i.v.
13 [t]	Cyclophosphamide: 200 mg/m^2 i.v.
15	Vincristine: 0.5–0.7 mg/m^2 i.v.
17	Doxorubicin: 25 mg/m^2 i.v.
19	Vincristine: 0.5–0.7 mg/m^2 i.v.
21 [b]	Cyclophosphamide: 200 mg/m^2 i.v.
23	Vincristine: 0.5–0.7 mg/m^2 i.v.
25 [d]	Doxorubicin: 25 mg/m^2 i.v.

19.11 University of Wisconsin–Madison combination chemotherapy protocol for cats with lymphoma. [a] Prednisone (1 mg/kg orally) is continued every other day from this point on. [b] If renal or CNS lymphoma is present, substitute cytarabine (600 mg/m^2 s.c. q12h over 2 days) at these treatments. [c] If the patient is in complete remission at week 9, continue to week 11. [d] If the patient is in complete remission at week 25, therapy is discontinued and the cat is rechecked monthly for recurrence. **Note:** A CBC should be performed before each chemotherapy treatment. If the neutrophil count is <1500 cells/µl, the clinician should wait 5–7 days and then repeat the CBC; the drug is administered if the neutrophil count has risen above the 1500 cell/µl cutoff.

Controversy exists as to the usefulness of doxorubicin for treating lymphoma in cats. Cats are less tolerant of doxorubicin than are dogs and a lower dose (either 25 mg/m^2 or 1 mg/kg i.v.) is generally employed. Several large studies have shown that the addition of doxorubicin to COP-based protocols has shown superior results to COP alone in the cat and these CHOP-based protocols are currently used by the author (Moore *et al.*, 1996; Vail *et al.*, 1998). Two smaller studies using single-agent doxorubicin documented complete responses in only one-quarter to one-half of treated cases; however, young Siamese cats with mediastinal lymphoma were over-represented in one of these studies and would not be expected to respond well as they are usually positive for FeLV (Peaston and Maddison, 1999; Kristal *et al.*, 2001). That being said, there is a subset of Siamese cats that develop FeLV-negative mediastinal lymphoma that have a more favourable prognosis (Teske, 2002).

A report in Europe documented response rates and durations with a COP combination that rival those reported for CHOP in American studies (Teske *et al.*, 2002). Ideally, a prospective randomized head-to-head trial will be necessary to settle the matter.

Reinduction or rescue therapy

Ultimately, most cats with lymphoma successfully treated with chemotherapy have a relapse of their disease. Often this relapse is accompanied by significantly more drug-resistant disease. The principles discussed above for dogs also apply to cats.

Radiation therapy

Radiation therapy has been used effectively to treat localized lymphoma in cats. Most cats will achieve a complete remission of local disease following radiation and this modality is especially useful for the treatment of nasal lymphoma. Complete response is usual and median remission durations of 1–2 years can be expected in FeLV-negative cats with disease confined to nasal and paranasal cavities. This appears to be superior to cats with nasal tumours treated with chemotherapy alone, where reported median remission durations are 6 months to a year. It is of course important to stage cats thoroughly, to ensure that their disease is localized before contemplating local therapy in the absence of systemic therapy. Some have advocated combinations of both chemotherapy and radiation therapy for cats with nasal tumours (Sfiligoi *et al.*, 2007) but it has been the author's experience that, if disease is confined to the nasal passage, systemic therapy can be withheld until such time as systemic disease is documented.

Prognosis

In general, cats with lymphoma experience lower response rates and remission and survival durations than dogs. Complete response rates vary between 50 and 70% following combination chemotherapy and overall median remission and survival durations are approximately 4 and 7 months, respectively. However, a significant proportion of cats (30–35%) that achieve a complete response with combination chemotherapy enjoy longer overall remission and survival times (i.e. >1 year). Thus initial response to treatment appears to be a strong prognostic indicator. Additionally, cats with low-grade intestinal lymphoma (see below) enjoy significantly longer remissions.

Response rates and lengths of response vary according to the presence or absence of several prognostic factors. The wide variations in frequency and the great variability of anatomical forms of lymphoma encountered in cats make specific prognoses more difficult than in dogs. Most reports have grouped anatomical types to produce overall response durations and, in general, the number of animals with any one specific anatomical form is too small for statistical analysis to be useful. That being said, it appears that the factors most strongly associated with a more positive prognosis in cats are:

- Complete response to therapy (unfortunately this cannot be determined prior to therapy)
- Small-cell low-grade histologies (particularly the alimentary forms)
- Negative FeLV status
- Early clinical stage
- Substage a (however, most cats are substage b)
- Anatomical location
- Addition of doxorubicin to the treatment protocol.

Unlike in the dog, the T-cell immunophenotype has not been established as an independent negative prognostic index in the cat. In general, FeLV-negative cats that achieve a complete response on multi-agent chemotherapy protocols have a high likelihood of long-term survival, with approximately 35% alive at 18 months after diagnosis.

The anatomical site of lymphoma in cats also can suggest prognosis.

- In high-grade alimentary lymphoma, median survivals of 7–10 months are expected with chemotherapy that includes doxorubicin. Cats with small-cell low-grade alimentary lymphoma in general do much better (median survivals of approximately 2 years).
- Mediastinal lymphoma is associated with the poorest prognosis; survival times of approximately 3 months are expected with chemotherapy.
- Cats with nasal lymphoma have a relatively good prognosis, as local radiation therapy results in excellent control, with median survivals approaching 18 months.
- Renal lymphoma is associated with shorter survival times, with median survival times ranging from 3 to 6 months.
- Few studies have reported on the results of cats with spinal lymphoma, but the reports that do exist reveal a generally poor prognosis, with median survivals of only a few months.

Hodgkin's-like lymphoma

A form of Hodgkin's-like lymphoma has been reported in the cat (Day *et al.*, 1999; Walton and Hendrick, 2001). This uncommon and distinct form of nodal lymphoma involves solitary or regional nodes of the head and neck and histologically closely resembles Hodgkin's lymphoma in human patients. Cases have usually been found to be an immunophenotypically heterogenous T-cell rich, B-cell lymphoma admixed with a population of bizarre giant or multinucleate cells, and none has been associated with either FeLV or FIV. Little is known about treatment outcome of this form of nodal lymphoma in cats, but the clinical course in most cases is prolonged.

The typical scenario is that of a solitary mandibular (Figure 19.12) or cervical node. Following staging to rule out systemic involvement, surgical excision of the affected node often effects control for several months whereupon a recurrence is discovered in a regionally draining node. It is currently unknown whether the addition of chemotherapy at initial diagnosis in combination with node extirpation will prolong or prevent recurrence. Eventually,

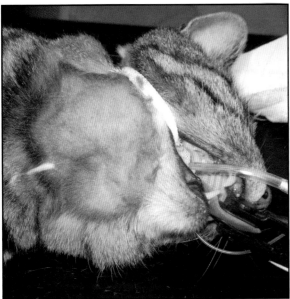

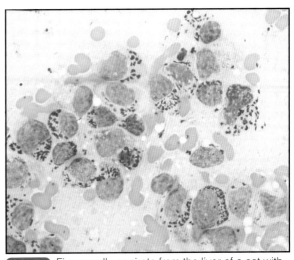

19.13 Fine-needle aspirate from the liver of a cat with large granular lymphoma. The normal hepatic architecture is effaced by a monotonous population of immature LGLs. (Wright's–Giemsa stain; original magnification X1000). (Courtesy of Kristen Friedrics, University of Wisconsin–Madison)

19.12 Massive mandibular lymph node enlargement in a cat with Hodgkin's-like lymphoma.

chemotherapy may be indicated if multiple nodes are involved, though the responsiveness of this form of lymphoma in cats is not well known at present. Occasionally, a more aggressive clinical course has been observed.

Small-cell alimentary tract lymphoma

While most alimentary tract forms of lymphoma in the cat are of intermediate or high grade, a significant subset of 'small-cell' or low-grade lymphomas have been identified and have important treatment and prognostic significance. Consequently, a less aggressive approach to systemic therapy is recommended for cases of small-cell lymphoma involving the intestinal tract, liver and mesenteric lymph nodes. Most cats will respond well to oral chlorambucil (20 mg/m² q2wk) and prednisone or prednisolone (5 mg orally q24h for 14 days, then q48h). Long-term survival is the norm for this disease, with median survival typically approaching 2 years (Kiselow *et al.*, 2008).

Large granular lymphoma

A less commonly reported but distinct form of alimentary lymphoma has been described and is classified as large granular lymphoma (LGL) (Wellman *et al.*, 1992; Drobatz *et al.*, 1993; McEntee *et al.*, 1993; Darbes *et al.*, 1998; Roccabianca *et al.*, 2006; Krick *et al.*, 2008). These tumours represent granulated round cell tumours and have been termed either 'globule leucocyte tumours' or 'large granular lymphocyte lymphoma', although they are probably variations of the same disease. Large granular lymphocytes (LGLs) are characterized by abundant cytoplasm with prominent azurophilic granules (Figure 19.13). This population of cells includes natural killer cells and cytotoxic T cells based on immunophenotypic analysis.

The tumours commonly originate in the small intestine, especially the jejunum or mesenteric lymph nodes. Most cases present with extension to many sites, including liver, lung, myocardium, salivary gland and spinal cord. Leukaemia has also been reported with this disease. Affected cats are generally negative for FeLV and FIV.

LGLs must be differentiated from several other granular cell types that may be found in the small intestine, including the enterochromaffin cells, mast cells and eosinophils. Cats with LGL tumours tend to respond poorly to chemotherapy, with median survival of approximately 1.5 months, though long-term responses have been occasionally reported.

Leukaemia and myeloproliferative disorders

Leukaemia, which may be classified as lymphoid or non-lymphoid, is defined as a neoplastic proliferation of haemopoietic cells originating within the bone marrow. The myeloproliferative disorders (MPDs) are a group of neoplastic diseases of bone marrow where unregulated proliferation of cells derived from haemopoietic stem cells occurs. These include myeloid, neutrophil, basophil, eosinophil, monocyte, lymphoid, megakaryocyte, and erythrocyte lineages. The characteristics of MPDs are shown in Figure 19.14.

The leukaemias and MPDs can also be classified according to the degree of cell differentiation:

- Well differentiated leukaemias are usually referred to as *chronic* leukaemias
- Poorly differentiated leukaemias are usually referred to as *acute* leukaemias.

This distinction is very important in the therapeutic management and prognosis of feline and canine leukaemias.

Type	Subtype	Cell lineage	Characteristics	Therapy	Prognosis
Acute	Acute myelogenous leukaemia (AML)	Myeloblasts	All are rare. Some mixed forms possible. Rapid disease course. Often require immunophenotypic and immunohistochemical diagnosis. Accumulations of blasts in bone marrow and/or peripheral blood. Clinical signs related to myelophthisis and resulting cytopenias. Sepsis or haemorrhage may result	Aggressive chemotherapy to decrease tumour burden and open up marrow. Aggressive supportive care for infection, thrombocytopenia and anaemia. Often unrewarding	Poor; even with aggressive therapy remissions are not durable
	Acute myelomonocytic leukaemia (AMML)	Myeloblasts/monoblasts			
	Acute monocytic leukaemia (AmoL)	Monoblasts			
	Acute megakaryoblastic leukaemia (AmkL)	Megakaryoblasts			
	Erythroleukaemia	Erythroblasts			
	Acute undifferentiated leukaemia	Untyped precursors			
Chronic	Chronic myelogenous leukaemia (CML)	Neutrophils, late precursors	Excessive differentiated bone marrow cells. Slower, insidious disease course. Patients can live for many months to years. Can eventually progress to a 'blast crisis' and revert to an acute disorder with a rapid clinical course	Therapy may not be warranted unless clinical signs present or significant secondary cytopenias. Hydroxycarbonamide is the drug of choice. Phlebotomy and radiophosphorus can also be used for primary erythrocytosis	Guarded. However, remissions can be achieved for many months or even years
	Primary/essential thrombocythaemia	Platelets			
	Basophilic leukaemia	Basophils and precursors			
	Eosinophilic leukaemia	Eosinophils and precursors			
	Polycythaemia vera	Erythrocytes			

19.14 Characteristics of myeloproliferative disorders in dogs and cats.

Lymphocytic leukaemia

Incidence and aetiology
Lymphocytic leukaemia is more common than non-lymphocytic leukaemia and other MPDs. The true incidence is not known. The median age is approximately 5 years and males may be over-represented. There may also be a breed predilection for German Shepherd Dogs.

Well differentiated or chronic lymphocytic leukaemia (CLL) is seen less frequently than acute lymphoblastic leukaemia (ALL) (Figure 19.15). The median age for CLL is higher than for ALL (approximately 11 years) and, again, males are over-represented.

Retroviruses have been implicated in cats: approximately two-thirds of cats with ALL are FeLV-antigenaemic (FeLV-positive), while most cats with CLL are FeLV-negative. However, there is no clear evidence implicating a retroviral cause in dogs.

Pathology
In ALL, the blast cells always infiltrate the bone marrow, resulting in variable degrees of anaemia, thrombocytopenia and neutropenia. Infiltration of the spleen and liver is common and extramedullary sites such as the nervous system, bone and gastrointestinal tract may be involved as well. Some animals may have lymph node involvement and develop generalized lymphadenopathy, but the nodal enlargement is typically not marked.

The lymphocytes of CLL are virtually indistinguishable morphologically from normal small lymphocytes. In CLL, the marrow is infiltrated with mature lymphocytes and the extent of marrow infiltration is generally less that that seen with ALL or MPD. Despite the well differentiated appearance of the lymphocytes in CLL, these cells function abnormally. Some animals with CLL have an accompanying monoclonal gammopathy.

Investigations have immunophenotyped cells from dogs with ALL and CLL (Vernau and Moore, 1999; Williams et al., 2008). Interestingly, the majority of CLLs were associated with a CD8 T-cell phenotype, which is different to the case in humans where most CLL are of B-cell derivation. In dogs, the CD34 immunophenotype is thought to be a marker of ALL, though some B- and T-cell immunophenotypes have been documented. Most cases of dogs with circulating B-cell lymphoblasts likely represent stage V lymphoma rather than ALL, as they are usually associated with marked peripheral lymphadenopathy and respond much better to treatment than true ALL. The majority of ALL in cats are of T-cell type.

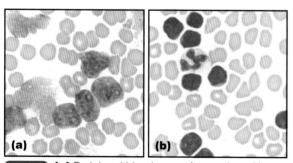

19.15 **(a)** Peripheral blood smear from a dog with acute lymphoblastic leukaemia, showing the characteristic morphologically immature lymphoblasts. **(b)** Peripheral blood smear of a dog with chronic lymphocytic leukaemia, showing morphologically mature lymphocytes. (Wright's–Giemsa stain, original magnification X1000) (Courtesy of Karen Young, University of Wisconsin–Madison)

Presentation and clinical signs

Acute lymphoblastic leukaemia: Animals with ALL usually have a history of anorexia, weight loss, polyuria/polydipsia and lethargy. Splenomegaly is common and other physical abnormalities may include haemorrhage, lymphadenopathy and hepatomegaly. Anaemia, thrombocytopenia and an elevated white blood cell (WBC) count are commonly detected on a complete blood count (CBC). The anaemia may be severe and is usually characterized as normocytic and normochromic (non-regenerative). WBC counts are usually elevated, despite the presence of a neutropenia, owing to an increased number of circulating lymphoblasts. Some dogs may be leucopenic. Infiltration of bone marrow by neoplastic lymphoblasts may be extensive, with resultant depression of normal haemopoietic elements.

Chronic lymphocytic leukaemia: In CLL, mild lymphadenopathy and mild to marked splenomegaly may be present. CBC shows that most dogs and cats are anaemic (PCV <35%) and mildly thrombocytopenic. The WBC count is usually >30 × 10⁹/l but can be as high as >300 × 10⁹/l, owing to an increase in circulating mature lymphocytes. Lymphocytosis is usually persistent and granulocytes are usually present in normal numbers. In some animals, the disease is identified incidentally while the patient is undergoing evaluation for another reason.

Clinical approach

Infiltration of neoplastic lymphoid cells into the bone marrow is the hallmark of both ALL and CLL. Therefore, careful examination of peripheral blood and bone marrow by an experienced cytopathologist is essential in establishing a diagnosis of lymphocytic leukaemia.

If diagnostic bone marrow cannot be obtained by aspiration, bone marrow core biopsy should be performed. In ALL, lymphoblasts predominate in the marrow and are also present in peripheral blood. In many cases, these cells cannot be easily distinguished from blast cells of other haemopoietic lineages without the use of immunophenotypic marker analysis. The presence of 30% or more lymphoblasts in the bone marrow is considered diagnostic. Approximately 10% of ALL cases are classified as 'aleukaemic' leukaemia because bone marrow infiltration is present but peripherally circulating lymphoblasts are absent. ALL may be further differentiated clinically from stage V multicentric lymphoma by its more rapid progression, lack of significant lymphadenopathy in approximately 50% of cases, poor chemoresponsiveness, short survival times and confirmation of CD34 immunophenotype (Williams *et al.*, 2008). The infiltration of bone marrow by lymphoblasts is accompanied by a decrease in the myeloid, erythroid and megakaryocytic cell lines.

The lymphocytes in CLL are small mature cells that occur in excessive numbers in bone marrow (>30% of nucleated cells) early in the disease.

Infiltration becomes more extensive as the disease slowly progresses and eventually the neoplastic cells replace normal marrow.

All cats with leukaemia should be tested for FeLV.

Management

Acute lymphoblastic leukaemia: Like other infiltrative bone marrow malignancies, ALL causes morbidity by suppressing normal bone marrow function. Neutropenia, thrombocytopenia and anaemia may be severe. Patients need supportive therapy such as fresh whole blood, broad-spectrum antibiotics, fluid therapy and nutritional support. Patients must be carefully monitored for bleeding and thrombosis that may signal the development of disseminated intravascular coagulation. The treatment of ALL requires aggressive chemotherapy and the standard CHOP protocols (outlined earlier) are often employed.

Chronic lymphocytic leukaemia: Because of the indolent nature of CLL in many animals, it is controversial whether or not all dogs with this disease should be treated. The clinician may elect to observe the patient if the discovery of CLL is incidental and if there are no accompanying physical or clinical signs and no significant haematological abnormalities. Treatment is generally reserved for those animals that are anaemic or thrombocytopenic, have significant lymphadenopathy or hepatosplenomegaly, or have an excessively high white blood cell count (lymphocytes >100 × 10⁹/l).

The treatment of choice for CLL is chlorambucil. This is given orally at a dose of 0.2 mg/kg or 6 mg/m² q24h for 7–14 days in dogs and cats. The dose can then be reduced to 0.1 mg/kg or 3 mg/m² q24h. For long-term maintenance, dosing every other day may be sufficient. The dose should be adjusted according to clinical response and bone marrow tolerance. The anti-tumour activity of chlorambucil combined with prednisone/prednisolone is better than that of chlorambucil alone. When chlorambucil is no longer effective, the choice of treatment is combination chemotherapy, such as the CHOP or COP protocols. The treatment of CLL is rarely curative and eventually most patients go on to evolve into ALL.

Prognosis

In general, the prognosis of ALL in the dog and cat is poor. The majority of animals do not achieve a complete remission and, when they do, this is not long lasting (<4 months). In the dog, cell size, cell number and immunophenotype can predict prognosis: large cells with CD21 expression, counts >30,000/µl and expression of CD34 have been associated with a more negative prognosis (Williams *et al.*, 2008).

As stated earlier, CLL is a slowly progressive disease, and some animals will not require therapy initially. In dogs undergoing chlorambucil and prednisone therapy, the median survival time is approximately 18 months after the initiation of therapy. Accurate figures on survival are not available in the cat, as CLL is a very rare disease in this species.

Non-lymphoid leukaemias and myeloproliferative disorders

Non-lymphoid MPDs are also classified according to cell lineage and degree of differentiation (i.e. acute or chronic) (see Figure 19.14).

Acute myeloproliferative disorders

Acute MPDs are rare in both dogs and cats and are characterized by the accumulation of immature blast cells in the bone marrow and peripheral blood. These cells may also infiltrate other organs, such as the lymphatic vessels, liver, spleen and central nervous system. The clinical course of the acute MPDs is rapid and generally fatal, due to the sequelae of bone marrow effacement (myelophthisis) by the immature blasts; this leads to profound anaemia, neutropenia and thrombocytopenia. Uncontrolled haemorrhage and sepsis are common outcomes. It is often difficult or impossible to classify the cell lineage involved by standard light microscopy alone; immunophenotypic, immunocytochemical and histochemical techniques are often necessary to determine the cell of origin. The classification of the various acute MPDs based on these techniques is beyond the scope of this chapter and the reader is referred to a recent review (Vail and Young, 2007).

Chronic myeloproliferative disorders

Chronic MPDs are characterized by an overproliferation of mature or well differentiated cells of bone marrow origin such as erythrocytes, granulocytes or platelets. The clinical course of the chronic MPDs can be prolonged and treatment may not be necessary in the early stages. Ultimately, the proliferating cells may result in myelophthisis and related sequelae, or a 'blast crisis' may occur where the chronic MPD shifts to an immature acute MPD and results in a rapid and fatal outcome.

Management and prognosis

As with the lymphoid leukaemias, the prognosis for animals with chronic MPDs is better than for those with acute MPDs. The acute MPDs rarely respond to available chemotherapy protocols; if they do, response durations are short. Chronic myelogenous leukaemia and primary erythrocytosis (polycythaemia vera) can enjoy significant remissions with hydroxycarbamide (hydroxyurea) chemotherapy. Hydroxycarbamide is used at a dose rate of 20–50 mg/kg orally q24h for 10 days, and is then reduced to 15 mg/kg q24h. Alternatively, polycythaemia vera can be managed with intermittent phlebotomies or, if available, radiophosphorus (^{32}P).

Plasma cell tumours

Plasma cell tumours are defined as neoplastic proliferations of cells of the B-lymphocyte plasma cell lineage. The proliferations are, in most instances, monoclonal (i.e. derived from a single cell), as they typically produce homogenous immunoglobulin. Plasma cell tumours include:

- Multiple myeloma
- IgM (Waldenström's) macroglobulinaemia
- Solitary plasmacytoma (including solitary osseous plasmacytoma and extramedullary plasmacytoma).

Multiple myeloma is the most clinically important plasma cell neoplasm, based on incidence and severity.

Multiple myeloma

Multiple myeloma (MM) represents 8% of all haemopoietic tumours in the dog. While the incidence in cats is unknown, it is diagnosed much less frequently in this species. MM occurs in older dogs and cats; no breed or sex predilection has been consistently reported.

In most cases, the malignant plasma cells produce an overabundance of a single type of, or component of, immunoglobulin, which is referred to as the M-component. Less commonly, biclonal immunoglobulin production has been reported. The M-component can represent any class of immunoglobulin, or only a portion of the molecule. This may be the light chain (Bence-Jones protein) or heavy chain ('heavy chain disease') of the molecule.

Aetiology

The aetiology of MM is unknown. In humans, genetic/epigenetic predispositions, viral infections, chronic immune stimulation and exposure to carcinogens have all been suggested as contributing factors. MM has not been associated with either FeLV or FIV infections in cats.

Pathophysiology

Tumour infiltration of organ systems (including bone marrow) and/or the presence of abnormally high circulating M-component results in a wide array of possible pathological abnormalities and related clinical syndromes (Matus et al., 1986). Feline myeloma, sometimes referred to as 'myeloma-related disorders', while involving the bone marrow in the majority of cases, appears to involve extramedullary sites (e.g. skin, abdominal viscera) more commonly than in dogs (Hanna, 2005; Patel et al., 2005; Mellor et al., 2006, 2008).

Presentation and clinical signs

Clinical signs with MM are variable and are due to the wide range of pathophysiological effects outlined in Figure 19.16. Clinical signs in dogs with MM, in decreasing order of frequency, are lethargy and weakness, lameness, bleeding, fundoscopic abnormalities, polyuria, polydipsia and CNS deficits. Anorexia and weight loss are the most common clinical signs in the cat and there may be a history of chronic respiratory infections. Skeletal lesions were thought not to occur commonly in cats, but most recent reports have found them to be common. Organomegaly due to organ infiltration with tumour is frequent.

Clinical syndrome	Aetiology	Clinical consequences	Frequency
Hyperviscosity syndrome (HVS)	High serum viscosity from elevated M-component results in sludging of blood in small vessels, ineffective delivery of oxygen and nutrients and coagulation abnormalities	Bleeding diathesis. Neurological signs. Ophthalmic abnormalities. Cardiomyopathy	Dogs: 20% Cats: 10–25%
Hypercalcaemia	In decreasing order of likelihood: production of osteoclast activating factor or other cytokines; elevation of N-terminal parathyroid hormone-related protein; may be secondary to associated renal disease	PU/PD. Hypercalcaemic nephrosis. Neurological signs. Cardiac arrhythmias	Dogs: 20% Cats: 10–20%
Renal disease	Can result from any of the following: Bence–Jones (light chain) proteinuria; tumour infiltration into renal tissue; hypercalcaemia; amyloidosis; diminished perfusion due to HVS; dehydration; urinary tract infections	Renal failure. Glomerulonephropathies with proteinuria	Dogs: 30–50% Cats: one-third
Immunocompromised patient	Depressed normal immunoglobulin levels. Leucopenias due to bone marrow infiltration (myelophthisis)	Immune deficiencies lead to secondary infections	The majority of patients are immunocompromised to some degree
Anaemia/leucopenia/thrombocytopenia	Blood loss from coagulation disorders. Anaemia of chronic disease. Erythrocyte destruction secondary to HVS. Myelophthisis	Risk of sepsis. Weakness. Haemorrhage	Dogs and cats: two-thirds anaemic; one-third leucopenic; one-third thrombocytopenic
Bleeding diathesis	M-components may: inhibit platelet aggregation; release platelet factor-3; absorb minor clotting proteins; generate abnormal fibrin polymerization. May also be due to: functional decrease in calcium; thrombocytopenia (myelophthisis); loss of clotting factors due to glomerulonephropathies	Haemorrhage (epistaxis, gingival bleeding). Anaemia. Weakness	Dogs: about one-third have active bleeding Cats: 10–15%
Lameness/bone pain	Bone lysis secondary to tumour lysis of long bones and vertebrae	Pathological fractures. Transverse myelopathy due to vertebral body fracture	Dogs: almost half Cats: 15–50%

19.16 Features of clinical syndromes associated with multiple myeloma in dogs and cats.

Clinical approach

A diagnosis of MM depends upon the demonstration of all or most of the following:

- Bone marrow plasmacytosis
- Presence of osteolytic bone lesions
- Serum or urine myeloma proteins (M-component)
- Organ infiltration with malignant plasmacytes.

In the absence of osteolytic bone lesions or organ infiltration, a diagnosis can also be made if marrow plasmacytosis is associated with a progressive increase in M-component.

A CBC, platelet count, serum biochemistry profile and urinalysis should be performed in all animals suspected of having MM and particular attention should be paid to renal function and serum calcium levels. Serum electrophoresis, immunoelectrophoresis and quantification determine the presence of a monoclonal gammopathy and categorize the class of immunoglobulin involved (Figure 19.17). In the dog, the M-component consists of IgA or IgG immunoglobulin (the author's experience is that the majority are IgA), while the majority of cases reported in the cat involve IgG. If IgM constitutes the M-component, the term Waldenström's macroglobulinaemia is applied.

Bicolonal gammopathy has also been reported in both species and cryoglobulinaemia (requiring specialized serum collection techniques) has been reported occasionally in dogs. Heat precipitation and electrophoresis of urine are necessary to detect the

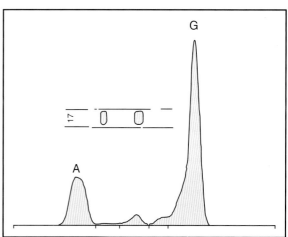

19.17 Serum protein electrophoresis from a dog with multiple myeloma. A, albumin. G, large M-component spike representing an IgA monocolonal gammopathy.

presence of Bence–Jones proteinuria; commercial urine dipstick methods are not capable of this determination.

Definitive diagnosis usually requires a bone marrow aspirate (Figure 19.18) or core biopsy. Normal marrow contains <5% plasma cells, while myelomatous marrow will typically have a much greater number. Marrow involvement can be location-dependent and some marrow compartments may appear normal cytologically; areas with obvious radiographic evidence of cortical lysis or osteoporosis are more

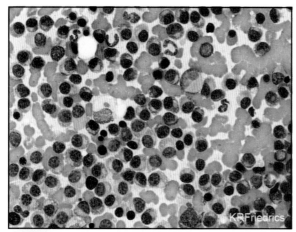

19.18 Bone marrow aspirate from a dog with MM, showing near effacement of normal marrow by plasma cells with eccentric nuclei and pale perinuclear Golgi areas. (Wright's–Giemsa stain, original magnification X1000). (Courtesy of Kristen Friedrics, University of Wisconsin–Madison)

likely to be effaced. The degree of differentiation and therefore the microscopic appearance of malignant plasma cells can vary from that of normal plasma cells to those in early stages of differentiation.

The presence and extent of osteolytic lesions (Figure 19.19) should be determined by skeletal survey radiography, as they have diagnostic, prognostic and therapeutic implications. Rarely, biopsy of these osteolytic lesions (i.e. Jamshidi bone core biopsy) is necessary for diagnosis. In macroglobulinaemia, malignant cells are more likely to infiltrate the spleen, liver and lymph tissue than bone. Bones engaged in active haemopoiesis (e.g. vertebrae, ribs, pelvis, skull and proximal long bones) are more commonly affected. All animals should undergo a careful fundoscopic examination; abnormalities may include retinal haemorrhage, venous dilatation with sacculation and tortuosity, retinal detachment and blindness.

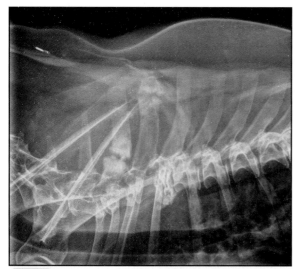

19.19 Lateral thoracic radiograph of a dog with MM, showing multiple expansile lytic lesions and pathological fractures in the axial skeleton, most apparent in the spinous processes of the vertebrae and in a collapse fracture of the third thoracic vertebral body.

Disease syndromes other than MM that can be associated with monoclonal gammopathies and should be considered in any list of differentials include:

- Other lymphoreticular tumours (e.g. lymphoma, CLL, ALL)
- Chronic infections (e.g. erhlichiosis, leishmaniasis, FIP)
- Monocolonal gammopathy of unknown significance (MGUS).

MGUS (benign, essential or idiopathic monoclonal gammopathy) is a benign monoclonal gammopathy that is not associated with osteolysis, bone marrow infiltration or Bence–Jones proteinuria.

Management

Therapy should be directed at both the tumour cell mass and the secondary systemic effects caused by the elevated M-component.

Chemotherapy: Chemotherapy is highly effective in reducing myeloma cell burden, relieving bone pain (unless significant pathological fracture is present), initiating skeletal healing and reducing levels of serum immunoglobulins in dogs. Complete elimination of neoplastic myeloma cells is rarely achieved; but significant decrease in the tumour load is achieved, which significantly extends both the quality and quantity of most patients' lives. While MM remains a gratifying disease to treat, eventual relapse is to be expected.

The treatment of choice for MM in dogs is a combination of the alkylating agent melphalan and prednisone/prednisolone. The initial starting dose of melphalan is 0.1 mg/kg orally q24h for 10 days; it is then reduced to 0.05 mg/kg q24h continuously. Prednisone is initiated at a dosage of 0.5 mg/kg orally q24h for 10 days, then reduced to every other day thereafter. Therapy is continued until clinical relapse occurs or melphalan-associated myelosuppression, in particular thrombocytopenia, necessitates a dose reduction or drug holiday. CBC, including platelet counts, should be performed every 2 weeks for 2 months following initiation of therapy and monthly thereafter.

An alternative pulse-dosing regimen for melphalan (7 mg/m^2 orally q24h for 5 consecutive days every 3 weeks) has been used successfully in a small number of cases where thrombocytopenia resulted from the use of more conventional continuous low-dose therapy. Melphalan plus prednisone/prednisolone has also been used in cats with MM, but response rates are lower and durations of response are shorter than in dogs.

Cyclophosphamide has been advocated as an alternative alkylating agent for the treatment of MM, though there is no evidence to suggest that it is superior to melphalan. In the author's practice, cyclophosphamide is limited to those cases presenting with severe hypercalcaemia or with widespread systemic involvement, where a faster-acting alkylating agent would theoretically alleviate systemic effects more quickly. In those situations, cyclophosphamide is given at a dosage of 250 mg/m² i.v. once. At the same time, oral melphalan therapy is initiated.

Chlorambucil, another alkylating agent, has also been used successfully for the treatment of IgM macroglobulinaomia in dogs at a dosage of 0.2 mg/kg orally q24h.

Evaluations of response to therapy should be based on improvement of clinical signs, clinicopathological parameters and radiographic improvement of skeletal lesions. Subjective improvement in bone pain, lameness, lethargy and anorexia should be evident in 2–4 weeks. Objective laboratory improvement, including reduction in serum immunoglobulin or Bence–Jones proteinuria, is usually noted in 4–6 weeks (curiously, an initial increase in M-component in the first 2 weeks of treatment has been noted on several occasions by the author). Improvement in osteolytic bone lesions may occur as early as a few weeks into therapy, but complete resolution of bone lesions may take months and may only be partial.

Since complete resolution of MM rarely occurs with therapy, a reduction in measured M-component to at least 50% of pre-treatment values would be classified as a good response. Quantification of serum immunoglobulin or urine Bence–Jones protein should be performed monthly until a good response is noted and then every 2–3 months. Bone marrow aspiration is repeated if M-component levels rise or if clinical signs recur. Additionally, if cytopenias (particularly thrombocytopenia) occur during therapy, a bone marrow aspirate is indicated to differentiate between tumour myelophthisis and chemotherapy-induced myelosupression.

Ancillary treatments: Hypercalcaemia, hyperviscosity syndrome (HVS), bleeding diatheses, renal disease, immunosuppression and pathological skeletal fractures often complicate the presentation and indeed the treatment of MM. Therapy directed more specifically at these complications may be indicated in the short term.

- Plasmapheresis is used for managing clinically significant HVS. Whole blood is collected from the patient, plasma is separated off from the packed cells, and the red cells are then re-suspended in normal saline and reinfused back into the patient.
- Bleeding diatheses will usually resolve along with HVS; however, platelet-rich plasma transfusions may be necessary.
- Pathological fractures of weight-bearing long bones and/or vertebrae (resulting in spinal cord compression) may require immediate surgical intervention in conjunction with systemic chemotherapy. Orthopaedic stabilization of fractures and spinal cord decompression should be undertaken where necessary and may be followed with external beam radiotherapy. Radiation therapy can be used for the initial control of bone pain in long bones. The use of bisphosphonates (e.g. pamidronate, zoledronate) to inhibit bone resorption in patients with MM is currently being investigated but is still controversial.

Rescue therapy: Rescue therapy is treatment that is initiated when melphalan/prednisone combinations eventually become ineffective, or in cases that are initially resistant to standard therapy. The author has had, in a few cases, success with a combination of doxorubicin (30 mg/m² i.v. every 21 days), vincristine (0.7 mg/m² i.v. on days 8 and 15) and prednisone (1.0 mg/kg orally q24h), given in 21-day cycles. Most dogs respond initially to this rescue protocol although the response tends to be short lived, lasting only a few months. High-dose cyclophosphamide (300 mg/m² i.v. every 21 days) has also been used with limited success.

Prognosis

In the short term, the prognosis for dogs with MM is good for initial control of the tumour and a return to a good quality of life. Long-term survival is usual, with a median of 1.5 years reported, but recurrence is expected. Eventually, the tumour is no longer responsive to available chemotherapeutic agents and death follows from renal failure, sepsis or euthanasia (due to intractable bone or spinal pain). Hypercalcaemia, Bence–Jones proteinuria and extensive bony lysis are known to be negative indices in the dog.

The prognosis for MM is guarded in cats, as response rates and durations are less than those reported in dogs. Most cats respond to melphalan/prednisone or cyclophosphamide-based protocols. However, responses are not long-lasting and most animals succumb within 2–3 months of diagnosis, though some case series report median survivals from 6 to 12 months (Hanna, 2005; Mellor *et al.*, 2006).

Less is understood about the prognosis for dogs with IgM macroglobulinaemia, but long-term responses to chlorambucil have occurred.

Solitary plasmacytoma

Solitary collections of monoclonal plasmacytic tumours can originate in bone or soft tissues and are referred to as solitary osseous plasmacytoma (SOP) and extramedullary plasmacytoma (EMP), respectively. The majority of SOPs eventually progress to systemic MM.

The biological behaviour of EMP varies with anatomical location. Cutaneous and oral cavity EMPs are typically benign disorders in the dog; there is an exception for multiple cutaneous plasmacytoma, a rare biologically aggressive form of the disease. In contrast, non-cutaneous EMPs in particular alimentary tract locations are associated with a much more aggressive natural behaviour and have been reported to involve the oesophagus, stomach and intestine. While bone marrow involvement and gammopathies are less common in these alimentary cases, metastasis to associated lymph nodes does occur. Colonic EMP tends to be an exception to the rule; it often remains solitary and is amenable to surgical resection, with resulting long-term survival.

Presentation and clinical signs

Clinical signs associated with solitary plasmacytomas reflect the anatomical location of involvement or, in those rare cases with significant elevations in M-component, hyperviscosity syndromes. SOP is usually associated with pain and lameness if the appendicular skeleton is affected, or neurological signs if vertebrae are involved. The more benign cutaneous form of EMP usually has no related clinical signs (see Chapter 12). In contrast, alimentary EMP often presents with signs suggestive of gastrointestinal disease. Ataxia and seizure activity have been associated with EMPs secondary to tumour-associated hypoglycaemia.

Clinical approach

A tissue biopsy for histological assessment is necessary for the diagnosis of SOP and EMP. Immunohistochemical studies may be helpful in confirming a diagnosis in more poorly differentiated tumours. In addition, PCR techniques can be used to determine the clonality of the immunoglobin heavy-chain variable region gene. Thorough staging of the disease is required in these cases, including bone marrow aspiration, serum electrophoresis and skeletal survey radiography, to ensure that the disease is confined to a single site prior to initiation of therapy.

Management

If thorough clinical staging fails to identify systemic involvement, animals with solitary forms of plasma cell tumours may be treated by local therapy, without the need for systemic chemotherapy. Local therapy can include surgical excision or external beam radiotherapy; these may be used alone, or in combination.

As most dogs with SOP and non-cutaneous EMP eventually develop systemic MM, controversy exists as to whether systemic chemotherapy should be initiated concurrently with local therapy. In human patients with solitary plasmacytomas, systemic spread may not occur for many months to years beyond diagnosis, and studies reveal that no benefit is derived from the initiation of systemic chemotherapy prior to the documentation of subsequent systemic spread. It is the author's opinion that the same approach should be applied to veterinary patients and, following local control, a regular follow-up schedule should be implemented in order to recognize both recurrence of disease and systemic spread. At that time, systemic therapy is warranted, as described above for MM.

Prognosis

Dogs with cutaneous and oral plasmacytomas are usually cured by surgical excision. Fewer reports exist for cutaneous plasmacytomas in cats but, while some are controlled with surgical excision, the potential to be a component of widespread systemic involvement is more likely. Dogs with SOP or EMP of the alimentary tract that are treated by surgical excision, in combination with systemic chemotherapy once systemic disease is documented, have survival times of more than 1 year in the majority of cases.

References and further reading

Avery PR and Avery AC (2004) Molecular methods to distinguish reactive and neoplastic lymphocyte expansions and their importance in transitional neoplastic states. *Veterinary Clinical Pathology* **33**,196—207

Backgren AW (1965) Lymphatic leukaemia in dogs. An epizootiological clinical and haematological study. *Acta Veterinaria Scandinavica* 6, Suppl.1

Bertone ER, Snyder LA and Moore AS (2002) Environmental tobacco smoke and risk of malignant lymphoma in pet cats. *American Journal of Epidemiology* **156**, 268–273

Breen M and Modiano JF (2008) Evolutionarily conserved cytogenetic changes in hematological malignancies of dogs and humans – man and his best friend share more than companionship. *Chromosome Research* **16**,145–154

Bridgeford EC, Marini RP, Feng Y *et al.* (2008) Gastric Helicobacter species as a cause of feline gastric lymphoma: a viable hypothesis. *Veterinary Immunology and Immunopathology* **123**, 106–113

Bronden LB, Rutteman GR, Flagstad A *et al.* (2003) Study of dog and cat owners' perceptions of medical treatment for cancer. *Veterinary Record* **152**,77–80

Darbes J, Majzoub M, Breuer W *et al.* (1998) Large granular lymphocyte leukemia/lymphoma in six cats. *Veterinary Pathology* **35**, 370–379

Day MJ, Kyaw-Tanner M, Silkstone MA *et al.* (1999) T-cell-rich B-cell lymphoma in the cat. *Journal of Comparative Pathology* **120**, 155–167

Dobson JM, Samuel S, Milstein H, Rogers K and Wood JLN (2002) Canine neoplasia in the UK: estimates of incidence rates from a population of insured dogs. *Journal of Small Animal Practice* **43**, 240–246

Drobatz KJ (1993) Globule leukocyte tumor in six cats. *Journal of the American Animal Hospital Association* **29**, 391–397

Gabor LJ, Canfield PJ and Malik R (1999) Immunophenotypic and histological characterization of 109 cases of feline lymphosarcoma. *Australian Veterinary Journal* **77**, 436–441

Hanna F (2005) Multiple myelomas in cats. *Journal of Feline Medicine and Surgery* **7**, 275–287

Kaiser HE (1981) Animal neoplasms: a systemic review. In: *Neoplasms – Comparative Pathology in Animals, Plants and Man*, ed. HE Kaiser, pp. 747–812. William & Wilkins, Baltimore

Kiselow MA, Rassnick KM, McDonough SP *et al.* (2008) Outcome of cats with low-grade lymphocytic lymphoma: 41 cases (1995–2005). *Journal of American Veterinary Medical Association* **232**, 405–410

Krick EL, Little L, Patel R *et al.* (2008) Description of clinical and pathological findings, treatment and outcome of feline large granular lymphocyte lymphoma (1996–2004). *Veterinary and Comparative Oncology* **6**, 102–110

Kristal O, Lana SE, Ogilvie GK *et al.* (2001) Single agent chemotherapy with doxorubicin for feline lymphoma: a retrospective study of 19 cases (1994–1997). *Journal of Veterinary Internal Medicine* **15**, 125–130

Lana S, Plasa S, Hampe K *et al.* (2006) Diagnosis of mediastinal masses in dogs by flow cytometry. *Journal of Veterinary Internal Medicine* **20**, 1161–1165

Louwerens M, London CA, Pedersen NC *et al.* (2005) Feline lymphoma in the post-feline leukemia virus era. *Journal of Veterinary Internal Medicine* **19**, 329–335

Matus RE, Leifer CE, MacEwen EG *et al.* (1986) Prognostic factors for multiple myeloma in the dog. *Journal of the American Veterinary Medical Association* **188**, 1288–1292

McEntee MF, Horton S, Blue J *et al.* (1993) Granulated round cell tumor of cats. *Veterinary Pathology* **30**,195–203

Mellanby RJ, Herrtage ME and Dobson JM (2003) Owners' assessments of their dog's quality of life during palliative chemotherapy for lymphoma. *Journal of Small Animal Practice* **44**, 100–103

Mellor PJ, Haugland S, Murphy S *et al.* (2006) Myeloma-related disorders in cats commonly present as extramedullary neoplasms in contrast to myeloma in human patients: 24 cases with clinical follow-up. *Journal of Veterinary Internal Medicine* **20**, 1376–1383

Mellor PJ, Haugland S, Smith KC *et al.* (2008) Histopathologic, immunohistochemical, and cytologic analysis of feline myeloma-related disorders: further evidence for primary extramedullary development in the cat. *Veterinary Pathology* **45**, 159–173

Modiano JF, Breen M, Burnett RC *et al.* (2005) Distinct B-cell and T-cell lymphoproliferative disease prevalence among dog breeds indicates heritable risk. *Cancer Research* **65**, 5654–5661

Moore AS, Cotter SM, Frimberger AE *et al.* (1996) A comparison of doxorubicin and COP for maintenance of remission in cats with lymphoma. *Journal of Veterinary Internal Medicine* **10**, 372–375

Patel RT, Caceres A, French AF *et al.* (2005) Multiple myeloma in 16 cats: a retrospective study. *Veterinary Clinical Pathology* **34**, 341–352

Peaston AE and Maddison JE (1999) Efficacy of doxorubicin as an induction agent for cats with lymphosarcoma. *Australian Veterinary Journal* **77**, 442–444

Ponce F, Magnol J-P, Ledieu D *et al.* (2004) Prognositc significance of morphological subtypes in canine malignant lymphomas during chemotherapy. *Veterinary Journal* **167**, 158–166

Reif JS, Lower KS and Ogilvie GK (1995) Residential exposure to magnetic fields and risk of canine lymphoma. *American Journal of Epidemiology* **141**, 352–359

Risbon RE, de Lorimier LP, Skorupski K *et al.* (2006) Response of canine epitheliotropic lymphoma to lomustine (CCNU): a retropective study of 46 cases (1999–2004). *Journal of Veterinary Internal Medicine* **20**, 1389–1397

Roccabianca P, Vernau W, Caniatti M *et al.* (2006) Feline large granular lymphocyte (LGL) lymphoma with secondary leukemia: primary intestinal origin with predominance of a CD3/CD8(alpha)(alpha) phenotype. *Veterinary Pathology* **43**, 15–28

Rosol TJ, Nagode LA, Couto CG *et al.* (1992) Parathyroid hormone (PTH)-related protein, PTH, and 1,25-dihydroxyvitamin D in dogs with cancer-associated hypercalcemia. *Endocrinology* **131**, 1157–1164

Sauerbrey ML, Mullins MN, Bannink EO *et al.* (2007) Lomustine and prednisone as a first-line treatment for dogs with multicentric lymphoma: 17 cases (2004–2005). *Journal of the American Veterinary Medical Association* **230**, 1866–1869

Sfiligoi G, Theon AP and Kent MS (2007) Response of 19 cats with nasal lymphoma to radiation therapy and chemotherapy. *Veterinary Radiology and Ultrasound* **48**, 388–393

Simon D, Moreno SN, Hirschberger J *et al.* (2008) Efficacy of a continuous, multiagent chemotherapeutic protocol versus a short-term single-agent protocol in dogs with lymphoma. *Journal of the American Veterinary Medical Association* **232**, 879–885

Teske E, Sraten GV, van Noort R and Rutteman GR (2002) Chemotherapy with cyclophosphamide, vincristine and prednisolone (COP) in cats with malignant lymphoma: new results with an old protocol. *Journal of Veterinary Internal Medicine* **16**, 179–186

Tzannes S, Hammond MF, Murphy S *et al.* (2008) Owners 'perception of their cats' quality of life during COP chemotherapy for lymphoma. *Journal of Feline Medicine and Surgery* **10**, 73–81

Vail DM (2007a) Feline lymphoma and leukemias. In: *Small Animal Clinical Oncology, 4th edn*, ed. SW Withrow and DM Vail, pp. 733–755. Saunders/Elsevier, St Louis, Missouri

Vail DM (2007b) Plasma cell tumors. In: *Small Animal Clinical Oncology, 4th edn*, ed. SW Withrow and DM Vail, pp. 769–784. Saunders/Elsevier, St Louis, Missouri

Vail DM (2007c) Feline lymphoma and leukemias. In: *Small Animal Clinical Oncology, 4th edn*, ed. SW Withrow and DM Vail, pp. 733–755. Saunders/Elsevier, St Louis, Missouri

Vail DM, Moore AS, Ogilvie GK *et al.* (1998) Feline lymphoma (145 cases): proliferation indices, CD3 immunoreactivity, and their association with prognosis in 90 cats. *Journal of Veterinary Internal Medicine* **12**, 349–354

Vail DM and Young KM (2007) Canine lymphoma and lymphoid leukemias. In: *Small Animal Clinical Oncology, 4th edn*, ed. SW Withrow and DM Vail, pp. 699–732. Saunders/Elsevier, St Louis, Missouri

Valli VE, Jacobs RM, Norris A *et al.* (2000) The histologic classification of 602 cases of feline lymphoproliferative disease using the National Cancer Institute working formulation. *Journal of Veterinary Diagnostic Investigation* **12**, 295–306

Valli VE, Jacobs RM, Parodi AL *et al.* (2002) *Histologic Classification of Hematopoietic Tumors of Domestic Animals, 2nd series, Volume VIII.* Armed Forces Institute of Pathology in cooperation with the American Registry of Pathology and The World Health Organization Collaboration Center for Worldwide Reference on Comparative Oncology, Washington, DC

Vernau W and Moore PF (1999) An immunophenotypic study of canine leukemias and preliminary assessment of clonality by polymerase chain reaction. *Veterinary Immunology and Immunopathology* **69**, 145–164

Walton RM and Hendrick MJ (2001) Feline Hodgkin's-like lymphoma: 20 cases (1992–1999). *Veterinary Pathology* **38**, 504–511

Wellman ML, Hammer AS, DiBartola SP *et al.* (1992) Lymphoma involving large granular lymphocytes in cats: 11 cases (1982–1991). *Journal of the American Veterinary Medical Association* **201**, 1265–1269

Williams LE, Rassnick KM, Power HT *et al.* (2006) CCNU in the treatment of canine epitheliotropic lymphoma. *Journal of Veterinary Internal Medicine* **20**, 136–143

Williams MF, Avery AC, Lana SE *et al.* (2008) Canine lymphoproliferative disease characterized by lymphocytosis: immunophenotypic markers of prognosis. *Journal of Veterinary Internal Medicine* **22**, 596–601

Zwahlen CH, Lucroy MD, Kraegel SA and Madewell BR (1998) Results of chemotherapy for cats with alimentary malignant lymphoma: 21 cases (1993–1997). *Journal of the American Veterinary Medical Association* **213**, 1144–1149

Tumours of the spleen

Jane M. Dobson

Introduction

Although tumours of the haemopoietic system often involve the spleen, this reticuloendothelial organ is also an important site for the development of non-lymphoid primary tumours and a site for metastasis. Most of these tumours are covered elsewhere in this manual, but splenic haemangiosarcoma and splenic sarcoma in the dog and visceral mast cell tumours (MCTs) in the cat warrant individual consideration.

Canine splenic tumours

Splenomegaly, or a splenic mass, is quite a common clinical finding in dogs and reports suggest that 43–75% of these cases are caused by neoplasia (Frey and Betts, 1977; Day *et al.*, 1995). Tumours affecting the spleen in dogs are summarized in Figure 19.20.

Primary tumours
• Haemangioma • Haemangiosarcoma • Sarcoma (various)
Secondary or multicentric tumours
• Lymphoproliferative and myeloproliferative conditions (e.g. lymphoma) • Malignant histiocytosis/disseminated histiocytic sarcoma • Haemangiosarcoma • Mast cell tumour • Other malignant tumours with widespread metastases (e.g. melanoma)
Non-neoplastic causes of splenomegaly or splenic mass
• Nodular hyperplasia • Haematoma • Thrombosis and infarction • Congestion • Extramedullary haemopoiesis • Torsion

19.20 Tumours and masses of the canine spleen.

Haemangiosarcoma is the most common tumour of the canine spleen. It affects older dogs (9–10 years) and the German Shepherd Dog is at greater risk than other breeds (Ng and Mills, 1985). Non-angiomatous mesenchymal tumours ('splenic sarcoma', including histiocytic sarcoma – see below) are

also recognized in the spleen of older dogs, especially those of the retriever breeds (Spangler *et al.*, 1994).

The aetiology of splenic tumours is not known. German Shepherd Dogs, Golden Retrievers and Labrador Retrievers are over-represented in some case series and such breed predispositions might suggest genetic factors. Angiogenic growth factors are strongly expressed in haemangiosarcoma cells, implicating dysregulated stimulation of one or more of these factor receptors in tumour development. Mutations in the tumour suppressor gene *PTEN* have also been implicated in the pathogenesis of canine haemangiosarcoma (Dickerson *et al.*, 2005).

Presentation and clinical signs

For low-grade and benign tumours, abdominal distension due to the enlarging tumour mass may be the presenting sign. Alternatively, the mass may be detected during routine clinical examination, as such tumours can reach a large size without causing clinical signs.

Splenic sarcomas may cause non-specific signs of malaise, but are also often detected on clinical examination, radiography or ultrasonography, or at the time of exploratory laparotomy.

The presenting signs of splenic haemangiosarcoma may be dramatic, with acute collapse following rupture of, or bleeding from, the primary mass, leading to a haemoperitoneum. Less specific signs of lethargy, weakness, pallor and anorexia may be detected prior to a major abdominal bleed. Some dogs may have a history of transient periods of weakness or collapse in the days or weeks preceding an acute collapse and it is postulated that these episodes represent abdominal bleeds from which the dog may recover due to auto-transfusion. Haemorrhagic diatheses due to disseminated intra-vascular coagulation (DIC) may be a presenting sign in some cases. However, splenic haemangiosarcoma may also be detected as an incidental finding in the absence of overt clinical signs.

Splenic neoplasia may be associated with cardiac dysrhythmias such as ventricular premature contractions.

Clinical approach

Haematology
A number of haematological abnormalities may be detected in dogs with splenic haemangiosarcoma:

- Anaemia – regenerative if due to blood loss; or microangiopathic if due to fragmentation of red blood cells during passage through a meshwork of fibrin in the microvascular network of the tumour
- Acanthocytes (damaged red cells; Figure 19.21) and schistocytes (red blood cell fragments) – highly indicative of haemangiosarcoma
- Thrombocytopenia – may be due to bleeding, sequestration of platelets within the microvascular network of the tumour, or DIC.

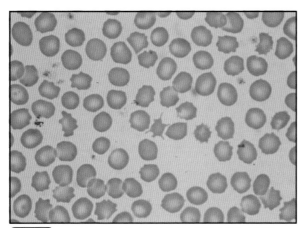

19.21 These erythrocytes are acanthocytes, which have rounded projections of variable length due to membrane damage. (Modified Wright's–Giemsa stain, original magnification X1000) (Courtesy of C Sommerey, Clinical Pathology, Department of Veterinary Medicine, University of Cambridge)

In cases with DIC, clotting studies reveal abnormalities in both primary and secondary haemostasis, fibrin degradation products are elevated, and fibrinogen and anti-thrombin III are decreased.

A haemophagocytic variant of histiocytic sarcoma has been described that consistently involves the spleen and is associated with a Coombs' test-negative regenerative anaemia, thrombocytopenia and hypoalbuminaemia (Dobson *et al.*; 2006; Moore *et al.*, 2006).

Imaging

Splenomegaly or a splenic mass may be detected on plain radiographs of the abdomen and these may also show evidence of abdominal fluid in cases with haemorrhage.

Ultrasonography can provide useful information about the structure of a splenic mass (or masses) and its relationship with normal splenic tissue. The vascular nature of haemangiosarcoma may be seen as a mixed or non-homogenous mass with echolucent areas, in contrast to the more homogenous denser structure of normal spleen.

Contrast-enhanced ultrasonography using microbubble contrast media has been used to improve characterization between benign and malignant focal or multifocal lesions in the spleen (Rossi *et al.*, 2008). Contrast-enhanced computed tomography can also provide significant differences in imaging characteristics between benign and malignant splenic lesions (Fife *et al.*, 2004).

Radiography of the thorax and ultrasonography of other abdominal organs, especially the liver and kidneys, are indicated to detect metastases.

Cytology and biopsy

Fine-needle aspiration (FNA) may assist in cytological diagnosis in cases of generalized splenomegaly (e.g. associated with lymphoma or MCTs in the cat), or where splenic lesions appear solid on ultrasonography.

> **WARNING**
> It is not advisable to attempt FNA in cases where splenic lesions have a vascular appearance on ultrasonography. It is unlikely that the resulting samples would be of diagnostic quality, as blood is usually all that is collected from such lesions. More importantly, the procedure carries a risk of causing haemorrhage into the abdomen and possible seeding of tumour cells.

Splenic biopsy may be indicated in cases with diffuse splenomegaly or multinodular splenic disease. Needle biopsy techniques may be used under ultrasound guidance (though they still carry a risk of bleeding), or incisional biopsy samples may be collected at laparotomy. The latter allows visualization of the whole spleen and thus better selection of representative lesions for biopsy specimens.

In cases where there is a distinct mass in the spleen, performing an excisional biopsy by splenectomy is preferable. Not only is this technically easier to perform, but it also provides the pathologist with sufficient material to achieve the correct diagnosis. This is particularly important for differentiation between splenic haematoma, haemangioma and haemangiosarcoma. Sufficient material should always be presented for histopathology. Either the whole spleen can be submitted, or sections that the clinician considers representative. However, if 'representative' pieces are submitted, it is always advisable to keep the rest of the spleen in case the clinical picture does not fit with the diagnosis.

Haemangiosarcoma and haemangioma

Haemangiosarcoma is the most important tumour of the canine spleen. Haemangioma and haematoma may also affect the spleen and it can be difficult to differentiate these conditions clinically and histopathologically, for example, when haemorrhage occurs within a haemangiosarcoma. It may be necessary to examine multiple histological sections from the lesion before a certain diagnosis can be reached. Collapse and presence of haemoperitoneum are significantly more common in dogs with splenic haemangiosarcoma than those with splenic haematoma (Prymak *et al.*, 1988) and in one study dogs with haemangiosarcoma had lower total protein concentrations and platelet counts than dogs with other splenic masses at the time of admission (Hammond and Pesillo-Crosby, 2008).

Haemangioma and haemangiosarcoma (Figure 19.22a) may each present as either a single mass or

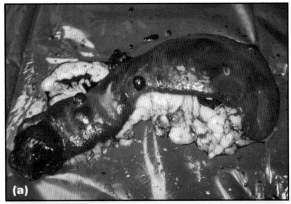

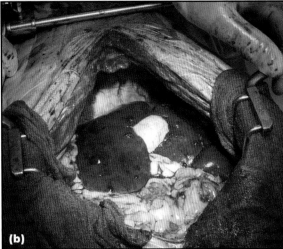

19.22 **(a)** Splenic haemangiosarcoma removed from a 6-year-old neutered female Mastiff. **(b)** The primary tumour has ruptured, but secondary masses can be seen in the spleen and liver. (Courtesy of Duncan Lascelles)

T – Primary tumour		
T0 = No evidence of tumour		
T1 = Tumour confined to primary site		
T2 = Tumour confined to primary site but ruptured		
T3 = Tumour invading adjacent structures		
N – Lymph nodes		
N0 = No evidence of lymph node involvement		
N1 = Regional lymph node involvment		
N2 = Distant lymph node involvement		
M – Metastasis		
M0 = No evidence of metastatic disease		
M1 = Metastasis in same body cavity as primary tumour		
M2 = Distant metastasis		
Stage grouping		
Stage 1 = T0 or T1, N0, M0		
Stage II = T1 or T2, N0 or N1, M1		
Stage III = T2 or T3, N1 or N2, M2		

19.23 Clinical staging for canine haemangiosarcoma.

multiple nodules within the spleen. Haemangiosarcoma arising in other tissues or organs may also metastasize to the spleen. It is debatable whether the heart or the spleen is the more common site for the development of haemangiosarcoma in the dog. In some patients with widespread tumour metastases, it is difficult to be certain which location is the primary focus, or whether the tumour might be multicentric.

Haemangiosarcoma is a highly malignant tumour, with haematogenous metastasis occurring early in the course of the disease (Figure 19.22b). Rupture of the primary tumour can lead to acute and fatal haemorrhage. Primary and metastatic tumours may be associated with DIC. In contrast, haemangioma of the spleen is a slowly growing tumour that can attain large proportions before diagnosis. Metastasis does not occur.

Staging

A clinical staging system for canine haemangiosarcoma has been described (Figure 19.23). In splenic haemangiosarcoma, the extent of the tumour within the spleen is of less importance than whether the tumour has invaded through the splenic capsule. Nodal metastases are uncommon, but radiography and ultrasonography are required to evaluate the patient for haematogenous metastases.

Management and prognosis

Surgery: Surgical removal of the tumour by splenectomy is the treatment of choice for splenic haemangioma and haemangiosarcoma. Preoperative considerations include correction of haematological or coagulation abnormalities with blood products if necessary and circulatory support with appropriate fluids. Dogs undergoing splenectomy are at risk of developing ventricular arrhythmias during and up to 24–48 hours after surgery and should be monitored by electrocardiography during surgery and postoperatively during the risk period. At the time of splenectomy the abdomen should be explored for signs of metastases and any suspicious lesions excised and submitted for histopathology. Care should be taken to ensure that vessels are ligated and ligatures are well placed. However, care should be taken not to ligate the branch of the splenic artery supplying the pancreas.

Chemotherapy: Postoperative chemotherapy is indicated in an attempt to prevent or delay the progression of micrometastatic disease. Single-agent or combination doxorubicin-based chemotherapy protocols are most often used following splenectomy, but median survival times are relatively short, in the order of 141–179 days for combination protocols (Hammer *et al.*, 1991; Sorenmo *et al.*, 1993), with <10% of dogs surviving >12 months. Doxorubicin used as a single agent has been reported to achieve similar survival times (Ogilvie *et al.*, 1996), as has low-dose continuous chemotherapy with cyclophosphamide, etoposide and piroxicam (Lana *et al.*, 2007). A recent study using epirubicin postoperatively suggested that dogs with stage I disease survived significantly longer than those with either stage II or stage III disease (median 345 days *versus* 93 and 68 days, respectively) (Kim *et al.*, 2007).

Prognosis: The prognosis for dogs with splenic haemangiosarcoma is poor. Haemangiosarcoma typically metastasizes early in the course of the disease and, in most cases, micrometastases will be present at the time of diagnosis of the primary tumour. These progress rapidly and are the reason for poor survival times following splenectomy, which range from 19 to 86 days (Wood *et al.*, 1998). The owners of dogs with haemoperitoneum should be advised, before any surgery, of the possibility of a poor prognosis if the mass is found to be splenic haemangiosarcoma.

Splenic sarcoma

Primary tumours of mesenchymal origin ('sarcomas') may arise within the spleen, giving rise to splenomegaly or a splenic mass. Some such tumours are well differentiated and can be classified according to their morphology. However, many lack clear differentiation, leading to diagnoses of 'undifferentiated sarcoma'. When more detailed immunohistochemical staining is performed on these tumours, it appears that they, along with splenic fibrosarcoma and leiomyosarcoma, might have a common origin from smooth muscle or splenic myofibroblasts (Spangler *et al.*, 1994), though some might now be classified as histiocytic sarcoma (see below).

Primary mesenchymal tumours of the spleen can be divided into three categories on the basis of their biological behaviour (Spangler *et al.*, 1994):

- Benign, non-invasive tumours (leiomyoma, lipoma): these do not metastasize and are associated with long patient survival times
- Intermediate tumours (mesenchymoma): these have a median survival period of 12 months
- Malignant tumours (fibrosarcoma, leiomyosarcoma, undifferentiated sarcoma): these tumours are capable of metastasis and are associated with relatively short postoperative survival times (median survival 4 months; 80–100% mortality after 12 months).

Management

Surgery: Surgical removal of the tumour by splenectomy is the treatment of choice for splenic sarcoma. Unfortunately, this is not a curative treatment for malignant splenic sarcomas.

Chemotherapy: As with splenic haemangiosarcoma, postoperative chemotherapy would be a logical treatment for dogs with malignant splenic sarcoma, but less is known about the chemosensitivity of such tumours. Larger-scale clinical trials are required to define the role of chemotherapy in the management of such tumours.

Prognosis: The prognosis for malignant splenic sarcoma is poor and a median survival time of 4 months has been reported, with metastases being a frequent reason for euthanasia (Spangler *et al.*, 1994). The mitotic index has been shown to be of prognostic importance in this group of tumours: those tumours with a mitotic index <9 showed significantly longer survival than those with a mitotic index >9 (Spangler *et al.*, 1994).

Histiocytic sarcoma

Histiocytic sarcoma may be localized or disseminated (see Chapter 14) but quite frequently involves the spleen. A haemophagocytic variant has recently been described in which the spleen is consistently involved. Affected animals have a diffuse splenomegaly with ill-defined masses within the spleen (Figure 19.24). Lesions may also be found in the liver, lung and bone marrow (Dobson *et al.*, 2006; Moore *et al.*, 2006). On cytological or histological examination the malignant histiocytes show marked erythrophagia, which is the cause of the accompanying anaemia (see above), but areas of extramedullary haemopoiesis are often found in the adjacent splenic tissue, which can complicate diagnosis by FNA cytology. These tumours have been shown to arise from splenic red pulp and bone marrow macrophages and express MHC class II and the beta 2 integrin CD11d (Moore *et al.*, 2006).

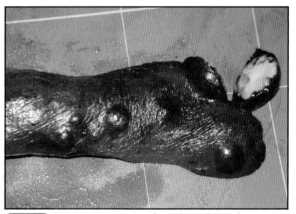

19.24 Histiocytic sarcoma from the spleen of a Flat-coated Retriever.

Management and prognosis

In the cases described to date the prognosis is grave, with most animals being euthanized or dying at the time of diagnosis due to widespread metastasis. Cases where the tumour is localized to the spleen might benefit from postoperative chemotherapy. Lomustine (CCNU) has recently been shown to have some efficacy in treatment of histiocytic sarcoma (Skorupski *et al.*, 2007), but no trials have yet been conducted to validate its use specifically in splenic histiocytic sarcoma.

Feline splenic tumours

Tumours of the spleen are less common in cats than in dogs. As with dogs forms of leukaemia and lymphoma may affect the feline spleen, but a splenic form of mast cell tumour (lymphoreticular or visceral MCT) accounts for 15% of 'splenic disease' in the cat (Spangler and Culbertson, 1992). Tumours and tumour-like conditions of the feline spleen are listed in Figure 19.25.

Primary tumours
• Mast cell tumour • Haemangiosarcoma • Sarcoma (various)

Secondary or multicentric tumours
• Lymphoproliferative and myeloproliferative conditions (e.g. lymphoma) • Haemangiosarcoma • Other malignant tumours with widespread metastases (e.g. adenocarcinoma)

Non-neoplastic causes of splenomegaly or splenic mass
• Nodular hyperplasia • Haematoma • Congestion • Extramedullary haemopoiesis

19.25 Tumours and masses of the feline spleen.

Feline visceral mast cell tumours

There are three distinct forms of MCT in cats: cutaneous (see Chapter 12), intestinal (see Chapter 15) and visceral. The principal site of development of the latter is the spleen, which accounts for >85% of visceral MCTs. Other organs and sites may have visceral MCTs, such as the liver, kidney, visceral lymph nodes, intestine, bone marrow and, occasionally, the mediastinum and lung. While it is possible for cutaneous MCT to spread to viscera, this is uncommon in the cat.

Presentation

Cats with visceral MCT present most commonly with anorexia, chronic vomiting and malaise. This is thought to be due to gastroduodenal ulceration resulting from the effects of histamine on gastric H2 receptors. Gastric ulcers may eventually perforate, leading to peritonitis and death. Splenic rupture has also been reported.

Cats with visceral MCT may be anaemic, due to blood loss from gastric or duodenal ulcers or due to bone marrow infiltration. Other cytopenias may also occur in cases with bone marrow infiltration. Circulating mast cells may be seen on blood smears; bone marrow aspiration is indicated in cats suspected of having visceral MCT.

Management and prognosis

Despite the fact that cats with visceral MCT often have signs of systemic involvement, or at least involvement of other organs, splenectomy appears to be the treatment of choice.

The prognosis for cats with visceral MCT is fair following splenectomy. In one report of seven cases, survival ranged from 2 to 34 months, with a median of 12 months. Resolution of haematological abnormalities was reported following splenectomy in these cats that received no other therapy (Liska *et al.*, 1979). It has been postulated that this response to splenectomy may involve the cat's immune system, hence the use of postoperative corticosteroids in these animals is controversial.

References and further reading

Brown NO, Patnaik AK and MacEwan EG (1985) Canine haemangiosarcoma. *Journal of the American Veterinary Medical Association* **186**, 56–58

Day MJ, Lucke VM and Pearson H (1995) A review of pathological diagnoses made from 87 canine splenic biopsies. *Journal of Small Animal Practice* **36**, 426–433

Dickerson EB, Thomas R, Fosmire SP *et al.* (2005) Mutations of phosphate and tensin homolog deleted from chromosome 10 in canine haemangiosarcoma. *Veterinary Pathology* **42**, 618–632

Dobson JM, Villiers E, Roulois A *et al.* (2006) Histiocytic sarcoma of the spleen in flat-coated retrievers presenting with regenerative anaemia and hypoproteinaemia. *Veterinary Record* **158**, 825–829

Fife WD, Samil VF, Drost WT, Matton JS and Hoshaw-Woodard S (2004) Comparison between malignant and non-malignant splenic masses in dogs using contrast-enhanced computed tomography. *Veterinary Radiology and Ultrasound* **45**, 289–297

Frey AJ and Betts CW (1977) A retrospective survey of splenectomy in the dog. *Journal of the American Animal Hospital Association* **13**, 730–734

Hammer AS, Couto CG, Filippi J *et al.* (1991) Efficacy and toxicity of VAC chemotherapy (vincristine, doxorubicin and cyclophosphamide) in dogs with haemangiosarcoma. *Journal of Veterinary Internal Medicine* **5**, 160–166

Hammond TN and Pesillo-Crosby SA (2008) Prevalence of hemangiosarcoma in anaemic dogs with a splenic mass and hemoperitoneum requiring transfusion: 71 cases (2003–2005). *Journal of the American Veterinary Medical Association* **232**, 553–558

Kerline RL and Hendrick MJ (1996) Malignant fibrous histiocytoma and malignant histiocytosis in the dog – convergent or divergent phenotypic differentiation? *Veterinary Pathology* **33**, 713–716

Kim SE, Liptak JM, Gall TT, Monteith GJ and Woods JP (2007) Epirubicin in the adjuvant treatment of splenic haemangiosarcoma in dogs: 59 cases (1997–2004) *Journal of the American Veterinary Medical Association* **231**, 1550–1557

Lana S, U'ren L, Plaza S *et al.* (2007) Continuous low-dose oral chemotherapy for adjuvant therapy of splenic haemangiosarcoma in dogs. *Journal of Veterinary Internal Medicine* **21**, 764–769

Liska WD, MacEwen EG, Zaki FA and Garvey M (1979) Feline systemic mastocytosis: a review and results of splenectomy in seven cases. *Journal of the American Animal Hospital Association* **15**, 589–597

Moore PF, Affolter VK and Vernau W (2006) Canine haemophagocytic histiocytic sarcoma: a proliferative disorder of CD11d+ macrophages. *Veterinary Pathology* **43**, 632–645

Ng CY and Mills JN (1985) Clinical and haematological features of haemangiosarcoma in dogs. *Australian Veterinary Journal* **62**, 1–4

Ogilvie GK, Powers BE, Mallinckrodt CH *et al.* (1996) Surgery and doxorubicin in dogs with hemangiosarcoma. *Journal of Veterinary Internal Medicine* **6**, 370–384

Prymak C, McKee LJ, Goldschmidt MH and Glickman LT (1988) Epidemiologic, clinical pathologic, and prognostic characteristics of splenic hemangiosarcoma and splenic hematoma in dogs: 217 cases (1985). *Journal of the American Veterinary Medical Association* **193**, 706–712

Rossi F, Leone VF, Vignoli M, Laddaga E and Terragni R. (2008) Use of contrast-enhanced ultrasound for characterization of focal splenic lesions. *Veterinary Radiology and Ultrasound* **49**, 154–164

Skorupski KA, Clifford CA, Paoloni MC *et al.* (2007) CCNU for the treatment of dogs with histiocytic sarcoma. *Journal of Veterinary Internal Medicine* **21**, 121–126

Sorenmo KU, Jeglum KA and Helfand SC (1993) Chemotherapy of canine haemangiosarcoma with doxorubicin and cyclophosphamide. *Journal of Veterinary Internal Medicine* **7**, 370–376

Spangler WL and Culbertson MR (1992) Prevalence and type of splenic diseases in cats: 455 cases (1985–1991). *Journal of the American Veterinary Medical Association* **201**, 773–776

Spangler WL, Culbertson MR and Kass PH (1994) Primary mesenchymal (nonangiomatous/nonlymphomatous) neoplasms occuring in the canine spleen: anatomic classification, immunohistochemistry and mitotic activity correlated with patient survival. *Veterinary Pathology* **31**, 37–47

Wood CA, Moore AS, Gliatto JM *et al.* (1998) Prognosis for dogs with Stage I or II splenic haemangiosarcoma treated by splenectomy alone: 32 cases (1991–1993). *Journal of the American Animal Hospital Association* **34**, 417–421

20

Endocrine tumours

J. Catharine R. Scott-Moncrieff

Introduction

Common endocrine tumours in dogs and cats include tumours of the thyroid gland, parathyroid gland, pituitary gland, adrenal gland and endocrine pancreas (Figure 20.1).

Thyroid gland tumours

The majority of cases of feline hyperthyroidism are due to benign adenoma or adenomatous hyperplasia. Unlike feline thyroid tumours, most clinically significant canine thyroid tumours are malignant carcinomas. The diagnosis and treatment of benign functional feline thyroid tumours has been extensively reviewed elsewhere. This chapter will focus on malignant thyroid cancers in the cat and dog.

Thyroid tumours in cats

Malignant thyroid neoplasia is diagnosed in approximately 1–2% of cases of cats with hyperthyroidism (Peterson and Becker, 1995). Most malignant thyroid tumours in the cat are functional tumours, with follicular carcinomas being most common. Rarely are cats diagnosed with non-functional thyroid tumours.

Clinical features

Age ranges from 6 to 18 years and males are over-represented. Many cats have a history of prior thyroidectomy. Weight loss, polydipsia and polyuria, polyphagia and hyperactivity are the most common historical findings. Tachycardia, hyperactivity, heart murmur, dyspnoea, polypnoea, moist pulmonary rales and tremor are common physical examination findings. Voice change has also been reported. Palpable cervical masses are present in 71% of cases; cervical masses may be attached to underlying or overlying tissues.

Diagnosis

Common abnormalities on blood tests are similar to those in cats with benign thyroid disease and include increased haematocrit and mean corpuscular volume, a stress leucogram, high liver enzyme activity, azotaemia and occasionally hypercalcaemia. Radiographic abnormalities may include cardiomegaly, evidence of congestive heart failure, mediastinal masses and evidence of pulmonary metastasis. The electrocardiogram may show increased R-wave amplitude, tachycardia and arrhythmias. Echocardiographic changes may include ventricular hypertrophy, thickening of the interventricular septum, and left atrial and ventricular dilatation.

The majority of cats with thyroid carcinoma have increased basal serum thyroxine (T4) concentrations. No differences have been identified in the range of serum T4 concentrations in cats with benign and malignant thyroid tumours. In cats with early hyperthyroidism, or those with concurrent disease, measurement of free T4, a T3 suppression test or thyroid scintigraphy may be helpful in confirming the diagnosis. A non-functional tumour should be suspected if a thyroid tumour is identified but T4 concentration is normal and there are no clinical signs of hyperthyroidism.

Nuclear scintigraphy using sodium pertechnetate is valuable in the evaluation of cats with suspected malignant thyroid tumours. Sodium pertechnetate (^{99m}Tc) is actively concentrated in all functional thyroid tissue. In cats with thyroid carcinoma, a ^{99m}Tc

Endocrine gland	Benign tumours	Malignant tumours
Thyroid	Thyroid adenoma	Thyroid carcinoma
Parathyroid	Parathyroid adenoma	Parathyroid carcinoma
Pituitary	Adenoma of somatotrophs or corticotrophs	Pituitary carcinoma
Adrenal	Adrenocortical adenoma Phaeochromocytoma	Adrenocortical carcinoma
Endocrine pancreas		Insulinoma Gastrinoma

20.1 Endocrine tumours of the dog and cat.

scan may demonstrate patchy or irregular uptake of isotope, extension of isotope uptake down the neck (Figure 20.2) and into the mediastinum, and evidence of distant metastasis; however, in some cats, scintigraphic findings in carcinoma may be similar to those for cats with thyroid adenomatous hyperplasia or adenoma. Also, scans that reveal uptake by multiple masses in the cervical region or masses extending into the cranial mediastinum may be a result of benign ectopic tissue. Scintigraphy alone cannot definitively distinguish between adenomatous hyperplasia and thyroid carcinoma. Bronchogenic carcinoma may have scintigraphic findings that may be confused with those of thyroid tumours. Non-functional thyroid tumours may or may not take up ^{99m}Tc, depending upon the degree of differentiation of the tumour.

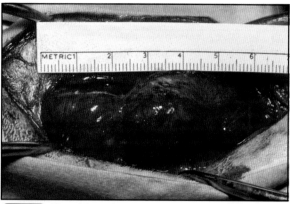

20.3 Thyroid carcinoma in a cat prior to surgical resection. Note the size and irregular shape of the tumour.

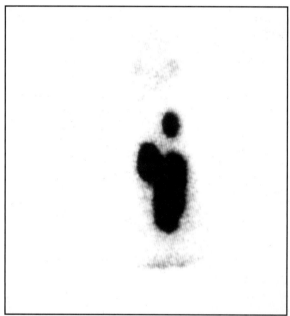

20.2 Ventrodorsal view from a technetium scan in a cat with thyroid carcinoma, showing irregular uptake of isotope into three thyroid masses in the cervical region.

Definitive diagnosis of thyroid carcinoma requires histopathological examination of excised tissue. Since the majority of feline thyroid tumours are benign, thyroid carcinoma may not be suspected on the initial evaluation. Factors that should increase the index of suspicion for thyroid carcinoma include recurrence of hyperthyroidism after previous thyroidectomy or radioiodine therapy, presence of multiple palpable cervical nodules (Figure 20.3) and cervical nodules that are firmly attached to underlying or overlying structures. Large palpable thyroid masses that compress surrounding structures may be due to either thyroid carcinoma or benign thyroid cyst. Thyroid carcinoma should also be suspected if scintigraphy reveals multiple areas of radionuclide uptake and irregular or patchy isotope uptake.

Cytological characteristics are usually unhelpful in differentiation of benign from malignant thyroid tumours, because pleomorphism, anaplasia and increased mitotic rate are not consistent features. Features that distinguish malignant from benign tumours include local tissue invasion, regional lymph node involvement and distant metastasis. Metastasis has been reported to occur in up to 71% of feline thyroid carcinomas.

Treatment

Therapeutic options for treatment of cats with hyperthyroidism due to benign disease include anti-thyroid drugs (e.g. methimazole, carbimazole), ^{131}iodine (^{131}I) or thyroidectomy.

Anti-thyroid drugs: While cats with thyroid carcinoma may show clinical improvement when treated with anti-thyroid drugs, these drugs are not recommended for several reasons. Thyroxine exerts a negative feedback effect on the anterior pituitary gland, resulting in decreased release of thyroid-stimulating hormone (TSH). Anti-thyroid drugs may increase release of TSH from the anterior pituitary gland by decreasing secretion of thyroxine and exacerbate tumour growth due to the tropic effects of TSH. Furthermore, anti-thyroid drugs are not cytotoxic and will slow neither progression of local tumour growth nor metastasis to distant organs. The only indication for using anti-thyroid drugs in the management of thyroid carcinoma is for the purpose of initial clinical stabilization prior to ^{131}I therapy or thyroidectomy.

Beta blockers: Beta blockers such as propanolol or atenolol are useful in hyperthyroid cats that require stabilization of cardiac disease prior to surgery or ^{131}I therapy. Beta blockers decrease the cardiotoxic effects of thyroid hormones but are contraindicated in patients with overt heart failure, asthma, or chronic bronchiolar disease. Atenolol, a beta-1-selective antagonist, may be a safer choice than propranolol in patients with respiratory disease and needs to be given only once a day.

Surgery: Thyroidectomy is the initial treatment of choice in cats with suspected thyroid carcinoma, because the diagnosis must be confirmed by histopathology and because complete excision can be curative. The thyroid tumour should be completely excised if possible; however, thyroid biopsy, followed by adjunctive therapy, may be more appropriate in cats with invasive or infiltrative masses. Preservation of the parathyroid glands is more difficult in cats with invasive thyroid carcinomas treated surgically, and postoperative monitoring of serum calcium concentrations is essential for cats undergoing bilateral thyroidectomy. A cat exhibiting signs of hypocalcaemia after thyroidectomy (e.g. muscle tremors, tetany, or convulsions) should be treated with appropriate calcium and vitamin D supplementation (see later for approach to treatment of hypocalcaemia).

Even if all visible tumour is removed, many thyroid carcinomas will recur within weeks to months. Thus, in histopathologically confirmed thyroid carcinoma, thyroid scintigraphy should be repeated 4–8 weeks after thyroidectomy in order to evaluate the success of surgical removal. If tumour recurrence is confirmed, treatment with high-dose ^{131}I is recommended. Following treatment with ^{131}I, periodic re-evaluation of serum T4 concentrations and ^{99m}Tc scans should be performed every 3–6 months. If recurrence is not detected in these follow-up evaluations after 1 year, the period between evaluations can progressively be lengthened.

Iodine treatment: Treatment with ^{131}I is indicated in cats with non-resectable thyroid carcinoma, evidence of metastasis, or recurrence after thyroidectomy. Higher doses (10–30 mCi) are required for thyroid carcinoma than for adenoma. A combination of surgical resection and postoperative treatment with high doses of ^{131}I is an effective approach. Surgical removal followed by administration of 30 mCi ^{131}I in seven cats with thyroid carcinoma resulted in survival times ranging from 10 to 41 months, and none of the cats died due to thyroid carcinoma (Guptill *et al.*, 1995). Higher doses of ^{131}I necessitate longer hospitalization to allow the isotope time to decay to activity levels compatible with discharge to the home environment. The majority of cats treated with higher doses of ^{131}I become permanently hypothyroid and require supplementation with levothyroxine.

Thyroid tumours in dogs

Clinically significant canine thyroid tumours are usually large, non-functional, unilateral, invasive and malignant. While one-third of all canine thyroid neoplasms detected at necropsy are small adenomas, these benign lesions rarely result in significant clinical signs. Malignant thyroid tumours account for 70–100% of clinically detected thyroid tumours in dogs and most are carcinomas. The majority of affected dogs are euthyroid; however, approximately 20% of thyroid carcinomas are functional, producing clinical signs of hyperthyroidism. Hypothyroidism due to destruction of normal thyroid tissue by the tumour has been reported in 6–20% of malignant thyroid tumours (Marks *et al.*, 1994; Théon *et al.*, 2000).

Most canine thyroid carcinomas arise from follicular cells, but parafollicular C-cell (medullary) carcinomas also occur. Canine thyroid carcinoma is characterized by local tissue invasion and a high rate of metastasis, particularly to the lungs, retropharyngeal lymph nodes and the liver. Other less common sites of metastasis include the base of the heart, spleen, kidney, bone marrow, prostate, adrenal gland, bones and spinal cord.

Clinical features

Canine thyroid carcinomas are most common in middle-aged and older animals, with a mean age of 10 years. Breeds at increased risk include Boxer, Beagle and Golden Retriever. Clinical signs due to the presence of a space-occupying cervical mass are the most common. Affected dogs may exhibit dyspnoea, coughing, dysphagia, retching, anorexia, facial oedema and dysphonia. Other clinical signs include vomiting, listlessness and weight loss. In dogs with functional thyroid tumours, polyuria and polydipsia, restless behaviour, polyphagia, weight loss, diarrhoea and tachycardia may be observed. Signs of hypothyroidism may be present in dogs that are hypothyroid. Physical examination findings include a firm, usually asymmetrical mass in the cervical region (Figure 20.4) and often submandibular lymphadenopathy. Dyspnoea, cachexia and neck pain occur less commonly. Cardiac arrhythmias or murmurs may be detected in hyperthyroid dogs.

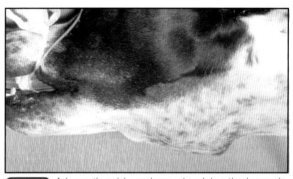

20.4 A large thyroid carcinoma involving the larynx in an 8-year-old neutered male English Pointer.

Diagnosis

Non-specific abnormalities, such as mild normocytic normochromic anaemia, leucocytosis, mild azotaemia and elevations in serum liver enzyme activities are typical findings on the minimum blood work database. Hypercalcaemia has been reported in dogs with thyroid carcinoma and may be due to either concurrent primary hyperparathyroidism or a paraneoplastic phenomenon. Some dogs with primary thyroid neoplasia have evidence of other primary endocrine tumours, in particular parathyroid tumours and adrenal tumours.

Thoracic and abdominal radiography and abdominal ultrasonography may identify heart-based, pulmonary, hepatic or other visceral metastases. Up to 60% of dogs with thyroid carcinoma have radiographic evidence of pulmonary metastasis at the time of diagnosis. Cervical ultrasonography and computed tomography (CT) may be useful in determining the extent of tumour invasion. Thyroid testing (T4, free T4, TSH) should be performed to determine thyroid status. Increased serum thyroid hormone concentrations due to the presence of autoantibodies to tri-iodothyronine (T3) or T4 are an important differential for canine hyperthyroidism.

Fine-needle aspiration cytology may be useful in differentiating a thyroid tumour from an abscess, cyst, salivary mucocele, or enlarged lymph node, but cytology is not helpful in definitively differentiating benign from malignant thyroid neoplasia. Aspirates are frequently non-diagnostic due to peripheral blood contamination. Use of larger biopsy instruments, such as a large-bore needle or Tru-cut biopsy needle, is not recommended, because most thyroid tumours are highly vascular. A surgical biopsy is necessary for differentiation between a thyroid adenoma and carcinoma. If the mass is clearly not amenable to complete surgical excision, an incisional wedge biopsy should be performed.

Nuclear imaging is useful in the diagnostic evaluation of dogs with thyroid tumours, and sodium pertechnetate is the isotope of choice. In a study of 29 dogs with thyroid carcinoma, ^{99m}Tc scans were abnormal in all dogs (Marks *et al.*, 1994) and location of the tumour at surgery correlated well with scintigraphic findings. Dogs with non-functional thyroid carcinomas tend to have poorly circumscribed heterogenous isotope uptake (Figure 20.5). Dogs with functional carcinomas usually have intense well circumscribed and homogenous uptake of isotope on ^{99m}Tc scan (Figure 20.6). Scintigraphy is no more sensitive than thoracic radiography for detection of pulmonary metastases.

Treatment

Surgery: Surgical resection is the initial treatment of choice for dogs with thyroid tumours, regardless of the functional status of the tumour. Thyroid adenomas are generally well encapsulated and more amenable to surgical resection than thyroid carcinomas. Even if complete removal of the tumour is not possible, surgical debulking provides tissue samples for histopathological evaluation and may also alleviate some of the clinical signs (e.g. dyspnoea, dysphagia, dysphonia) associated with the tumour. Surgery is best performed by an experienced surgeon because of the vascularity of thyroid tumours and the risk of damage to the recurrent laryngeal nerves, parathyroid glands and major blood vessels. Thyroid tumours that are mobile and well circumscribed are the best surgical candidates. Successful outcome after thyroidectomy has been reported in 20/82 of dogs with thyroid carcinoma (Klein *et al.*, 1995). Dogs were preselected for surgery based on the presence of a freely movable mass and the absence of evidence of metastasis. Median survival time (MST) was >36 months. In dogs with extensive local tumour infiltration or with distant metastases, however, surgical resection is strictly palliative. When the tumour is >100 cm³, the probability of metastasis is extremely likely, even if not clinically apparent. Adjunctive chemotherapy, palliative radiation therapy, or radioiodide therapy should be considered in these patients.

Chemotherapy: Chemotherapy alone is unlikely to result in total remission of thyroid carcinoma. Doxorubicin, cisplatin and combination therapy utilizing doxorubicin, cyclophosphamide and vincristine

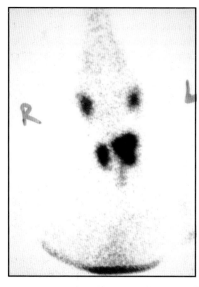

20.5 Ventrodorsal view from a technetium scan of a dog, showing heterogenous uptake (shape and density) into a thyroid mass. Histopathology of the excised mass indicated thyroid adenocarcinoma.

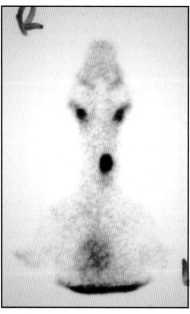

20.6 Ventrodorsal view from a technetium scan of a hyperthyroid dog, showing homogenous uptake into a thyroid mass. Histopathology of excised tissue was consistent with a well differentiated thyroid carcinoma.

have been used empirically to treat thyroid carcinoma in the dog, with MSTs ranging from 3 to 9 months. There is no strong evidence base to support the use of chemotherapy for canine thyroid carcinoma.

Radiotherapy: External beam radiation therapy is effective for local control of unresectable thyroid tumours, but is ineffective in prevention of metastatic disease. An 80% 1-year survival rate has been reported in 25 dogs with unresectable thyroid carcinomas (Théon, 2000); 28% of the dogs developed metastasis. Maximal reduction in tumour size reduction was observed at 8–22 months. Acute complications of external beam radiation include changes in vocalization, dysphagia, skin changes, oesophagitis, pharyngitis, laryngitis and hypothyroidism.

Iodine treatment: In dogs with unresectable thyroid carcinomas that concentrate radioiodine based on nuclear scintigraphy, treatment with ^{131}I is a viable alternative to external beam irradiation. In a retrospective case series of 39 dogs with non-resectable thyroid carcinoma treated with ^{131}I, MST ranged from 366 days in dogs with metastatic disease to 839 days in dogs with local disease (Turrel *et al.*, 2006). Although 50% of the dogs were hyperthyroid, there was no association between the pre-treatment T4 concentration and survival. In a second study, 43 dogs were treated with ^{131}I at doses ranging from 55 to 185 mCi, either alone or as an adjunct to surgery (Worth *et al.*, 2005). MSTs were 34 months in the dogs treated with surgery and ^{131}I, and 30 months in the dogs treated with ^{131}I alone, compared with 3 months in untreated dogs. These studies suggest that ^{131}I is a viable treatment in dogs with unresectable thyroid carcinoma and that the benefit of ^{131}I is not limited to dogs with functional thyroid.

Prognosis
Canine thyroid carcinoma has a much more guarded prognosis than feline thyroid carcinoma due to the propensity for both local tissue invasion, metastasis to distant sites and relative resistance to ^{131}I treatment.

Parathyroid gland tumours

Parathyroid gland tumours cause primary hyperparathyroidism (PHPT) due to autonomous production of parathyroid hormone (PTH) by neoplastic parathyroid 'chief' cells. A solitary parathyroid adenoma/hyperplasia is the most common cause of PHPT and parathyroid carcinoma is rare. Excess PTH secretion from the parathyroid gland causes hypercalcaemia through direct and indirect actions of the hormone. PTH increases renal conservation of calcium in the distal tubules and collecting ducts, decreases proximal tubular resorption of phosphorus and enhances osteoclastic activity, promoting release of calcium and phosphorus from bone. PTH also facilitates renal conversion of 25-hydroxycholecalciferol to 1,25-dihydroxycholecalciferol. Activated vitamin D increases intestinal absorption of calcium and phosphorus. Bone resorption and intestinal absorption of phosphorus promote increased serum phosphorus concentrations, but this is insufficient to counteract renal phosphorus loss, resulting in a net decrease in serum phosphorus concentrations. Increased calcium concentration results in a negative feedback effect on PTH secretion, quickly returning calcium levels to normal. In animals with primary hyperparathyroidism, neoplastic parathyroid tissue is insensitive to increasing serum concentrations of calcium, and synthesis and secretion of PTH continues despite persistent hypercalcaemia.

Parathyroid tumours in dogs

Clinical features
Primary hyperparathyroidism affects mainly older dogs. The mean age of onset in dogs is 11 years (range 6–17 years) and there is no sex predisposition (Feldman *et al.*, 2005). Primary hyperparathyroidism is inherited as an autosomal dominant trait in the Keeshond but the mutation locus has not yet been identified (Goldstein *et al.*, 2007). Fifty per cent of dogs with PHPT present due to clinical signs of urolithiasis or urinary tract infection. Signs directly attributable to hypercalcaemia occur in <50% of affected dogs and include polyuria, polydipsia, weakness, decreased activity, inappetence, weight loss, muscle atrophy, vomiting, shivering and trembling. Other rarer manifestations include seizures, lameness and bone pain. Hypercalcaemia is an incidental finding in >30% of dogs with PHPT. The physical examination is usually normal. Muscle atrophy, weakness and thin body condition occur in some dogs.

The most consistent laboratory abnormalities in dogs with PHPT are hypercalcaemia, hypophosphataemia and low urine specific gravity (SG). Hypercalcaemia may be mild to marked, with total calcium ranging from 12.1 to 23.0 mg/dl (3.03–5.75 mmol/l). Mild increases in total serum calcium concentrations may be secondary to hyperalbuminaemia, because approximately 50% of total calcium is protein-bound. Ionized serum calcium concentration is unaffected by changes in plasma protein concentration and is useful for confirmation of mild hypercalcaemia. The majority of dogs with PHPT have a serum phosphorus level either within or below the reference range. Most dogs with primary hyperparathyroidism have urine SG <1.030. Renal failure is present in <4% of dogs with PHPT, most likely because hypercalcaemia typically occurs in conjunction with a normal or low phosphorus concentration. Increased activity of alkaline phosphatase is found in 40% of dogs with PHPT secondary to osteolysis. Approximately 30% of dogs have cystic calculi (calcium phosphate or calcium oxalate), most likely due to hypercalciuria secondary to increased glomerular filtration of calcium, though other factors may play a role.

Diagnosis
Diagnosis of PHPT is by ruling out other more common causes of hypercalcaemia such as non-parathyroid neoplasia (Figure 20.7) (see also Chapter 4), in conjunction with documentation of an inappropriate PTH concentration (normal or high) in the presence of hypercalcaemia and a low or normal serum phosphorus concentration (Figure 20.8). PTH concentration should be below the reference range in dogs with hypercalcaemia and thus a normal PTH does not exclude PHPT. In one study, PTH concentrations were within the laboratory reference range in 73% of 210 dogs with PHPT (Feldman *et al.*, 2005).

- Primary hyperparathyroidism (due to parathyroid hyperplasia, adenoma, carcinoma)
- Hypercalcaemia of malignancy (lymphoma, apocrine gland adenocarcinoma, multiple myeloma, melanoma, carcinomas)
- Chronic renal failure
- Hypoadrenocorticism
- Vitamin D toxicosis
- Nutritional secondary hyperparathyroidism
- Granulomatous diseases (e.g. blastomycosis, histoplasmosis, schistosomiasis)
- Idiopathic hypercalcaemia (cats only)
- Haemoconcentration
- Laboratory error

20.7 Causes of increased blood calcium levels in dogs and cats.

Serum measurement	Primary hyperparathyroidism	Hypercalcaemia of malignancy	Chronic renal failure	Hypervitaminosis D
Total calcium	↑	↑	↑ or N or ↓	N or ↑
Ionized calcium	↑	↑	N or ↓	↑
Phosphorus	N or ↓	N or ↓	↑ or N	↑ or N
Parathyroid hormone (PTH)	↑ or N	↓	↑ or N	↓
PTH-related peptide (PTH-rP)	↓	↑ or N	↑ or N	↓
Vitamin D	↑ or N	↓	↓	↑

20.8 Interpretation of diagnostic testing in dogs with hypercalcaemic disorders. ↑ = raised; N = normal; ↓ = decreased

Cervical ultrasonography may be useful to confirm the presence of one or more enlarged parathyroid glands in dogs with suspected PHPT. Affected dogs usually have one round or oval mass in close association with one thyroid lobe. Parathyroid gland tumours ranging from 3 mm to 23 mm in diameter have been identified in PHPT (Figure 20.9). Ultrasound findings correlate well with findings at surgery, but ultrasound is subjective and dependent on the skill of the operator. About 10% of dogs with PHPT have bilateral parathyroid gland involvement (Rasor *et al.*, 2007).

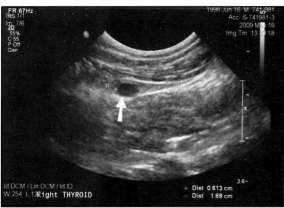

20.9 Ultrasound image of a single parathyroid gland adenoma (arrowed) in a 10-year-old neutered male Long-haired Dachshund.

Treatment

Treatment of parathyroid neoplasia should include both acute medical management of hypercalcaemia (if warranted) and ablation of abnormal parathyroid gland tissue. Hypercalcaemia should be treated medically if increased serum calcium concentrations cause clinical signs (see Chapter 4). Parathyroidectomy results in long-term control of hypercalcaemia and provides tissue for a definitive diagnosis.

Diuretic therapy: Correction of fluid deficits and saline diuresis will promote renal excretion of calcium. Diuretic therapy should be initiated only after fluid deficits are corrected. Loop diuretics, such as furosemide, inhibit calcium reabsorption in the thick ascending limb of the loop of Henle, enhancing calciuresis. If saline diuresis and concomitant diuretic

therapy fail to decrease serum calcium concentrations effectively, glucocorticoids may be used to decrease calcium concentrations in patients with primary hyperparathyroidism. Glucocorticoid treatment should be avoided until all diagnostic samples have been collected.

Surgery and heat ablation: Definitive therapy by surgical parathyroidectomy or ultrasound-guided heat ablation is recommended, even in dogs with mild hypercalcaemia, because the severity of hypercalcaemia tends to worsen with time and because of the risk of urolithiasis. Tumours may be located in either the internal or external parathyroid glands. Bilateral disease has been reported with primary hyperparathyroidism, particularly with parathyroid gland hyperplasia. If the internal parathyroid gland is involved, the associated thyroid gland should also be removed. Ultrasound-guided heat ablation is an acceptable alternative to parathyroidectomy but availability of the equipment is currently very limited and success is highly dependent upon the skill of the operator (Rasor *et al.*, 2007). Chemical ablation using ultrasound-guided ethanol injection has a lower success rate and this technique has largely been replaced by the heat ablation technique.

Treatment of postoperative hypocalcaemia: Because of the low incidence of malignancy, the long-term prognosis in patients with PHPT is good with appropriate and early surgical treatment. The most common and potentially life-threatening complication is postoperative hypocalcaemia due to atrophy of normal parathyroid tissue. Hypocalcaemia typically occurs between 24 hours and 6 days after surgery. Mild hypocalcaemia without clinical signs is common and does not require treatment. Clinically symptomatic hypocalcaemia is most likely in dogs that have a calcium concentration >14 mg/dl (3.5 mmol/l) prior to surgery, so prophylactic treatment with calcitriol and calcium supplementation immediately following recovery from anaesthesia is recommended in these patients.

Parenteral calcium supplementation (10% calcium gluconate at a dose of 0.5–1.5 ml/kg as an intravenous infusion over 10–30 minutes) should be the initial approach to treatment of clinical hypocalcaemia.

Electrocardiographic monitoring is recommended during calcium administration. Once serum calcium concentrations are at the lower end of normal, treatment with calcitriol and oral calcium supplementation should be initiated; in the meantime normocalcaemia should be maintained by intravenous or subcutaneous administration of calcium gluconate (diluted 50:50 with 0.9% sodium chloride) approximately every 6–8 hours until vitamin D and oral calcium supplementation becomes effective (1–4 days). Calcitriol has a fast onset of action (1–4 days) and a short half-life (<24 hours). The recommended dose for calcitriol in both the dog and cat is 20–30 ng (**nanograms**) per kg per day. Calcium carbonate is the oral calcium preparation of choice because of its high concentration of elemental calcium. Calcium supplementation should provide 50–100 mg/kg/day of elemental calcium. Serum calcium concentrations should be maintained at the lower end of the normal range (8–10 mg/dl) (2.0–2.5 mmol/l).

After vitamin D and calcium supplementation have been initiated, serum calcium concentrations should be monitored daily until they stabilize in the lower end of the normal range; then weekly until a stable dose regimen is achieved. The dose of vitamin D can be reduced in 25% decrements every 2–4 weeks until vitamin D therapy is completely discontinued, with serum calcium concentrations measured after each dose adjustment. Calcium supplementation may then be slowly withdrawn.

The most important complication associated with therapy for hypocalcemia is hypercalcaemia. Owners should be advised to watch for recurrence of signs of hypercalcaemia, such as polyuria and polydipsia. If hypercalcaemia occurs, supplemental therapy should be discontinued immediately and saline diuresis and furosemide treatment should be instituted if hypercalcaemia is severe. Persistent elevations in serum calcium concentrations despite withdrawal of vitamin D and calcium supplementation suggest recurrence of hyperparathyroidism.

Prognosis
Appropriate medical and surgical management of PHPT results in a good to excellent prognosis. Non-reversible renal disease, identification of a metastatic parathyroid carcinoma and inadequate attention to calcium and vitamin D supplementation are factors that contribute to a less favourable outcome.

Parathyroid tumours in cats
Primary hyperparathyroidism is rare in cats. Parathyroid adenoma, hyperplasia and carcinoma have all been reported in cats. In contrast to dogs with hyperparathyroidism and hypercalcaemia, the most common presenting signs in the cat are anorexia, lethargy and constipation, with polyuria and polydipsia occurring less frequently. The enlarged parathyroid glands may be palpable in some cats. Calcium concentrations ranging from 11.1 to 22.8 mg/dl (2.8–5.7 mmol/l) have been reported in cats with PHPT. Diagnosis and treatment of PHPT in cats are similar to those described for dogs.

Pituitary gland tumours

Pituitary tumours in dogs and cats may be either functional or non-functional. Functional tumours may secrete either growth hormone, causing acromegaly, or adrenocorticotrophic hormone (ACTH), causing hyperadrenocorticism (Cushing's disease).

Feline acromegaly (hypersomatotropism)
Acromegaly is caused by excess secretion of growth hormone (GH) from a pituitary adenoma. Excess circulating GH causes increased secretion of insulin-like growth factor I (IGF-1) from the liver. Increased GH causes insulin resistance, carbohydrate intolerance, hyperglycaemia and diabetes mellitus. The anabolic effects of IGF-1 cause proliferation of bone, cartilage and soft tissues, with organomegaly. Feline acromegaly is believed to be a rare condition, though recent studies suggest that it may be a more common cause of insulin resistance in diabetic cats than has been previously recognized.

Clinical features
Most cats with acromegaly are middle-aged or older (median 10 years, range 4–17) and 90% are male. Clinical signs include polyuria, polydipsia, polyphagia (due to insulin-resistant diabetes mellitus), large body size, weight gain (despite poor glycaemic control) and enlargement of the head and extremities (Figures 20.10 and 20.11). All reported cases have had concurrent diabetes mellitus (Niessen *et al.*, 2007). Central nervous system signs, including lethargy, circling, seizures and dementia, can occur due to extrasellar expansion of the pituitary tumour.

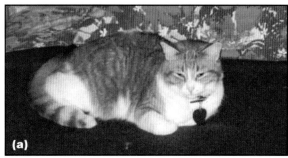

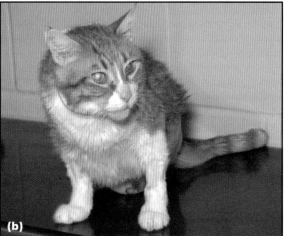

20.10 A 10-year-old castrated male cat **(a)** before and **(b)** after development of acromegaly.

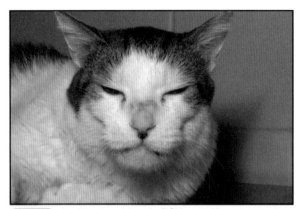

20.11 An 11-year-old male DSH cat with acromegaly, demonstrating enlargement of the head and mild prognathia inferior.

Physical examination may reveal abdominal organomegaly, inferior prognathia, cataracts, clubbed paws, broad facial features, cardiac murmurs or arrhythmias, respiratory stridor, lameness, peripheral neuropathy and central neurological signs attributable to an enlarging pituitary mass. Although weight loss due to poorly regulated diabetes mellitus may occur initially, a key finding in acromegalic cats is weight gain or a stable weight in a diabetic cat with other indicators of poor glycaemic control. Some cats with acromegaly may be phenotypically indistinguishable from normal cats.

Diagnosis

A tentative diagnosis of acromegaly is based on the presence of insulin-resistant diabetes mellitus, clinical signs and growth hormone and IGF-1 concentrations. The most common abnormalities on blood and urine testing are hyperglycaemia and glucosuria. Other laboratory abnormalities include hyperproteinaemia, hypercholesterolaemia and hyperphosphataemia. Mild to severe azotaemia, proteinuria, increased liver enzyme activity and erythrocytosis may also be present. Thoracic radiographs may reveal cardiomegaly or other signs of congestive heart failure in more severely affected cats. Echocardiographic evaluation may demonstrate thickening of the intraventricular septum and the left ventricular caudal wall. Radiography of affected joints may reveal evidence of degenerative joint disease with osteophyte formation, soft tissue swelling or joint space collapse. Other radiographic abnormalities may include organ enlargement (hepatomegaly and renomegaly), thickening of the bony ridges of the calvarium, inferior prognathism and spondylosis deformans.

Measurement of IGF-1 is a good screening test for acromegaly. The assay has a specificity of 92% and sensitivity of 84% (Berg et al., 2007). Some poorly controlled diabetic cats have increased IGF-1 concentrations, but in most cases these increases are not as high as in those cats with documented acromegaly. Most cats with acromegaly have increased serum GH concentration, though in some cases GH concentration may be normal because of short half-life and episodic secretion. A tentative diagnosis of acromegaly based on measurement of

GH or IGF-1 should be confirmed by either contrast-enhanced CT or MRI of the brain (Figure 20.12) to document the presence of a pituitary mass. In one case of confirmed acromegaly, acidophil proliferation within the pituitary gland did not result in a detectable mass on CT or MRI. Thus even negative MRI findings do not preclude a diagnosis of acromegaly (Niessen et al, 2007).

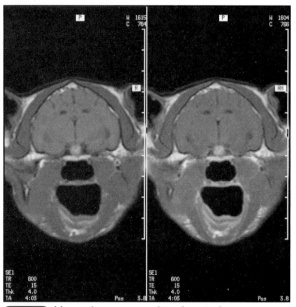

20.12 Magnetic resonance imaging study demonstrating a pituitary mass in a cat with acromegaly.

Treatment

Treatment modalities that have been effective for cats with acromegaly include radiation therapy and hypophysectomy. Radiation therapy may improve neurological signs in cats with pituitary tumours and result in decreased insulin requirements or diabetic remission in cats with acromegaly (Mayer et al., 2006; Dunning et al., 2009). Unfortunately the cost and availability of radiation therapy often limit access to treatment. Although hypophysectomy is feasible in cats, it is not routinely performed in most parts of the world. In cats in which definitive treatment of the tumour is not possible, long-term control of clinical signs of diabetes mellitus may be achieved using high doses of insulin. Because of the profound insulin resistance associated with acromegaly, hypoglycaemic complications using this approach are unusual. Mean survival of 20 months was reported in a study of 14 cats with acromegaly, despite the fact that only 2 cats were treated with radiation therapy (Peterson et al., 1990). Cause of death in acromegalic cats is most commonly due to renal failure and/or congestive heart failure.

Hyperadrenocorticism

Hyperadrenocorticism (Cushing's syndrome) is an endocrine disorder caused by overproduction of cortisol from the adrenal cortex due to the presence of either a pituitary or an adrenal gland tumour.

Secretion of cortisol by the adrenal gland is under the control of the hypothalamic–pituitary–adrenal axis. The hypothalamus produces corticotropin-releasing hormone (CRH) which stimulates the production of adrenocorticotrophic hormone (ACTH) by the pituitary gland. ACTH stimulates the adrenal cortex to produce cortisol. Cortisol decreases ACTH and CRH production by the pituitary and hypothalamus by negative feedback. In pituitary-dependent hyperadrenocorticism (PDH), cortisol inhibition is inadequate to inhibit the production of ACTH by an autonomously functioning pituitary tumour, resulting in adrenal hyperplasia and increased concentrations of plasma cortisol. With a functional adrenal tumour (AT), hypercortisolaemia is caused by increased synthesis and secretion of cortisol by the tumour that is no longer dependent on the presence of ACTH to stimulate cortisol production. The numerous gluconeogenic, lipolytic, catabolic, anti-inflammatory and immunosuppressive effects of glucocorticoids result in the clinical signs of hyperadrenocorticism.

Hyperadrenocorticism in dogs

Eighty five per cent of cases of canine hyperadrenocorticism are due to PDH and 15% are due to a functional AT. Pituitary tumours are usually benign adenomas. Fifty per cent of adrenal tumours are benign and 50% are malignant. Dogs with concurrent PDH and AT have been described.

Clinical features

Hyperadrenocorticism affects middle-aged and older dogs. The median age is 11 years. It has been diagnosed in numerous breeds, with Poodles, Dachshunds, Beagles, German Shepherd Dogs, Boston Terriers and Boxers being over-represented. There is a slightly increased predisposition for females (55–65%). Larger breeds may be affected more frequently with AT than smaller breeds.

Clinical signs include polydipsia, polyuria, polyphagia, hepatomegaly, muscle weakness, panting, exercise intolerance, lethargy and development of a pendulous abdomen. Dermatological abnormalities such as bilaterally symmetrical alopecia (Figure 20.13), thin skin, easy bruising, pyoderma, calcinosis cutis, cutaneous hyperpigmentation and seborrhoea are also common. Other clinical manifestations include reproductive abnormalities, pulmonary thromboembolism, systemic hypertension, proteinuria, increased susceptibility to infections (especially of the urinary tract), and insulin resistance. Neurological abnormalities may include pseudomyotonia, facial nerve paralysis, and central nervous system signs. Stupor, seizures, circling, ataxia, and blindness are suggestive of an enlarging pituitary tumour.

Diagnosis

Common abnormalities on blood testing include leucocytosis, monocytosis, eosinopenia, lymphopenia and mild polycythaemia. Increased levels of alkaline phosphatase (ALP) are found in 95% of dogs with hyperadrenocorticism. Serum alanine aminotransferase (ALT) concentrations are more mildly increased. Other biochemical changes include hypercholesterolaemia, hyperglycaemia, hypophosphataemia, hypernatraemia and hypokalaemia. Urinalysis may reveal low urine SG, glucosuria and evidence of urinary tract infection. Because urinary tract infection may be occult, urine culture and sensitivity should be performed routinely in dogs with suspected hyperadrenocorticism.

A diagnosis of hyperadrenocorticism should be confirmed by the low-dose dexamethasone suppression (LDDS) test, ACTH stimulation test, or both. An increased urine cortisol:creatinine (C:Cr) ratio in a dog with obvious clinical signs of hyperadrenocorticism is also very supportive of the diagnosis. PDH must then be differentiated from AT, by a combination of the low- and high-dose (HDDS) dexamethasone suppression tests, measurement of endogenous ACTH concentrations, abdominal radiography and abdominal ultrasonography.

ACTH stimulation test: This test relies on the assumption that hyperplastic or neoplastic adrenals have abnormally large reserves of cortisol and therefore hyper-respond to maximal stimulation by ACTH (Figure 20.14). Plasma samples are collected prior

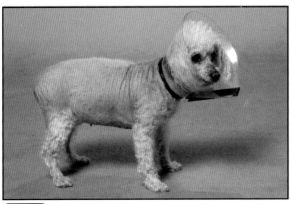

20.13 A poodle showing clinical manifestations of hyperadrenocorticism. Note the alopecia and thin skin.

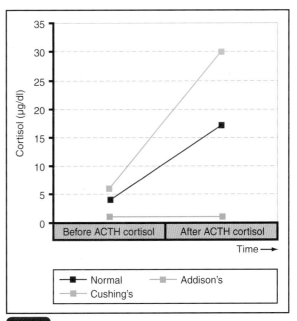

20.14 ACTH stimulation test results.

to, and 1 hour following, administration of synthetic ACTH (5 μg/kg i.m. or i.v.). The ACTH stimulation test is abnormal in 85–90% of PDH cases and in 50% of AT. The ACTH stimulation test allows differentiation of iatrogenic from spontaneous hyperadrenocorticism and is less affected by stress and concurrent disease than the LDDS test. The ACTH stimulation test does not distinguish between AT and PDH. Because of the low sensitivity of this test, a diagnosis of hyperadrenocorticism should not be excluded based on a normal ACTH stimulation test result.

LDDS test: This test is more sensitive for hyperadrenocorticism and is abnormal in 95% of dogs. It does not distinguish spontaneous from iatrogenic hyperadrenocorticism. Plasma samples are collected prior to and 8 hours following administration of dexamethasone (0.01 mg/kg i.v.). An additional sample collected at 4 hours after dexamethasone administration may help to differentiate dogs with PDH from those with AT. Administration of dexamethasone should suppress production of ACTH from the normal pituitary and decrease cortisol secretion (Figure 20.15). Suppression persists in the normal dog for 24–48 hours. Since dexamethasone is not detected by the assay for cortisol, the decrease in cortisol can be measured despite dexamethasone administration. Adrenal tumours function independently of ACTH, while a hyperplastic or neoplastic pituitary gland is relatively resistant to negative feedback from circulating steroids. In either disorder, there is a lack of cortisol suppression 8 hours after dexamethasone administration.

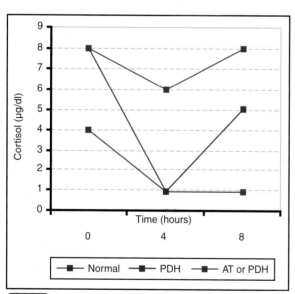

20.15 Low-dose dexamethasone suppression test results.

Urinary cortisol:creatinine ratio: The urine C:Cr is an estimate of 24-hour cortisol production. The measurement is made on a voided morning urine sample collected at home, so it is a very convenient initial screening test. The C:Cr ratio is a sensitive test for diagnosis of hyperadrenocorticism but has low specificity. A C:Cr ratio within the reference range is helpful in ruling out hyperadrenocorticism, but many

non-adrenal diseases also increase the C:Cr ratio and so the result should be interpreted with care. In dogs with a positive result, a second test should be performed to confirm the diagnosis.

It is important to be aware that false-positive test results may occur with all adrenal function tests, especially in dogs with other concurrent illness. Testing for hyperadrenocorticism should only be performed in dogs with appropriate clinical signs that are systemically well.

Tests to differentiate PDH from AT

The most useful endocrine tests for distinguishing AT from PDH are the HDDS and LDDS tests and measurement of endogenous ACTH concentration.

LDDS and HDDS tests: These tests rely on the fact that secretion of cortisol by adrenal tumours is unaffected by administration of dexamethasone, while in PDH the pituitary gland retains some response to the feedback effects of dexamethasone. The protocol for the high-dose (HDDS) test is the same as the low-dose test except that a 4-hour blood sample is not required and the dexamethasone dose is higher (0.1 mg/kg). Suppression is defined as a 4- or 8-hour plasma cortisol concentration after dexamethasone administration <50% of the baseline sample. Suppression of cortisol concentrations is diagnostic for PDH (see Figure 20.15) but lack of suppression is not diagnostic for AT, because 20% of PDH cases fail to suppress with the higher dose of dexamethasone. If suppression >50% is seen at 4 or 8 hours on an LDDS, an HDDS test is unnecessary.

Endogenous ACTH concentration: Dogs with functional adrenal tumours have low ACTH concentrations. Levels within or above the reference range are consistent with a diagnosis of PDH. ACTH concentrations are low or borderline in some dogs with PDH, possibly due to episodic secretion of ACTH; therefore, a low ACTH concentration alone is not enough to confirm a diagnosis of adrenal tumour. ACTH concentrations are higher in dogs with larger pituitary tumours and those with neurological signs (Kipperman *et al.*, 1992; Bosje *et al.*, 2002; Granger *et al.*, 2005). Endogenous ACTH is susceptible to rapid enzymatic degradation *in vitro* and so handling recommendations from the laboratory should be followed carefully.

Imaging: Approximately 57% of adrenal tumours are identified on abdominal radiography as a soft tissue mass or a mineralized opacity, compared with 72% with ultrasonography (Reusch and Feldman, 1991). Other radiographic findings may include hepatomegaly, osteopenia, dystrophic mineralization and distension of the urinary bladder. Thoracic radiographs may reveal evidence of metastasis, pulmonary thromboembolism or mineralization.

In dogs with PDH, ultrasonography of the adrenal glands typically reveals bilaterally symmetrical enlargement of the adrenal glands with preservation of normal adrenal architecture (Figure 20.16). The glands may not be identical in size but the difference

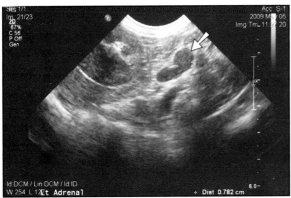

20.16 Ultrasound image of the left adrenal gland in an 8-year-old neutered male Labrador with pituitary-dependent hyperadrenocorticism. The adrenal gland is enlarged (arrowed) but has normal architecture.

in thickness is usually <5 mm (Grooters *et al.*, 1996) The size of the adrenal glands may be within the normal range in some dogs with PDH. In dogs with a functional adrenal tumour there is unilateral adrenal gland enlargement with abnormal adrenal gland architecture (Figure 20.17). Evidence of tumour thrombus within the vena cava is detected by ultrasonography in 11% of dogs with adrenocortical tumours (Kyles *et al.*, 2003) and evidence of distant metastasis to the liver, kidneys and other abdominal organs may be present. Bilateral adrenal tumours and macronodular hyperplasia of the adrenal gland in dogs with PDH may complicate the interpretation of ultrasound findings.

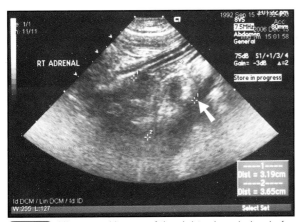

20.17 Ultrasound image of the right adrenal gland of a 5-year-old neutered female Australian Shepherd Dog with bilateral adrenal tumours. Note the rounded appearance (arrowed) and abnormal adrenal architecture.

CT is also a useful tool for evaluating the adrenal glands, especially in dogs with adrenal tumours (Figure 20.18). MRI or CT of the brain is helpful in determining pituitary tumour size in dogs with PDH. Approximately 70% of dogs with PDH have a detectable pituitary tumour on CT or MRI (Bertoy *et al.*, 1995).

Treatment of PDH

Options for treatment of dogs with PDH include either medical management with mitotane or trilostane, or surgical hypophysectomy. Radiation therapy

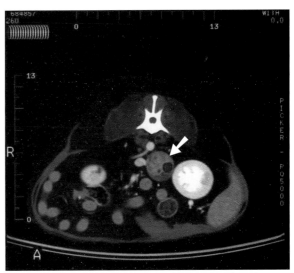

20.18 CT image of a 10-year-old neutered female mixed-breed dog with a left adrenal tumour. Note the adrenal mass (arrowed) medial to the left kidney (bright due to contrast medium).

is used for treatment of dogs with pituitary tumours that are causing neurological signs.

Medical management: Trilostane is a synthetic hormonally inactive steroid analogue that is a competitive inhibitor of the 3 β-hydroxysteroid dehydrogenase system (Neiger *et al.*, 2002). Trilostane blocks synthesis of a number of adrenal steroids, including cortisol and aldosterone. Trilostane is rapidly absorbed orally and suppression of plasma cortisol concentrations is short lived (<20 hours). The drug is well tolerated in dogs and is effective in controlling clinical signs of hyperadrenocorticism in most patients. Current recommendations are to start at a dose of 2–6 mg/kg q24h and then increase or decrease the dose based on evaluation of ACTH stimulation tests performed 4–6 hours after drug administration. Twice-a-day therapy at lower doses of 1–3 mg/kg may result in good control of clinical signs at a lower total daily dose with less risk of adverse effects than higher doses administered once a day (Vaughan *et al.*, 2008). ACTH stimulation testing should be performed 10, 30 and 90 days after start of treatment and 30 days after each dose adjustment. Adverse effects are usually mild and self-limiting and include diarrhoea, vomiting and lethargy in up to 63% of treated dogs. Both isolated glucocorticoid deficiency and overt hypoadrenocorticism occur occasionally due to trilostane treatment and in some cases resolution may take weeks to months. Adrenal necrosis (possibly secondary to high ACTH concentrations) may be the cause of hypoadrenocorticism in some dogs and there have been reports of acute death during treatment.

Mitotane (o,p'-DDD) is directly cytotoxic to the zona fasciculata and reticularis of the adrenal cortex and has been widely prescribed for the medical management of both PDH and AT. Treatment consists of an induction period, typically 7–10 days, followed by a lifelong maintenance protocol. Mitotane is initially administered at a dose of 50 mg/kg q24h, divided twice daily with food, which improves intestinal absorption. Common side effects of mitotane include weakness, vomiting, anorexia, diarrhoea and ataxia. The goal of induction is to decrease both basal and post-ACTH plasma cortisol concentrations to within normal resting ranges. The ACTH stimulation test is usually performed between days 7 and 10 of induction, or earlier if clinical signs of hyperadrenocorticism are resolving or if the dog is exhibiting signs suggestive of mitotane toxicity. If a dog still has an exaggerated response to ACTH stimulation after 10 days of induction therapy, the induction period should be continued for an additional 3–10 days, with repeat ACTH stimulation tests performed until a low post-ACTH response is achieved. Some dogs with PDH will take considerably longer than 10 days to achieve this goal.

Once adrenocortical reserve has been reduced satisfactorily, mitotane is administered at a maintenance dose of 50 mg/kg/week, divided into two or more doses. ACTH stimulation tests should be performed following 1, 3 and 6 months of therapy (or earlier, if necessary) and every 3–6 months thereafter in order to assess the efficacy of therapy. If plasma cortisol concentrations after ACTH stimulation increase above the resting range, the mitotane dose should be increased. Side effects of mitotane administration during the maintenance period are similar to those observed during the induction period. If side effects are observed, temporary discontinuation of mitotane therapy may be necessary until adverse clinical signs resolve.

In a retrospective study of dogs treated with either mitotane ($n = 25$) or trilostane ($n = 123$), long-term survival was not statistically different between the groups (Barker et al., 2005). MST in the mitotane group was 708 days (range 33–1399) and in the trilostane group was 662 days (range 8–1971). Other drugs that have been reported to be effective in dogs with PDH include ketoconazole, l-deprenyl, retinoic acid and cabergoline.

Radiation therapy: Radiotherapy improves outcome in dogs with PDH that have associated neurological signs due to a pituitary tumour, and in dogs with pituitary tumours >0.8–1.0 cm in diameter. Neurological abnormalities attributed to the presence of a space-occupying pituitary mass include change in behaviour, inappetence, obtundation, aggressiveness, anisocoria, apparent blindness and seizures. Interestingly there is poor correlation between development of neurological signs in dogs with PDH and the presence of a pituitary tumour on CT or MRI scan (Wood et al., 2007).

Radiation therapy has been reported to increase survival and improve neurological signs in dogs with pituitary masses. Complications associated with radiation therapy include alopecia and leucotrichia. Resolution of associated endocrine signs after radiation therapy is not consistent and may be delayed for several months; therefore dogs with PDH may need continued medical treatment. Dogs that present with more severe neurological impairment (e.g. stupor, seizures) have a worse outcome than dogs

that present with signs of mild neurological impairment. Likewise, dogs with large tumours have a poorer prognosis than dogs with smaller tumours.

Transphenoidal hypophysectomy: Hypophysectomy has been used successfully to treat PDH in dogs, but the technical expertise required limits the availability of this treatment. In 150 dogs undergoing hypophysectomy for treatment of PDH, the 1- and 2-year survival rates were 84% and 76%, respectively (Hanson et al., 2005). Complications include procedure-related mortality, incomplete hypophysectomy, reduced tear production and central diabetes insipidus. The prognosis is worse for dogs with larger pituitary tumours.

Treatment for adrenal-dependent hyperadrenocorticism

Adrenalectomy: Surgical adrenalectomy is the treatment of choice for ATs because it can provide permanent resolution of hyperadrenocorticism. However, patient selection is important, because perioperative mortality is high (20%) (Kyles et al., 2003; Schwartz et al., 2008). Adrenalectomy should be reserved for patients that do not have extensive tumour invasion or metastasis and those that are not severely debilitated. Presurgical treatment with mitotane or trilostane for 1–3 months may be indicated in dogs with severe clinical signs of hyperadrenocorticism.

Patients with ATs require close monitoring during and immediately following surgery and must be adequately supported with careful intravenous fluid therapy, glucocorticoid supplementation and mineralocorticoid administration if necessary. Without adequate glucocorticoid supplementation, removal of a unilateral AT will result in life-threatening hypoadrenocorticism, because of atrophy of the contralateral adrenal gland. Glucocorticoid replacement can be provided with dexamethasone administered in intravenous fluids over 6 hours as soon as the tumour is identified. Alternatively, hydrocortisone as a continuous infusion will provide glucocorticoid and mineralocorticoid supplementation. Blood pressure, central venous pressure, electrolytes, blood urea nitrogen and blood glucose should be carefully monitored during and after surgery. If clinical or laboratory evidence for mineralocorticoid deficiency is evident following surgery, mineralocorticoid supplementation (desoxycorticosterone pivalate or fludrocortisone acetate) should be administered. After surgery, oral supplementation with prednisone can be initiated once the patient is bright, alert and eating. Glucocorticoid and mineralocorticoids should be gradually tapered over several months.

The prognosis for dogs undergoing adrenalectomy is good in those that survive the perioperative period. MSTs of 690–778 days have been reported (Anderson et al., 2001; Schwartz et al., 2008). Dogs with ATs that require concurrent nephrectomy (Figure 20.19) and cause intraoperative haemorrhage have a guarded prognosis. Immediate postoperative complications such as acute renal failure, pancreatitis, pneumonia, and pulmonary artery thromboembolism occur in up to 35% of patients.

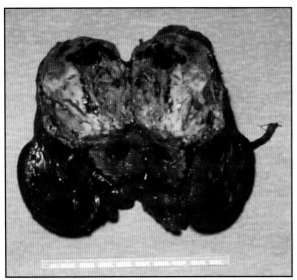

20.19 A large adrenal mass invading a kidney, seen after concurrent adrenalectomy and nephrectomy.

Medical management: This may be more appropriate for some dogs with ATs, such as dogs with large tumours, metastatic lesions in the lungs, liver, or other organs, and severely debilitated patients. Dogs with ATs generally improve in response to medical therapy with mitotane and the tumour may shrink during mitotane treatment. In most cases higher doses of mitotane are required to control clinical signs than in dogs with PDH. In a study of 32 dogs with ATs that were treated with mitotane, the MST was 12 months and final maintenance dosage ranged from 35 to 1275 mg/kg/week (Kintzer and Peterson, 1994). Some dogs had prolonged survival times and dogs without metastatic disease survived longer. The recommended initial induction dosage is 50–75 mg/kg q24h for 10–14 days with concurrent prednisone administration (0.2 mg/kg), followed by an initial maintenance dosage of 75–100 mg/kg/week.

Hyperadrenocorticism in cats

Clinical features

Cats with hyperadrenocorticism are middle-aged or older (median 10 years, range 5–16 years) and females are slightly over-represented. Most have diabetes mellitus at the time of diagnosis. Clinical signs include insulin-resistant diabetes mellitus (polyuria, polydipsia, polyphagia, weight loss and peripheral neuropathy), lethargy, abdominal enlargement or pot-bellied appearance, muscle atrophy, unkempt hair coat (Figure 20.20), bilaterally symmetrical alopecia, cutaneous fragility and recurrent abscess formation. The physical examination may reveal hepatomegaly, seborrhoea and cutaneous lacerations. Skin fragility may be so severe that tearing of the skin occurs during routine grooming (Figure 20.21). Virilization, oestrous behaviour and hyperaldosteronism may occur in cats with adrenal tumours that secrete adrenal steroids other than cortisol.

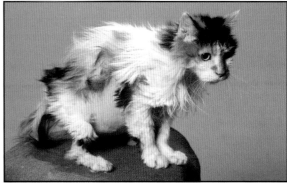

20.20 A 13-year-old neutered female DSH cat with PDH.

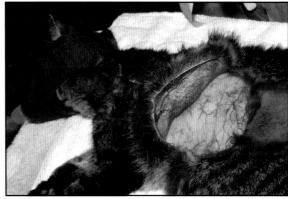

20.21 Skin laceration induced by grooming in a 10-year-old neutered male DSH cat with PDH.

Diagnosis

The results of a CBC, biochemical panel and urinalysis are usually typical of cats with diabetes mellitus. Increased ALP and ALT, hypercholesterolaemia, hyperglycaemia and low BUN are common. Endocrine tests used in diagnosis of feline hyperadrenocorticism include the ACTH stimulation test, the LDDS test and urine C:Cr ratio.

LDDS test: This is the test of choice for diagnosis of feline hyperadrenocorticism and is performed using a higher dose of dexamethasone (0.1 mg/kg i.v.) than in the dog. A baseline blood sample is collected and additional samples are collected at 4 and 8 hours after dexamethasone administration. Cortisol concentration will be suppressed (<1.5 µg/dl) (41.4 nmol/l) at 8 hours in normal cats but not in cats with hyperadrenocorticism. A few cats with hyperadrenocorticism will suppress normally on the LDDS. If the index of suspicion for hyperadrenocorticism is high, a second test using the lower dose of dexamethasone (0.01 mg/kg) can be performed but some normal cats will fail to suppress at this dose.

ACTH stimulation test: This test is less sensitive than the LDDS test. Synthetic ACTH is administered at a dose of 125 µg/cat either i.v. or i.m. Samples are at baseline, and then at 30 and 60 minutes after administration of ACTH. A post-ACTH cortisol of >15 µg/dl (414 nmol/l) at either 30 or 60 minutes after administration is consistent with a diagnosis of hyperadrenocorticism.

C:Cr ratio: This is a useful screening test for hyper-adrenocorticism. Urine for measurement of the C:Cr ratio should be collected at home to minimize the influence of stress. Hyperadrenocorticism is unlikely if the result is normal. Increased values occur in cats with hyperadrenocorticism, but increases may also occur in cats with other concurrent illness and so additional testing should be used for confirmation.

Tests to differentiate PDH from AT

PDH occurs in 85% of cats with spontaneous hyper-adrenocorticism, while 15% have functional ATs. Abdominal ultrasonography is the most useful diagnostic method for differentiation of PDH from AT. In equivocal cases, the HDDS test (1 mg/kg) or measurement of endogenous ACTH concentration may be helpful.

Treatment

Unfortunately medical management of hyperadreno-corticism is less successful in the cat than in the dog. Moreover, cats with hyperadrenocorticism are often poor surgical candidates. Thus the long-term prognosis in cats with hyperadrenocorticism is guarded.

Medical management: Trilostane is currently the most effective drug for medical management of cats with PDH (Neiger *et al.*, 2004). Treatment with trilostane may improve clinical signs but cats typically remain diabetic. The effective dose of trilostane ranges from 15 mg orally q24h to 60 mg orally q12h. ACTH stimulation tests should be used to titrate the dose, similar to the protocol for dogs.

Metyrapone, an 11b-hydroxylase inhibitor that blocks the conversion of 11-deoxycortisol to cortisol, has been used successfully to treat hyperadrenocorticism in the cat (Daley *et al.*, 1993; Moore *et al.*, 2000). The recommended dose is 65 mg/kg orally q8–12h. Side effects include depression, tremors, ataxia, hypocortisolaemia and severe hypoglycaemia (secondary to continuation of insulin administration in the face of resolving hyperglycaemia).

Results of treatment with mitotane and ketoconazole have been disappointing, with partial responses observed in only some cats.

Radiation therapy: Radiotherapy is another option for cats with PDH. Resolution of neurological signs, improved clinical signs and improved glycaemic regulation have been reported after radiation treatment (Kazer-Hotz, 2002; Mayer *et al.*, 2006). Improvement in endocrine function occurs within 1–5 months of completion of radiation therapy.

Surgery: In cats with functional ATs, adrenalectomy is the treatment of choice, but initial medical treatment may be necessary in severely debilitated cats. Bilateral adrenalectomy is also effective in cats with PDH that do not respond to medical therapy. As in dogs, intravenous fluid supplementation and gluco-corticoid administration are vital for successful post-operative management. Cats with diabetes mellitus require careful management of insulin requirements perioperatively. Cats undergoing bilateral adrenal-ectomy or with evidence of hypoadrenocorticism (hyperkalaemia, hyponatraemia) need supplemental mineralocorticoids (desoxycorticosterone pivalate or fludrocortisone). Postoperative complications include electrolyte derangements, skin lacerations, pancreatitis, hypoglycaemia, pneumonia, sepsis and venous thrombosis.

The long-term prognosis for cats with hyperadreno-corticism is fair to good following adrenalectomy. Of 10 cats treated by adrenalectomy, 3 died within 5 weeks of surgery of complications associated with sepsis or thromboembolism. The remaining 7 survived a median of 12 months (Duesberg *et al.*, 1995).

Other adrenal gland tumours

Non-cortisol-secreting adrenocortical tumours

In some dogs and cats with functional ATs, adrenal steroid hormones other than cortisol are the major secretory products of the tumour. Cortisol concentrations are low and do not increase after ACTH stimulation. Increased production of adrenal steroids other than cortisol may be due to deficiencies of enzymes involved in steroidogenic pathways, due to mutations in neoplastic adrenal tissue. Cortisol concentrations are hypothesized to be low because of suppression of the hypothalamic pituitary axis by elevated progestin concentrations. Most reported non-cortisol-secreting adrenocortical tumours in dogs and cats have been carcinomas.

Clinical signs are usually consistent with hyper-adrenocorticism, but some cases may demonstrate masculinization, or signs of hyperaldosteronism such as weakness, hypertension and hypokalaemia. Adrenocortical tumours are usually readily identified by imaging studies. Endocrine function tests do not demonstrate hypercortisolaemia and in most cases the response to ACTH is below the reference range. Hormones that have been reported to be increased in different combinations in affected dogs and cats include 17-hydroxyprogesterone, progesterone, oestradiol, testosterone and androstenedione. Increased concentrations of aldosterone and desoxycorticosterone, either alone in combination with other adrenal hormones, may also occur.

Canine phaeochromocytoma

Phaeochromocytomas are catecholamine-secreting tumours of neuroectoderm-derived chromaffin cells that usually arise from the adrenal medulla. Phaeo-chromocytomas are uncommon in the dog and rare in the cat. The catecholamines adrenaline and nor-adrenaline are synthesized by the hydroxylation and decarboxylation of phenylalanine and tyrosine. The rate-limiting step in the catecholamine synthetic pathway is the hydroxylation of tyrosine by tyrosine hydroxylase. Negative feedback inhibition of the activity of this enzyme by dopamine and noradrenaline normally controls catecholamine production. This normal control mechanism is disrupted in animals with phaeochromocytoma, resulting in the formation and secretion of excess noradrenaline and adrenaline.

Clinical features

Phaeochromocytomas usually occur in older dogs (mean age 10–12 years, range 3–16 years). There is no breed predisposition and males are slightly over-represented. Clinical signs may be due to excess catecholamine secretion and activation of adrenergic receptors, effects of distant tumour metastases, or tumour invasion of regional organs and the caudal vena cava.

The onset and duration of clinical signs associated with phaeochromocytoma are extremely variable and clinical signs may be acute or chronic. Dogs with phaeochromocytoma may die acutely, or present in cardiovascular collapse and die shortly thereafter, but in over 50% of dogs the tumour is an incidental finding during exploratory laparotomy or at necropsy (Gilson *et al.*, 1994; Barthez *et al.*, 1997). Concurrent neoplasia (particularly endocrine neoplasia) is detected in over 50% of affected dogs.

The most common clinical signs are weight loss, anorexia, lethargy, panting and weakness (Barthez *et al.*, 1997). Weakness may be due either to adverse cardiac effects (e.g. tachycardia or arrhythmias) from excess catecholamine secretion or to impaired blood flow from tumour invasion of the caudal vena cava. Other clinical signs include exercise intolerance, cutaneous flushing, abdominal distension (secondary to ascites or haemoperitoneum), polyuria, polydipsia, a palpable abdominal mass, dyspnoea, cough, cardiac abnormalities (tachycardia, arrhythmias, systolic murmur, signs of congestive heart failure), pale mucous membranes and acute collapse. Neurological abnormalities (e.g. seizures and paraparesis) may result secondary to metastasis or hypertension-induced haemorrhage in the central nervous system. A severe hypertensive episode may also cause epistaxis or a sudden onset of blindness from retinal haemorrhage and detachment. Phaeochromocytoma has been reported in six dogs with concurrent hyperadrenocorticism.

Diagnosis

While systemic hypertension is considered the hallmark sign of phaeochromocytoma, it may be episodic. In one study of 61 dogs with phaeochromocytoma, only 10 of 23 dogs tested were hypertensive (Barthez *et al.*, 1997). Dogs with suspected phaeochromocytoma should have several blood pressure determinations during the course of the diagnostic evaluation. A fundic examination is helpful to detect retinal haemorrhages that may have occurred during previous hypertensive episodes.

Blood tests are often unremarkable in dogs with phaeochromocytoma. Reported CBC abnormalities include neutrophilic leucocytosis, mild non-regenerative anaemia, or mild haemoconcentration. Serum biochemical abnormalities may include elevations in serum liver enzyme activities, mild uraemia, hypercholesterolaemia, proteinuria and hypoalbuminaemia.

A presurgical diagnosis is difficult to establish. Phaeochromocytomas are distinguished from adrenocortical tumours based on the lack of the characteristic clinical signs of hyperadrenocorticism and normal function testing of the adrenal cortex (ACTH stimulation, LDDS and HDDS tests). There is some overlap, however, in the spectrum of clinical signs, and adrenal function tests may be abnormal in dogs with underlying systemic illness (Kaplan *et al.*, 1995). Tests to document excessive concentrations of catecholamines and their metabolites in the plasma and urine have not been thoroughly investigated in the dog. Measurement of 24-hour secretion of urinary catecholamines and metabolites is the traditional approach to diagnosis in human medicine, but reference ranges for dogs have not been established. Reference ranges for urinary catecholamine and ratios of metanephrine to creatinine have been established in normal dogs and show promise for diagnosis of phaeochromocytoma.

Abdominal radiography may reveal the presence of a large adrenal mass or ascites. Abdominal ultrasonography may identify an adrenal mass, abdominal metastasis to other organs such as the liver, regional lymph nodes, spleen and kidneys. Invasion or encroachment of the caudal vena cava occurs in up to 50% of dogs with phaeochromocytoma. CT may be useful in identifying tumour extent and metastasis. Thoracic radiographs should be performed in dogs with suspected phaeochromocytoma to evaluate for cardiac enlargement, the presence and severity of signs compatible with congestive heart failure (pulmonary oedema, pleural effusion), the size of the caudal vena cava (enlargement may suggest the presence of an intracaval tumour thrombus), concurrent bronchopneumonia and pulmonary or cardiac metastases. Echocardiography may also be helpful in documenting left ventricular hypertrophy or tumour thrombi.

Treatment

Surgery: The treatment of choice for phaeochromocytoma is surgical removal. Even with metastasis, surgical debulking may be beneficial to increase the efficacy of medical management. Presurgical treatment with the alpha-1-adrenergic blocking vasodilator phenoxybenzamine (0.1–2.5 mg/kg q12h) is associated with improved perioperative mortality rate (Herrera, 2008). Phenoxybenzamine reverses vasoconstriction and hypovolaemia prior to surgery and controls fluctuations of blood pressure and heart rate during anaesthesia. The dose should be individualized for each patient with the aim of preventing hypertension without inducing hypotension.

Adrenalectomy is best performed by an experienced surgeon with access to good monitoring equipment and postoperative care. Blood pressure and the electrocardiogram should be monitored prior to induction of anaesthesia, throughout the surgical procedure and into the postoperative recovery period. Hypertension should be controlled with an alpha-1-adrenergic blocking agent such as phentolamine. Cardiac arrhythmias and severe tachycardia may be treated with a beta-adrenergic blocking agent, such as propranolol. However, propranolol should only be given following administration of an alpha-1-adrenergic blocker, in order to prevent severe hypertension occurring secondary to blockade of beta receptor-mediated vasodilatation of vascular smooth muscle. Hypotension may develop after the tumour is removed; strategies utilized to alleviate hypotension include decreasing or discontinuing phentolamine, vascular volume expansion with an appropriate colloid and treatment with dopamine. Manipulation of the tumour may exacerbate systemic hypertension and so care should be taken when handling the mass.

Medical management: If complete surgical resection of the tumour is not possible, or if surgery is not an option, medical management may be used to control systemic blood pressure and prevent life-threatening arrhythmias. Phenoxybenzamine or prazosin may be utilized to control hypertension, and propranolol can be administered to control tachycardia and cardiac arrhythmias.

Prognosis

The prognosis for phaeochromocytoma is guarded. More than 50% of canine phaeochromocytomas in one report were malignant, with local tumour invasion occurring in 26 of 50 dogs (52%), regional lymph node metastasis in 6 of 50 dogs (12%), and distant metastasis in 12 of 50 dogs (24%) (Gilson *et al.*, 1994).

Incidentally discovered adrenal masses

With the increased use of abdominal ultrasonography and CT imaging, adrenal masses may be an incidental finding. The approach to an incidentally discovered adrenal mass should include a detailed history and physical examination to investigate for clinical signs of hyperadrenocorticism, phaeochromocytoma or other neoplasia that could metastasize to the adrenal gland. A sensitive screening test for hyperadrenocorticism, retinal examination and multiple blood pressure measurements should be performed. Thoracic radiographs should be considered to screen for neoplasia. Depending upon the characteristics of the mass and the clinical findings a fine-needle aspirate of the mass may be considered.

Based on the diagnostic evaluation and the appearance of the adrenal mass (benign-appearing nodule *versus* adrenal mass with disruption of architecture and invasion of vessels), exploratory surgery or careful monitoring of the mass may be recommended. The percentage of these incidentally discovered adrenal masses that progress to become problem tumours has not been defined. In addition, evidence from human medicine suggests that about a third of 'masses' seen ultrasonographically are not grossly visible at exploratory surgery or histologically.

Endocrine cancers of the pancreas

The islets of Langerhans form the endocrine portion of the pancreas and secrete a number of polypeptide hormones. Beta cells secrete insulin, alpha cells secrete glucagon, delta cells secrete somatostatin,

F cells secrete pancreatic polypeptide and fetal islet cells secrete gastrin. Pancreatic endocrine tumours may secrete one or more of these specific hormones. Pancreatic endocrine tumours reported in dogs and cats include insulinomas, gastrinomas and glucagonomas. (Tumours of the exocrine pancreas are discussed in Chapter 15i.)

Canine insulinoma

Insulinomas are functional insulin-secreting tumours of the pancreatic beta cells. Insulin secretion is regulated primarily by the serum glucose concentration; as glucose concentrations increase, insulin secretion increases; in response, serum glucose concentration decreases due to glucose uptake by peripheral tissues and glycogen storage. As blood glucose decreases in response to the effects of insulin, insulin secretion also falls. In the presence of an insulinoma, insulin secretion is unresponsive to the regulating effect of serum glucose concentrations and insulin production continues in the presence of hypoglycaemia.

Clinical features

Insulinoma is most common in middle-aged to old dogs (average age 9 years, range 3–15 years) and certain breeds such as the Poodle, Fox Terrier, Irish Setter, German Shepherd Dog, Boxer, Golden Retriever and Labrador Retriever are over-represented. Clinical signs result from hypoglycaemia, which causes neuroglycopenia, and stimulation of the sympathetic nervous system, which results in elevated circulating catecholamine concentrations. Clinical signs are typically episodic and include seizures, weakness, collapse, ataxia, posterior paresis, muscle fasciculation, dementia, polyphagia and depression. Physical examination findings are generally non-specific. The most common findings are obesity (due to the anabolic effects of insulin) and neurological abnormalities. A peripheral polyneuropathy in dogs with insulinoma has been described and is believed to be a paraneoplastic effect.

Diagnosis

Hypoglycaemia is the hallmark sign of insulinoma. The CBC and urinalysis are usually unremarkable in animals. The most common findings are hypoglycaemia and sometimes increased serum liver enzyme activities. Other causes of hypoglycaemia in the dog are listed in Figure 20.22.

- Non-islet-cell tumours (hepatic, leiomyomas/leiomyosarcomas, other)
- Hypoadrenocorticism
- Hypopituitarism (growth hormone, ACTH)
- Toxicosis (e.g. xylitol)
- Sepsis/endotoxaemia
- Puppy/toy breed hypoglycaemia
- Glycogen storage diseases
- Insulin overdose
- *In vitro* consumption (polycythaemia, leucocytosis)
- Artefactual (prolonged storage, portable glucometers)

20.22 Other causes of hypoglycaemia in dogs.

Documentation of hypoglycaemia, neurological abnormalities secondary to hypoglycaemia and resolution of clinical signs by feeding or administering glucose are suggestive of insulinoma. The diagnosis can usually be confirmed by measurement of serum insulin concentration at a time when the serum glucose concentration is <60 mg/dl (<3.33 mmol/l). If the serum insulin concentration is in the high normal range or above the normal range, this is supportive of insulinoma; if the serum insulin concentration is below the normal reference range, insulinoma is unlikely.

Ratios such as the amended insulin:glucose ratio have poor specificity and may result in false-positive results in dogs that do not have insulinoma. If the serum insulin is in the borderline range, repeating the measurement up to four times in a 24-hour period may be useful. This increases the likelihood of detecting an insulin peak. If serum insulin concentrations are consistently below the reference range in the presence of hypoglycaemia, other causes of hypoglycaemia should be investigated. Provocative tests (e.g. glucagon, glucose and tolbutamide tolerance tests) have generally been disappointing in diagnosing insulinoma in the dog and are not recommended.

Thoracic radiographs are usually normal in dogs with insulinoma. Abdominal radiography and ultrasonography may be helpful in identifying large pancreatic tumours and metastatic masses. The most common sites of metastasis include regional lymph nodes and the liver. Abdominal radiography and ultrasonography have poor sensitivity for detection of small pancreatic masses or metastasis and only 35% of insulinomas are detected by abdominal ultrasonography. CT is more sensitive for detection of pancreatic masses, identifying in one study 10 of 14 pancreatic masses that were confirmed as insulinoma at surgery (Robben et al., 2005). Unfortunately there were many false positives for metastatic disease.

Somatostatin receptor activity is a promising new area for the localization of pancreatic and metastatic sites of insulinomas. Somatostatin receptors have been identified at the surface of most neuroendocrine cells and are present in abnormal density in islet cell tumours. Somatostatin receptors can be imaged in vivo by means of indium 111 pentetreotide (Octeoscan) scintigraphy. In a study of five dogs with insulinoma, an abnormal focus of activity was identified in four dogs, with one dog having equivocal results (Garden, 2005).

Treatment

Medical management: Indications for medical management of insulinoma include stabilization of patients prior to exploratory surgery, patients with obvious metastatic disease and postsurgical patients in which complete surgical removal of the tumour or metastases was not possible. In patients with clinical signs of hypoglycaemia, intravenous glucose should be administered (1–5 ml 50% dextrose i.v. slowly over 10 minutes). If clinical hypoglycaemia persists, continuous infusion of dextrose (2.5–5% dextrose in water i.v.) should be administered at 1½–2 times the maintenance rate. Higher concentrations of dextrose stimulate the pancreas and exacerbate hypoglycaemia and should be avoided. Dexamethasone (0.5–1.0 mg/kg over 6 hours) may be added to intravenous fluids if necessary. This dose can be repeated every 12–24 hours as needed.

Frequent feeding of a diet high in fat, protein and complex carbohydrates, but low in simple sugars, may control clinical signs for a period of time. Stress should be minimized and exercise limited. Once frequent feeding fails to control clinical signs, treatment with glucocorticoids is necessary.

- The starting dose for prednisone is 0.25 mg/kg q12h. The dose should be titrated upwards in order to control clinical signs as necessary. There is little benefit to increasing the dose >3 mg/kg/dose.
- Diazoxide inhibits insulin secretion from the pancreas, stimulates gluconeogenesis and glycogenolysis, and has a direct inhibitory effect on cellular uptake of glucose. The dose is 5–30 mg/kg q12h, starting at the lower end of the dose and increasing as necessary. Side effects include anorexia, vomiting, diarrhoea, hyperglycaemia, cataracts, tachycardia, bone marrow suppression, hypernatraemia, cardiac arrhythmias and pancreatitis.

If clinical signs of hypoglycaemia cannot be controlled by dextrose and glucocorticoid treatment, a glucagon constant-rate infusion should be added at a rate of 5–10 ng/kg/min (Fischer et al., 2000). Glucagon antagonizes the hypoglycaemic effects of insulin by directly stimulating hepatic gluconeogenesis and glycogenolysis. Octreotide, a somatostatin analogue, has also been used to treat dogs with insulinoma, but the results have been equivocal. In one report, octreotide at a dose of 2–4 µg/kg q24h was not efficacious in controlling either the clinical signs of hypoglycaemia or changing serum concentrations of glucose and insulin (Simpson et al., 1995), whereas others have reported resolution or improvement of clinical signs in dogs treated with octreotide at similar doses. Treatment with a single dose of octreotide (50 micrograms s.c.) decreased insulin concentrations and increased blood glucose concentrations in 11 dogs with insulinoma (Robben et al., 2006). Octreotide is expensive and most dogs become refractory over time.

Chemotherapeutic agents such as alloxan and streptozocin have direct toxicity for the beta cells of the pancreas, but both drugs are also nephrotoxic. Streptozocin (500 mg/m² q3wk combined with a diuresis protocol) is well tolerated in dogs and has been associated with resolution of paraneoplastic peripheral neuropathy and reductions in tumour size (Moore et al., 2002).

Surgery: Serum glucose concentrations should be maintained >40 mg/dl (>2.22 mmol/l) during surgery by intravenous infusion of 5% dextrose. The pancreas should be carefully inspected for evidence of a tumour (Figure 20.23). Most dogs have visible

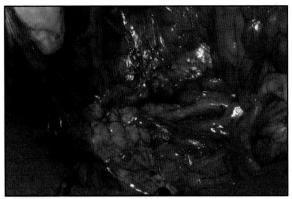

20.23 Insulinoma identified in the pancreas during surgery in a 10-year-old neutered male German Shorthaired Pointer with hypoglycaemia.

pancreatic masses, but a few may require gentle palpation of the organ to identify small tumours. Minimal handling of the pancreas is desirable, in order to prevent postoperative pancreatitis. Partial pancreatectomy or nodulectomy is performed to remove the affected tissue.

Intravenous fluids with dextrose should be continued and oral intake of food and water withheld for 24–48 hours following surgery, to minimize risk of postoperative pancreatitis. If the patient is not vomiting, gradual introduction of water and a bland diet should be initiated after this period. Other potential postoperative complications are hypoglycaemia or hyperglycaemia. Blood glucose concentrations should be evaluated twice daily for at least 3–4 days following surgery. Transitory diabetes mellitus may occur as a result of atrophy of the normal beta islet cells. Insulin administration is recommended only if hyperglycaemia persists for more than 2–3 days following discontinuation of dextrose. Postoperative hypoglycaemia should be treated with the feeding of small frequent meals. If it persists, more aggressive medical therapy should be instituted (see above). Persistent postoperative hypoglycaemia suggests that tumour resection is incomplete and is a poor prognostic indicator.

Prognosis
Insulinoma is a malignant tumour in dogs and the long-term prognosis is guarded to poor. Evidence of gross metastasis is present in at least one-third of dogs at the time of diagnosis. Survival times are longer for dogs treated surgically. In one study, MST for dogs treated surgically was longer at 381 days (range 20–1758 days), than for those treated medically (74 days, range 8–508 days) (Tobin *et al.*, 1999), though the dogs in the medical group may have received less aggressive therapy. In another study of 28 dogs with insulinoma, MST for 19 dogs treated with partial pancreatectomy and prednisone and diazoxide was 785 days (Polton *et al.*, 2007). The long-term prognosis for dogs with detectable metastatic disease is generally considered poor, but long survival times after aggressive surgical debulking of primary and metastatic nodules has been reported.

Canine gastrinoma (Zollinger–Ellison syndrome)
Pancreatic islet-cell tumours that secrete excessive amounts of gastrin are referred to as gastrinomas. Affected dogs have gastric acid hypersecretion, gastrointestinal ulceration and a gastrin-secreting pancreatic mass.

Clinical features
Gastrinomas are rare tumours in dogs. The most common clinical signs are chronic vomiting, diarrhoea, anorexia, depression, lethargy and weight loss. Melaena, haematemesis, haematochezia and pale mucous membranes may also occur secondary to gastrointestinal blood loss.

Diagnosis
The diagnosis is made by documentation of increased circulating gastrin concentrations followed by exploratory laparotomy and tumour resection or biopsy. Histopathology and immunohistochemical staining are necessary to confirm the diagnosis.

Treatment
Surgical exploration and partial pancreatectomy are required to establish a definitive diagnosis, resect perforating ulcers, manage peritonitis and remove or debulk the tumour. Gastrinomas are malignant tumours in dogs, and surgery is usually only palliative. For patients in which complete tumour resection is not possible, hypersecretion of gastric acid should be controlled with drugs that decrease gastric acid secretion, such as H_2 receptor antagonists (cimetidine, ranitidine, famotidine), proton pump inhibitors (omeprazole) and the somatostatin analogue octreotide.

Omeprazole (0.7–1.0 mg/kg orally q24h) is the drug of choice due to its longer duration of action and more effective blockade of both basal and stimulated gastric acid secretion, compared with H_2 receptor antagonists. Higher doses of H_2 receptor antagonists may be necessary to control clinical signs in dogs with gastrinoma. Other drugs, such as sucralfate and misoprostol, may also be of benefit.

Octreotide blocks gastric acid production by inhibiting gastrin secretion and by directly inhibiting parietal cell acid secretion. Octreotide (10–20 µg s.c. q8h) in combination with cimetidine and sucralfate was successfully used to treat a dog with gastrinoma that had failed to respond to cimetidine and sucralfate alone.

Prognosis
The long-term prognosis in dogs with gastrinomas is poor due to the high rate of metastasis at the time of diagnosis. Although complete surgical resection of the tumour may be unlikely, aggressive use of antisecretory drugs such as omeprazole may extend life expectancy.

Glucagonoma
Glucagonoma is a rare islet-cell tumour of the pancreas that secretes excessive quantities of glucagon. Clinical signs are hyperkeratosis of the

footpads and erythematous, erosive and crusting lesions affecting the muzzle, external genitalia, perineum and periocular region. Necrolytic migratory erythema associated with liver disease (hepatocutaneous syndrome; see Chapter 4) is a potential differential diagnosis for the cutaneous changes reported in dogs with glucagonoma.

References and further reading

Anderson CR, Birchard SJ, Powers BE *et al.* (2001) Surgical treatment of adrenocortical tumors: 21 cases (1990–1996). *Journal of the American Animal Hospital Association* **37**, 93–97

Barker EN, Campbell S, Tebb AJ *et al.* (2005) A comparison of the survival times of dogs treated with mitotane or trilostane for pituitary-dependent hyperadrenocorticism. *Journal of Veterinary Internal Medicine* **19**, 810–815

Barthez PY, Marks SL, Woo J *et al.* (1997) Pheochromocytoma in dogs: 61 cases (1984–1995). *Journal of Veterinary Internal Medicine* **11**, 272–278

Berg RIM, Nelson RW, Feldman EC *et al.* (2007) Serum insulin-like growth factor-I concentration in cats with diabetes mellitus and acromegaly. J*ournal of Veterinary Internal Medicine* **21**, 892–898

Bertoy EH, Feldman EC, Nelson RW *et al.* (1995) Magnetic resonance imaging of the brain in dogs with recently diagnosed but untreated pituitary-dependent hyperadrenocorticism. *Journal of the American Veterinary Medical Association* **206**, 651–656

Bertoy EH, Feldman EC, Nelson RW *et al.* (1996) One year follow-up evaluation of magnetic resonance imaging of the brain in dogs with pituitary-dependent hyperadrenocorticism. *Journal of the American Veterinary Medical Association* **208**, 1268–1273

Bosje JT, Rijnberk A, Mol JA *et al.* (2002) Plasma concentrations of ACTH precursors correlate with pituitary size and resistance to dexamethasone in dogs with pituitary-dependent hyperadrenocorticism. *Domestic Animal Endocrinology* **22**, 201–210

Daley CA, Zerbe CA, Schick RO *et al.* (1993) Use of metyrapone to treat pituitary-dependent hyperadrenocorticism in a cat with large cutaneous wounds. *Journal of the American Veterinary Medical Association* **202**, 956–960

Duesberg CA, Feldman EC, Nelson RW *et al.* (1995) Magnetic resonance imaging for diagnosis of pituitary macrotumors in dogs. *Journal of the American Veterinary Medical Association* **206**, 657–662

Duesberg CA, Nelson RW, Feldman EC *et al.* (1995) Adrenalectomy for treatment of hyperadrenocorticism in cats: 10 cases (1988–1992). *Journal of the American Veterinary Medical Association* **207**, 1066–1070

Dunning MD, Leather CA, Bexfield NJ *et al.* (2009) Exogenous insulin requirements following hypofractionated radiotherapy in cats with diabetes mellitus and acromegaly. *Journal of Veterinary Internal Medicine* **23**, 243–249

Feldman EC, Hoar B, Pollard R *et al.* (2005) Pretreatment clinical and laboratory findings in dogs with primary hyperparathyroidism: 210 cases (1987–2004). *Journal of the American Veterinary Medical Association* **227**, 756–761

Feldman EC and Nelson RW (2004) *Canine and Feline Endocrinology and Reproduction, 3rd edn.* WB Saunders, Philadelphia

Fischer JR, Smith SA and Harkin KR (2000) Glucagon constant-rate infusion: a novel strategy for the management of hyperinsulinemic–hypoglycemic crisis in the dog. *Journal of the American Animal Hospital Association* **36**, 27–32

Garden OA, Reubi C, Dykes NL *et al.* (2005) Somatostatin receptor imaging in vivo by planar scintigraphy facilitates the diagnosis of canine insulinomas. *Journal of Veterinary Internal Medicine* **19**, 168–176

Gilson SD, Withrow SJ, Wheeler SL *et al.* (1994) Pheochromocytoma in 50 dogs. *Journal of Veterinary Internal Medicine* **8**, 228–232

Goldstein RE, Atwater DZ, Cazolli DM *et al.* (2007) Inheritance, mode of inheritance, and candidate genes for primary hyperparathyroidism in Keeshonden. *Journal of Veterinary Internal Medicine* **21**, 199–203

Granger N, de Fornel P, Devauchelle P *et al.* (2005) Plasma pro-opiomelanocortin, pro-adrenocorticotropin hormone, and pituitary adenoma size in dogs with Cushing's disease. *Journal of Veterinary Internal Medicine* **19**, 23–28

Grooters AM, Biller DS, Theisen SK *et al.* (1996) Ultrasonographic characteristics of the adrenal glands in dogs with pituitary-dependent hyperadrenocorticism: comparison with normal dogs. *Journal of Veterinary Internal Medicine* **10**, 110–115

Guptill L, Scott-Moncrieff JCR, Janovitz EB *et al.* (1995) Response to high-dose radioactive iodine administration in cats with thyroid carcinoma that had previously undergone surgery. *Journal of the American Veterinary Medical Association* **207**, 1055–1058

Hanson JM, van't Hoofd MM, Voorhout G *et al.* (2005) Efficacy of transsphenoidal hypophysectomy in treatment of dogs with pituitary-dependent hyperadrenocorticism. *Journal of Veterinary Internal Medicine* **19**, 687–694

Herrera MA, Mehl ML, Kass PH *et al.* (2008) Predictive factors and the effect of phenoxybenzamine on outcome in dogs undergoing adrenalectomy for phaeochromocytoma. *Journal of Veterinary Internal Medicine* **22**, 1333–1339

Kallet AJ, Richter KP, Feldman EC *et al.* (1991) Primary hyperparathyroidism in cats: seven cases (1984–1989). *Journal of the American of the Veterinary Medical Association* **199**, 1767–1771

Kaplan AJ, Peterson ME and Kemmpainen RJ (1995) Effects of disease on the results of diagnostic tests for use in detecting hyperadrenocorticism in dogs. *Journal of the American Veterinary Medical Association* **207**, 445–451

Kaser-Hotz B, Rohrer CR, Stankeova S *et al.* (2002) Radiotherapy of pituitary tumors in five cats. *Journal of Small Animal Practice* **43**, 303–307

Kent MS, Bommarito D and Feldman E (2007) Survival, neurologic response, and prognostic factors in dogs with pituitary masses treated with radiation therapy and untreated dogs. *Journal of Veterinary Internal Medicine* **21**, 1027–1033

Kintzer PP and Peterson ME (1991) Mitotane (op'-DDD) treatment of 200 dogs with pituitary-dependent hyperadrenocorticism. *Journal of Veterinary Internal Medicine* **5**, 182–190

Kintzer PP and Peterson ME (1994) Mitotane treatment of 32 dogs with cortisol-secreting adrenocortical neoplasms. *Journal of the American Veterinary Medical Association* **205**, 54–61

Kipperman BS, Feldman EC, Dybdal NO *et al.* (1992) Pituitary tumor size, neurologic signs, and relation to endocrine test results in dogs with pituitary-dependent hyperadrenocorticism: 43 cases (1980–1990). *Journal of the American Veterinary Medical Association* **201**, 762–767

Klein MK, Powers BE, Withrow SJ *et al.* (1995) Treatment of thyroid carcinoma in dogs by surgical resection alone: 20 cases (1981–1989). *Journal of the American Veterinary Medical Association* **206**, 1007–1009

Kyles AE, Feldman EC, De Cock HEV *et al.* (2003) Surgical management of adrenal gland tumors with and without associated tumor thrombi in dogs: 40 cases (1994–2001). *Journal of the American Veterinary Medical Association* **223**, 654–662

Marks SL, Koblik PD, Hornof WJ *et al.* (1994) 99mTc-pertechnetate imaging of thyroid tumors in dogs: 29 cases (1980–1992). *Journal of the American Veterinary Medical Association* **204**, 756–760

Mayer MN, Greco DS and LaRue SM (2006) Outcomes of pituitary irradiation in cats. *Journal of Veterinary Internal Medicine* **20**, 1151–1154

Moore AS, Nelson RW, Henry CJ *et al.* (2002) Streptozocin for treatment of pancreatic islet cell tumors in dogs: 17 cases (1989–1999). *Journal of the American Veterinary Medical Association* **221**, 811–818

Neiger R, Ramsey I, O'Connor J *et al.* (2002) Trilostane treatment of 78 dogs with pituitary dependent hyperadrenocorticism. *Veterinary Record* **150**, 799–804

Neiger RN, Witt AL, Noble A *et al.* (2004) Trilostane therapy for treatment of pituitary-dependent hyperadrenocorticism in 5 cats. *Journal of Veterinary Internal Medicine* **18**, 160–164

Nelson RW, Feldman EC and Smith MC (1988) Hyperadrenocorticism in cats: seven cases (1978–1987). *Journal of the American Veterinary Medical Association* **193**, 245–250

Niessen SJM, Petrie G, Gaudiano F *et al.* (2007) Feline acromegaly: an underdiagnosed endocrinopathy? *Journal of Veterinary Internal Medicine* **21**, 899–905

Peterson ME and Becker DV (1995) Radioiodine treatment of 524 cats with hyperthyroidism. *Journal of the American Veterinary Medical Association* **207**, 1422–1428

Peterson ME, Taylor RS, Greco DS *et al.* (1990) Acromegaly in 14 cats. *Journal of Veterinary Internal Medicine* **4**, 192–201

Polton GA, White RN, Brearley MJ *et al.* (2007) Improved survival in a retrospective cohort of 28 dogs with insulinoma. *Journal of Small Animal Practice* **48**, 151–156

Rasor L, Pollard R, Feldman EC (2007) Retrospective evaluation of three treatment methods for primary hyperparathyroidism in dogs. *Journal of the American Animal Hospital Association* **43**, 70–77

Reusch CE and Feldman EC (1991) Canine hyperadrenocorticism due to adrenocortical neoplasia. *Journal of Veterinary Internal Medicine* **5**, 3–10

Robben JH, Pollak WEA, Kirpensteijn J *et al.* (2005) Comparisons of ultrasonography, computed tomography, and single emission computed tomography for the detection and localization of canine insulinoma. *Journal of Veterinary Internal Medicine* **19**, 15–22

Robben JH, van den Brom WR, Mol JA *et al.* (2006) Effect of octreotide on plasma concentrations of glucose, insulin, glucagon, growth hormone and cortisol in healthy dogs and dogs with insulinoma. *Research in Veterinary Science* **80**, 25–32

Schwartz P, Kovak JR, Koprowski A *et al.* (2008) Evaluation of prognostic factors in the surgical treatment of adrenal gland tumors in dogs: 41 cases (1999–2005). *Journal of the American Veterinary Medical Association* **232**, 77–84

Simpson KW, Stepien RL, Elwood CM *et al.* (1995) Evaluation of the long-acting somatostatin analogue octreotide in the management of insulinoma in three dogs. *Journal of Small Animal Practice* **36**, 161–165

Théon AP and Feldman E (1998) Megavoltage irradiation of pituitary macrotumors in dogs with neurologic signs. *Journal of the American Veterinary Medical Association* **13**, 225–231

Théon AP, Marks SL, Feldman ES *et al.* (2000) Prognostic factors and patterns of treatment failure in dogs with unresectable differentiated thyroid carcinomas treated with megavoltage irradiation. *Journal of the American Veterinary Medical Association* **216**, 1775–1779

Tobin RL, Nelson RW, Lucroy MD *et al.* (1999) Outcome of surgical versus medical treatment of dogs with beta cell neoplasia: 39 cases (1990–1997). *Journal of the American Veterinary Medical Association* **215**, 226–230

Turrel JM, Feldman EC, Nelson RW *et al.* (1988) Thyroid carcinoma causing hyperthyroidism in cats: 14 cases (1981–1986). *Journal of the American Veterinary Medical Association* **193**, 359–364

Turrel JM, McEntee MC, Burke BP *et al.* (2006) Sodium iodide ^{131}I treatment of dogs with nonresectable thyroid tumors: 39 cases (1990–2003). *Journal of the American Veterinary Medical Association* **229**, 542–548

Vaughan MA, Feldman EC, Hoar BR *et al.* (2008) Evaluation of twice-daily, low dose trilostane treatment administered orally in dogs with naturally occurring hyperadrenocorticism. *Journal of the American Veterinary Medical Association* **232**, 1321–1328

von Dehn BJ, Nelson RW, Feldman EC *et al.* (1995) Pheochromocytoma and hyperadrenocorticism in dogs: six cases (1981–1992). *Journal of the American Veterinary Medical Association* **207**, 322–324

Wood FD, Pollard RE, Ueling MR *et al.* (2007) Diagnostic imaging findings and endocrine test results in dogs with pituitary-dependent hyperadrenocorticism that did or did not have neurologic abnormalities. *Journal of the American Veterinary Medical Association* **231**, 1081–1085

Worth AJ, Zuber RM and Hocking M (2005) Radioiodide (^{131}I) therapy for the treatment of canine thyroid carcinoma. *Australian Veterinary Journal* **83**, 208–214

21

Tumours of the nervous system

Christopher Mariani

Introduction

Tumours affecting the nervous system may involve the central nervous system (CNS) (brain and spinal cord) or the peripheral nervous system (PNS) (peripheral and cranial nerves). Tumours are classified as primary if they arise from tissues or cell types normally present within the nervous system or meningeal tissues, or secondary if they arise from adjacent structures (e.g. nasal cavity, skull, vertebrae) or metastasize to the nervous system.

Intracranial tumours

Intracranial tumours are listed in Figure 21.1.

Tumour types and pathogenesis

Nervous system tumours may be described as extra-axial (arising from outside the brain parenchyma) or intra-axial (arising from within the parenchyma). Clinical signs related to intracranial tumours are caused by compression of nervous tissue and vasculature, impaired blood flow to nervous tissue, cerebral oedema, haemorrhage, or by direct invasion of brain parenchyma. The skull of mature animals is a rigid, non-expandable compartment. Increases in tissue (tumour) within this compartment increase the intracranial pressure (ICP), which causes impaired blood flow, ischaemia and shifts in brain tissue. Brain herniation under the tentorium cerebelli or through the foramen magnum leads to compression of vital midbrain and medullary centres, reduced consciousness, respiratory arrest and death.

The changes that result in seizures with brain tumours are incompletely understood. Although compression of nervous tissue and the resulting changes described above are involved in some cases, other factors such as proliferation of reactive astrocytes adjacent to the tumour likely play a role. Systemic metastasis of brain tumours is rare in small animals, but has been reported for meningiomas. Spread of tumour cells through the cerebrospinal fluid (CSF) ('drop metastasis') is seen with some tumours, notably choroid plexus carcinomas.

Dogs

Meningiomas are the most frequently recognized intracranial tumour in dogs, though gliomas (astrocytomas, oligodendrogliomas) and pituitary tumours

Primary tumours

• Meningeal tumours:
  o Meningioma
  o Granular cell tumours (rare)
  o Meningeal sarcoma (rare)
• Neuroepithelial tumours:
  o Astrocytoma
  o Oligodendroglioma
  o Choroid plexus tumours
  o Ependymoma
  o Primitive neuroectodermal tumours (PNETs)
  o Medulloblastoma (cerebellum only)
• Haemopoietic tumours: [a]
  o Lymphoma
  o Histiocytic sarcoma

Secondary tumours

• Pituitary tumours:
  o Pituitary adenoma
  o Pituitary carcinoma
• Nasal tumours:
  o Nasal adenocarcinoma
• Skull tumours:
  o Multilobular tumour of bone
  o Osteosarcoma
  o Chondrosarcoma
• Cranial nerve tumours:
  o Peripheral nerve sheath tumour
• Metastatic tumours

Non-neoplastic lesions
• Vascular hamartoma • Epidermoid, dermoid and arachnoid cysts • Granuloma or abscess • Encephalitis • Stroke

21.1 Classification of intracranial tumours. [a] Lymphoma and histiocytic sarcoma may be classified as either primary or secondary, depending on whether they arise primarily within the brain, arise adjacent to brain tissue, or occur as part of a systemic process.

(see Chapter 20) are also common. Choroid plexus tumours occur with some frequency and arise from within the ventricular system. Round cell tumours affecting the brain of canine patients include lymphoma and histiocytic sarcoma (see Chapter 19a). Both may occur as part of a systemic proliferation of neoplastic cells, as a primary CNS neoplasm, or with secondary extension from an extradural or extracranial process. Common metastatic brain tumours include haemangiosarcoma, melanoma and carcinomas (e.g. mammary, prostatic).

Boxers, Boston Terriers, Bulldogs and other brachycephalic breeds frequently develop gliomas, while dolichocephalic breeds appear to be at increased risk for the development of meningiomas. Poodles and Dachshunds frequently develop pituitary tumours. Bernese Mountain Dogs, Rottweilers, Golden Retrievers and Flat-coated Retrievers are at increased risk for histiocytic sarcoma, while Golden Retrievers were at increased risk for choroid plexus tumours in one study (Westworth *et al.*, 2008). Consistent gender predispositions have not been documented in dogs. Molecular aberrations contributing to the development, growth and invasion of nervous system tumours are just beginning to be elucidated in dogs. Similar to humans, recent studies show that canine brain tumours over-express receptor tyrosine kinases (Dickinson *et al.*, 2006a) and telomerase (Long *et al.*, 2006) and possess a number of other genetic aberrations involved in cytoskeletal rearrangement and cell transformation (Thomson *et al.*, 2005).

Cats

Meningiomas are the most frequent intracranial tumours in cats. Lymphoma (see Chapter 19a) and pituitary tumours (see Chapter 20) also occur relatively commonly (Troxel *et al.*, 2003; Tomek *et al.*, 2006), while astrocytomas, oligodendrogliomas, ependymomas and choroid plexus tumours are rare in this species. Risk factors have been poorly defined in cats. Most tumours occur in older animals, but cats with mucopolysaccharidosis type I appear to be at risk for the development of meningiomas at a young age. Male cats seem to be at increased risk for meningioma development.

Presentation and clinical signs

As with any disease of the nervous system, clinical signs depend on the specific anatomical region affected. Tumours involving the forebrain may lead to seizures, altered mentation, contralateral proprioceptive deficits, blindness and compulsive circling. Tumours involving the cerebellum may result in ataxia, dysmetria and intention tremors. Tumours involving the midbrain or medulla may cause altered mentation, ipsilateral or contralateral proprioceptive deficits, tetraparesis, ataxia and cranial nerve dysfunction. Common cranial nerves affected include the oculomotor (mydriasis, ophthalmoplegia), trigeminal (reduced facial sensation, atrophy of masticatory muscles), facial (droopy lip, absent palpebral reflex) and vestibular nerves (ataxia, head tilt, nystagmus). Neck pain is occasionally seen with intracranial neoplasia.

Dogs

Seizures are the most common clinical sign associated with brain tumours in the dog and often occur without any accompanying neurological deficits. As the tumour increases in size, and with the development of cerebral oedema, other signs of intracranial dysfunction may be noted. Meningiomas in the dog frequently arise in the olfactory and frontal regions and at the cerebellomedullary junction, leading to forebrain and vestibular signs, respectively. Gliomas frequently arise in the temporal or piriform lobes,

causing seizures. Pituitary tumours may be functional or non-functional, with or without associated endocrinopathies (see Chapter 20). These tumours often expand dorsally into the hypothalamus and thalamus, causing altered mentation (behavioural changes, decreased consciousness, head pressing, compulsive pacing) and blindness.

Cats

Cats with meningiomas typically present with altered mentation and behavioural changes, while seizures are relatively less common than in dogs (Tomek *et al.*, 2006). Clinical signs associated with other tumours are similar to those in dogs.

Clinical approach

A diagnosis of neoplasia affecting the CNS is often suspected based on the clinical signs and signalment of the patient, though a variety of other disease processes can present with identical signs. In the brain, the main differential diagnoses to consider are meningoencephalitis, cerebrovascular disease (stroke) and idiopathic (genetic) or acquired (cryptogenic, probably symptomatic) epilepsy. In addition, although the majority of intracranial tumours occur in older patients, these tumours can develop in young animals and this diagnosis should not be excluded based on age alone.

The initial diagnostic plan for animals with nervous system tumours usually includes a complete blood count (CBC), serum biochemistry and urinalysis. These tests rarely provide valuable diagnostic information pertaining to the tumour, but are useful in detecting comorbid disease, which is important for anaesthetic planning and may ultimately affect therapy. Exceptions may be seen with haematological malignancies such as lymphoma and multiple myeloma, which may have abnormalities present on blood and urine tests. Similarly, thoracic and abdominal imaging are helpful in staging disease and in detecting comorbid conditions prior to anaesthesia for more advanced diagnostics. Although nervous system tumours rarely metastasize to the lungs or other organ systems, metastatic disease affecting both the lungs and nervous system is a concern and animals with nervous system tumours frequently have a second primary tumour in another location (Snyder *et al.*, 2006, 2008). Specific diagnostic tests available to investigate brain disease include imaging, CSF analysis, electrodiagnostic tests and cytological or histopathological examination of biopsied tissue.

Diagnostic imaging

Conventional radiography is rarely useful in the examination of brain tumours, although tumours originating from or adjacent to the skull that cause bone lysis or proliferation can occasionally be detected (Figure 21.2). Hyperostosis of the skull is frequently seen with meningiomas, particularly in cats, and can sometimes be appreciated on plain radiographs.

Computed tomography (CT) or magnetic resonance imaging (MRI) is required to obtain adequate imaging of the brain parenchyma. CT utilizes X-rays in order to generate a series of transverse images of

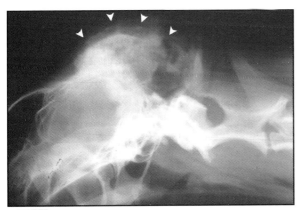

21.2 Lateral radiograph of the skull of a dog presented after the owner noticed a swelling on its head. Note the proliferative bony lesion on the caudodorsal surface of the skull (arrowed). The final diagnosis was multilobular tumour of bone.

the area of interest. Although image quality varies widely, depending on equipment and imaging software, MRI is almost always superior to CT in the imaging of lesions involving the brain, providing much better contrast between different soft tissues and highlighting pathological abnormalities. With both CT and MRI, images can be obtained before and after intravenous contrast administration to look for enhancing lesions characteristic of tumours. One particular limitation of CT is 'beam-hardening' artefact, which is produced by the thick petrous temporal bone in small animals, obscuring imaging of the adjacent brainstem.

Cerebrospinal fluid analysis

Analysis of CSF is a useful adjunct to imaging in patients with brain tumours. Parameters evaluated typically include cell counts, protein level and cytology. A definitive diagnosis is rarely obtained, though occasionally neoplastic cells may be detected on cytological examination (Figure 21.3). This occurs most frequently with lymphoma and choroid plexus carcinomas (Westworth *et al.*, 2008). More commonly, CSF analysis is useful to support or eliminate a diagnosis of meningoencephalitis, but interpretation must be made together with imaging and in the context of other patient information.

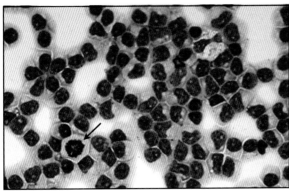

21.3 Cytospin preparation of CSF from a dog with CNS lymphoma that was presented for seizures. Note the population of large mononuclear cells consistent with lymphoblasts. A mitotic figure is also present (arrowed).

A common finding in animals with brain tumours is increased CSF protein without elevated white blood cell numbers (albuminocytological dissociation). Protein elevation is often marked in animals with choroid plexus tumours, particularly carcinomas (Westworth *et al.*, 2008). Pleocytosis may be seen with some tumours, notably meningiomas (Dickinson *et al.*, 2006b).

Although CSF can be collected safely in the majority of patients with intracranial neoplasia, animals with increased ICP may be at risk for sudden changes in pressure gradients and accompanying herniation of brain tissue with this procedure. Pretreatment with mannitol or hypertonic saline and collection of fluid from the lumbar cistern may help to prevent complications associated with CSF collection, but the risks may be considered too great in some patients (e.g. those with stupor, coma, or abnormal respiration). Diagnostic imaging should ideally be performed prior to CSF collection in order to identify existing brain herniation or other risk factors.

Electrodiagnostic tests

Although electrodiagnostic tests are used infrequently in the evaluation of animals with brain tumours, they can provide a functional correlation to the anatomical information obtained from diagnostic imaging. Brainstem auditory evoked response (BAER) testing may demonstrate dysfunction of the auditory nerve (VIII) or its ascending pathways in the brainstem. Electromyography and nerve conduction velocity may be used to investigate the integrity of cranial nerves with motor innervation (III, IV, V, VI, VII, IX, X, XI, XII). Electroencephalography may provide information regarding seizure activity, or dysfunction of regions of the brain affected by neoplastic disease.

Cytology and histology

Although histological examination of tumour tissue is the gold standard diagnostic technique for intracranial tumours, it is performed less frequently in patients with intracranial tumours than in those with neoplasms in other organs. This is due to difficulties with access and the perceived risks of obtaining the sample. Despite these challenges, a histological diagnosis is ideal before moving forward with expensive and potentially harmful definitive therapy.

Options for obtaining tissue include resection of tissue via an open craniotomy or craniectomy, or biopsy of tissue with a needle or similar device. A biopsy sample may be obtained 'freehand' after analysis of MRI or CT images, or may be guided by a variety of imaging techniques, including ultrasonography and CT. Stereotactic CT-guided biopsy of brain lesions is commonly performed in human patients with intracranial lesions and is available for veterinary patients at some centres (Koblik *et al.*, 1999). Cytological analysis of aspirates, touch preparations, or smear preparations from tumour tissue can provide a rapid diagnosis in many cases (Vernau *et al.*, 2001).

Management

Management of intracranial tumours can be aimed at either palliating clinical signs or definitively addressing neoplastic disease to maximize survival time. Definitive therapy for intracranial neoplasms, as with cancer in other organ systems, typically involves surgery, radiation therapy, chemotherapy, or a combination of these. The therapeutic plan depends on the species, signalment, type of tumour, tumour location, comorbid disease processes and financial concerns of the owner.

Palliative therapy

Palliation involves the administration of anticonvulsant medications to control seizures and of glucocorticoids to reduce tumour-associated cerebral oedema. Traditional anticonvulsant medications (phenobarbital, bromide) are usually quite effective in controlling seizures, but have substantial side-effect profiles. The main advantage of the newer anticonvulsant medications (levetiracetam, zonisamide, gabapentin, pregabalin) is a reduction of sedation and other side effects. Although experience with these drugs as sole therapy in veterinary patients is limited, they may prove very useful in animals with brain tumours where sedation may be compounded by existing mentation impairment. Glucocorticoid administration at anti-inflammatory doses is usually sufficient to reduce the vasogenic oedema associated with intracranial neoplasms, and few animals benefit from higher doses.

Definitive therapy

Surgery: A number of surgical approaches have been developed for the treatment of intracranial disease in small animals. Extra-axial tumours on the dorsal or lateral surfaces of the brain are the easiest to approach, while intra-axial, intraventricular and ventral skull-base tumours may be difficult or impossible to access safely. Potential complications of intracranial surgery include haemorrhage, postoperative infection and increases in ICP. Despite these risks, surgical intervention can yield a biopsy sample of tumour for definitive diagnosis, substantial debulking of tumour tissue or a chance for cure in some instances, and life-saving relief of ICP elevation in certain scenarios.

Radiation therapy: This is the most commonly utilized therapy for small animals with intracranial tumours and can be delivered in a variety of ways. Conventional fractionated radiotherapy is delivered at a variety of different time intervals, depending on facility and curative intent, usually to a total dose of 45–55 Gy. More precise modalities are available at some institutions and include intensity-modulated radiation therapy (IMRT) and stereotactic radiosurgery (SRS) (Lester *et al.*, 2001). Both techniques take advantage of advanced imaging techniques to deliver large doses of radiation to the tumour in a highly conformal manner. In the case of SRS, a large dose is delivered in a single fraction, which has considerable benefits in veterinary practice, allowing a single anaesthetic episode for treatment.

Side effects of conventional radiation therapy include alopecia, leucotrichia, moist dermatitis and ulceration of the oral cavity or external ear canal. In addition, as the CNS is a late-responding tissue (see Chapter 8), radiation injury to the brain can occur 6 months or longer after initiating therapy. These late effects are more likely with higher fraction doses, which should ideally be 3 Gy or less. Although orthovoltage protocols have been utilized with some success, megavoltage delivery with cobalt or a linear accelerator is preferred. Conformal therapies such as IMRT and SRS have fewer side effects than conventional radiation therapy.

Chemotherapy: Chemotherapy is the least investigated of the major anti-neoplastic modalities for intracranial tumours in small animals. Few studies exist and it is difficult to make recommendations, considering the paucity of efficacy data available. The medications most commonly used are lomustine (CCNU), hydroxycarbamide and cytarabine (Ara-C).

Meningioma

Dogs: Meningiomas are the most surgically accessible intracranial tumours in canine patients, due to their extra-axial location. However, in contrast to feline meningiomas, the demarcation between tumour tissue and normal brain is frequently difficult to appreciate. As a result, residual tumour tissue is commonly present after surgery and recurrence is frequent with surgical therapy alone. Although studies are limited, most reports of canine meningiomas treated with surgery alone describe median survival times of 1–7 months. However, several recent studies describing newer surgical techniques have reported dramatically improved survival times associated with more complete tumour removal (Greco *et al.*, 2006; Klopp and Rao, 2009).

A number of studies have examined survival times after radiation therapy of brain masses in dogs, with results typically ranging from about 1 to 1.5 years. Unfortunately, many of these studies did not have histological confirmation of the neoplasm, and definitive statements about radiation therapy for any brain tumour in small animals are difficult to make. However, the weight of the evidence suggests a beneficial effect of radiation for meningiomas in dogs, whether as a sole therapy or as adjunctive therapy after surgical debulking or incomplete excision.

Little information is available documenting the response of canine meningiomas to chemotherapeutic protocols. Anecdotal success has been reported with the use of hydroxycarbamide, lomustine and temozolomide.

Cats: Many meningiomas in cats are amenable to surgical therapy, as they tend to occur in superficial and easily accessible areas and are usually fairly well demarcated from adjacent brain tissue (Figure 21.4), facilitating complete removal. Surgery alone often leads to fairly long survival times and many cats die of unrelated causes without signs of tumour recurrence. Successful outcomes can also be achieved with surgical excision of multiple meningiomas (Forterre *et al.*, 2007). Incompletely resected

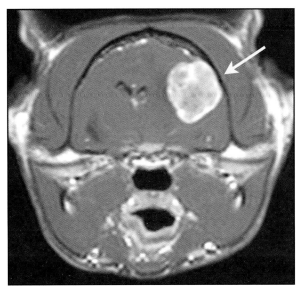

21.4 Meningioma in a cat. Transverse plane, post-contrast, T1-weighted MR image of the brain of a cat presenting for altered mentation. Note the large, extra-axial contrast-enhancing mass, with a broad dural attachment, characteristic of a meningioma (arrowed). The mass is causing compression of the ventricular system and deviation of the midline structures to the contralateral side.

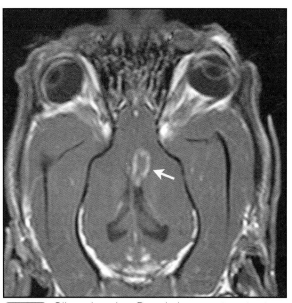

21.5 Glioma in a dog. Dorsal plane, post-contrast, T1-weighted MR image of the brain of a dog presented with seizures. Note the intra-axial, ring-enhancing mass adjacent to the lateral ventricle (arrowed), consistent with an aggressive glial cell tumour. The lesion is causing a mass effect, with deviation of the midline structures towards the contralateral side. The final diagnosis was anaplastic oligodendroglioma.

tumours or meningiomas in areas that are more difficult to access surgically (e.g. skull base, ventricle) may benefit from radiotherqpy. SRS has been performed successfully in cats with meningiomas, but this experience is quite limited to date. There are no reports of the use of chemotherapy in cats with meningiomas.

Neuroepithelial tumours

Dogs: The intra-axial location of gliomas (Figure 21.5) makes surgical excision more challenging, and reports of surgical therapy for gliomas are uncommon in the veterinary literature. Surgery may provide a definitive diagnosis, but is unlikely to result in complete excision, and adjunctive therapy is typically recommended. Similar to meningiomas, radiotherapy is commonly used alone or after surgical debulking of the tumour. Definitive conclusions are difficult to make in light of the frequent lack of a histological diagnosis, though most reports and anecdotal evidence suggest that radiation therapy is beneficial in these scenarios and extends survival in dogs with astrocytomas or oligodendrogliomas. The role of chemotherapy for these tumours is virtually unknown, but lomustine, carmustine, or temozolomide may provide some benefit.

The location and vascular nature of choroid plexus tumours make surgical excision challenging, though this has been successful in some cases. Very little information is available regarding radiotherapy or chemotherapy for these tumours. Before pursuing definitive therapy, careful examination and additional imaging of the entire CNS should be considered, as metastasis via the CSF is common. Definitive therapy for other tumours of neuroepithelial origin has been rarely described in the veterinary literature.

Patients may benefit from surgical debulking, if accessible, and adjunctive radiation therapy.

Cats: There is a paucity of data concerning therapy of these tumours in the cat and recommendations are generally made based on experience with canine patients.

Round cell tumours

Recommendations for the therapy of intracranial lymphoma in veterinary patients have not been widely discussed. Beyond obtaining a diagnosis, surgery typically plays a minor role in therapy. Chemotherapy is the cornerstone of lymphoma therapy (see Chapter 19a), as the process is usually assumed to be systemic. For animals with CNS involvement, inclusion of a drug that penetrates the blood–brain barrier and achieves high levels in the brain is recommended. Cytarabine meets these criteria and can be administered as an intravenous infusion, subcutaneously or intrathecally. Radiation therapy may also play an important role in patients with primary CNS lymphoma, or in those where rapid reduction of the size of the tumour is desirable due to life-threatening increases in ICP.

No data are available regarding the therapy of intracranial histiocytic sarcoma. Regardless of location in the body, this neoplasm has traditionally carried a very poor prognosis. However, a recent study suggests that lomustine may be efficacious (Skorupski *et al.*, 2007). Although intracranial tumours were not represented in this study, the ability of lomustine to penetrate the blood–brain barrier warrants further investigation of this drug for intracranial disease.

Pituitary tumours

Therapy of the functional aspects of pituitary tumours is discussed in Chapter 20. Surgical removal of the pituitary gland has been described in dogs and cats, and is available at a few select specialty centres (Meij *et al.*, 2002). This procedure is typically performed by accessing the gland through a trans-sphenoidal approach (i.e. through the palate), which limits the size of tumour that can be removed. Thus, many macroadenomas (Figure 21.6) are difficult to access and remove surgically. With these limitations, definitive therapy for most pituitary tumours involves radiation therapy, which has been shown to improve survival time when compared with dogs not receiving it (Kent *et al.*, 2007).

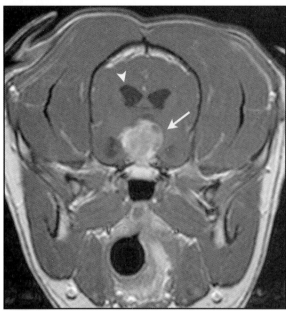

21.6 Pituitary tumour in a dog. Transverse plane, post-contrast, T1-weighted MR image of a dog presented with altered mentation. Note the large spherical contrast-enhancing mass lesion that appears to be originating from the sellar region, consistent with a pituitary tumour (arrowed). The mass is compressing the third ventricle, and there is mild to moderate dilatation of the lateral ventricles, consistent with obstructive hydrocephalus (arrowhead).

Tumours with secondary extension into the cranial vault

Tumours of the skull may be treated successfully in some cases with surgical removal (Figure 21.7). These tumours are often clearly demarcated from underlying brain, allowing a clear plane of dissection to be developed. The main limiting factor is the size of the tumour, as extensive skull involvement may require reconstructive surgery (cranioplasty). Incompletely excised tumours are likely to benefit from adjunctive radiation therapy. Nasal tumours may be debulked surgically, but radiation is typically an important part of definitive therapy. Adjunctive chemotherapy may be useful in preventing systemic metastases. Surgical therapy of tumours of cranial nerves in intracranial locations has been described, but is technically challenging and rarely performed. Some of these tumours may benefit from radiotherapy.

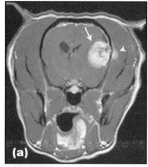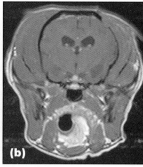

21.7 Skull tumour in a dog. Transverse plane, post-contrast, T1-weighted MR images of the brain of a dog presented for seizures. **(a)** Note the large spherical contrast-enhancing, extra-axial mass (arrowed). The lesion is causing a substantial mass effect, with compression of the lateral ventricle and deviation of the midline towards the contralateral side. A contrast-enhancing lesion is present within the temporal musculature adjacent to the intracranial lesion (arrowhead), suggestive of a lesion traversing the skull. **(b)** After craniectomy and mass removal, the brain has returned to its normal position, and no visible tumour remains. The final diagnosis was fibrosarcoma.

Metastatic tumours

Human patients often undergo surgical removal or targeted radiation therapy (e.g. SRS) of metastatic brain lesions in addition to systemic chemotherapy. This appears to provide a clear benefit in improving clinical signs and extending survival in many patients. Although such approaches may be considered, therapy for metastatic CNS tumours has been poorly documented to date in veterinary medicine.

Prognosis

Formulating a prognosis for veterinary patients with brain tumours is difficult, as there is a dearth of knowledge concerning the natural history of these diseases. Efforts are hindered by the delayed recognition of a mass lesion or failure to equate clinical signs (particularly seizures) with a structural brain lesion, the lack of a definitive histological diagnosis, variable therapeutic protocols and the lack of controlled trials comparing different therapies. However, some general statements and guidelines can be developed, even with these shortcomings.

- Animals with less severe clinical signs (e.g. intermittent seizures with a normal interictal neurological examination, subtle proprioceptive deficits) tend to do better and survive longer than those with more extensive intracranial signs (e.g. mentation changes, altered consciousness, moderate to severe paresis).
- Animals treated with palliative therapy (e.g. glucocorticoids, anticonvulsants) have shorter median survival times than those treated with definitive therapy. This is usually in the order of 1–6 months, though longer survival times (up to several years) are possible.
- Cats with meningiomas treated with surgical resection often have survival times of 2 years or longer. Even if surgical resection is not complete,

the slow-growing nature of these tumours often results in the death of the cat from other causes before intracranial signs recur.
- Dogs with meningiomas treated with surgical resection alone often have survival times in the range of 3–9 months. Death usually occurs due to regrowth of tumour. Complete tumour removal may result in dramatically increased survival.
- Dogs with meningiomas treated with radiation alone often have survival times in the range of 7–16 months.
- Dogs with meningiomas treated with surgical resection and adjunctive radiotherapy have median survival times in the range of 12–28 months.
- The prognosis for dogs and cats with intra-axial tumours (e.g. astrocytomas, oligodendrogliomas) is often less favourable. Although data are lacking, survival times of 3–12 months with definitive radiotherapy might be anticipated.
- Dogs with pituitary tumours treated with radiation therapy have prolonged survival when compared with untreated dogs (Kent *et al.*, 2007): survival times range from 5 months to 4 years.
- The prognosis for animals with primitive neuroectodermal tumours (PNET) and histiocytic sarcoma is generally unfavourable.
- Limited use of SRS in dogs suggests that it compares favourably with conventional radiotherapy in terms of survival times, with fewer side effects.

Spinal cord tumours

Tumour types and pathogenesis

Tumours involving the spinal cord can also be classified as primary or secondary (Figure 21.8), depending on whether they arise from CNS neural tissue or create spinal cord signs through extension from adjacent anatomical structures. Another useful classification system is one that describes the anatomical location of the tumour relative to the meninges and spinal cord. A lesion may be extradural, intradural but extramedullary (outside the spinal cord), or intramedullary:

- Extradural tumours may arise from the vertebrae, adjacent muscle or other soft tissue, or within the spinal canal (e.g. lymphoma)
- Intradural–extramedullary lesions may arise from the meninges, peripheral nerve or nerve root
- Intramedullary tumours include astrocytomas, oligodendrogliomas and ependymomas.

The main clinical problems associated with spinal and spinal cord tumours are pain and myelopathy. Pain may result from involvement of the vertebrae, nerve roots and meninges, but is often not associated with intramedullary lesions. Myelopathy may result from direct invasion of the tumour into the spinal cord or compression of the spinal cord by an adjacent tissue mass. Occasionally haemorrhage or pathological fractures of the vertebrae may occur secondary to neoplastic disease.

Primary tumours

- Meningeal tumours:
  o Meningioma
  o Meningeal sarcoma (rare)
- Neuroepithelial tumours:
  o Astrocytoma
  o Oligodendroglioma
  o Ependymoma
- Nephroblastoma
- Haemopoietic tumours:
  o Lymphoma [a]

Secondary tumours

- Vertebral tumours:
  o Osteosarcoma
  o Chondrosarcoma
  o Fibrosarcoma
  o Plasmacytoma and multiple myeloma
  o Metastatic tumours
- Peripheral nerve tumours:
  o Peripheral nerve sheath tumour
- Soft tissue sarcomas
- Metastatic tumours

Non-neoplastic lesions
- Vascular hamartoma - Dermoid or arachnoid cysts - Intervertebral disc disease (IVDD) - Syringohydromyelia - Granuloma or abscess - Myelitis - Fibrocartilaginous embolism (FCE)

21.8 Tumours involving the spinal cord. [a] As with intracranial tumours, lymphoma may occur as a primary or secondary neoplasm.

Dogs

The most common tumours causing spinal cord disease in the dog are vertebral tumours, soft tissue sarcomas, meningiomas, and tumours of the peripheral nerve and nerve root. Common vertebral tumours include osteosarcoma, multiple myeloma and metastatic carcinomas (e.g. prostate, mammary, squamous cell). Most peripheral nerve and nerve root tumours in the dog are classified as peripheral nerve sheath tumours (PNSTs) and typically display malignant behaviour. Intramedullary tumours are uncommon in dogs, but include astrocytomas, oligodendrogliomas, ependymomas, lymphoma and metastatic tumours.

Cats

Spinal cord tumours are less common in cats than in dogs, but include many of the same types of neoplasm. Lymphoma is relatively more common in feline patients and may occur as an extradural mass, or may directly infiltrate the nerve roots and spinal cord.

Presentation and clinical signs

Tumours involving the spinal cord cause varying degrees of paresis and ataxia, and possibly decreased segmental spinal reflexes if the brachial or lumbar plexuses are involved. Spinal pain is common and may be the only clinical sign in many patients. Clinical signs are typically chronic and progressive in nature, but acute presentations can be seen, particularly when associated with sudden haemorrhage or pathological fractures of the vertebrae. A chronic lameness with subsequent development of paresis is a classic presentation for PNST, which can invade the spinal cord (discussed below).

Clinical approach

For animals with potential spinal cord neoplasia, the main differential diagnoses are intervertebral disc disease (IVDD), discospondylitis, meningomyelitis and fibrocartilaginous embolism (FCE). The main tests available to differentiate these conditions are diagnostic imaging, CSF analysis and electrodiagnostic evaluation. As with intracranial disease, a CBC, serum biochemical analysis and urinalysis are typically the first steps in order to identify comorbid disease and to evaluate the suitability of the patient for anaesthesia, which is required for most neurodiagnostic tests. Similarly, imaging of the thoracic and abdominal cavities with radiographs and ultrasonography should be considered to screen for comorbid or metastatic disease.

Diagnostic imaging

Conventional radiographs are useful to visualize the vertebrae and may show lytic lesions with tumours arising from the vertebrae or invading from adjacent soft tissue structures (Figure 21.9). Rarely, expansile spinal cord tumours may be appreciated by remodelling and widening of the vertebral canal. Spinal radiographs are also useful to identify discospondylitis. However, considerable bony destruction must be present before it can be appreciated with survey radiographs and this modality does not allow direct visualization of the spinal cord, meninges, or nerve roots.

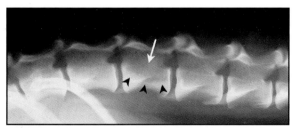

21.9 Lateral thoracolumbar spinal radiograph of a dog presented for back pain and ambulatory paraparesis. The body of the second lumbar vertebra shows reduced density, consistent with bony lysis (arrowheads). There is an absence of the thin discrete radiodense line that normally delineates the dorsal aspect of the vertebral body and the floor of the spinal canal (arrowed). The final diagnosis was osteosarcoma.

To compensate for the shortcomings inherent in conventional radiography, myelography was developed, which involves the injection of radiopaque contrast material into the subarachnoid space. Lesions identified with myelography are typically described as being extradural, intradural–extramedullary, or intramedullary (Figure 21.10). Although useful to document spinal cord compression, myelography has a number of potential limitations and side effects. Good quality images are dependent on adequate contrast

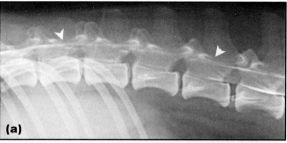

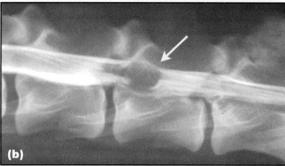

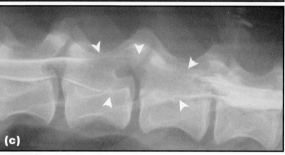

21.10 Myelographic patterns of compression. **(a)** Lateral myelogram of the thoracolumbar spine of a dog presented with back pain. There is attenuation of the ventral and dorsal contrast columns (arrowheads), consistent with an extradural lesion. **(b)** Lateral myelogram of the thoracolumbar spine of a dog presented with back pain and ataxia. There is a filling defect in the subarachnoid space, characterized by a large 'golf-tee' appearance (arrowed), consistent with an intradural–extramedullary lesion. **(c)** Lateral myelogram of the thoracolumbar spine of a dog presented with paraparesis. Note the attenuation of both the ventral and dorsal contrast columns, with apparent expansion of the spinal cord and spinal canal (arrowheads). This is consistent with an intramedullary lesion.

flow within the subarachnoid space, which can be impaired by marked compression occurring over multiple vertebral levels, contrast leakage into the epidural space, or operator inexperience. In addition, myelography can cause seizures or worsening of the spinal cord signs. As a result of these limitations, myelography is being supplanted in many specialty veterinary hospitals by more advanced diagnostic imaging techniques such as CT and MRI.

CT is much more sensitive than radiography in detecting alterations in the integrity of vertebrae (Figure 21.11) caused by bony or soft tissue tumours. In addition, CT allows improved contrast between soft tissue structures and some degree of visualization of the spinal canal. It can also be very useful after myelography to improve the identification of subarachnoid contrast and to delineate the exact location of a compressive lesion.

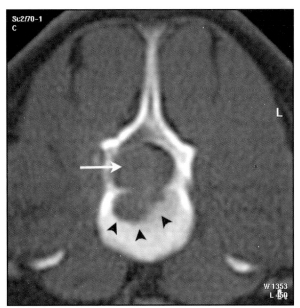

21.11 Transverse plane CT image of a lumbar vertebra in a dog presented for back pain and ataxia. Note the obvious lytic lesion of the vertebral body (arrowheads). The mass extends up into the spinal canal, and is compressing the spinal cord (arrowed). The final diagnosis was osteosarcoma.

MRI is the single best imaging modality available to evaluate spinal cord disease, and allows visualization of the spinal cord parenchyma and intramedullary lesions not detectable with other modalities (see Figures 21.12 and 21.13).

Cerebrospinal fluid analysis
Although the collection and analysis of CSF rarely provides a definitive diagnosis of spinal cord neoplasia, this test is often essential to support the diagnosis and to rule out other disease processes such as meningomyelitis. Neoplastic disease affecting the spinal cord often results in an increased CSF protein level with a normal cell count and cytology. A similar pattern is seen with many spinal cord diseases (e.g. IVDD, FCE), but meningomyelitis typically results in pleocytosis. In rare cases neoplastic cells may be identified on cytological examination.

Electrodiagnostic tests
Although rarely used in the investigation of spinal cord disease in small animals, tests such as spinal evoked potentials, cord dorsum potentials and magnetic motor evoked potentials may be useful to document spinal cord dysfunction in some scenarios. Electromyography and other electrodiagnostic techniques examining peripheral nerve function are useful to investigate peripheral nerve tumours, which may invade the spinal cord (discussed below).

Cytology and histology
Although a presumptive diagnosis of neoplastic disease may be made with imaging and CSF analysis, histological examination of a tissue sample of the mass lesion is ideal before initiating treatment. Samples of vertebral or paravertebral tumours can often be obtained with imaging guidance (ultrasound or CT) and used to plan definitive therapy. In some cases, laminectomy may be required in order to obtain a diagnostic tissue sample.

Management

Palliative therapy
Palliative therapy for tumours involving the spinal cord involves the control of pain and reduction of oedema and inflammation associated with the tumour. Glucocorticoids may reduce the vasogenic oedema associated with some tumours and improve paresis and other neurological signs. A reduction in inflammatory cells, particularly around nerve roots, may ameliorate the pain associated with the tumour. Other potentially useful medications include traditional analgesics such as non-steroidal inflammatory drugs (NSAIDs) and opioids, as well as NMDA receptor antagonists, bisphosphonates and some anticonvulsants.

Although NSAIDs and opioids can be beneficial in alleviating pain associated with bones or joints, they often function poorly in the control of neuropathic pain. Neuropathic pain involves alterations in molecular structure and signalling at the level of peripheral and central neurons. Gabapentin, pregabalin and NMDA receptor antagonists (ketamine, amantadine) may interfere with this aberrant neuronal signalling and improve pain control. Bisphosphanate drugs are potentially useful adjuncts in the management of lytic bone lesions. Tramadol is a unique drug with opioid, noradrenergic and serotonergic effects. Although any single drug may be useful in pain control, multimodal therapy is typically more effective and is usually recommended. Finally, palliative radiation therapy can be very effective in the management of spinal pain associated with vertebral tumours.

Definitive therapy
There are relatively limited options available for the definitive therapy of tumours involving the spinal cord. For most tumours, the treatment is centred around surgical excision or debulking, with or without adjunctive radiotherapy. The spinal cord is relatively sensitive to radiation and care must be taken when irradiating these tumours. The role of chemotherapy is poorly defined in the majority of these neoplasms.

Vertebral tumours and soft tissue sarcomas
Tumours of the vertebrae may be debulked surgically, which can provide some improvement and temporary relief of clinical signs. Most tumours originate from the vertebral body, and although complete removal of this structure (spondylectomy) has been described, this procedure is extremely challenging, carries a significant risk of mortality and is rarely performed. Adjunctive RT may prolong the time until recurrence of clinical signs. Soft tissue sarcomas are managed similarly, with debulking surgery and adjunctive radiotherapy. Round cell tumours of the vertebrae are treated differently (see below).

Round cell tumours
Plasmacytoma (Figure 21.12) and multiple myeloma typically arise from the bone marrow within vertebral

337

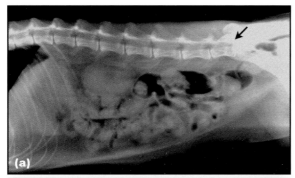

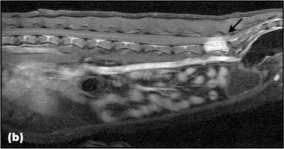

21.12 Vertebral tumour in a cat presented for spinal pain and paraparesis. **(a)** Lateral radiograph of the thoracolumbar spine. A questionable lytic lesion is present in the body of the seventh lumbar (L7) vertebra (arrowed). **(b)** Lateral plane, post-contrast, T1-weighted MR image. Note the obvious contrast-enhancing lesion involving L7 and extending dorsally into the spinal canal (arrowed). The final diagnosis was plasmacytoma.

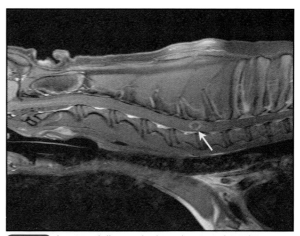

21.13 Intramedullary spinal cord tumour in a dog. Sagittal plane, post-contrast, T1-weighted MR image of the cervical spine of a dog presented for tetraparesis. Note the ring-enhancing, intramedullary lesion present over the sixth and seventh cervical vertebrae. The dog also had a large pulmonary mass. Final diagnosis was poorly differentiated metastatic sarcoma.

bodies, while lymphoma may occur within bone, as an extradural mass within the spinal canal, within nerve roots and meninges, or as an intramedullary mass. Surgery may be considered for rapid relief of signs in patients with severe compressive myelopathy, but systemic chemotherapy is the treatment of choice for most round cell neoplasms. Adjunctive radiation therapy may benefit animals with solitary lesions.

Meningiomas, peripheral nerve sheath tumours and nephroblastomas

Definitive therapy for these neoplasms is similar and consists of surgical excision with or without adjunctive radiation therapy. Debulking of the tumour often improves clinical signs and this improvement may be sustained for months, or even for several years in some cases. Occasionally tumours may be completely excised. For incompletely excised tumours, adjunctive radiotherapy should be considered.

Intramedullary tumours

Intramedullary tumours include astrocytomas, oligodendrogliomas, ependymomas, lymphoma and metastatic tumours (Figure 21.13). Therapy for these neoplasms has been infrequently described in the veterinary literature. Surgical debulking of these lesions is rarely undertaken, but may be beneficial in some cases. Radiation therapy provides a less invasive treatment that may be useful for some patients. Lymphoma is best treated with systemic chemotherapy with or without adjunctive radiotherapy.

Prognosis

The prognosis for animals with neoplasia involving the spinal cord must be considered guarded in the majority of cases, as cures are uncommon. Surgical excision may provide long-term benefit in many animals with meningiomas, nephroblastomas and low-grade PNST, with reported survival times in the range of 4 months to 4 years. One recent study found a benefit of adjunctive radiotherapy in dogs with spinal meningiomas over surgical therapy alone (Petersen *et al.*, 2008). Cats with multiple myeloma or lymphoma involving the spinal cord have a guarded prognosis. Dogs with multiple myeloma have a reasonable prognosis with systemic chemotherapy and often survive 1–3 years after diagnosis.

Peripheral nerve tumours

Tumour types

The majority of peripheral nerve tumours in small animals (Figure 21.14) are classified as peripheral nerve sheath tumours (PNSTs), which encompasses

Primary tumours
• Peripheral nerve sheath tumour (PNST)   • Lymphoma   • Peripheral neuroblastoma (rare)   • Paraganglioma (rare)
Secondary tumours
• Soft tissue sarcomas
Non-neoplastic lesions

• Neuritis
 • Myopathy
 • Focal neuropathy or radiculopathy:
    o Invertebral disc disease (IVDD)
    o Hypothyroidism

21.14 Peripheral nerve tumours.

schwannomas, neurofibromas and neurofibrosarcomas (Brehm *et al.*, 1995). These tumours affect large-breed dogs more frequently than small breeds and are rare in cats (Jones *et al.*, 1995). The brachial and lumbar plexuses are common sites of occurrence. Cranial nerve involvement is relatively uncommon, although trigeminal nerve (CN V) tumours are occasionally seen (Bagley *et al.*, 1998). In small animals PNSTs usually behave aggressively, with local tissue invasion and malignant histology, but systemic metastasis is rare. Other tumours arising from within the peripheral nervous system, including paragangliomas and peripheral neuroblastomas, have been described, but are very rare in small animals. Lymphoma can arise from within or around peripheral nerves, nerve roots or cranial nerves in both dogs and cats and occasionally affects multiple nerves or nerve roots.

Presentation and clinical signs

Tumours involving peripheral nerves cause clinical signs referable to the nerve involved, including lameness, reflex deficits, paresis, reduced muscle tone and muscle atrophy (Brehm *et al.*, 1995; Jones *et al.*, 1995). Chronic thoracic limb lameness is a common presenting complaint in larger dogs with tumours involving the brachial plexus. Although osteoarthritis or other orthopaedic disease is often suspected, these patients usually have a poor response to NSAIDs. Additional clinical signs such as atrophy of the musculature on the affected limb and pain with deep palpation of the axillary region may increase the suspicion of a brachial plexus tumour. Occasionally a mass may be palpated in the axilla or on rectal examination. With time, invasion of the spinal cord may occur, with accompanying paresis of the affected limb and pelvic limbs. Animals with trigeminal nerve sheath tumours usually present for unilateral atrophy of the masticatory muscles. Lymphoma may cause unilateral or bilateral dysfunction of single or multiple cranial nerves, without evidence of CNS signs.

Clinical approach

Focal peripheral nerve signs in an older animal are highly suggestive of neoplastic disease affecting the nerve. Other potential diagnoses include neuritis, myopathic disease, or a focal peripheral neuropathy or radiculopathy (e.g. nerve root compression secondary to IVDD or spondylosis deformans, hypothyroidism). Diagnostic tests to consider include imaging of the affected nerve or body region, electrodiagnostic evaluation of the affected nerve(s) and muscle, and potentially nerve and muscle biopsy. Routine blood tests should be considered to rule out metabolic neuropathies and as a pre-anaesthetic screen.

Diagnostic imaging

MRI (Figure 21.15) is the preferred modality for imaging the peripheral nerves (Kraft *et al.*, 2007), although CT and ultrasonography (Rose *et al.*, 2005) may be useful in some cases. Myelography may be able to detect tumours invading the spinal cord, which often cause a characteristic 'golf-tee' appearance of the

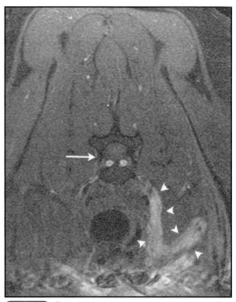

21.15 Brachial plexus tumour in a dog. Transverse plane, post-contrast, T1-weighted MR image of the cervical spine and brachial plexus of a dog presented with a chronic thoracic limb lameness. Note the contrast enhancement and marked thickening of the peripheral nerve on the right side (arrowheads). The spine is indicated by the white arrow. The final diagnosis was peripheral nerve sheath tumour.

contrast material due to their intradural location. Routine radiographic imaging is usually of limited value in the diagnosis of these neoplasms, though it may be helpful in ruling out osteoarthritis or tumours involving the bone.

Cerebrospinal fluid analysis

Although CSF analysis is normal in animals with exclusive PNS involvement, peripheral nerve tumours invading the brain or spinal cord may show CSF changes, most commonly elevations in protein. Analysis of CSF should be considered if lymphoma is a possibility, as neoplastic lymphocytes may be found in some patients.

Electrodiagnostic testing

Electromyography (EMG) often shows neuropathic changes in animals with PNSTs, which can be very helpful in supporting this diagnosis over other causes of chronic lameness (e.g. orthopaedic disease). However, this is not specific for neoplasia and may be abnormal with other peripheral neuropathies, although focal involvement of a single limb or cranial nerve is unusual with these diseases.

Cytology and histology

Examination of muscle and nerve tissue can be useful in confirming a diagnosis of peripheral neuropathy and may be supportive of non-neoplastic neuropathic or myopathic disease in some cases. Histological confirmation of the tumour is ideal before initiating definitive therapy. Therefore, an incisional or needle biopsy of a palpable mass should be considered and may be aided with ultrasound guidance in some cases (da Costa *et al.*, 2008).

Management

The best opportunity for long-term therapeutic success with PNSTs lies in complete excision of the neoplasm with wide margins. Unfortunately, this is often impossible by the time a diagnosis is made, as these tumours tend to invade proximally, often infiltrating multiple nerve roots and potentially spinal cord or brainstem (Brehm *et al.*, 1995). As a result, aggressive therapy consisting of limb amputation with laminectomy and sectioning of nerve roots at the level of the meninges may be the best chance of tumour cure, but is still unsuccessful in some cases. Likewise, PNST involving cranial nerves may be addressed successfully with surgery (Bagley *et al.*, 1998), but such treatment is usually extremely challenging and may not be possible in many animals. Patients with incomplete tumour excision may benefit from adjunctive RT.

Due to the propensity for recurrence, palliative therapy is chosen by many clients and consists mainly of analgesics. Gabapentin (and likely pregabalin), tramadol and amantadine are helpful drugs to address neuropathic pain in these patients. Although NSAIDs are often ineffective as sole therapy, they may provide a useful contribution in a multimodal analgesic protocol. Lymphoma affecting peripheral or cranial nerves may benefit from systemic chemotherapy and local radiation therapy.

Prognosis

PNSTs occurring in distal nerves that can be completely excised may have a good prognosis. However, PNSTs involving the brachial and lumbar plexuses have a guarded prognosis, due to the tendency for these tumours to invade multiple nerve roots, with resulting difficulties in complete resection (Brehm *et al.*, 1995). Recurrence of signs or the development of new spinal cord signs typically occurs within several months. Dogs with lymphoma treated with chemotherapy with or without local radiotherapy may have a reasonable prognosis, with many animals surviving 1–2 years after diagnosis.

References and further reading

Bagley RS, Wheeler SJ, Klopp L *et al.* (1998) Clinical features of trigeminal nerve-sheath tumor in 10 dogs. *Journal of the American Animal Hospital Association* **34**, 19–25

Brehm DM, Vite CH, Steinberg HS *et al.* (1995) A retrospective evaluation of 51 cases of peripheral nerve sheath tumors in the dog. *Journal of the American Animal Hospital Association* **31**, 349–359

da Costa RC, Parent JM, Dobson H *et al.* (2008) Ultrasound-guided fine needle aspiration in the diagnosis of peripheral nerve sheath tumors in 4 dogs. *Canadian Veterinary Journal* **49**, 77–81

Dickinson PJ, Roberts BN, Higgins RJ *et al.* (2006a) Expression of receptor tyrosine kinases VEGFR-1 (FLT-1), VEGFR-2 (KDR), EGFR-1, PDGFRα and c-Met in canine primary brain tumours. *Veterinary and Comparative Oncology* **4**, 132–140

Dickinson PJ, Sturges BK, Kass PH *et al.* (2006b) Characteristics of cisternal cerebrospinal fluid associated with intracranial meningiomas in dogs: 56 cases (1985–2004). *Journal of the American Veterinary Medical Association* **228**, 564–567

Forterre F, Tomek A, Konar M *et al.* (2007) Multiple meningiomas: clinical, radiological, surgical, and pathological findings with outcome in four cats. *Journal of Feline Medicine and Surgery* **9**, 36–43

Greco JJ, Aiken SA, Berg JM *et al.* (2006) Evaluation of intracranial meningioma resection with a surgical aspirator in dogs: 17 cases (1996–2004). *Journal of the American Veterinary Medical Association* **229**, 394–400

Jones BR, Alley MR, Johnstone AC *et al.* (1995) Nerve sheath tumours in the dog and cat. *New Zealand Veterinary Journal* **43**, 190–196

Kent MS, Bommarito D, Feldman E *et al.* (2007) Survival, neurologic response, and prognostic factors in dogs with pituitary masses treated with radiation therapy and untreated dogs. *Journal of Veterinary Internal Medicine* **21**, 1027–1033

Klopp LS and Rao S (2009) Endoscopic-assisted intracranial tumor removal in dogs and cats: long-term outcome of 39 cases. *Journal of Veterinary Internal Medicine* **23**, 108–115

Koblik PD, LeCouteur RA, Higgins RJ *et al.* (1999) CT-guided brain biopsy using a modified Pelorus Mark III stereotactic system: experience with 50 dogs. *Veterinary Radiology and Ultrasound* **40**, 434–440

Kraft S, Ehrhart EJ, Gall D *et al.* (2007) Magnetic resonance imaging characteristics of peripheral nerve sheath tumors of the canine brachial plexus in 18 dogs. *Veterinary Radiology and Ultrasound* **48**, 1–7

Lester NV, Hopkins AL, Bova FJ *et al.* (2001) Radiosurgery using a stereotactic headframe system for irradiation of brain tumors in dogs. *Journal of the American Veterinary Medical Association* **219**, 1562–1567

Long S, Argyle DJ, Nixon C *et al.* (2006) Telomerase reverse transcriptase (TERT) expression and proliferation in canine brain tumours. *Neuropathology and Applied Neurobiology* **32**, 662–673

Meij B, Voorhout G and Rijnberk A (2002) Progress in transsphenoidal hypophysectomy for treatment of pituitary-dependent hyperadrenocorticism in dogs and cats. *Molecular and Cellular Endocrinology* **197**, 89–96

Petersen SA, Sturges BK, Dickinson PJ *et al.* (2008) Canine intraspinal meningiomas: imaging features, histopathologic classification, and long-term outcome in 34 dogs. *Journal of Veterinary Internal Medicine* **22**, 946–953

Rose S, Long C, Knipe M *et al.* (2005) Ultrasonographic evaluation of brachial plexus tumors in five dogs. *Veterinary Radiology and Ultrasound* **46**, 514–517

Skorupski KA, Clifford CA, Paoloni MC *et al.* (2007) CCNU for the treatment of dogs with histiocytic sarcoma. *Journal of Veterinary Internal Medicine* **21**, 121–126

Snyder JM, Lipitz L, Skorupski KA *et al.* (2008) Secondary intracranial neoplasia in the dog: 177 cases (1986–2003). *Journal of Veterinary Internal Medicine* **22**, 172–177

Snyder JM, Shofer FS, Van Winkle TJ *et al.* (2006) Canine intracranial primary neoplasia: 173 cases (1986–2003). *Journal of Veterinary Internal Medicine* **20**, 669–675

Thomson SAM, Kennerly E, Olby N *et al.* (2005) Microarray analysis of differentially expressed genes of primary tumors in the canine central nervous system. *Veterinary Pathology* **42**, 550–558

Tomek A, Cizinauskas S, Doherr M *et al.* (2006) Intracranial neoplasia in 61 cats: localisation, tumour types and seizure patterns. *Journal of Feline Medicine and Surgery* **8**, 243–253

Troxel MT, Vite CH, Van Winkle TJ *et al.* (2003) Feline intracranial neoplasia: retrospective review of 160 cases (1985–2001). *Journal of Veterinary Internal Medicine* **17**, 850–859

Vernau KM, Higgins RJ, Bollen AW *et al.* (2001) Primary canine and feline nervous system tumors: intraoperative diagnosis using the smear technique. *Veterinary Pathology* **38**, 47–57

Westworth DR, Dickinson PJ, Vernau W *et al.* (2008) Choroid plexus tumors in 56 dogs (1985–2007). *Journal of Veterinary Internal Medicine* **22**, 1157–1165

22

Ocular tumours

David Gould

Introduction

In all cases of ocular and periocular tumours, it is important to carry out a thorough general physical examination in addition to a detailed ophthalmic examination. Haematology and serum biochemistry profiles may be indicated. Where malignancy is suspected, chest radiography and abdominal ultrasonography should be performed.

Tumours of the orbit

Differential diagnosis

Space-occupying lesions of the orbit may be neoplastic or non-neoplastic; Figure 22.1 lists the major differential diagnoses.

Primary tumours
• Osteosarcoma
• Fibrosarcoma
• Chondrosarcoma
• Myxosarcoma
• Meningioma
• Neurofibrosarcoma
• Adenoma
• Adenocarcinoma
• Melanoma
• Lipoma
• Histiocytoma
• Mast cell tumour
Secondary tumours
• Lymphoma
• Squamous cell carcinoma (SCC)
• Nasal adenocarcinoma
• Cerebral meningioma
Non-neoplastic orbital masses
• Abscessation
• Cellulitis
• Foreign body
• Pseudotumour
• Haemorrhage
• Zygomatic mucocele
• Masticatory myositis
• Extraocular muscle myositis
• Lacrimal gland cyst

22.1 Orbital space-occupying lesions.

Neoplastic lesions may be primary or secondary. Primary tumours may arise from the bony orbital walls or from the soft tissue contents of the orbit. A wide range of tumour types has been reported. Primary tumours tend to be slow to metastasize but are often locally invasive. Secondary tumours may enter the orbit by local extension (e.g. from the nasal cavity, paranasal sinuses, cranial cavity, oral cavity or skin) or by metastatic spread.

General considerations

Neoplasia is a common cause of orbital disease in middle-aged to older dogs. The average age of affected dogs is around 8 years and there is no apparent breed or sex predilection.

Orbital neoplasia is less common in cats, although it remains a significant cause of feline orbital disease. The average age of affected cats is around 9 years; again there is no breed or sex predilection.

In both dogs and cats >90% of orbital tumours are malignant. In dogs, the majority of orbital tumours are primary, whereas in cats secondary causes predominate.

Presentation and clinical signs

Exophthalmos (Figure 22.2) is the major presenting sign of an orbital mass. Associated signs include reduced globe retropulsion, a widened palpebral fissure, chemosis, exposure keratitis and epiphora. In cases where the mass lies outside the muscle cone formed by the retractor bulbi muscles, third-eyelid protrusion and strabismus may be seen. If the mass lies within the muscle cone formed by the retractor bulbi muscles, globe protrusion is axial and third-eyelid protrusion may be minimal.

Secondary orbital tumours that arise in the adjacent nasal passages (e.g. nasal adenocarcinoma or squamous cell carcinoma, SCC) may be associated with nasal signs including sneezing, stertor, nasal discharge (Figure 22.3) or epistaxis, and may also be associated with facial distortion.

Most orbital tumours are slowly progressive and painless. However, some may be associated with pain due to local compressive or inflammatory effects. For this reason the presence or absence of pain cannot reliably be used to distinguish an orbital tumour from orbital abscessation (the major other differential diagnosis in exophthalmos).

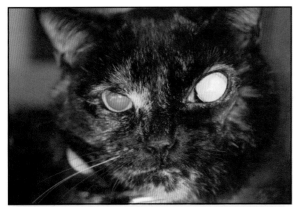

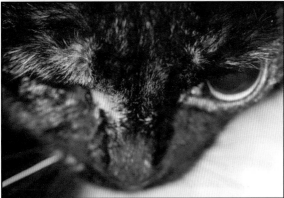

22.2 Left exophthalmos due to orbital meningioma in a 9-year-old cat. The exophthalmos was most readily evident when viewed from above: note the prominent left cornea shown in comparison with the right eye. An MRI scan showed that the tumour invaded the orbit from the brain.

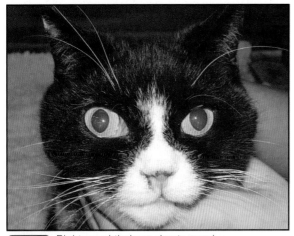

22.3 Right exophthalmos due to nasal adenocarcinoma invading the orbit. Note the ipsilateral nasal discharge.

Clinical approach

A detailed ophthalmic examination should be performed. Masses that involve cranial nerves within the orbit (II, III, IV, VI and ophthalmic branch of V) may lead to detectable cranial nerve defects such as blindness, reduced pupillary light reflexes, abnormal globe position or mobility, and reduced corneal sensation. Masses close to the globe can cause indentation of the posterior sclera, which may be visualized by ophthalmoscopy. Masses that impinge on the optic nerve sheath may induce papilloedema (Figure 22.4).

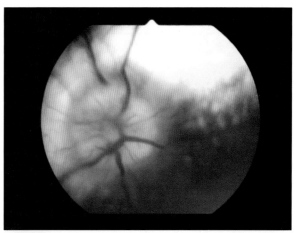

22.4 Papilloedema due to compression of the optic nerve by an orbital tumour in a dog. The optic nerve head protrudes into the vitreous, and the retinal blood vessels can be seen to change direction as they follow its course. The retina appears out of focus due to the narrow depth of field of the fundus camera.

Ultrasonography

Orbital ultrasonography is an appropriate first-line approach for imaging the orbit. Most commonly, real-time B-mode ultrasonography is performed using a 7.5 MHz scanner. This can be done on a conscious animal via a transcorneal approach, following topical corneal anaesthesia.

A major limitation of orbital ultrasonography is that it may not reveal the true extent of the mass or accurately identify its margins. This is particularly true for deep or extensive orbital disease, for example masses extending intracranially or into adjacent soft tissues. For such suspected cases, advanced imaging techniques are more appropriate.

Ultrasound-guided fine-needle aspiration (FNA) under general anaesthesia may allow cytological diagnosis of orbital neoplasia in around 50% of cases. Extreme care must be taken during this procedure to avoid inadvertent trauma to the globe.

Radiography

Skull radiography may be useful where there is bone involvement. It should include the orbit, nasal and paranasal sinuses and maxilla. A combination of lateral, dorsoventral, ventrodorsal and oblique views is required. A skyline view is useful where frontal sinus involvement is suspected; and a dorso-ventral intraoral view is also useful to identify conditions involving the nasal turbinate bones. However, the complexity of skull anatomy and the superimposed images of its structures make interpretation of radiographic images difficult. Chest radiography is indicated for staging purposes.

Advanced imaging techniques

Magnetic resonance imaging (MRI) and computed tomography (CT) provide excellent detail of orbital structures. CT provides better visualization of bony structures of the orbit, whereas MRI is superior for soft tissue visualization. These modalities are indicated when ultrasonographic results are inconclusive, when there is a possibility of extensive orbital or extra-orbital involvement, or in cases in which orbital surgery is to be considered (Dennis, 2000; Boroffka *et al.*, 2007).

Management and prognosis

Surgical resection
Surgical resection is the treatment of choice for primary orbital tumours. Small and discrete tumours may be removed via an orbitotomy, so that the globe and associated structures can be preserved (Ramsey and Fox, 1997). However, orbitotomy is a complex surgical procedure and should be performed only by experienced surgeons with knowledge of orbital anatomy and an appreciation of potential complications. Large or infiltrative tumours usually require exenteration (removal of the entire orbital contents, including the globe).

Secondary orbital tumours in general are poorly amenable to surgical resection. The surgical techniques of partial or full orbitectomy in dogs and cats have been described and can result in complete local resection.

Radiotherapy
Radiotherapy as a sole treatment for orbital neoplasia is not usually performed, because of the sensitivity of the eye to radiation. However, it may be indicated as adjunctive therapy following exenteration. It may also be used as a primary treatment for nasal or paranasal tumours with orbital extension, though such treatment is palliative and is associated with radiation-induced ocular damage.

Chemotherapy
Most orbital tumours are not amenable to chemotherapy. An exception is orbital lymphoma, which may be responsive to chemotherapeutic agents.

Prognosis
In dogs, the prognosis for orbital neoplasia is guarded to poor. In a retrospective study of 44 cases, only 19% survived for >1 year (Hendrix and Gelatt, 2000). In cats the prognosis is grave: in one study, mean survival time following diagnosis of orbital tumour was just 1.9 months (Gilger *et al.*, 1992). Another study reported a mean survival time of 10 months in dogs and <1 month in cats (Attali-Soussay *et al.*, 2001).

Tumours of the eyelid

Differential diagnosis
Non-neoplastic eyelid masses and erosive eyelid disease that may mimic erosive eyelid tumours are listed in Figure 22.5.

General considerations
Eyelid tumours are very common in dogs. With the exception of viral papilloma, they usually affect dogs older than 9 years. Eyelid tumours occur infrequently in cats.

In dogs most eyelid tumours are benign. The three most common types are:

Non-neoplastic eyelid masses

- Dermoid
- External hordeolum (abscessation or inflammation of Zeiss or Moll glands within the eyelid skin)
- Internal hordeolum (abscessation of a meibomian gland within the palpebral conjunctiva)
- Chalazion (granuloma formation following rupture of an impacted meibomian gland)
- Meibomian cyst
- Cutaneous histiocytosis
- Nodular fasciitis
- Cutaneous nodular leishmaniasis

Erosive eyelid disease that may mimic erosive eyelid tumours

- Pemphigus vulgaris
- Pemphigus erythematosus
- Systemic lupus erythematosus
- Viral blepharitis (feline pox or feline herpesvirus-1)
- Feline eosinophilic blepharitis

 22.5 Conditions to be differentiated from eyelid tumours.

- Sebaceous gland adenoma (accounting for 60% of all canine eyelid tumours)
- Benign melanoma (17% of cases)
- Squamous papilloma (11% of cases).

Other tumour types are uncommon and together account for <10% of all canine eyelid neoplasms. However, some of these may be malignant. They include malignant melanoma, sebaceous adenocarcinoma, histiocytoma, mast cell tumour (MCT), lymphoma and basal cell tumour. Malignant eyelid tumours are usually locally invasive rather than metastatic. An exception to this is malignant melanoma, which may metastasize (Roberts *et al.*, 1986).

In cats, eyelid tumours are more likely to be malignant:

- SCC is the most common eyelid neoplasm, accounting for up to 65% of cases (McLaughlin *et al.*, 1993). Major predisposing factors are exposure to ultraviolet light and lack of cutaneous pigmentation. It is locally invasive and late to metastasize.
- Other malignant tumour types in cats include fibrosarcoma, adenocarcinoma, lymphoma and haemangiosarcoma.
- Benign eyelid masses in cats include basal cell carcinoma, MCT, papilloma and apocrine hidrocystoma.

Presentation and clinical signs
Sebaceous adenomas arise from the meibomian glands and present as focal masses on the eyelid margin. Their frond-like appearance means that they are commonly clinically mistaken for papilloma. However, diagnosis is straightforward, because eversion of the eyelid will reveal swelling of the meibomian gland beneath the palpebral conjunctiva (Figure 22.6). They may be associated with ocular discomfort due to corneal irritation, which may lead to keratitis and corneal ulceration.

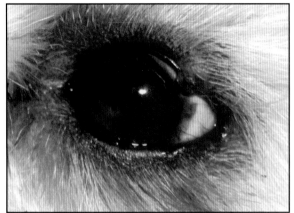

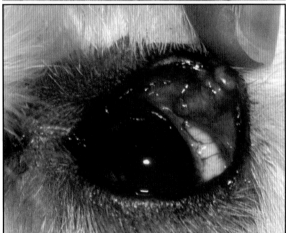

22.6 Canine sebaceous adenoma affecting the left eye of an 8-year-old West Highland White Terrier. This type of tumour arises from the meibomian gland opening on the eyelid margin. Eversion of the eyelid revealed swelling of the meibomian gland beneath the palpebral conjunctiva. (Courtesy of SM Crispin)

Other eyelid tumours in both dogs and cats present as focal, erosive or infiltrative masses of varying size (Figures 22.7 and 22.8).

Apocrine hidrocystoma in cats present as single or multiple round pigmented eyelid masses, which may be unilateral or bilateral (Figure 22.9). Histopathological examination shows that these are cystic adenomas of the apocrine sweat glands. They are more common in the Persian and Himalayan breeds.

Clinical approach

In many cases a presumptive diagnosis is made on clinical examination. Impression smears are poorly diagnostic for most eyelid tumours. FNA is usually more rewarding, though cytology does not allow tumour grading. Biopsy is the diagnostic modality of choice and excisional biopsy is usually possible for small masses.

Management and prognosis

Surgical resection
Surgical resection is the treatment of choice for most cases of eyelid neoplasia. Since there is only a finite amount of eyelid margin, it is advisable to remove eyelid tumours at an early stage, especially

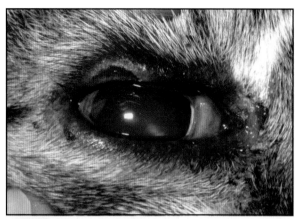

22.7 Erosive basal cell carcinoma of the right upper eyelid in a 6-year-old cat.

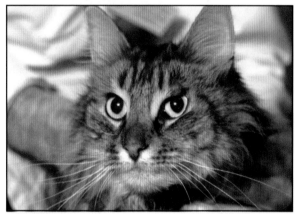

22.8 Mast cell tumour of the left upper eyelid in a 3-year-old cat.

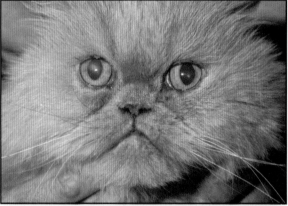

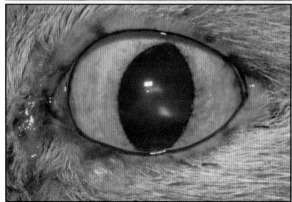

22.9 Multiple bilateral apocrine hidrocystomas affecting the lower eyelid in a 10-year-old Persian cat.

if they are enlarging. Preoperative consideration of how to achieve primary closure following mass excision is imperative. In dogs, direct primary closure of the eyelid margin can be achieved following removal of up to 25% of the eyelid margin. In cats (which have more tightly apposed eyelids) and in dogs in which >25% of the eyelid margin is removed, additional reconstructive blepharoplasty techniques are usually required to achieve primary closure of the eyelid margin. A large number of techniques have been described; these may be complex and it may be advisable to seek specialist advice.

For small tumours involving the eyelid margin, a full-thickness wedge excision is performed, followed by a two-layer closure. However, benign tumours involving only the skin and superficial subcutaneous layers may be removed by a partial thickness excision that spares the conjunctival layer (Gelatt and Gelatt, 2003).

The margin of excision required depends on tumour type. For benign masses a 1–2 mm margin of excision should be achieved where possible. For suspected malignant masses, FNA or biopsy followed by histological tumour grading is recommended prior to surgery to aid surgical planning.

Surgical resection of canine eyelid MCTs poses a particular problem, since it is impossible to achieve the 2 cm margin of excision recommended as surgical treatment for grade I–II MCTs of the skin (Fulcher et al., 2006) without losing eyelid function. Surgical resection with as wide a margin of excision as possible whilst still maintaining eyelid function is advisable. This will usually involve an additional reconstructive blepharoplasty procedure such as a pedicle advancement flap, rotational skin graft, sliding Z-plasty, full-thickness lid graft or lip-to-lid technique (Petersen-Jones, 2002; Gelatt and Gelatt, 2003).

Surgery may also be combined with adjunctive treatments such as chemotherapy in such cases, although it should be noted that there is little published information on the effectiveness of chemotherapy in treatment of MCTs and to date treatment regimes remain somewhat empirical (Dobson and Scase, 2007). Neoadjuvant therapy with prednisolone may be beneficial at this site (Stanclift and Gilson, 2008). For possible chemotherapeutic options, see Chapter 12.

Grade III MCTs require radical surgical excision including exenteration.

Cryosurgery

Cryosurgery may be performed on small eyelid tumours. Thermal coupling within and adjacent to the mass is recommended during the freezing process, and generous application of a petrolatum-based ocular lubricant to the corneal surface prior to treatment will reduce the risk of iatrogenic corneal freezing during the procedure. In studies comparing surgery and cryosurgery for treatment of eyelid tumours, recurrence rates were not significantly different but cryotherapy led to earlier tumour recurrence (Roberts et al., 1986; Collins and Collins, 1994).

Other modalities

- Brachytherapy, using radioactive gold[198] seeds, has been used successfully in the treatment of feline eyelid SCC (Hardman and Stanley, 2001).
- Carbon dioxide laser therapy has been reported for treatment of meibomian gland adenomata in dogs (Bussieres et al., 2005).
- Photodynamic therapy has been reported for the treatment of early superficial eyelid SCC in cats, although 7 of 11 treated cases (64%) subsequently recurred (Stell et al., 2001).
- Chemotherapy is indicated for lymphoma involving the eyelids. Chemotherapy may also be useful as an adjunct to surgical resection of MCTs.
- Histiocytic-type MCTs in cats (in particular the Siamese breed) may require no treatment, as these tumours may regress spontaneously.
- Apocrine hidrocystoma in cats may require no treatment, unless it causes local ocular irritation.
- External beam radiotherapy is not used in the treatment of eyelid neoplasia, because of the sensitivity of the eye to radiation.

Prognosis

The prognosis following removal of benign eyelid tumours is very good, though some (in particular, canine sebaceous adenoma) carry a significant risk of local recurrence. The prognosis following removal of malignant eyelid tumours depends on the tumour type and stage of malignancy.

- Because of its low rate of metastasis, early SCC in both dogs and cats carries a favourable prognosis.
- Invasive SCC has a more guarded prognosis, as it may be difficult to achieve adequate margins of excision.
- Malignant melanoma of the eyelids may be associated with metastatic disease and therefore carries a guarded prognosis in both dogs and cats.
- Canine MCTs of the eyelids should carry a guarded prognosis in view of the difficulty in achieving a satisfactory margin of excision, but published follow-up data on such cases are scant.
- Feline MCTs are usually benign and may regress spontaneously, particularly in the Siamese breed (Wilcock et al., 1986).
- Apocrine hidrocystomas are benign and carry a good prognosis, but recurrence or development of multiple masses is common (Cantaloube et al., 2004).

Tumours of the conjunctiva, third eyelid and external globe

Differential diagnosis

Non-neoplastic masses are listed in Figure 22.10.

Some examples of non-neoplastic ocular surface masses are shown in Figures 22.11 and 22.12.

- Dermoid
- Nodular granulomatous episclerokeratitis (NGE)
- Necrotizing or non-necrotizing sclerokeratitis
- Systemic histiocytosis
- Proliferative keratoconjunctivitis
- Nodular fasciitis
- Idiopathic sterile granulomatosis
- Staphyloma
- Subconjunctival orbital fat prolapse
- Parasitic granuloma
- Lacrimal gland cyst
- Conjunctival cyst
- Corneal epithelial cyst
- Iris prolapse
- Foreign body

22.10 Non-neoplastic masses of the conjunctiva, third eyelid and globe.

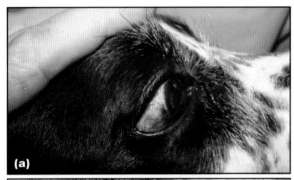

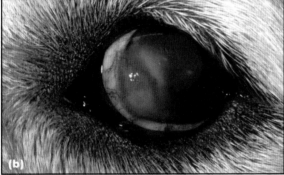

22.11 Two examples of a group of immune-mediated conditions of the canine globe that may mimic tumours: **(a)** nodular granulomatous episclerokeratitis in a 4-year-old English Springer Spaniel; **(b)** necrotizing sclerokeratitis in a 2-year-old Golden Retriever. Definitive diagnosis is by biopsy.

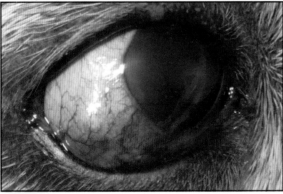

22.12 Staphyloma affecting the right eye of a 7-year-old crossbreed dog. This condition represents a focal area of scleral thinning with exposure of underlying choroidal pigment. The lesion can mimic ocular melanoma.

General considerations

Tumours of the conjunctiva, third eyelid or external globe are uncommon in dogs and cats. Reported types include melanoma, SCC, lymphoma, MCT, papilloma, adenocarcinoma, haemangioma, haemangiosarcoma, fibrosarcoma, histiocytoma, transmissible venereal tumour, lobular orbital adenoma, angioendothelioma, angiokeratoma and epithelioma.

Because of the large differential diagnosis list, biopsy is recommended if there is any doubt as to the nature of the mass under investigation.

Presentation and clinical signs

Conjunctival and third-eyelid tumours usually present as a visible mass or erosive lesion. They may be associated with secondary conjunctivitis and ocular discharge, which may mask the underlying disease. Diffuse conjunctival lymphoma may mimic chronic conjunctivitis (Figure 22.13), as may conjunctival MCTs. Melanoma usually presents as a focal dark swelling of varying size, most commonly arising from the limbus or epibulbar region (Figure 22.14). Intraocular tumours may extend externally through the limbus to mimic limbal melanoma (Figure 22.15).

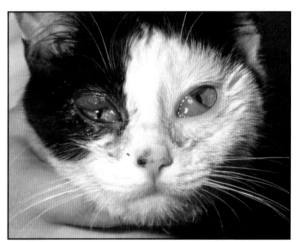

22.13 Lymphoma infiltrating the right dorsal palpebral conjunctiva in a 4-month-old FeLV-positive DSH cat. This condition can mimic chronic conjunctivitis. Conjunctival biopsy is usually diagnostic.

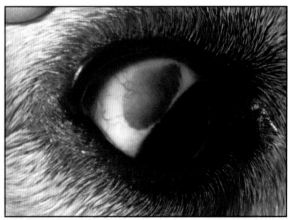

22.14 Canine epibulbar melanoma in a 6-year-old Golden Retriever. Epibulbar and limbal melanomas involve the episclera, not the overlying conjunctiva; note how the conjunctival blood vessels pass over the tumour and not into it.

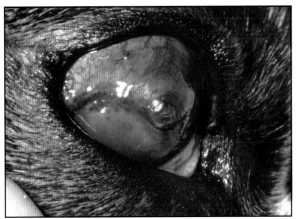

22.15 Canine anterior uveal melanoma in an 8-year-old Boxer dog, showing extraocular extension through the limbus. It is important to differentiate this from limbal melanoma.

Clinical approach

Ophthalmic examination
A thorough ophthalmic examination should be performed. For limbal melanoma, this should include gonioscopy (examination of the iridocorneal drainage angle) to check for intraocular involvement. Gonioscopy is a specialist technique and referral to a veterinary ophthalmologist should be considered in such cases.

Imaging
Ocular and orbital ultrasonography is indicated if local invasion of tissues is suspected. Chest radiography is indicated for conjunctival or third-eyelid tumours if there is a possibility of malignant disease. Diagnostic imaging is not usually indicated for canine limbal melanoma. However, thoracic radiography and abdominal ultrasonography may be advisable for feline limbal melanoma in view of the possibility of distant metastasis.

Biopsy
Biopsy is indicated in most cases. It is particularly useful to distinguish neoplasia from inflammatory conditions such as nodular granulomatous episclerokeratitis. For small masses, excisional biopsy is often possible.

Management and prognosis

Limbal and epibulbar melanomas
In dogs, limbal or epibulbar melanoma is nearly always benign. German Shepherd Dogs may be predisposed. In cats, limbal melanoma is also usually benign, although metastatic disease has been reported (Day and Lucke, 1995; Betton et al., 1999). In middle-aged to older dogs, in which these tumours are usually very slow growing, regular monitoring may be sufficient. In young dogs, however, limbal or epibulbar melanoma may grow rapidly and therefore early treatment is recommended. Likewise, in cats (in which the tumour may be malignant), early intervention is advisable.

Surgical excision followed by cryosurgery is usually curative. Laser photocoagulation has also been reported, but recurrence rates were slightly higher than for combined excision/cryosurgery (Sullivan et al., 1996).

Conjunctival melanoma
Conjunctival melanoma at a site distant to the limbus is uncommon, but is important to recognize because its behaviour may be aggressive. In a case series of 12 dogs, local recurrence after excision was reported in 6 cases and metastasis in 2 cases (Collins et al., 1991). In cats, there have only been a few reports of conjunctival melanoma, but from these reports it seems to be malignant in the majority of cases, with local recurrence and distant metastasis likely (Patnaik and Mooney, 1988; Cook et al., 1995; Schobert and Dubielzig, 2008). However, benign feline conjunctival melanoma has been reported (Payen et al., 2008).

In both dogs and cats, wide surgical excision in combination with cryosurgery is advised following distant staging.

Conjunctival or third-eyelid MCT
In dogs, case reports of conjunctival MCTs indicate that they are histopathologically and clinically benign (Johnson et al., 1988). A recent retrospective study of 35 conjunctival MCTs in dogs indicated a breed predisposition in the Labrador Retriever. Around 90% of the tumours were grade I or II, and follow-up data up to 24 months showed that no dogs died of MCT-related disease (Fife et al., 2007).

A single report of a third-eyelid MCT in a cat stated that surgical excision with a narrow margin of excision was curative (Larocca, 2000).

Third-eyelid adenocarcinoma
The treatment of choice is removal of the entire third eyelid, because of the risk of local invasion. If the tumour has invaded the orbit, exenteration is required.

Squamous cell carcinoma
Accurate determination of tumour margins is important, because SCC of the third eyelid or conjunctiva is often associated with extension from the eyelids, and the tumour may also invade into the orbit. Surgical excision, possibly in combination with other modalities, may be indicated. If local invasion is extensive, exenteration may be indicated.

Prognosis

- Third-eyelid adenocarcinoma and SCC are locally invasive, rather than metastatic, and have a good prognosis if treated early (Wilcock and Peiffer, 1988).
- MCTs of the conjunctiva or third eyelid in dogs and cats seem to carry a good prognosis following local excision (Gilger et al., 2007).
- Limbal melanoma in dogs has a good prognosis following surgical removal. In cats the prognosis is also good but it should be borne in mind that

distant metastasis has been documented in this species (Day and Lucke, 1995; Betton *et al.*, 1999).
- Conjunctival melanoma has a guarded prognosis in dogs and a poor prognosis in cats, in view of the risk of local recurrence and of metastasis (Collins *et al.*, 1991; Patnaik and Mooney, 1998).

Intraocular tumours

Differential diagnosis
Non-neoplastic intraocular masses are listed in Figure 22.16.

- Benign iris pigmentation
- Ocular melanosis
- Foreign body
- Uveal cyst
- Inflammatory masses

22.16 Non-neoplastic intraocular masses.

General considerations
Intraocular tumours may be primary or secondary. The two most common primary tumour types are uveal melanoma and iridociliary epithelial tumour. Other primary tumours are rare but reported types include sarcoma (cats only), medulloepithelioma, astrocytoma, glioma, ciliary body haemangioma, iridal haemangiosarcoma, iridal leiomyosarcoma, iridal myxoid leiomyoma, primary ocular osteosarcoma and anterior uveal spindle-cell tumour.

The most common secondary intraocular tumour is lymphoma (see Chapter 19a). Other types reported include haemangiosarcoma, metastatic adenocarcinoma, metastatic carcinoma, metastatic melanoma, malignant histiocytosis, seminoma, transmissible venereal tumour, sarcoma, fibrosarcoma, rhabdomyosarcoma, phaeochromocytoma and histiocytic sarcoma.

Uveal melanoma
Melanoma is the most common primary intraocular tumour of dogs and cats. It usually arises from the anterior uveal tract (iris or ciliary body); choroidal melanoma is rare. In both species, older animals are most commonly affected. A breed predisposition in Labrador Retrievers and Persian cats has been suggested, though this remains unproven.

The behaviour of anterior uveal melanoma is different in dogs and cats. The majority of canine anterior uveal melanomas are benign and only around 5% metastasize. Nonetheless, even benign melanomas may be locally invasive (Giuliano *et al.*, 1999). In contrast, feline anterior uveal melanoma is very aggressive, with local invasion and metastasis the norm. It has a reported metastatic rate of up to 63% (Patnaik and Mooney, 1988).

Iridociliary epithelial tumours
Ciliary body adenoma and adenocarcinoma are the next most common primary intraocular tumours of dogs, but are rare in cats. Middle-aged to older dogs are predisposed. Adenomas are well differentiated, slow growing and, although they may infiltrate the ciliary body or iris stroma, do not invade the sclera. Adenocarcinomas are less well differentiated, show increased numbers of mitotic figures and are locally invasive. The metastatic potential of both adenoma and adenocarcinoma is extremely low, but metastasis to the lungs has been documented on occasion.

Medulloepithelioma arising from the undifferentiated non-pigmented epithelium of the ciliary body has been reported (Klosterman *et al.*, 2006).

Sarcoma
Intraocular sarcoma is the second most common primary intraocular tumour of cats after anterior uveal melanoma. Previous ocular trauma is a major predisposing factor (Dubielzig *et al.*, 1990). Older cats are most at risk and the time from traumatic injury to diagnosis of sarcoma averages 5 years. Secondary uveitis or glaucoma is common. The tumour is highly malignant and both local invasion and metastatic disease are common.

Glioma
Non-neuronal CNS tissue tumours reported to involve the retina or optic nerve head include astrocytoma and oligodendroglioma (Naranjo *et al.*, 2008). The metastatic potential is low.

Secondary tumours
With the exception of lymphoma, secondary intraocular tumours are uncommon. They may invade the eye by haematogenous spread or by local extension. Local extension is rare, because the tough fibrous coat of the globe offers a formidable physical barrier, but intracranial tumours such as meningioma may invade the posterior segment via the optic nerve sheath. Haematogenous spread accounts for most secondary tumours and these include lymphoma, haemangiosarcoma, carcinoma/adenocarcinoma, osteosarcoma and oral malignant melanoma, amongst others. In one study, 37% of dogs with lymphoma had ocular involvement, making ocular disease the second most common presenting sign of lymphoma after lymphadenopathy (Krohne *et al.*, 1994).

Presentation and clinical signs
All intraocular tumours, whether benign or malignant, may cause severe intraocular pathology due to space-occupying effects, local infiltration and release of local immunogenic and angiogenic factors. Common complications include intraocular haemorrhage, uveitis, retinal detachment and glaucoma. The presence of these may mask the underlying tumour.

Melanoma
Canine anterior uveal melanoma affecting the iris usually presents as a discrete nodular mass on the surface of the iris (Figure 22.17). Secondary changes such as haemorrhage, uveitis, retinal detachment and glaucoma are common and may mask the underlying tumour. Differential diagnosis includes benign iris melanosis and anterior uveal cyst (Figure 22.18). In the Cairn Terrier a major differential diagnosis is diffuse ocular melanosis (Petersen-Jones *et al.*, 2007, 2008).

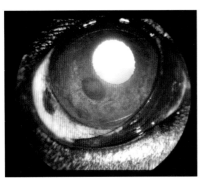

22.17 Benign anterior uveal melanoma affecting the iris in a 7-year-old crossbreed dog.

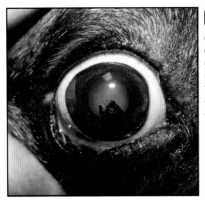

22.18 Anterior uveal cyst in a 4-year-old crossbreed dog. Transillumination using focal illumination demonstrates its cystic nature.

Feline iris melanoma usually presents as progressive diffuse infiltration of the iris (Figure 22.19) rather than a nodular mass. The main differential diagnoses are benign iris melanosis (Figure 22.20) and chronic uveitis, and it may be impossible to distinguish these conditions by clinical examination alone. Clues that a pigmented iris lesion may be neoplastic include:

- Progressive and insidious iris pigmentation
- Iris thickening
- Increased intraocular pressure relative to the contralateral eye
- Abnormalities in pupil size or motility
- Pigment shedding into the anterior chamber when viewed by a slit-lamp
- Pigment invasion of the iridocorneal drainage angle when viewed by gonioscopy.

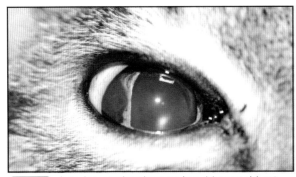

22.19 Anterior uveal melanoma in a 14-year-old cat. Note the pupil distortion and pigment deposition on the anterior lens capsule, both of which imply potential malignancy. Thickening of the iris was also evident on slit-lamp examination, and the intraocular pressure was elevated relative to the contralateral eye. In addition, gonioscopy revealed progression of the pigmented tumour towards the iridocorneal drainage angle (see Figure 22.26).

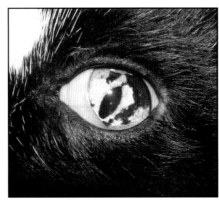

22.20 Benign ocular melanosis in a 4-year-old cat.

Iridociliary epithelial tumours

These usually present as pink or red intraocular masses that may protrude through or distort the pupil (Figure 22.21). Occasionally pigmented iridociliary tumours are encountered that may mimic anterior uveal melanoma (Figure 22.22). Secondary intraocular changes such as haemorrhage, uveitis, retinal detachment and glaucoma may occur.

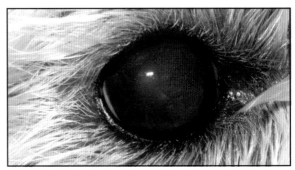

22.21 Ciliary body adenoma in a 10-year-old West Highland White Terrier. The mass protrudes through and distorts the pupil medially. In this case, FNA of the mass allowed cytological diagnosis.

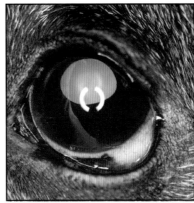

22.22 Rarely, pigmented iridociliary tumours are seen that may mimic anterior uveal melanoma. In this 11-year-old Staffordshire Bull Terrier, ophthalmic examination suggested an iris melanoma. However, histopathological examination following enucleation revealed a pigmented iridociliary tumour. (below, courtesy of J Mould)

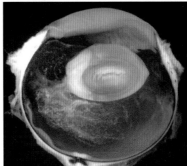

Retinal tumours
Primary tumours of the retina, choroid or optic nerve are very rare.

Secondary tumours
These may present as bilateral ocular disease or concurrent systemic disease. Uveitis, intraocular haemorrhage and secondary glaucoma are common and may mask the underlying tumour. In canine lymphoma, neoplastic lymphocytes may infiltrate the cornea, creating a characteristic dense white circumcorneal band (Figure 22.23).

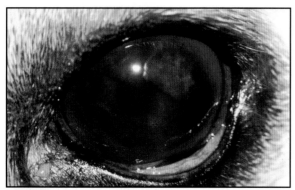

22.23 Multicentric lymphoma causing anterior uveitis in a 5-year-old Labrador Retriever. In this case chronic uveitis has caused extensive adhesions between the iris and lens capsule, leading to iris bombé and secondary glaucoma. Note the dense white circumcorneal band.

Clinical approach

Ophthalmic examination
A complete ophthalmic examination should be performed, including tonometry to measure the intraocular pressure and gonioscopy to examine the iridocorneal drainage angle. These two diagnostic techniques are especially important in the investigation of anterior uveal melanomas, which may invade the iridocorneal drainage angle and cause secondary glaucoma.

Tonometry should be performed with minimal restraint. Particular care must be taken to avoid pressure on the patient's neck, since obstruction of the jugular veins will transiently raise intraocular pressure. The patient should be conscious, standing or in sternal recumbency (Figure 22.24). Applanation

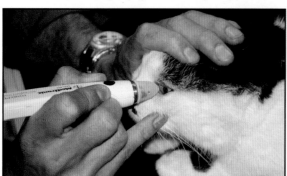

22.24 Tonometry using an applanation tonometer. Care must be taken to avoid pressure on the neck, as this can artificially elevate intraocular pressure readings.

tonometry or rebound tonometry (e.g. using a Tonopen or Tonovet, respectively) are the most accurate methods in veterinary patients. When measuring intraocular pressures, left and right eyes should be compared. If there is a difference in intraocular pressure of 8 mmHg or more, this may be considered significant (Ollivier *et al.*, 2007).

Gonioscopy describes the examination of the iridocorneal drainage angle. For anatomical reasons, direct visualization of the drainage angle is difficult and a variety of goniolenses have been developed to facilitate examination (Figure 22.25). The goniolens is placed on the corneal surface following application of topical anaesthesia and the drainage angle is then visualized through the goniolens with the aid of a slit-lamp (Figure 22.26). Gonioscopy is a specialist technique and referral to a veterinary ophthalmologist trained in its use is recommended. Following gonioscopy, it is important to dilate the pupil with a mydriatic and examine the posterior segment in detail.

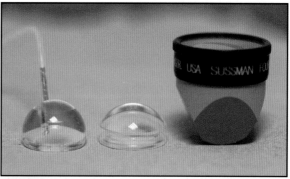

22.25 Barkan-Lovac, Koeppe and Sussman goniolenses.

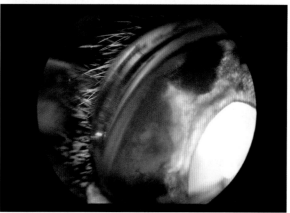

22.26 Gonioscopy of the eye shown in Figure 22.19 using a Koeppe goniolens revealed pigmented tissue extending towards the pectinate fibres of the iridocorneal drainage angle.

Haematology/serum biochemistry
This is generally not indicated in the investigation of intraocular tumours, except when secondary neoplasia is suspected (in particular, lymphoma).

Diagnostic imaging
Ocular ultrasonography is indicated for all intraocular tumours in order to assess the size and location of the intraocular mass. Thoracic and abdominal radiography and abdominal ultrasonography are indicated

for malignant neoplasia. MRI or CT scanning may be helpful in determining the extent of locally invasive tumours (in particular, feline intraocular sarcoma).

Aqueocentesis

Cytology of an aqueocentesis sample may be diagnostic for ocular lymphoma, but is not helpful in the diagnosis of other intraocular tumours as cell shedding into the aqueous humour is usually minimal. The technique should be performed under sterile surgical conditions with the patient under general anaesthesia and with the aid of a strong light source. A 25–27 G needle attached to a 1 ml syringe is passed via the limbus into the anterior chamber (Figure 22.27). Fine tissue forceps are required to stabilize the globe during passage of the needle. Magnification in the form of surgical head loupes aids visualization during the procedure, and extreme care must be taken to avoid iatrogenic damage to the iris or lens. A 0.2 ml sample of aqueous humour is slowly and carefully withdrawn and placed in an EDTA tube. If cytological examination is not to be performed immediately, a drop of formalin in the collection tube will aid cell preservation. Because of the relatively low cell yield from a sample of aqueous humour, cytospin analysis following collection of the sample is recommended prior to cytological examination.

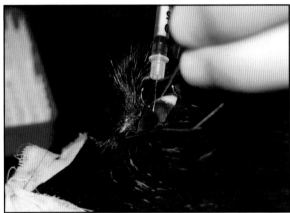

22.27 Aqueocentesis technique. This can aid diagnosis of ocular lymphoma when suggestive anterior segment signs such as anterior uveitis are present. It is rarely useful for diagnosis of other tumour types, since there is minimal cell shedding from most types of anterior segment tumours.

Biopsy/FNA

FNA of anterior segment tumours is not routinely performed, because it has a low diagnostic yield. Furthermore, the technique carries a risk of severe intraocular complications such as haemorrhage and traumatic lens rupture. Biopsy of anterior segment tumours is performed occasionally, but wet-field cautery is required because of the high risk of intraocular haemorrhage; only clinicians experienced in intraocular surgery should perform this technique.

Histopathological examination of excised tumour tissue gives a guide to its malignant potential. For anterior uveal melanoma, mitotic index is the most reliable indicator of malignancy in both dogs and cats (Bussanich *et al.*, 1987; Day and Lucke, 1995). For epithelial tumours, specialized staining

techniques can be used to differentiate primary epithelial tumours from secondary metastatic disease (Dubielzig *et al.*, 1998).

Management and prognosis

Surgery

Surgical excision is possible for some small iris tumours, but experience of intraocular surgery and access to wet-field cautery is required. In many cases enucleation is indicated. Following removal, all tumour tissue should be submitted for histopathological evaluation.

Other modalities

- Regular monitoring of canine primary intraocular tumours may be sufficient in view of their benign behaviour. Enucleation should be considered if they progress to cause local mass effects such as glaucoma, or if malignancy is suspected.
- Diode laser photocoagulation has been used to treat presumed iris melanoma in dogs (Cook and Wilkie, 1999). This has the major benefit of preserving the globe and vision and may be useful in the early stages of disease. To date, there are no published reports of its use in the treatment of feline anterior uveal melanoma.
- Radiation therapy may have a palliative role in advanced ocular sarcoma.
- Chemotherapy is indicated for lymphoma with ocular involvement.

Prognosis

Prognosis depends on tumour type and species.

- Generally, canine primary intraocular tumours carry a very good prognosis following removal, though histologically malignant anterior uveal melanoma is associated with a shorter life expectancy (Giuliano *et al.*, 1999).
- Feline anterior uveal melanoma carries a guarded prognosis, with a shortened life expectancy and a high risk of metastatic disease to lungs and liver (Patnaik and Mooney, 1988; Kalishman *et al.*, 1998).
- Feline intraocular sarcoma carries a very poor prognosis, with mortality rate exceeding 90% (Peiffer *et al.*, 1999).
- In dogs, lymphoma with ocular involvement carries a poor prognosis. Ocular involvement in animals with lymphoma indicates stage V disease, and dogs presenting with ocular involvement have a life expectancy that is 60–70% of that of dogs presenting without ocular signs (Krohne *et al.*, 1994).

Ocular paraneoplastic signs

Paraneoplastic signs within the eye may be seen with some extraocular tumours; therefore, a complete ophthalmic examination is warranted in all cases where neoplasia is suspected.

- Multiple myeloma may cause serum hyperviscosity.
- Examination of the retinal blood vessels may demonstrate grossly dilated and tortuous retinal blood vessels. Intraretinal haemorrhage and retinal detachment may also be observed.
- Brain tumours may cause visual deficits or cranial nerve abnormalities, depending on their location. Brain tumours may also be associated with swelling of the optic nerve head (papilloedema), due to raised intracranial pressure (Figure 22.28).
- Uveitis may be seen in a variety of systemic tumours, in particular lymphoma.
- Feline leukaemia virus (FeLV) may cause abnormalities in pupil shape (D-shaped pupil) due to infiltration of tumour cells into the oculomotor nerve or iris. FeLV infection may also be associated with nystagmus, intraretinal haemorrhage and anterior uveitis (Brightman *et al.*, 1986).
- In cats, the eye appears to be a preferential site for metastasis of primary lung carcinoma, in a similar way that metastasis to the digits has been documented in such tumours. Tumour cells may block end-stage blood vessels within the choroid, leading to an ischaemic chorioretinopathy. The resultant chorioretinal necrosis gives a characteristic ophthalmoscopic appearance of areas of tan discoloration in the tapetal fundus (Cassotis *et al.*, 1999). The tumour cells infiltrate not only the blood vessels but also all intraocular surfaces, yet interestingly they do not form discrete masses in any of these sites (Mould and Billson, 2002).

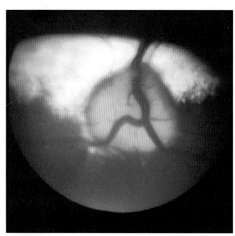

22.28 Papilloedema in association with an intracranial mass in a 12-year-old West Highland White Terrier.

References and further reading

Attali-Soussay K, Jegou JP and Clerc B (2001) Retrobulbar tumors in dogs and cats: 25 cases. *Veterinary Ophthalmology* **4**, 19–27

Betton A, Healy LN, English RV and Bunch SE (1999) Atypical limbal melanoma in a cat. *Journal of Veterinary Internal Medicine* **13**, 379–381

Billson M, Miller-Michau T, Mould JRB and Davidson MG (2006) Idiopathic sclerosing pseudotumour in seven cats. *Veterinary Ophthalmology* **9**, 45–51

Boroffka SAED, Verbruggen A-M, Grinwis GCM, Voorhout G and Barthez PY (2007) Assessment of ultrasonography and computed tomography for the evaluation of unilateral orbital disease in dogs.

Journal of the American Veterinary Medical Association **230**, 671–680

Brightman AH, Ogilvie GK and Tompkins M (1986) Ocular disease in FeLV-positive cats: 11 cases (1981–1986). *Journal of the American Veterinary Medical Association* **198**, 1049–1051

Brooks DE (1999) Ocular imaging. In: *Textbook of Veterinary Ophthalmology, 3rd edn*, ed. KN Gelatt, pp. 467–482. Williams and Wilkins, Philadelphia

Bussanich NM, Dolman PJ, Rootman J and Dolman CL (1987) Canine uveal melanomas: series and literature review. *Journal of the American Animal Hospital Association* **23**, 415–422

Bussieres M, Krohne SG, Stiles J and Townsend WM (2005) The use of carbon dioxide laser for ablation of meibomian gland adenomas in dogs. *Journal of the American Animal Hospital Association* **41**, 227–234

Cantaloube B, Raymond-Letron I and Regnier A (2004) Multiple eyelid apocrine hidrocystomas in two Persian cats. *Veterinary Ophthalmology* **7**, 121–125

Cassotis NJ, Dubielzig RR, Gilger BC and Davidson MG (1999) Angioinvasive pulmonary carcinoma with posterior segment metastasis in four cats. *Veterinary Ophthalmology* **2**, 125–131

Chaitman J, van der Woerdt A and Bartick TE (1999) Multiple eyelid cysts resembling apocrine hidrocystomas in three Persian cats and one Himalayan cat. *Veterinary Pathology* **36**, 474–476

Collins BK, Collier LL, Miller MA and Linton LL (1991) Biological behaviour and histological characteristics of canine conjunctival melanoma. *Progress in Veterinary and Comparative Ophthalmology* **3**, 135–139

Collins LL and Collins BK (1994) Excision and cryosurgical ablation of severe periocular papillomatosis in a dog. *Journal of the American Veterinary Medical Association* **204**, 881–885

Cook CS and Wilkie DA (1999) Treatment of presumed iris melanoma in dogs by diode laser photocoagulation. *Veterinary Ophthalmology* **2**, 217–225

Cook CS, Rosenkrantz W and Peiffer RL (1995) Malignant melanoma of the conjunctiva in a cat. *Journal of the American Veterinary Medical Association* **186**, 505–506

Day MJ and Lucke VM (1995) Melanocytic neoplasia in the cat. *Journal of Small Animal Practice* **36**, 207–213

Dennis R (2000) Use of magnetic resonance imaging for the investigation of orbital disease in small animals. *Journal of Small Animal Practice* **41**, 145–155

Dobson JM and Scase TJ (2007) Advances in the diagnosis and management of cutaneous mast cell tumours in dogs. *Journal of Small Animal Practice* **48**, 424–431

Dubielzig RR, Everitt J, Shadduck JA et al. (1990) Clinical and morphological features of post traumatic ocular sarcomas in cats. *Veterinary Pathology* **27**, 62–65

Dubielzig RR, Steinberg H, Garvin H, Deehr AJ and Fischer B (1998) Iridociliary epithelial tumours in 100 dogs and 17 cats: a morphological study. *Veterinary Ophthalmology* **1**, 223–231

Fife MM, Blocker T, Dubielzig RR, Fife T and Dunn K (2007) Retrospective evaluation of canine conjunctival mast cell tumours. *ACVO 2007 Abstracts, Veterinary Ophthalmology* **10**, 398

Fulcher RP, Ludwog LL, Bergman PJ et al. (2006) Evaluation of a two-centimeter lateral surgical margin for excision of grade I and grade II cutaneous mast cell tumours in dogs. *Journal of the American Veterinary Medical Association* **228**, 210–215

Gelatt KN and Gelatt JP (2003) Surgery of the eyelids. In: *Small Animal Ophthalmic Surgery: Practical Techniques for the Veterinarian*, pp. 74–124. Butterworth Heinemann, Edinburgh

Gilger BC, Bentley E and Ollivier FJ (2007) Diseases and surgery of the canine cornea and sclera. In: *Veterinary Ophthalmology, 4th edn*, ed. KN Gelatt, pp. 690–752. Blackwell Publishing, Ames, Iowa

Gilger BC, McLaughlin SA, Whitley RD and Wright JC (1992) Orbital neoplasms in cats: 21 cases (1974–1990). *Journal of the American Veterinary Medical Association* **201**, 1083–1086

Giuliano EA, Chappell R, Fischer B and Dubielzig RR (1999) A matched observational study of canine survival with primary intraocular melanocytic neoplasia. *Veterinary Ophthalmology* **2**, 185–190

Glaze MB and Gelatt KN (1999) Feline ophthalmology. In: *Textbook of Veterinary Ophthalmology, 3rd edn*, ed. KN Gelatt, pp. 997–1052. Williams and Wilkins, Philadelphia

Grahn BH, Peiffer RL, Cullen CL and Haines DM (2006) Classification of feline intraocular neoplasms based on morphology, histochemical staining, and immunohistochemical labeling. *Veterinary Ophthalmology* **9**, 395–403

Hardman C and Stanley R (2001) Radioactive gold-198 seeds for the treatment of squamous cell carcinoma in the eyelid of a cat. *Australian Veterinary Journal* **79**, 604–608

Headrick JF, Bentley E and Dubielzig RR (2004) Canine lobular orbital adenoma: a report of 15 cases with distinctive features. *Veterinary Ophthalmology* **7**, 47–51

Hendrix DVH (1999) Diseases and surgery of the canine conjunctiva. In: *Textbook of Veterinary Ophthalmology, 3rd edn*, ed. KN Gelatt, pp. 619–634. Williams and Wilkins, Philadelphia

Hendrix DVH (2007) Diseases and surgery of the canine anterior uvea. In: *Textbook of Veterinary Ophthalmology, 4th edn,* ed. KN Gelatt, pp. 812 858. Blackwell Publishing, Ames, Iowa

Hendrix DVH and Gelatt KN (2000) Diagnosis, treatment and outcome of orbital neoplasia in dogs: a retrospective study of 44 cases. *Journal of Small Animal Practice* **41,** 105–108

Johnson BW, Brightman AH and Whiteley HE (1988) Conjunctival mast cell tumour in two dogs. *Journal of the American Animal Hospital Association* **37,** 557–562

Kalishman JB, Chappell R, Flood LA and Dubielzig RR (1998) A matched observational study of survival in cats with enucleation due to diffuse iris melanoma. *Veterinary Ophthalmology* **1,** 25–29

Kern TJ (1985) Orbital neoplasia in 23 dogs. *Journal of the American Veterinary Medical Association* **186,** 489–491

Klosterman E, Colitz CMH, Chandler HL *et al.* (2006) Immunohistochemical properties of ocular adenomas, adenocarcinomas and medulloepitheliomas. *Veterinary Ophthalmology* **9,** 387–394

Kneissl S, Konar M, Fuchs-Baumgartinger A and Nell B (2007) Magnetic resonance imaging features of orbital inflammation with intracranial extension in four dogs. *Veterinary Radiology and Ultrasound* **48,** 403–408

Krohne SG, Henderson NM, Richardson RC and Vestre WA (1994) Prevalence of ocular involvement in dogs with multicentric lymphoma: prospective evaluation of 94 cases. *Veterinary and Comparative Ophthalmology* **4,** 127–135

Larocca RD (2000) Eosinophilic conjunctivitis, herpes virus and mast cell tumor of the third eyelid in a cat. *Veterinary Ophthalmology* **3,** 221–225

Mason DR, Lamb CR and McLellan GJ (2001) Ultrasonographic findings in 50 dogs with retrobulbar disease. *Journal of the American Animal Hospital Association* **37,** 557–562

Mauldin EA, Deehr AJ, Hertzke D and Dubielzig RR (2000) Canine orbital meningiomas: a review of 22 cases. *Veterinary Ophthalmology* **3,** 11–16

McLaughlin SA, Whitley RD, Gilger BC, Wright JC and Lindley DM (1993) Eyelid neoplasms in cats: a review of demographic data. *Journal of the American Animal Hospital Association* **29,** 63–67

Mould JRB and Billson FM (2002) 'Lung–eye syndrome' in the cat. In: *BSAVA Scientific Proceedings, 45th Annual Congress,* Birmingham, p. 614

Naranjo C, Dubielzig R and Friedrichs KR (2007) Canine ocular histiocytic sarcoma. *Veterinary Ophthalmology* **10,** 178–185

Naranjo C, Schobert C and Dubielzig R (2008) Canine ocular gliomas: a retrospective study. *Veterinary Ophthalmology* **11,** 356–362

Narfstrom K and Petersen-Jones S (2007) Diseases of the canine ocular fundus. In: *Veterinary Ophthalmology, 4th edn,* ed. KN Gelatt, pp. 944–1025. Blackwell Publishing, Ames, Iowa

O'Brien MG, Withrow SJ, Straw RC, Posers BE and Kirpenstein JK (1996) Total and partial orbitectomy for the treatment of periorbital tumours in 24 dogs and 6 cats: a retrospective study. *Veterinary Surgery* **25,** 471–479

Ollivier FJ, Plummer CE and Barrie KP (2007) Ophthalmic examination and diagnostics. Part 1: The eye examination and diagnostic procedures. In: *Textbook of Veterinary Ophthalmology, 4th edn,* ed. KN Gelatt, pp. 812–858. Blackwell Publishing, Ames, Iowa

Patnaik AK and Mooney S (1988) Feline melanoma: a comparative study of ocular, oral, and dermal neoplasms. *Veterinary Pathology* **25,** 105–112

Payen G, Estrada M, Clerc B and Chahory S (2008) A case of conjunctival melanoma in a cat. *Veterinary Ophthalmology* **11,** 401–405

Peiffer RL, Wilcock BP, Dubielzig RR, Render JA and Whiteley HE (1999) Fundamentals of veterinary ophthalmic pathology. In: *Textbook of Veterinary Ophthalmology, 3rd edn,* ed. KN Gelatt, pp. 355–425. Williams and Wilkins, Philadelphia

Petersen-Jones SM (2002) The eyelids and nictitating membrane. In: *BSAVA Manual of Small Animal Ophthalmology, 2nd edn,* ed. S Petersen-Jones and S Crispin, pp 78–104. BSAVA Publications, Gloucester

Petersen-Jones SM, Forcier J and Mentzer AL (2007) Ocular melanosis in the Cairn Terrier: clinical description and investigation of mode of inheritance. *Veterinary Ophthalmology* **10** (Supplement 1), 63–69

Petersen-Jones SM, Mentzer AL, Dubielzig RR *et al.* (2008) Ocular melanosis in the Cairn Terrier: histopathological description of the condition, and immunohistological and ultrastructural characterization of the characteristic pigment-laden cells. *Veterinary Ophthalmology* **11,** 260–268

Ramsey DT and Fox DB (1997) Surgery of the orbit. *Veterinary Clinics of North America, Small Animal Practice* **27,** 1215–1264

Roberts SM, Severin GA and Lavach JD (1986) Prevalence and treatment of palpebral neoplasms in the dog: 200 cases (1975–1983). *Journal of the American Veterinary Medical Association* **189,** 1355–1359

Schobert CS and Dubielzig RR (2008) Feline conjunctival melanoma: histopathological characteristics and clinical outcomes. ACVO 2008 Abstracts. *Veterinary Ophthalmology* **11,** 415

Stades FC and Gelatt KN (2007) Diseases and surgery of the canine eyelid. In: *Veterinary Ophthalmology, 4th edn,* ed. KN Gelatt, pp. 563–317. Blackwell Publishing, Ames, Iowa

Stanclift RM and Gilson SD (2008) Evaluation of neoadjuvant prednisolone administration and surgical excision in treatment of canine mast cell tumours. *Journal of the American Veterinary Medical Association* **232,** 53–62

Stell AJ, Dobson JM and Langmack K (2001) Photodynamic therapy of feline squamous cell carcinoma using topical 5-aminolaevulinic acid. *Journal of Small Animal Practice* **42,** 164–169

Stiles J and Townsend WM (2007) Feline ophthalmology. In: *Veterinary Ophthalmology, 4th edn,* ed. KN Gelatt, pp. 1095–1164. Blackwell Publishing, Ames, Iowa

Sullivan TC, Nasisse MP, Davidson MG and Glover TL (1996) Photocoagulation of limbal melanoma in dogs and cats: 15 cases (1989–1993). *Journal of the American Veterinary Medical Association* **208,** 891–894

Wilcock BP (1993) The eye and ear. In: *Pathology of Domestic Animals, 4th edn,* ed. KVF Jubb *et al.,* pp. 441–529. Academic Press, San Diego

Wilcock BP and Peiffer R (1988) Adenocarcinoma of the gland of the third eyelid in seven dogs. *Journal of the American Veterinary Medical Association* **193,** 1549–1550

Wilcock BP, Yager JA and Zink MC (1986) The morphology and behaviour of feline cutaneous mastocytomas. *Veterinary Pathology* **23,** 320–324

Williams LW, Gelatt KN and Gwin RM (1981) Ophthalmic neoplasms in the cat. *Journal of the American Animal Hospital Association* **17,** 999–1008

Index

Index

Index

Index

Index

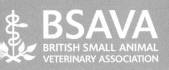

BSAVA

BRITISH SMALL ANIMAL VETERINARY ASSOCIATION

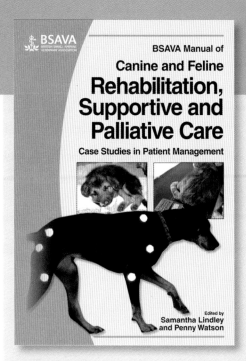

BSAVA Manual of
Canine and Feline
Rehabilitation,
Supportive and
Palliative Care
Case Studies in Patient Management

Edited by

Samantha Lindley and Penny Watson

Companion animals are undergoing previously uncontemplated treatments and surviving what would once have been rapidly fatal conditions. This NEW Manual is aimed at the whole veterinary team, drawing on all their skills to help patients achieve as full a function and quality of life as possible after surgery, trauma or disease, and to manage chronic conditions effectively for the benefit of animal, owner and the practice team.

Part One discusses the principles of rehabilitation, supportive and palliative care. The science behind pain and its management, clinical nutrition and physical therapies is explored, and clinical applications reviewed with reference to published evidence of efficacy and/or effectiveness.

In Part Two, this truly innovative Manual presents a collection of Case Studies across a range of canine and feline patients – from discospondylitis to glaucoma in dogs and from triaditis to leg amputation in cats. The following are considered for every case, with expert assessment from the contributors to Part One of the book:

- Acute and chronic pain management
- Fear, stress and conflict concerns
- Nutritional requirements
- Physiotherapy
- Hydrotherapy
- Acupuncture
- Nursing and supportive care
- Owner advice and homecare recommendations.

Contents:
Part 1: Principles Introduction; Acute pain: assessment and management; Chronic pain; Fear, anxiety and conflict in companion animals; Principles of clinical nutrition; Obesity and weight management; Immune-modulating dietary components and nutraceuticals; An introduction to physical therapies; Physiotherapy and physical rehabilitation; Hydrotherapy; Acupuncture in palliative and rehabilitative medicine. **Part 2: Case Studies** Patients undergoing soft tissue surgery; Patients with neurological disorders; Patients with orthopaedic disease; Patients with neoplastic disease; Patients with cardiac disease; Patients with respiratory disease; Patients with urogenital disease; Patients with gastrointestinal, liver or pancreatic disease; Patients with oral or dental disease; Patients with ocular disease; Patients with dermatological disease; Appendix; Index

ORDERING DETAILS

British Small Animal Veterinary Association
Woodrow House, 1 Telford Way, Waterwells Business Park,
Quedgeley, Gloucester GL2 2AB

Tel:	01452 726700
Fax:	01452 726701
Email:	administration@bsava.com
Web:	www.bsava.com

BSAVA reserves the right to change these prices at any time

Published September 2010
416 pages
ISBN   978 0 905319 20 6

Price to non-members: £75.00

MEMBER PRICE: £49.00

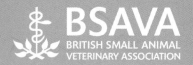

BSAVA Manual of Canine and Feline
Gastroenterology
2nd edition

Edited by Edward Hall, James Simpson and David Williams

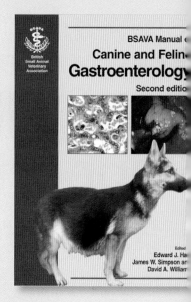

- Diagnostic approach
- Common presenting complaints
- Standard format within chapters aids information retrieval
- New sections on critical care, assisted feeding and therapeutics

'...an excellent reference manual...' **European Journal of Companion Animal Practice**

Published 2005
344 pages
Extensively illustrated in colour
ISBN   978 0 905214 73 3

Price to non-members: £75.00

MEMBER PRICE: £49.00

BSAVA Manual of Canine and Feline
Nephrology and Urology
2nd edition

Edited by Jonathan Elliott and Gregory Grauer

- New features:
  - Clinical staging of kidney disease
  - Blood pressure measurement
  - Cystoscopy
  - Lithotripsy
  - Dialysis

'This second edition has been thoroughly revised, reviewed and updated by an international panel of 26 experts... making this new edition an immediate standard in the field.' **Veterinary Information Network**

Published 2007
312 pages
Extensively illustrated in colour
ISBN   978 0 905214 93 1

Price to non-members: £75.00

MEMBER PRICE: £49.00

ORDERING DETAILS

British Small Animal Veterinary Association
Woodrow House, 1 Telford Way, Waterwells Business Park, Quedgeley, Gloucester GL2 2AB

Tel: 01452 726700   Fax: 01452 726701
Email: administration@bsava.com   Web: www.bsava.com

BSAVA reserves the right to change these prices at any time

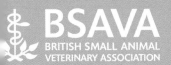
BSAVA Manual of Canine and Feline
Abdominal Surgery

Edited by John Williams and Jacqui Niles

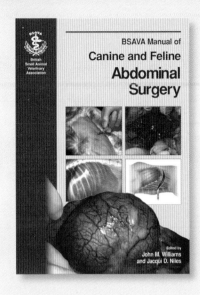

Principles and equipment
Systems and conditions
GDV
Step-by-step Operative Techniques
Postoperative care

Published 2005; 352 pages
Extensively illustrated in colour
ISBN   978 0 905214 81 8
Price to non-members: £75.00
MEMBER PRICE: £49.00

BSAVA Manual of Canine and Feline
Head, Neck and Thoracic Surgery

Edited by Daniel Brockman and David Holt

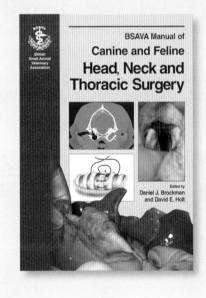

Principles and equipment
Systems and conditions
Emergency tracheostomy
Step-by-step Operative Techniques
Postoperative care

Published 2005; 240 pages
Extensively illustrated in colour
ISBN   978 0 905214 82 5
Price to non-members: £67.00
MEMBER PRICE: £44.00

BSAVA Manual of Canine and Feline
Wound Management and Reconstruction
2nd edition

Edited by John Williams
and Alison Moores

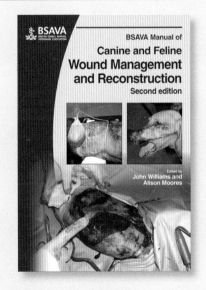

Wound healing and management
Skin and muscle flaps
Skin grafting
Practical decision-making
Step-by-step Operative Techniques

Published 2009; 288 pages
Extensively illustrated in colour
ISBN   978 1 905319 09 1
Price to non-members: £70.00
MEMBER PRICE: £49.00

BSAVA Member Benefits

We stick together to get ahead

The British Small Animal Veterinary Association exists to promote excellence in small animal practice through education and science. More than 6000 members in the UK and overseas benefit from the widest range of practical and scientific benefits, including...

BSAVA Congress
Nowhere else in the UK can you access such high-quality CPD over four days delivered by world-renowned experts. Member rates subsidised.

MP3s & Online Tools
With the congress podcast archive, members now have access to hundreds of hours of CPD with BSAVA Congress MP3s available online, as well as a range of other vital resources online at www.bsava.com

BSAVA Manuals
Members save around one third off our highly regarded series of Manuals designed for the busy practitioner, covering canine and feline medicine and surgery, diagnostic techniques, exotic pets, and veterinary nursing.

BSAVA Small Animal Formulary and *BSAVA Guide to Procedures in Small Animal Practice*
Members receive a complimentary copy of each of these indispensible practice tools.

Journal of Small Animal Practice
Members benefit from a free subscription so they remain informed and engaged with the latest ideas, techniques and research through high-quality original articles.

companion
The latest free subscription for BSAVA members delivers relevant, indispensible and practical features, essential for everyone in veterinary practice.

CPD
As a not-for-profit organisation, we can subsidise our courses for members whilst still delivering quality CPD with leading international specialists, offering you choice, value and excellence throughout the UK and in your region.

© Molnia | Dreamstime.com

Living and working outside Britain?
Join BSAVA as an overseas member at special rates to receive all your benefits online. See www.bsava.com for details.

Join Now
For more information about BSAVA and member benefits visit www.bsava.com, email administration@bsava.com, or call 01452 726700.

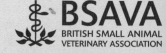

BSAVA
BRITISH SMALL ANIMAL
VETERINARY ASSOCIATION